Automatic Ventilation of the Lungs

SBN 632 03050 X

FIRST PUBLISHED 1959
SECOND EDITION 1969

GERMAN EDITION 1962

Printed in Great Britain

TO OUR PARENTS

THE MAGNITUDE OF OUR DEBT TO WHOM WE ONLY FULLY
REALIZE WITH THE PASSAGE OF TIME.
THEIR EXAMPLE OF INTEGRITY AND INDUSTRY
IS A CONSTANT INSPIRATION

Contents

APPENDICES

Preface

One of the striking advances in anaesthesia is the attention and skill now devoted to the attainment of proper ventilation of the patient's lungs by means of controlled respiration. Spontaneous breathing may become seriously depressed and inadequate as a result of anaesthesia. It may be deliberately abolished altogether, by a range of relaxants and narcotic drugs, in order to make intrathoracic and many other operations feasible or more safe—circumstances which occur daily in every hospital where surgery and anaesthesia of high standard are practised. The remarkable capacity of simple rhythmic squeezing of a bag by hand to maintain life has led to the transfer of this procedure to circumstances apart from anaesthesia, in which respiratory insufficiency threatens the patient's life. Controlled respiration is now regarded as an important part of the treatment of, for example, certain forms of poliomyelitis, of tetanus, of narcotic poisoning, of crush injury of the chest, and a number of other conditions, either of disease or injury, of the central nervous or respiratory systems. In all these, respiratory insufficiency is commonly present and is a frequent cause of death.

The rhythmic squeezing of a bag was, and still is, the basic method of performing controlled respiration. A demand, born of clinical needs and satisfied by man's mechanical ingenuity, has brought into being a large number of automatic ventilators of increasing complexity. One type after another, each claiming to have advantages over its fellows, has made its appearance during the last two decades. Like most anaesthetists, we have often been perplexed about these devices and questions have come readily to our minds; How do they work? How should they work? What should they be able to do? What are the clinical effects, good or bad, that are associated with their use?—and many other questions too. A few of these can be answered and this we attempt to do here.

The ventilators with which we have concerned ourselves are of direct interest to the anaesthetist. In the main they have been designed specially for use during anaesthesia or are adaptable for that purpose. However, several were designed for ward use to maintain artificial ventilation in respiratory insufficiency and these are included though they may not be immediately suitable for use during anaesthesia. We regretfully came to the conclusion that the extra space and effort which would be needed for those automatic devices designed primarily for emergency resuscitation could not be justified. These instruments have therefore been omitted.

We are actively engaged in the field of clinical anaesthesia and we address our book principally to our anaesthetic colleagues. Others, too, may find something of value though it is possible that no one section of this book will satisfy experts in that section.

Respiratory physiologists may become still more aware of some of the clinical, mechanical, and physical problems which beset the anaesthetist in the operating theatre and the ward, and of the urgent need to communicate, in both directions, the accumulating knowledge of this subject in a terminology which is not too far removed from everyday clinical usage.

Physicians called upon to treat cases of severe respiratory insufficiency may now at long last lose their distrust of what is still to many of them an unfamiliar technique. They will be convinced of the need for a clear, albeit basic, understanding of both natural and artificial respiration in the competent handling of patients with respiratory failure, irrespective of the underlying cause of the respiratory difficulty; their expert knowledge of the latter has not in the past always enabled them to deal successfully with the former.

Surgeons may come to view even more kindly, and now with understanding, the efforts of the anaesthetist on their patients' behalf. The squeezing of a bag or the manipulation of a ventilator's controls must not be empiric, for it is largely based on knowledge which ranges over various fields, and must include respiratory physiology. An appreciation of this will extend the confidence already reposed by them in their anaesthetists.

Engineers and instrument makers may perhaps be moved to temper their inventive skill to the present state of knowledge of the clinical effects of controlled respiration, and to the traumatic and far-from-scientific environments of the operating theatre and ward in which their products will be used. Their ingenuity may well have already outstripped the clinical and physiological knowledge which alone can clarify what is wanted from a ventilator.

Our own colleagues, the anaesthetists, will see the need for the collaboration of a widening range of experts, physiological, mechanical, electrical, and pneumatic, if the ventilators of to-day are to satisfy the requirements of the knowledge of to-morrow. The present task of the anaesthetist is clearly to study the patient, in the operating room and ward, ever more closely in order that changes in ventilator action can be correlated with changes in the patient. Only then will it be possible to adjust with intelligence and confidence the various ventilatory parameters such as positive pressure, negative pressure, respiratory frequency, the ratio of inspiratory to expiratory times, and the rest, to the individual patient's needs. It is not more ventilators that are needed but more understanding of the effects of the ones available and of their clinical use.

The text of our first edition has been almost entirely re-written. Our understanding of the physical aspects of artificial ventilation has advanced. New ventilators have appeared and old ones become obsolete. The accounts of the modes of action of many of the ventilators have been expanded in the light of our own original laboratory experiments. The interaction of controls has, wherever possible, been clarified.

The complexity of mechanical, pneumatic, and electrical design of ventilators has now reached a point at which classification on some rational basis is no longer easy. We have therefore described the ventilators in alphabetical order.

Our own knowledge of the clinical aspects of controlled respiration and of automatic ventilators derives from long clinical experience. Many of the ventilators described were made available to us for inspection and for detailed laboratory study. Others we could only read about. In all cases we have had to rely on the manufacturers for a great deal of constructional detail. They were generous to an embarrassing degree in supplying information of every sort. We thank them most sincerely for information, charts, drawings, and photographs about their products. We also thank the editors of the numerous journals listed and the authors of the various papers for permission to reproduce material.

In most cases photographs of the ventilators are included. The reason is not so much to give information of detail, but to give the reader a general idea of what the ventilators look like, of their bulk, and to what extent they are experimental, or developed commercial products. The difference between a mental picture of a ventilator, derived from a stylized diagram of the working parts, and the real thing can be startling.

This preface is signed by the senior author alone to enable him to pay tribute to his co-authors for their amiability and competency in joining him once again in preparing this edition. In particular he welcomes W.W.Mapleson, PH.D., Senior Lecturer (Physics) in this Department, whose name now appears in the main-authors list. He now brings to the whole book his knowledge as a physicist, and particularly his unique knowledge of the physics of automatic ventilators.

Great praise is due to E.K.Hillard, L.I.B.S.T., Chief Technician in this Department, who was at our side throughout this revision. He not only put his long experience in the design and construction of anaesthetic equipment at our disposal, but also his remarkable skill as an artist and draughtsman. With very few exceptions the diagrams and graphs were drawn by him.

We also received much help from R.J.Marshall, A.I.B.P., F.R.P.S., Director of the Department of Medical Illustration of the United Cardiff Hospitals, and Lecturer in Medical Illustration in the Welsh National School of Medicine, whose personal skill, and that of his staff, was of invaluable assistance. We are also grateful to our anaesthetic colleagues in Cardiff who helped to clarify and crystallize our views over the years, to our surgical friends for their forbearance when recording instruments sometimes limited their working space, and, above all, to the University of Wales, through the Welsh National School of Medicine, for providing the academic atmosphere and facilities in which ideas germinate, studies progress, and literary projects come to fruition. A special word of thanks is also due to our publishers, and especially to our friend Per Saugman, for continual encouragement and help through what has proved to be a prolonged labour. The lavish way this book is illustrated is proof of their agreement with us that illustrations are indispensable if a difficult and unfamiliar field is to be made clear.

Lastly, but not least, we thank our secretary, Miss W.R.Davies, and her assistants, who have typed, re-typed, and re-typed our numerous and bulky manuscripts cheerfully and accurately.

Cardiff, 1969. W.W.M.

CHAPTER I

Physiological Aspects of Controlled Respiration

INTRODUCTION

Controlled respiration is the term with which anaesthetists have become familiar for the process more properly referred to as artificial ventilation of the lungs. Both terms are synonymous with the more limited, if descriptive, Intermittent-Positive-Pressure Respiration (I.P.P.R.). Because we are anaesthetists we have therefore retained the term controlled respiration (see Glossary, p. 814). This procedure was suggested in 1934[1] as a means of providing a quieter operating field in abdominal surgery. Little interest was aroused at the time and it remained for the demands of thoracic surgery to bring the method to the fore. Controlled respiration has now been in daily routine use in anaesthesia for some thirty years.[2] At first it was the means of preventing the harmful effects of the open chest and thus solving what had been known for nearly a century as the 'pneumothorax problem'; later it was the means of counteracting the paralysing effects of curare and other relaxants on the respiratory muscles. By now many millions of patients have been successfully ventilated by this means with little evidence of harmful result. It can therefore be safely concluded that controlled respiration is a very effective method of ventilating the lungs in respiratory insufficiency.

The efficacy of this method of ventilation in oxygenating the blood is strikingly demonstrated by the speed with which a patient, cyanosed through respiratory insufficiency, flushes a brilliant pink when controlled respiration is started, so long as the cardiovascular system is not in any way seriously interfered with or depressed.

The adequacy of carbon-dioxide removal is shown by the speed with which a raised blood pressure, sweating, tachycardia, and wound bleeding respond in a patient previously suffering from respiratory insufficiency. For example, patients may suffer from carbon-dioxide accumulation, leading even to narcosis, as a result not only of underventilation during anaesthesia[3] but of disease such as cor pulmonale, emphysema, or bronchopneumonia.[4] In such cases controlled respiration, with a canister of soda-lime interposed between the reservoir bag or automatic ventilator and the patient, produces effective and rapid carbon-dioxide elimination as shown by the soda-lime becoming very hot in a short time, and by the rapid recovery of the patient. Nowadays blood-gas analysis confirms these clinical observations.

The possible harmful effects of controlled respiration are described later (see p. 9). They lie principally in the directions of cardiovascular depression because of interference with the venous return to the heart and of disturbances in the distribution of blood and gases through the lungs during ventilation. However, it can be said here that when the mean pressure in the lungs is not excessive, and when the gas flows through the respiratory tract are within normal limits, and when disease of the lungs with consequent alteration in local areas of compliance and resistance is not gross, the harmful effects, if any, in healthy subjects, are so small that they can be neglected.

Nevertheless, it is essential to understand, from a physiological point of view, the basis of the effectiveness and of the high degree of safety of controlled respiration, and the mechanisms underlying the harmful effects which may, in certain circumstances, be produced. Only with such an understanding can those who use automatic ventilators* make use of the more-exact controls provided by them and employ controlled respiration in such a way that their patients will derive the full benefit thereof, whilst any harmful effects are minimized. Furthermore, with this knowledge it is possible to establish, on a rational basis, criteria for the design of automatic ventilators.[5]

We therefore discuss first the physiological factors which affect the volume exchange produced by controlled respiration, the differences between controlled and spontaneous respiration, the possible harmful effects of controlled respiration, and the means whereby these effects may be minimized.

PHYSIOLOGICAL FACTORS AFFECTING VOLUME EXCHANGE

Compliance[6–28]

The relationship between the volume and the pressure of the gas in the alveoli when both are measured as changes from their resting levels is determined by the elastic properties of the lungs and chest wall. The term 'compliance' expresses this relationship. It is defined as the volume increase which corresponds to each unit pressure increase in the alveoli. Normally this is given in litres per centimetre of water (litres/cmH_2O). Thus, if an increase in alveolar pressure of 10 cmH_2O occurs with a volume increase within the alveoli of 500 ml (0·5 litre), the compliance is $0{\cdot}5/10 = 0{\cdot}05$ litre/cmH_2O.

Once the compliance is known, the increase in alveolar pressure which corresponds to a given increase in volume can be easily calculated. Conversely, given the increase in pressure, the increase in volume necessarily accompanying it can likewise be calculated.

The actual value of the compliance varies considerably in different individuals and

* This term replaces 'respirator' which should more properly be reserved for apparatus designed to filter contaminants from the inspired air.

in different circumstances in the same individual. The range of the published figures is wide. In supine anaesthetized relaxed patients the total compliance varies from 0·02 litre/cmH_2O to 0·14 litre/cmH_2O. In this book we have taken 0·05 litre/cmH_2O as a typical value. The value for conscious individuals is usually quoted as 0·1 litre/cmH_2O; this higher value may be partly due to imperfect relaxation, and the inability to refrain from some spontaneous inspiration during inflation. However, more recently it has become evident that compliance is indeed reduced under anaesthesia and can be raised, although only temporarily, towards the level for conscious individuals by a few extra-large tidal volumes or 'sighs'. A few ventilators are now available which will deliver such 'sighs' at regular intervals.

The total compliance has two components: that of the chest wall and that of the lungs. Again values vary, but we have taken the compliance of the lungs alone in anaesthetized patients to be 0·1 litre/cmH_2O, although this may be a little high, and 0·2 litre/cmH_2O in the conscious subject. When the chest is opened, the influence of the thoracic wall becomes very small and the total compliance is virtually equal to the compliance of the lungs alone. In clinical practice the compliance may be modified considerably from moment to moment by such factors as the degree of muscular relaxation, posture, assistants leaning on the chest, retractors pushing against the lungs or diaphragm,[7, 12, 29] and, of course, by the occlusion of branch bronchi or bronchioles during, say, thoracic surgery.

Airway resistance[30–45]

The airway resistance expresses the relationship between the pressure difference across the airway (between the mouth and the alveoli) and the rate at which gas is flowing through the airway. It is expressed as pressure difference per unit flow and is usually measured in centimetres of water pressure per litre per second (cmH_2O/(litre/sec)).
For example,

if the airway resistance is	2 cmH_2O/(litre/sec)
then a gas flow through the airway of	30 litres/min(0·5 litre/sec)
is accompanied by a pressure difference of	$2 \times 0{\cdot}5 = 1$ cmH_2O
Conversely, if it is known that a flow through the airway of	30 litres/min(0·5 litre/sec)
is accompanied by a pressure difference of	1 cmH_2O
it may be deduced that the airway resistance is	$1/0{\cdot}5 = 2$ cmH_2O/(litre/sec)

In addition to airway resistance there is also 'viscous' tissue resistance to expansion of the lungs. The viscous resistance arises from the lobes sliding against each other, the mediastinal structures such as the heart, and the chest wall. The sum of airway resistance and tissue resistance is referred to as respiratory resistance.

In normal conscious subjects, this is about 4 cmH_2O/(litre/sec).* The value of the airway resistance is increased during anaesthesia. This may arise due to both a narrowing and an elongation of the bronchi, and to the presence of apparatus such as an endotracheal tube. Thus, during anaesthesia, the respiratory resistance from the carina downward is of the order of 4 cmH_2O/(litre/sec). With an endotracheal tube in place the total airway resistance is commonly of the order of 6 cmH_2O/(litre/sec). We have therefore used the latter figure in the 'standard conditions' when studying the mode of action of ventilators and giving their functional analyses, and for the numerical examples given below. Furthermore, to simplify the argument, we have assumed that the 6 cmH_2O/(litre/sec) is all airway resistance and that the tissue resistance is negligible. The presence of disease may increase the respiratory resistance. For example, in conscious subjects, figures of from 3 to 15 cmH_2O/(litre/sec) in emphysema, and 13 to 18 cmH_2O/(litre/sec) in asthma have been found. Still higher values may be expected in gross respiratory obstruction.

During inflation of the lungs the pressure at the mouth must be greater than the pressure in the alveoli or no gas would flow from one to the other. Conversely, during the expiratory phase the pressure in the alveoli must be the greater, and there is therefore at least an instant of time between the two phases when the pressure is the same throughout the respiratory tract and no gas flows in either direction. The differences in pressure depend on, and are an indication of, the magnitude of the respiratory resistance. During inflation the actual pressure at the mouth at any moment is the sum of the pressure drop across the airway resistance and the alveolar pressure, which corresponds to the volume of gas in the lungs at that moment.

Thus, consider a ventilator from which gas flows steadily at the rate of	0·5 litre/sec	(1)
into a patient whose compliance is	0·05 litre/cmH_2O	(2)
and whose airway resistance is	6 cm H_2O/(litre/sec)	(3)
for a period of	1 second	(4)

Then,

from (1) and (3), the pressure difference across the airway is constant at	3 cmH_2O	(5)

and,

from (1) and (4), the volume increase in the alveoli is	0·5 litre	(6)

* The figures for resistance given in this paragraph are for a particular flow rate (0·5 litre/sec). The resistance is not constant for a given airway, but increases slightly with increase in flow rate due to the development of turbulence.[46] For the sake of simplicity, however, the respiratory resistance will here be taken as constant.

Therefore,

from (2) and (6), the pressure in the alveoli at the end of the period is 10 cmH_2O (7)

and,

from (1) and (3), the pressure at the mouth at the start of inflation (due to airway resistance) is 3 cmH_2O (8)

and,

from (7) and (8), the pressure at the mouth just before the end of inflation (due to airway resistance and alveolar pressure) is 13 cmH_2O (9)

In this example the difference between the alveolar and mouth pressures is appreciable. If a higher flow rate is used, or the airway resistance is much higher, considerably larger differences can result.

A clear distinction must therefore always be drawn between the pressure registered at the mouth and the alveolar pressure. In practice during automatic ventilation the manometer is almost invariably situated on the ventilator. However, resistance between the ventilator and the patient's mouth, and hence the pressure difference between the two, is usually negligible. Therefore, for all practical purposes, the pressure at the ventilator can usually be taken to be the same as that at the mouth.

Fig. 1.1 illustrates a state of affairs which could well occur in clinical practice. The pressure as recorded at the 'mouth' rises rapidly to 20 cmH_2O. At the end of the inspiratory phase when, say, 700 ml have entered the 'lungs' and the flow has fallen to zero, the pressures at the mouth and in the alveoli are the same (14 cmH_2O), the compliance in this case being 0·05 litre/cmH_2O. Assuming a free path for expiration, the pressure at the 'mouth' now falls rapidly to zero whilst that in the 'alveoli' does the same more slowly. Since the pressure at the mouth is equal to the sum of the alveolar pressure and the pressure difference across the airway resistance, a high flow into the lungs, or a high airway resistance, and hence a high pressure difference across the airway, can lead to a peak pressure at the mouth much in excess of the final peak pressure in the alveoli.

The biggest difference in pressure between the mouth and alveoli (A in fig. 1.1) occurs when the flow into the lungs is highest. As the end of the inspiratory phase is approached the difference becomes gradually smaller until, at the end of the phase, no flow occurs and the pressure is the same throughout the respiratory tract. The peak pressure at the mouth is higher (B) than the peak pressure reached in the alveoli and it occurs some time (C) before the latter which marks the end of the inspiratory phase. It is possible, by watching a manometer registering mouth pressure, to note the highest pressure reached there, but not the point (D), at which the mouth pressure is the same as the alveolar pressure. The anaesthetist must therefore exercise caution in translating a manometer reading of pressure at the mouth into volume transferred to the lungs. Figures for compliance relate changes in the volume and pressure in the *alveoli.*

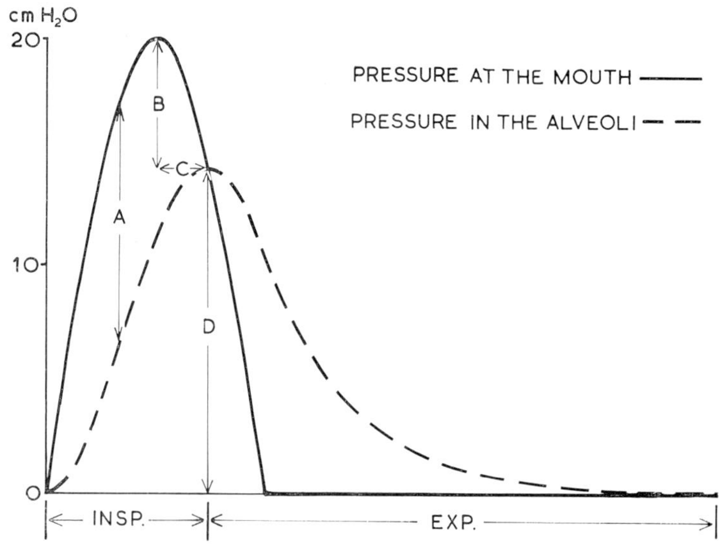

Fig. 1.1. Graph showing the difference that can exist between 'pressure at the mouth' and 'pressure in the alveoli'. Reproduced from recordings made during a laboratory experiment with an 'artificial lung' having a compliance = 0·05 litre/cmH_2O and an airway resistance = 2 cmH_2O/(litre/sec). Controlled respiration was by squeezing a bag, the pattern being a quick and forceful inspiratory phase followed by a longer expiratory phase.

The resistance of an unobstructed airway is small and, with a slow rhythm of ventilation, the pressure at the mouth during the inspiratory phase is little more than about 4–6 cmH_2O higher than that in the alveoli. In these circumstances a practical approximation to the volume exchange can be made from the manometer reading if the compliance of the chest is known or assumed. A higher pressure at the mouth then indicates that a correspondingly larger volume has been transferred to the patient, and this may well be in excess of his normal tidal volume and undesirable.

There are other occasions, however, when a high pressure at the mouth may be needed to produce a tidal volume within the normal range. For example, the airway resistance may be high or the compliance low. A fall in the tidal exchange resulting from an increase in the airway resistance due to such causes as organic obstruction, increased secretions, or kinks in the tubing can be overcome to a large extent by increasing the pressure at the mouth, thereby maintaining a sufficient flow of gas, so that a volume within the range desired is again transferred into the lungs in the required time. Needless to say, in such circumstances the pressure in the alveoli, being determined only by the compliance and the volume transferred, is within normal limits. Since in such a case expiration will be impeded by the respiratory obstruction and the pressure difference across the airway at the beginning of the expiratory phase is less than that applied at the beginning of the inspiratory phase, either extra time must be allowed for the lungs to empty or negative pressure applied during this phase to increase the pressure difference between lungs and mouth and so speed up the flow of gas out of the lungs.

We have already drawn attention to the need for caution in translating manometer readings on the ventilator into tidal volumes. A similar caution is also necessary in respect of volume readings taken from a calibrated reservoir bag. The volume expelled from the bag may differ considerably from the volume entering the patient's lungs. Losses may occur due to the distension of the breathing tubes and also the compression of the gas within them. In addition the entry and escape of fresh gas into and from the patient circuit are responsible for further differences between the two volumes. This latter effect is fully discussed in Chapter 4, and attention is drawn to it in the functional analyses of individual ventilators. From a clinical point of view it should be borne in mind that this latter phenomenon occurs in most ventilators in which the reservoir bag of the ventilator takes the place of the reservoir bag of a carbon-dioxide absorption apparatus. In these circumstances the volume of gas entering the patient may be either greater or less than the volume leaving the reservoir bag of the ventilator. Whether it is greater or less, and the magnitude of the difference, depend on the rate of fresh-gas supply and the arrangements for admitting fresh gas and disposing of excess. A careful study of both the ventilator mechanism and of its physical characteristics is essential if the magnitude of the volume transfer to the patient is to be accurately estimated. A reliable ventilation meter (see p. 47) will give an unambiguous measure of tidal and minute volumes.

THE DIFFERENCES BETWEEN CONTROLLED AND SPONTANEOUS RESPIRATION

Introduction

The respiratory muscles, principally the diaphragm, enlarge the size of the thoracic cavity, the specific volume of the gas[47] within it increases, and the pressure within the thorax falls. The difference between the intrapleural and alveolar pressures overcomes the elasticity of the lungs: the difference between the pressure in the alveoli and the exterior overcomes the airway resistance. The magnitudes of these two pressure differences differ from each other; that across the airway, even at the height of gas flow, is small, say 2 cmH_2O, so long as the airway is unobstructed. That between pleura and alveoli is larger, ranging from -10 cmH_2O at the end of inspiration to -5 cmH_2O at the end of expiration.

Intrapulmonary pressure

During spontaneous respiration air flows from the outside atmosphere to the inside of the lungs because a pressure difference is created between the exterior and the alveoli.

This pressure difference is of comparatively small magnitude since it has only to overcome airway resistance, the main effort of the respiratory muscles being used to overcome the elasticity of the lungs. The pressure difference in a conscious subject breathing quietly is of the order of 1 to 2 cmH_2O (fig. 1.2) and since the pressure at the mouth is atmospheric, the pressure in the alveoli during inspiration must be sub-atmospheric by this amount. By the end of inspiration the pressure within the alveoli has become atmospheric again. When expiration starts, the pressure in the alveoli rises a few cmH_2O above atmospheric and gradually falls to atmospheric again as the lungs empty.

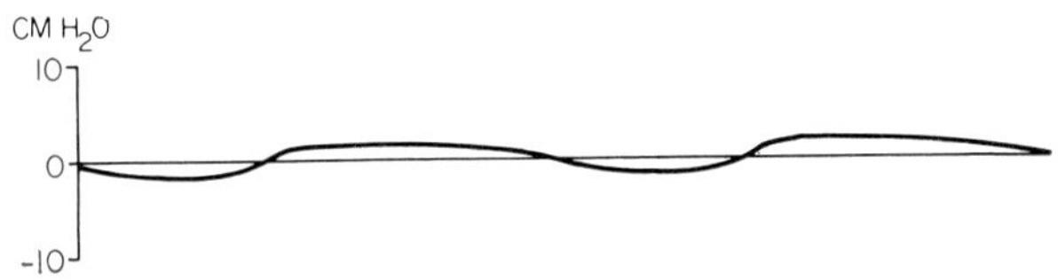

Fig. 1.2. The calculated changes in pressure in the alveoli of a conscious patient breathing spontaneously. Tidal volume = 800 ml; compliance of lungs and thorax = 0·1 litre/cmH_2O; compliance of lungs alone = 0·2 litre/cmH_2O; airway resistance = 2 cmH_2O/(litre/sec); respiratory frequency = 15/min.

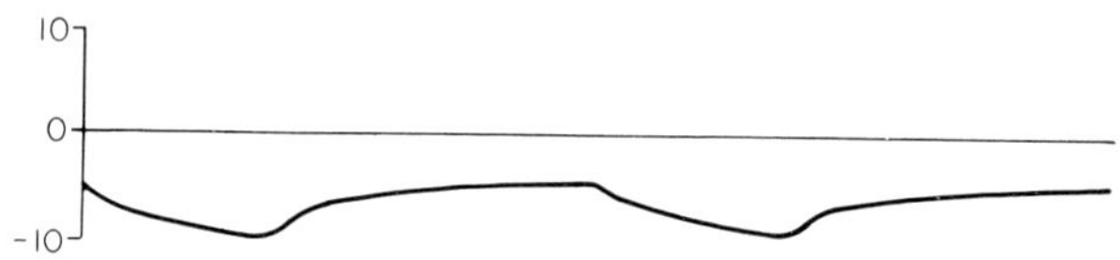

Fig. 1.3. The calculated changes in intrapleural pressure in the same circumstances as fig. 1.2.

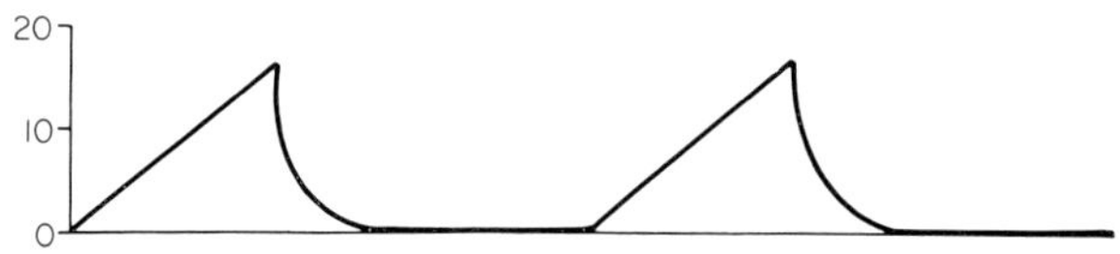

Fig. 1.4. The calculated changes in pressure in the alveoli of a patient with intermittent-positive-pressure ventilation. Tidal volume = 800 ml; compliance of lungs and thorax = 0·05 litre/cmH_2O; compliance of lungs alone = 0·1 litre/cmH_2O; resistance (including apparatus) = 4 cmH_2O/(litre/sec); respiratory frequency = 15/min.

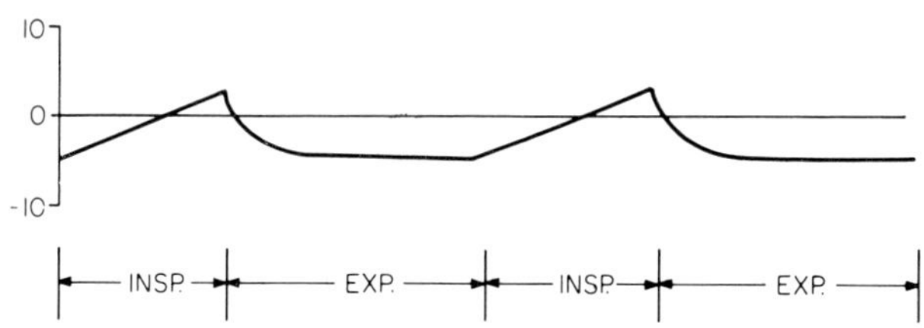

Fig. 1.5. The calculated changes in intrapleural pressure in the same circumstances as fig. 1.4.

In contrast to this, during controlled respiration (fig. 1.4) with positive pressure alone, the pressure in the alveoli rises from atmospheric to, say, +16 cmH_2O (for a volume of 800 ml, assuming a compliance of 0·05 litre/cmH_2O). During the expiratory phase the pressure falls to atmospheric as the lungs empty.

Intrapleural pressure

The intrapleural pressure also reflects the considerable difference between the two types of respiration.

During spontaneous breathing the intrapleural pressure is normally about −5 cmH_2O[48, 49] at the end of expiration. During inspiration a further fall occurs to about −10 cmH_2O returning to −5 cmH_2O during expiration (fig. 1.3).

In controlled respiration (fig. 1.5) under the same conditions (tidal volume 800 ml, compliance 0·05 litre/cmH_2O) the intrapleural pressure rises during the inspiratory phase from −5 cmH_2O to +3 cmH_2O, falling to −5 cmH_2O again during expiration. The rise of 8 cmH_2O is half that in the lungs because it has been assumed that the compliance of the lungs alone is double that of the lungs and chest wall (see p. 3).

HARMFUL EFFECTS OF CONTROLLED RESPIRATION

In spite of the striking efficacy and safety of controlled respiration, the method involves considerable deviation from the normal physiological mechanism of respiration.[50] When used improperly, or on patients incapable of compensating for the almost inevitable though usually minor upsets which result from interference with normal bodily processes, controlled respiration may be harmful to a significant degree.

A. Cardiovascular Effects

Over the past twenty-five years much information[51–97] has been gathered about the cardiovascular effects of intermittent-positive-pressure respiration, the main features of which are summarized here.

The connexion between the venous return and the intrathoracic pressure was recognized by Valsalva[98, 99, 100] in the seventeenth century. His 'experiment' of trying to expire against a closed glottis raises the intrathoracic pressure to a positive level, interferes with the venous return, and causes marked distension of the peripheral veins especially in the head and neck; the blood pressure falls, and, if the experiment is persisted with, the subject may lose consciousness as a result of cerebral ischaemia.

The abolition of the 'thoracic pump' mechanism

The fall in pressure within the thorax during spontaneous inspiration not only sucks air into the lungs, but also blood from outside the thorax into the great thoracic veins and the heart.[101,102,103] The interference with, and the modification of, the sub-atmospheric pressure changes by controlled respiration disturb this important mechanism. The normal pressure gradient between the intrathoracic veins and those outside is upset because the positive pressure within the lungs is transmitted in part to the structures within the thorax as seen in figs. 1.4 and 1.5. During spontaneous breathing (fig. 1.3) the pressure within the thorax, i.e. the intrapleural pressure, at the height of inspiration is, say, -10 cmH_2O.[49,103] During controlled respiration (fig. 1.5) this becomes $+3$ cmH_2O. Only during the quiescent part of the expiratory phase is the negative intrapleural pressure the same in both spontaneous and controlled respiration.

During spontaneous breathing the venous return is therefore greatest during inspiration. During controlled respiration this situation is reversed and the venous return rises during the expiratory phase (figs. 1.6[94] and 1.7[73]).

At the end of the inspiratory phase of controlled respiration the central venous pressure is raised (fig. 1.8) and the venous gradient decreased. The venous return to the

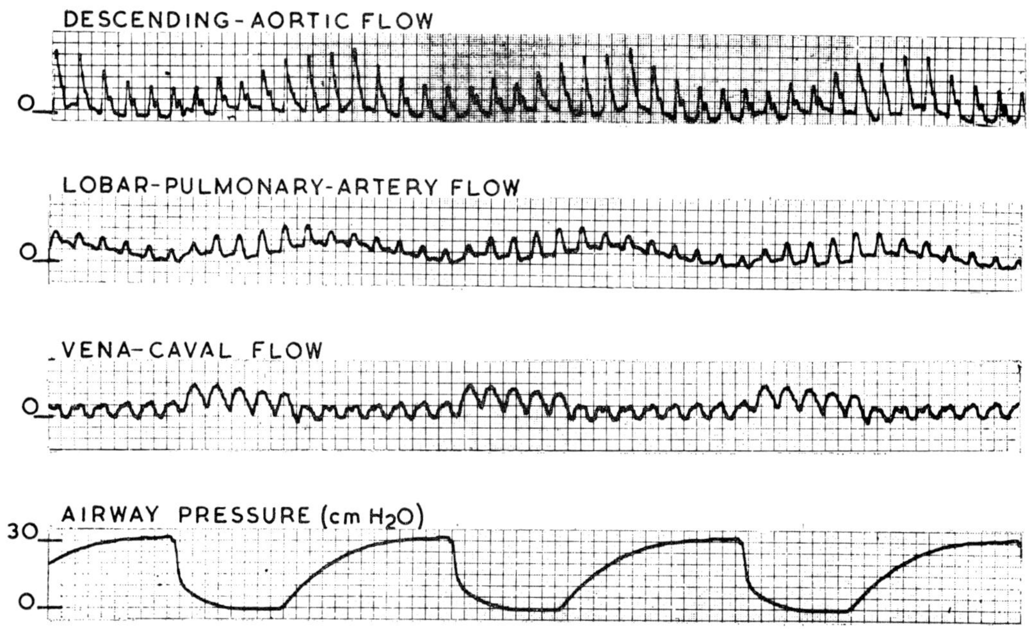

Fig. 1.6. Effects of intermittent-positive-pressure ventilation on the descending-aortic, lobar-pulmonary-artery, and vena-caval flows in dogs.

Courtesy of *Anesthesiology*[94] and Dr B.C. Morgan.

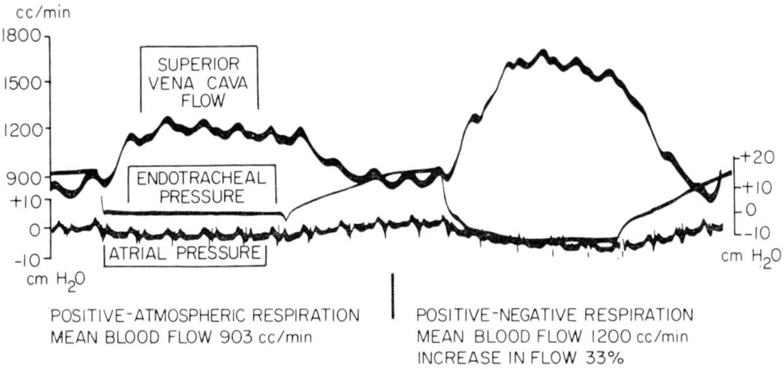

Fig. 1.7. The effect of a negative-pressure phase in increasing the venous return to the heart (after Hubay *et al.*[73]).

The tracing is from a dog. The substitution of negative pressure during the expiratory phase, instead of atmospheric, increased the blood-flow in the superior vena cava by 33 per cent.

Courtesy of *Anesthesiology*.

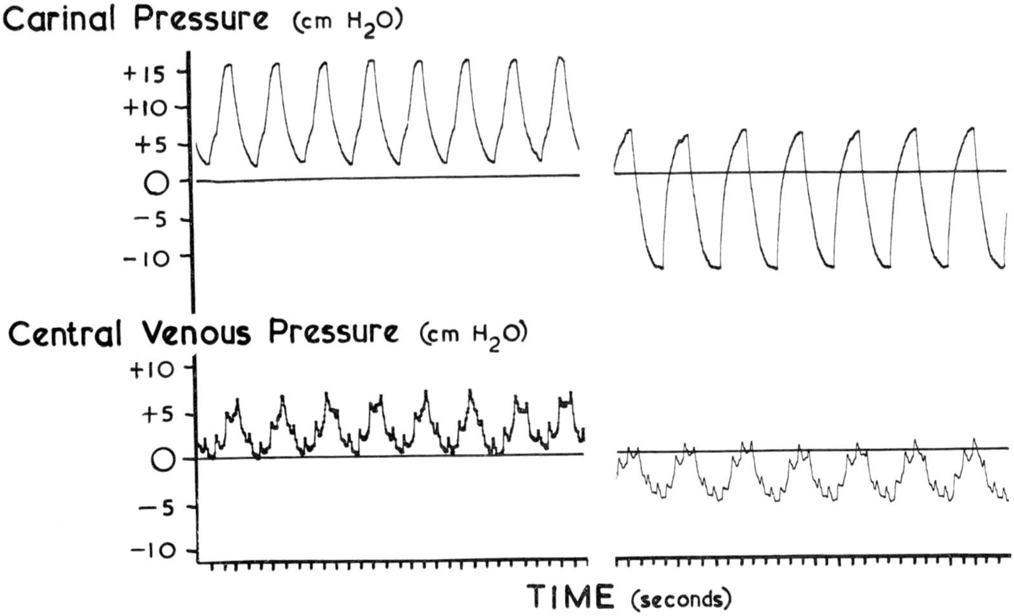

Fig. 1.8. Recordings of the carinal and central venous pressures in man during intermittent-positive-atmospheric-pressure ventilation and intermittent-positive-negative-pressure ventilation.

Courtesy of Dr S.Galloon.

heart (figs. 1.6 and 1.7) and hence the cardiac output (figs. 1.6 and 1.9[94]) are reduced, and the blood pressure falls. Normally, however, this is rapidly compensated for by a rise in peripheral venous pressure which reconstitutes the venous gradient and so re-establishes the venous return to its former level. The restoration of the venous gradient is essential if an adequate cardiac output during controlled respiration is to be maintained. It is dependent upon the capacity to adjust the distribution of blood between the vascular compartments by changes in vascular tone, and on the presence of a normal circulating blood volume.

Should either of these factors be interfered with, or the inspiratory phase be unduly prolonged, then the untoward circulatory effects of the positive pressure in the lungs will become marked. For example, severe haemorrhage markedly reduces the volume of circulating blood. In such a patient extensive vasoconstriction may have already occurred to counteract the hypovolaemia, and further compensation be impossible; the effect of controlled respiration may then be disastrous.

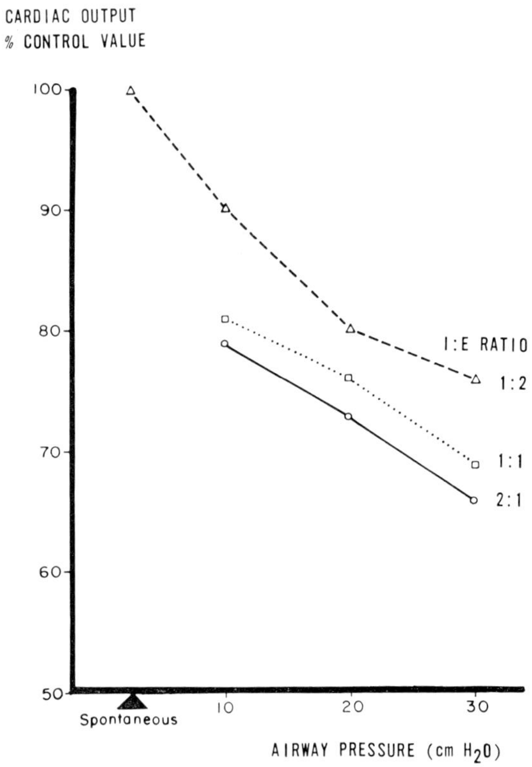

Fig. 1.9. Effects of increasing the airway pressure and the inspiratory-expiratory ratio on cardiac output in dogs.

Courtesy of *Anesthesiology*[94] and Dr B.C.Morgan.

'Tamponade' of the heart

During the inspiratory phase of controlled respiration the heart itself is compressed to some extent between the inflating lungs, as a result of which its output suffers. By comparing the graphs in figs. 1.3 and 1.5 it can be seen that at the end of the inspiratory phase the heart is subjected, in controlled respiration, to a slight positive pressure, whereas in spontaneous breathing the intrapleural pressure is then at its lowest level. The higher the peak pressure and the longer the time during which it acts (i.e. the higher the I : E ratio) the greater is the cardiac tamponade and the interference with the cardiac output (see figs. 1.9 and 1.10).

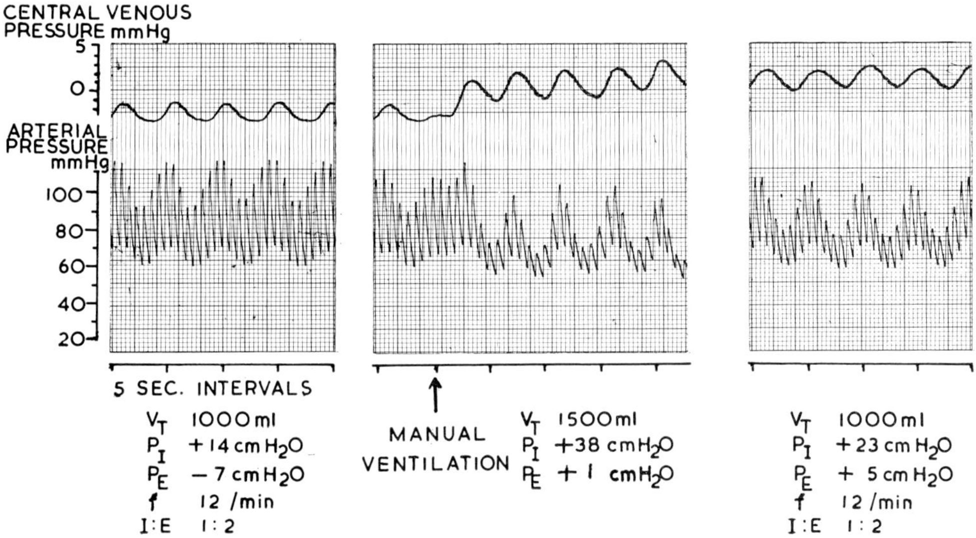

Fig. 1.10. Recordings of the arterial and central venous pressures in man under different circumstances of artificial ventilation.

Interference with pulmonary blood flow

The pulmonary capillary blood pressure is about 12 cmH_2O.[104] The capillaries will therefore suffer compression in part or whole as the alveolar pressure rises above atmospheric. Even pressures as low as 6·5 cmH_2O in the lungs decrease the pulmonary capillary circulation and throw an extra burden on the right ventricle. If the patient is on the verge of decompensation, even such a low pressure in the lungs as this might be sufficient to precipitate right-heart failure.

In considering the relative importance of these three ways in which controlled respiration interferes with the cardiovascular system, it should be borne in mind that while they are all of considerable importance in patients with an intact thorax, the circumstances alter when the chest is opened. The thoracic pump now no longer operates because the chest is open, while any cardiac tamponade, if it occurs, will be mainly surgical in origin. The interference with the pulmonary blood flow is now the most important adverse effect directly due to the controlled respiration, and may in itself be sufficient to interfere seriously with cardiac ouput.

B. Damage to the Lungs[105–125]

The possibility of rupture of the alveoli is remote in properly-conducted controlled respiration, unless a condition such as bullous emphysema is present. Rupture even then is probably no more likely to occur during controlled respiration with properly-limited positive pressure than during normal life. Each act of coughing produces an intrapulmonary pressure which may be as high as 80–90 cmH_2O, while straining at defaecation may give rise to still higher pressures.

The pressure required to rupture the exposed and unsupported lungs of various mammals has been found to be about 40–80 cmH_2O. When the lungs are supported by the thoracic cage and the abdominal musculature of the living animal a pressure of 80–140 cmH_2O is needed. The maximum safe intrapulmonary pressure in the intact mammal is about 70 cmH_2O. The pressure developed by squeezing the thin rubber reservoir bag commonly found on anaesthetic apparatus can rarely be made to exceed 40–60 cmH_2O (see p. 96 and fig. 3.12). Nevertheless, as more complex devices capable of producing higher inflating pressures are brought on to the market, the possibility of damage to the lungs must be borne in mind.

The rupture in experimental animals is usually into the mediastinum with passage of air up the fascial planes into the cervical region. At higher pressures this is sometimes accompanied by air embolism and haemorrhages into the lung tissues. If an external equalizing pressure is applied to the thorax and abdomen, protection from overdistension is obtained, and in these circumstances pressures as high as 230 cmH_2O have been tolerated without damage.

Rupture of the lungs in man leads to interstitial emphysema spreading up the pulmonary vascular sheaths into the mediastinum (fig. 1.11).[125] Rupture of the pleura in these cases is probably a secondary event, the primary process being the 'stretching away' of the alveoli from the inelastic pulmonary vascular sheaths lying between them. Subsequent break-through of air from the mediastinum to the intrapleural space may occur.

C. Uneven Ventilation

It is evident from the foregoing section that the risk of rupture of the alveoli during controlled respiration seems to be very small. This is so even in patients with pulmonary disease in which a high airway resistance and a low lung compliance call for the use of high pressure at the mouth during the inspiratory phase. However, it should be borne in

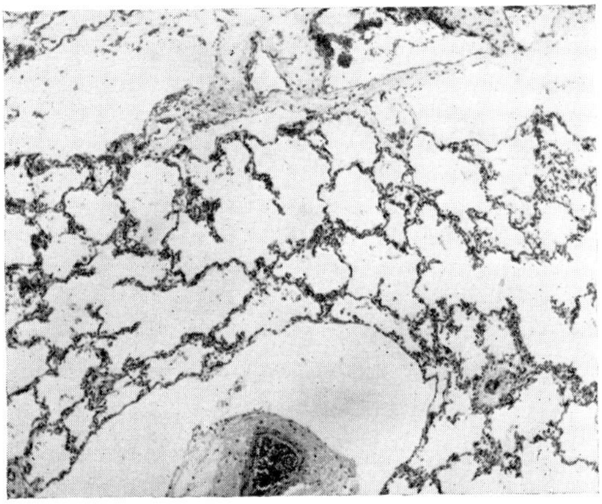

Fig. 1.11. Microphotograph of a section of lung taken from an infant who did not survive operative repair of a congenital diaphragmatic hernia. The disruption of the alveolar walls produced by overinflation of the unsupported lung and the consequent perivascular spread of air are well illustrated.

Courtesy of Blackwell Scientific Publications.[125]

mind that in many patients the distribution of the inflating gas within the lungs is not uniform. When this occurs the normal relationship that must exist between the ventilation of the lungs and the perfusion of the lungs with blood is disturbed. The full implications of uneven ventilation are complex [31] and may be exaggerated during inexpert controlled ventilation. The most serious result of this is the perfusion of insufficiently-ventilated parts of the lungs with venous blood, and therefore insufficient oxygenation of this blood. The condition is that of a venous shunt from the right side of the heart to the left. In otherwise healthy individuals uneven distribution of gas eventually results in a diminution of blood flow through the less-well-ventilated parts of the lungs, and any venous shunt is thereby minimized. Another possible effect of importance is the ventilation of insufficiently-perfused parts of the lung; such ventilation is largely 'wasted' and represents an increase in the physiological dead-space. In such circumstances a 'normal' total ventilation may result in a raised arterial P_{CO_2}.

Uneven distribution may be due to localized changes in elasticity or in the patency of the small airways such as are found in asthma, chronic bronchitis and emphysema. Apart from pathological causes within the patient, the lateral posture causes uneven ventilation by decreasing ventilation of the dependent lung. Surgical retractors and packs may also cause uneven ventilation by limiting the expansion of small or even extensive parts of the lung. The localized accumulation of secretions will also have the same effect.

In any of these circumstances of uneven ventilation, an added risk of alveolar damage exists. For example, the anaesthetist, unaware that a deterioration in the patient's condition is due to uneven ventilation (i.e. a disturbed ventilation/perfusion ratio), may make vigorous efforts to increase the tidal volume in the belief that increased ventilation is the patient's only requirement.

In other cases the high inspiratory flow, which may occur when a short inspiratory period is aimed at in order to reduce the mean lung pressure (see p. 22), may produce a considerable difference of pressure between adjacent alveoli, even when the extent of any concomitant pathology is comparatively minor. Thus, whenever either the inspiratory flow is increased, or the pressure at the mouth raised to a high level, any tendency to uneven distribution of gas in the lungs is exaggerated. It is then that, at some point in the respiratory cycle, differences of pressure exist between neighbouring alveoli or parts of the lung, and unequal forces act across the alveolar septa tending to rupture them. Although clinical reports have not drawn attention to this type of damage, perhaps because of the difficulty in recognizing it *in vivo*, it may be more common than is suspected. That vigorous ventilation within clinical limits can produce widespread alveolar damage is shown by case reports [124,125] in which the lungs were examined histologically after death.

The possibility of damage to the lungs resulting from uneven ventilation must be regarded as to some extent speculative and it should not deter the anaesthetist in his attempt to ventilate his patient adequately. The maintenance of effective alveolar ventilation on which life depends is of paramount importance, though the manner in which this is achieved is often capable of variation within wide limits. The special circumstances, such as ventilation of small children (see Chapter 6), in which particular problems occur when deciding on an optimum pattern of ventilation are discussed later.

D. Metabolic[126, 127, 128]

The acid-base balance of the blood will be disturbed with any deviation of alveolar ventilation from the normal. Over-ventilation will cause a fall in the P_{CO_2} and a rise in the pH, i.e. an alkalaemia. Conversely, under-ventilation will lead to a rise in the P_{CO_2} and a fall in the pH, i.e. an acidaemia. Ideally the normal equilibrium should be maintained as being part of the optimum physiological environment. However there is no lack of evidence that retention of carbon dioxide in the body, as indicated by a rise of P_{CO_2} and a fall in pH, is to be avoided since it leads not only to general depression of the body, including the central nervous system, ending in coma, but also to important undesirable effects on individual organs. On the heart, for example, it enhances the toxic action of many drugs and of such procedures as hypothermia, giving rise to an increased irritability and liability to arrhythmias, and ultimately to ventricular fibrillation and cardiac arrest. The sensitivity of the heart and other organs, including the liver, to hypoxia is likewise increased in the presence of a raised carbon-dioxide level.

There is less certainty of the harm of over-ventilation. At any rate, short periods, such as occur during surgery, seem to be harmless from a purely metabolic point of view, though the risk of lung damage should always be remembered. Inasmuch as over-ventilation will, in general, make certain of good oxygenation and carbon-dioxide elimination, it is to be preferred to under-ventilation. However, like under-ventilation it also produces changes in tissue activity. The attention of anaesthetists is directed, for example, to the alteration in activity of various drugs, the most important of which is that of the muscle relaxants.

E. Cerebral Vasoconstriction[129–135]

Over-ventilation undoubtedly leads to cerebral vasoconstriction and to a potentiation of anaesthesia, if not to a state resembling anaesthesia itself. There is little doubt that the triumphs of modern anaesthesia, brought about by the widespread use of relaxants, controlled respiration, and small doses of anaesthetic agents, could hardly have occurred without over-ventilation being a common, if not a usual, accompaniment of the technique. The mechanism whereby over-ventilation causes cerebral vasoconstriction is not completely understood, though it is to a large extent dependent on the reduction of the level of carbon dioxide in the blood. This effect was first shown by Kety and Schmidt;[133] it is well demonstrated in fig. 1.12.[134]

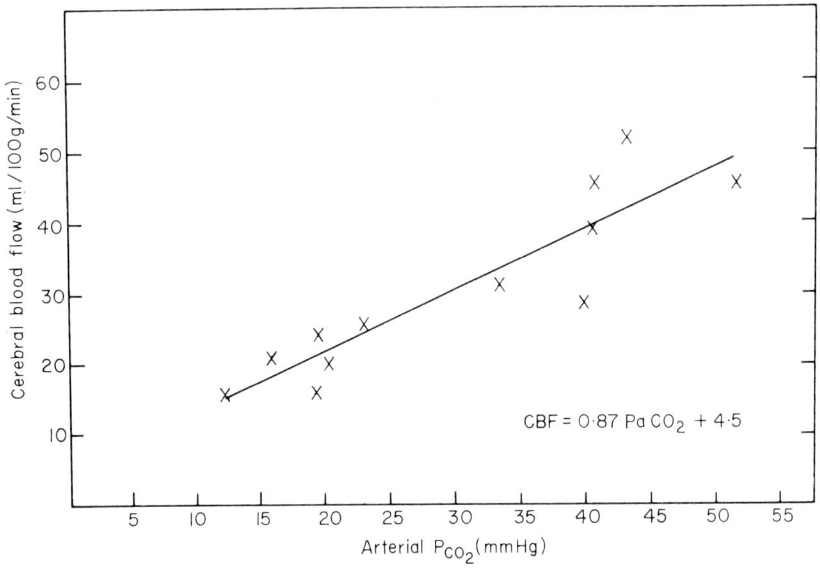

Fig. 1.12. The relationship between the arterial P_{CO_2} and the cerebral blood-flow in man during anaesthesia.

Courtesy of *Anesthesiology*[134] and Dr H.Wollman.

F. Other Harmful Effects

Certain other effects may be associated with controlled respiration particularly if carried out with a face-mask instead of an endotracheal tube. Then, the possibility of accidental 'inflation of the stomach' arises. The pressure at the mouth in these circumstances should therefore be carefully limited; thus while pressures of up to 15 cmH_2O rarely distend the stomach, pressures over 20 cmH_2O invariably do so. If this occurs the stomach dilates and may present a hindrance to the surgeon performing an abdominal operation. In addition, unless the gas in the stomach is evacuated by means of a tube the patient may suffer acute discomfort in the post-operative period. Rupture of the eardrums has also been reported during controlled ventilation.

MINIMIZING THE HARMFUL CARDIOVASCULAR EFFECTS OF CONTROLLED RESPIRATION

Any harmful cardiovascular effects of controlled respiration are basically the result of the abnormally-high positive pressure within the lungs. This eliminates in part or whole the sub-atmospheric pressure normally present within the thorax. Both the magnitude of the positive pressure and the time during which it acts are of importance; these two factors are combined in the term 'mean pressure'. The lower the mean intrapulmonary pressure during the respiratory cycle, the less marked these cardiovascular effects will be.[60, 70, 73, 136]

Some definition is here necessary of the term 'mean pressure' within the lungs. This does not imply the arithmetical mean between the highest and lowest pressures in the respiratory cycle. It is, in fact, the mean of a very large number of equally-spaced instantaneous readings of the pressure within the lung during one respiratory cycle (fig. 1.13). To determine the mean it is necessary to take the sum of all the instantaneous readings of pressure and divide it by the number of readings. The former is proportional to the area between the pressure curve and the line of zero pressure; the number of readings is proportional to the length of the base line which represents the duration of one cycle (5 secs in figs. 1.13 and 1.14). Put in another way, therefore, the mean pressure

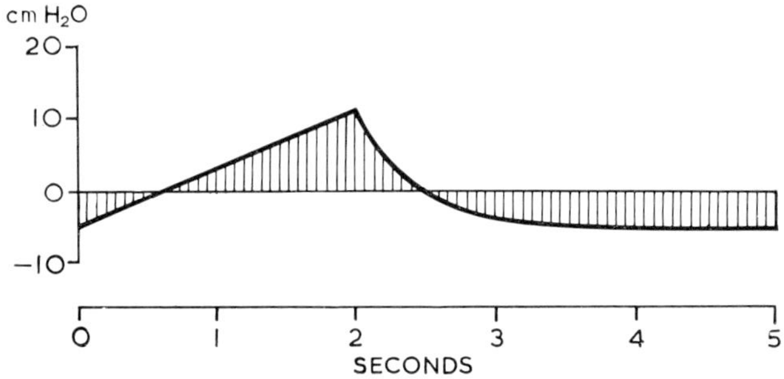

Fig. 1.13. Graph illustrating the determination of mean pressure by taking many equally-spaced measurements of the height of the curve over one respiratory cycle.

Sum of positive heights $= 163{\cdot}4$ cmH_2O
Sum of negative heights $= -170{\cdot}3$ cmH_2O
Net sum of heights $= -6{\cdot}9$ cmH_2O
Number of heights $= 70$

$$\text{Therefore, mean pressure} = -\frac{6{\cdot}9}{70} = -0{\cdot}1 \text{ cmH}_2\text{O}$$

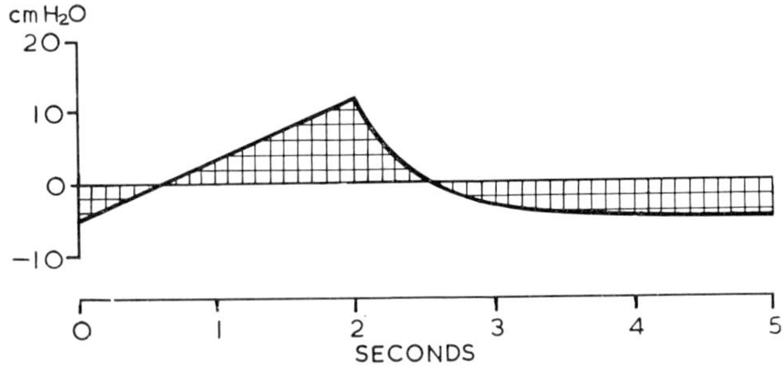

Fig. 1.14. Graph illustrating the determination of mean pressure by estimating the area under the curve over one respiratory cycle.

Number of positive squares	= 55
Number of negative squares	= −57·5
Net number of squares	= −2·5
'Area' of one square	= 2 cmH_2O × 0·1 sec
Therefore, area of −2·5 squares	= −0·5 cmH_2O . sec
Duration of cycle	= 5 sec
Therefore, mean pressure	= −0·1 cmH_2O

is equal to the area enclosed between the pressure curve and the line of zero pressure for one respiratory cycle, divided by the duration of the cycle (fig. 1.14). Should there be any negative pressure in the lungs during the respiratory cycle the pressure curve will fall below the zero line. Areas enclosed by the pressure curve below the zero line should be taken as negative and subtracted from the area enclosed by the pressure curve above the zero line.

Figs. 1.15–1.19 exemplify the use and importance of the term 'mean pressure'. The pressure curves illustrated might have occurred during automatic ventilation on five different occasions in the same patient. Although in each case the range of alveolar pressure, and hence the volume exchange, and the frequency of ventilation are the same, the mean pressure varies widely from −0·5 cmH_2O to + 8·3 cmH_2O. However, whatever modifications are made in the intrapulmonary pressure curve, the over-riding need for an adequate volume exchange should always be borne in mind (see p. 36).

Reduction of the mean intrapulmonary pressure

The ways in which the mean pressure in the lungs may be kept low are as follows.

Positive pressure should not be maintained for longer than is necessary to effect the desired volume exchange

Once the required volume has entered the lungs expiration should be allowed to begin. In healthy lungs it is unlikely that any important additional gaseous exchange with the blood occurs once the volume exchange has taken place. The maintenance of a

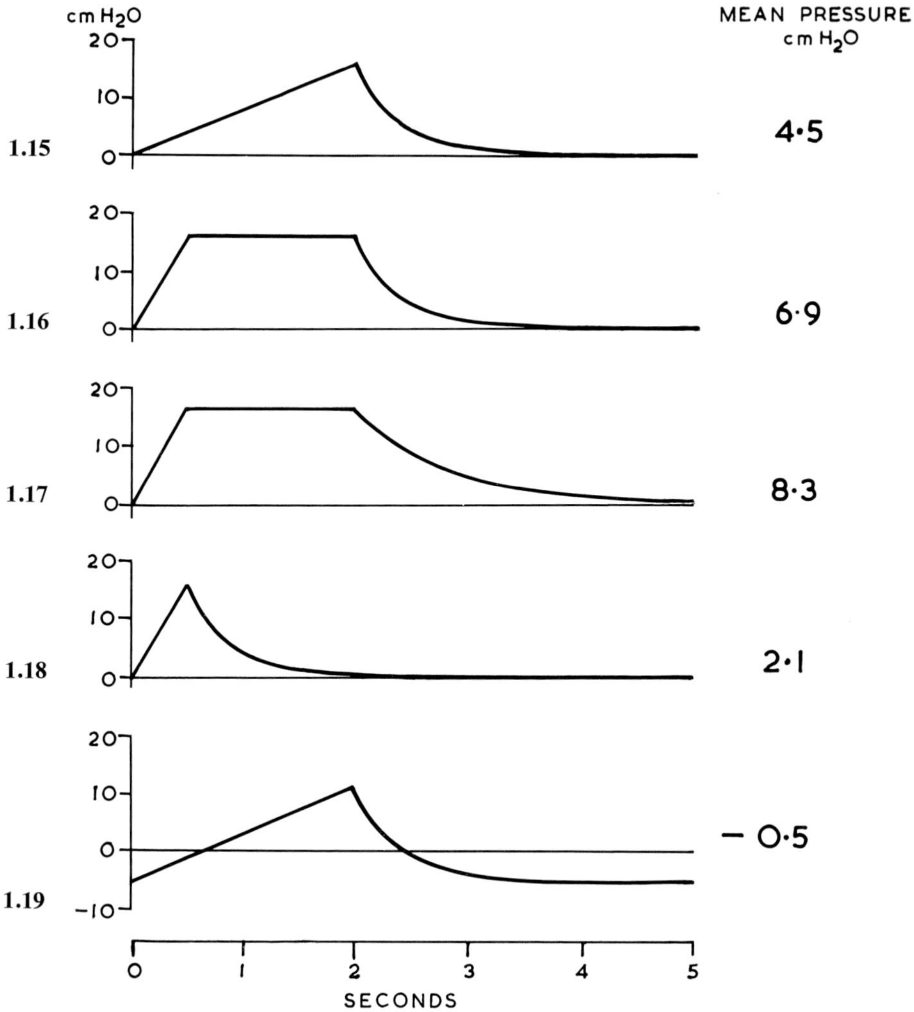

Figs. 1.15, 1.16, 1.17, 1.18, and 1.19. Diagrams illustrating the meaning of the term 'mean pressure in the lungs' during artificial ventilation. In each case the total respiratory cycle lasts 5 seconds; the tidal volume is 800 ml and the compliance is 0·05 litre/cmH_2O. Hence the pressure range is 16 cmH_2O. The airway resistance is taken as 6 cmH_2O/(litre/sec). However, possible changes in other variables produce a wide range of mean pressures.

Fig. 1.15. Inflation is slow (flow of inflating gas is 24 litres/min). Expiration is 'free.' The resistance of the apparatus is taken as 2 cmH_2O/(litre/sec).
The mean pressure is 4·5 cmH_2O.

Fig. 1.16. Inflation is rapid (flow of inflating gas is 96 litres/min) at the beginning of the inspiratory phase. The lungs are then held inflated for some time so that the inspiratory phase lasts for 2 seconds, as in fig. 1.15. Expiration is again 'free'.
The mean pressure is 6·9 cmH_2O.

'plateau' in the pressure curve (figs. 1.16 and 1.17) after the volume exchange has occurred may aid the more-even distribution of the inflating gas in patients with pulmonary disease. However, this benefit will, to some extent, be offset by the circulatory embarrassment (fig. 1.20) which will also result.

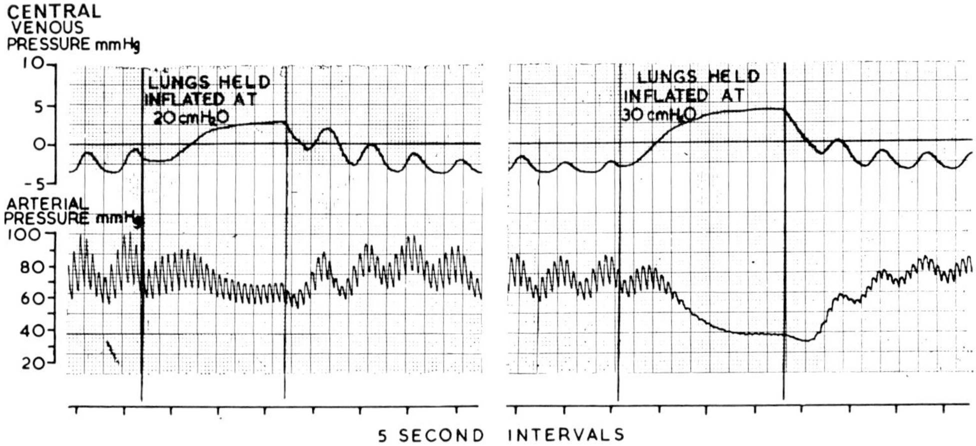

VENTILATOR SETTINGS

V_T 1000 ml
P_I + 14 cm H_2O
P_E −7 cm H_2O
f 12 /min
I:E 1:2

Fig. 1.20. Recordings of the arterial and central venous pressures in man during artificial ventilation to show the effect of holding the lungs inflated.

Inspiration should be shorter than expiration

The foregoing paragraph stresses the importance of a release of pressure once the volume exchange has occurred. Just as important is the limitation of the time taken for the volume exchange. The inspiratory phase should occupy less than half of the total respiratory cycle.[57, 59, 60, 61, 72, 77, 137, 138, 139] A longer positive-pressure phase will tend to cause

---

Fig. 1.17. The inspiratory phase follows the same course as in fig. 1.16, but expiration is impeded by an apparatus resistance of 10 cmH_2O/(litre/sec).
The mean pressure is 8·3 cmH_2O.

Fig. 1.18. Inflation is rapid (flow of inflating gas is 96 litres/min) and is followed immediately by the 'free' expiration.
The mean pressure is 2·1 cmH_2O.

Fig. 1.19. Inflation is slow (flow of inflating gas is 24 litres/min) and again occupies 2 seconds. During the expiratory phase a steady negative pressure (−5 cmH_2O) is introduced. Expiration is 'free'.
The mean pressure is −0·5 cmH_2O.

reduction of cardiac output. Many ventilators allow the ratio of inspiratory to expiratory time to be varied between 1 : 1 and 1 : 4. In one case (the 'Barnet II', see p. 286) the ratio can be varied from 9 : 1 to 1 : 9! A common setting is about 1 : 2.

An important benefit of a long expiratory phase is that it allows the lungs to deflate so that the intrapulmonary pressure falls to zero. The heart is free from tamponade and its output rises, the intrathoracic pressure falls, and the great veins and heart fill. If the expiratory period is too short these events are curtailed and the next inflation commences while the lung is still partially inflated; the heart is subjected to continuous tamponade, the venous return is continuously hampered, and the pulmonary circulation continuously impeded. The mean pressure within the lungs is raised, and, even in a healthy adult, a short expiratory period may cause gradually-increasing cardiovascular embarrassment. In chronic bronchitic and emphysematous patients in whom there is already a degree of cardio-respiratory failure a too-short expiratory period may cause even further deterioration in cardiovascular function.

On the other hand, there is reason for not using an inspiratory-expiratory ratio which is too small. There is evidence that, at least in the case of pressure generators, when the inspiratory period is reduced to about 0·5 sec, i.e. the inspiratory-expiratory ratio approaches about 1 : 6, the physiological dead-space may exceed 50% of the tidal volume.

The lungs should be inflated with rapid flows of gas

The faster the flow of gas into the lungs the shorter the inspiratory phase can be. Limits, however, are set to this by mechanical design problems, by the danger of alveolar rupture in circumstances of uneven ventilation, and even by the development of uneven ventilation itself by virtue of the resultant short inspiratory period. However, in general terms, the tendency should be to use higher rather than lower flows during inflation.[78]

The magnitude of the inflating flow can be determined in the following manner.

Respiratory frequency	= 20 per min
One respiratory cycle	= 3 sec
If ratio of inspiration : expiration	= 1 : 2
then, time of inspiration	= 1 sec

For a tidal volume of 500 ml in 1 second, flow must be 30 litres/min.

In circumstances where the anaesthetist is mainly concerned to reduce the mean alveolar pressure, a more extreme I : E ratio may be desired. Calculation along the above lines will show that a higher inflating flow will be needed. The same result will follow the use of an increased ventilation.

Expiratory resistance should be low

In some ventilators a control is fitted which introduces an adjustable resistance to expiration, which is claimed to produce more-even distribution of gas. However, any resistance to the outflow of gas from the lungs, unless it is more than compensated for by negative pressure, will delay the fall of pressure during the expiratory phase and hence raise the mean intrapulmonary pressure (fig. 1.17).

The dead space should be small

The dead space may be reduced by the insertion of an endotracheal or tracheostomy tube, and by careful design of the connexions between ventilator and patient. By taking these steps the tidal volume needed to produce a given alveolar ventilation at a given respiratory frequency can be reduced. This will reduce the peak, and hence the mean, intrapulmonary pressure.

Negative pressure may be applied during the expiratory phase[70,71,73,74,82,136]

The application of negative pressure during the expiratory phase lowers the mean intrapulmonary pressure in two different ways.

(a) A particular volume exchange during the inspiratory phase requires a certain pressure difference between mouth and alveoli depending on the patient's compliance and on his airway resistance. If the inspiratory phase starts with a negative pressure of a few cmH_2O in the lungs, the required pressure difference, and hence volume exchange, occurs with a lower peak of positive pressure (fig. 1.19). This is what occurs in automatic ventilators in which a negative pressure is maintained throughout the expiratory phase.

(b) A negative-pressure phase can also accelerate the fall in pressure in the lungs during expiration. This is of particular importance when either the airway resistance is raised by disease, e.g. asthma and growths, and hence cannot readily be lowered, or when the apparatus resistance is high, e.g. heavily-loaded expiratory valves and badly-designed equipment. However, a negative-pressure phase has disadvantages which are discussed below.

In practice most or all of these various methods of reducing the mean intrapulmonary pressure and maintaining the venous return are employed in the same patient. That the patient suffers least cardiovascular harm if his ventilatory requirements are satisfied with as low a mean pressure in his lungs as possible, is not in doubt. Whether one factor is more important than another is still not clear.

Other aspects of negative pressure in the expiratory phase

In addition to reducing the mean intrapulmonary pressure, a negative-pressure phase will have some direct effect in increasing the venous return to the heart (figs. 1.7 and 1.10). The mechanism of this effect seems to be a restoration of a suction effect during the expiratory phase in contradistinction to the natural 'thoracic pump' accompanying spontaneous breathing, which is mainly effective during inspiration. Negative pressure during the expiratory phase is transmitted to the intrathoracic structures, including the great veins, and causes an increased venous-pressure gradient during the time of its action. The increased venous return which occurs when a negative-pressure phase is introduced does not take place when the chest is widely-opened for then the negative pressure cannot be transmitted to the intrathoracic structures since they are all exposed to the atmosphere. From this point of view there seems little advantage in employing a negative-pressure phase during these operations.

In spite of the advantages set out here of a negative-pressure phase there are circumstances in which it may be harmful. As a result of the pathological changes in the lungs of patients with emphysema, the lung compliance is high and the airway resistance is high. In addition, the wall structure of the smaller airways becomes weaker and more-easily collapsed than normal. As a result, when the pressure difference between alveoli and mouth exceeds a certain value, the well-known 'check valve' or 'trapping' mechanism[34, 140, 141, 142] comes into play: the small airways tend to collapse and expiration slows down considerably.

This is well-illustrated in the diagrammatic representation of the expiratory phase in a normal patient and in an emphysematous patient (figs. 1.21 and 1.22).[141] In the normal

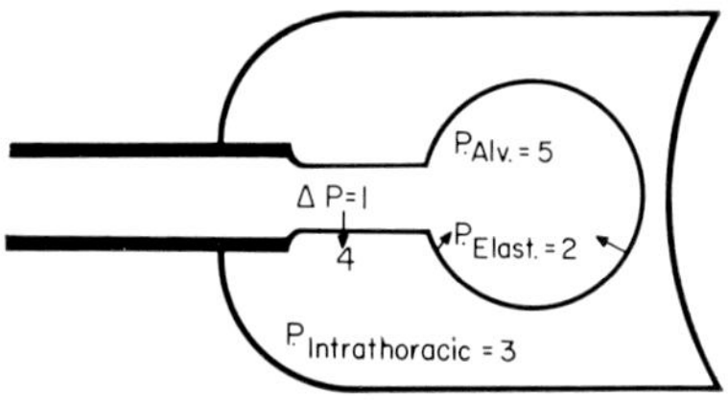

Fig. 1.21. Diagrammatic representation of the forces acting on the alveoli and small airways in a normal patient.

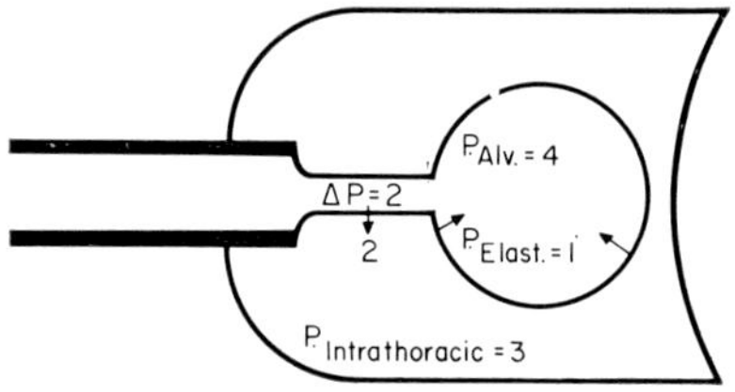

Fig. 1.22. Diagrammatic representation of the forces acting on the alveoli and small airways in an emphysematous patient.

Courtesy of John Sherratt & Son[141] and Dr E.J.M.Campbell.

patient (fig. 1.21) the alveolar-mouth pressure difference of 5 units is made up of 2 units of pressure derived from the elastic recoil of the lungs and 3 units derived from the elastic recoil of the thorax. The pressure drop of 1 unit occurring in the smaller airways still leaves the intraluminal pressure greater (4 units) than the intrathoracic pressure (3 units). The smaller airways remain patent, and the expiratory flow is unimpeded. In the emphysematous patient (fig. 1.22) the alveolar-mouth pressure difference is now only 4 units since there is only 1 unit deriving from the lowered elasticity of the lung structure and hence the higher compliance. The smaller unsupported airways are more narrowed than in the normal, and the pressure drop is therefore greater (2 units). The intraluminal pressure is now smaller (2 units) than the intrathoracic pressure (3 units) and the small airways tend to be restricted if not actually collapsed. The expiratory flow is therefore impeded, or even arrested. This effect is known as 'trapping'. This effect occurs not only when the conscious patient spontaneously tries to speed up the rate of his expiration, by voluntarily raising his intrathoracic pressure and so creating a high pressure difference, but also during controlled respiration when negative pressure is applied during the expiratory phase in an attempt to speed up expiratory flow by creating a high pressure difference.

The same sequence of events occurs even in healthy patients when negative pressure is applied during the expiratory phase. There is now clear evidence[142] that in this circumstance the airway resistance is increased with a consequent tendency towards a smaller ventilation and impairment of gas exchange.

A negative-pressure phase should only therefore be employed with great caution in emphysematous patients. In extreme cases such a patient can be reduced to a state of asphyxial collapse by the use of a high pressure difference, whether this is the result of a high positive pressure in the alveoli at the end of the inspiratory period without a negative pressure in the expiratory phase, or a lower positive pressure in the alveoli and a negative pressure in the expiratory phase.

A further disadvantage of a negative-pressure expiratory phase which has recently come to light is the increase in physiological dead-space which accompanies it.[143]

An additional need for caution is in operations on the head and neck, in which large veins may be opened, and also in other circumstances where air can enter the veins. The increased negative pressure in the thorax as a result of the negative-pressure phase may be transmitted both to a further distance and to a greater extent than usual, and the danger of air embolism is very real. These factors are particularly important in the head-up position.

The application of negative pressure during the expiratory phase should not be confused with the use of suction for the removal of secretions. The negative pressure produced by an automatic ventilator rarely exceeds -15 cmH_2O, whereas the negative pressure at the tip of a suction catheter is commonly of the order of half an atmosphere, i.e. -500 cmH_2O. Negative pressure of the latter magnitude, particularly when the suction catheter is large enough to prevent a free flow of air from the exterior to its tip, can cause widespread atelectasis and acute dilatation of the heart.[144]

REFERENCES

1 GUEDEL A.E. and TREWEEK D.N. (1934) Ether apnoeas. *Curr. Res. Anesth. Analg.* **13**, 263.

2 MUSHIN W.W. and RENDELL-BAKER L. (1953) *Principles of thoracic anaesthesia*, p. 14. Oxford: Blackwell.

3 SCURR C. (1956) Controlled respiration: standardization of ventilation. *Br. J. Anaesth.* **28**, 23.

4 HUGH-JONES P. (1958) Oligopnoea. *Proc. R. Soc. Med.* **51**, 104.

5 THOMPSON P.W. (1966) Classification and function of automatic ventilators. *Abstracts; Second European Congress of Anaesthesiology, Copenhagen* (1966), p. 118.

6 Fry D.L., Ebert R.V., Stead W.W. and Brown C.C. (1954) The mechanics of pulmonary ventilation in normal subjects and in patients with emphysema. *Am. J. Med.* **16**, 80.

7 Nims R.G., Conner E.H. and Comroe J.H. jr. (1955) The compliance of the human thorax in anaesthetized patients. *J. clin. Invest.* **34**, 744.

8 Brownlee W.E. and Allbritten F.F. (1956) The significance of the lung-thorax compliance in ventilation during thoracic surgery. *J. thorac. Surg.* **32**, 454.

9 Butler J. and Smith B.H. (1957) Pressure-volume relationships of the chest in the completely relaxed anaesthetised patient. *Clin. Sci.* **16**, 125.

10 Campbell E.J.M., Howell, J.B.L. and Peckett B.W. (1957) The pressure-volume relationships of the thorax of anaesthetized human subjects: a comparison of the effects of expiratory resistance and positive pressure inflation. *J. Physiol., Lond.* **136**, 563.

11 Howell J.B.L. and Peckett B.W. (1957) Studies of the elastic properties of the thorax of supine anaesthetized paralysed human subjects. *J. Physiol., Lond.* **136**, 1.

12 Bromage P.R. (1958) Total respiratory compliance in anaesthetized subjects and modifications produced by noxious stimuli. *Clin. Sci.* **17**, 217.

13 Elam J.O., Kerr J.H. and Janney C.D. (1958) Performance of ventilators; effect of changes in lung-thorax compliance. *Anesthesiology*, **19**, 56.

14 Agostoni E. (1959) Volume-pressure relationships of the thorax and lung in the newborn. *J. appl. Physiol.* **14**, 909.

15 Newman H.C., Campbell E.J.M. and Dinnick O.P. (1959). A simple method of measuring the compliance and the non-elastic resistance of the chest during anaesthesia. *Br. J. Anaesth.* **31**, 282.

16 Opie L.H., Spalding J.M.K. and Stott F.D. (1959) Mechanical properties of the chest during intermittent positive-pressure respiration. *Lancet*, **1**, 545.

17 Safar P. and Aguto-Escarraga L. (1959). Compliance in apneic anesthetized adults. *Anesthesiology*, **20**, 283.

18 Emerson P.A., Torres G.E. and Lyons H.A. (1960) The effect of intermittent positive pressure breathing on the lung compliance and intrapulmonary mixing of gases. *Thorax*, **15**, 124.

19 Gliedman M.L., Sellers R.D., Timmes J.L., Vestal B.L. and Karlson K.E. (1962) Pressure-volume relationships of the single lung. *Anesthesiology*, **23**, 41.

20 Watson W.E. (1962) Some observations on dynamic lung compliance during intermittent positive pressure respiration. *Br. J. Anaesth.* **34**, 153.

21 Watson W.E. (1962) Observations on the dynamic lung compliance of patients with respiratory weakness receiving intermittent positive pressure respiration. *Br. J. Anaesth.* **34**, 690.

22 Chu J.S., Dawson P., Klaus M. and Sweet A.Y. (1964) Lung compliance and lung volume measured concurrently in normal full-term and premature infants. *Pediatrics, Springfield*, **34**, 525.

23 Laver M.B., Morgan J., Bendixen H.H. and Radford E.P. jr. (1964) Lung volume, compliance and arterial oxygen tension during controlled ventilation. *J. appl. Physiol.* **19**, 725.

24 Gold M.I. and Helrich M. (1965) Pulmonary compliance during anesthesia. *Anesthesiology*, **26**, 281.

25 Larson C.P. (1965) Pulmonary compliance in anesthetized man. *Anesthesiology*, **26**, 710.

26 Mittman C., Edelman N.H., Norris A.H. and Shock N.W. (1965) Relationship between chest wall and pulmonary compliance with age. *J. appl. Physiol.* **20**, 1211.

27 Garzon A.A., Lichtenstein S. and Karlson K.E. (1966) The effect of position and thoracotomy on the pressure required to inflate each lung. *Dis Chest*, **50**, 142.

28 Okinaka A.J. (1966) Postoperative pattern of breathing and compliance. *Archs Surg., Chicago*, **92**, 887.

29 BROWNLEE W.E. and ALLBRITTEN F.F. (1957) The work of breathing during surgical operations. *Archs Surg., Chicago*, **74**, 846.

30 OTIS A.B., FENN W.O. and RAHN H. (1950) Mechanics of breathing in man. *J. appl. Physiol.* **2**, 592.

31 COMROE J.H. jr., FORSTER R.E., DUBOIS A.B., BRISCOE W.A. and CARLSEN E. (1962) *The lung: Clinical physiology and pulmonary function tests.* 2nd ed. Chicago: Year Book Medical Publishers.

32 ATTINGER E.O., MONROE R.G. and SEGAL M.S. (1956) The mechanics of breathing in different body positions in normal subjects. *J. clin. Invest.* **35**, 904.

33 MARSHALL R. and DUBOIS A.B. (1956) The measurement of the viscous resistance of the lung tissues in normal man. *Clin. Sci.* **15**, 161.

34 CAMPBELL E.J.M. (1958) Mechanism of airway obstruction in emphysema and asthma. *Proc. R. Soc. Med.* **51**, 108.

35 NEWMAN H.C., CAMPBELL E.J.M. and DINNICK O.P. (1959) A simple method of measuring the compliance and the non-elastic resistance of the chest during anaesthesia. *Br. J. Anaesth.* **31**, 282

36 OPIE L.H., SPALDING J.M.K. and STOTT F.D. (1959) Mechanical properties of the chest during intermittent positive-pressure respiration. *Lancet*, **1**, 545.

37 WELLS R.E. (1959) Mechanics of respiration in bronchial asthma. *Am. J. Med.* **26**, 384.

38 BODMAN R.I. (1963) Clinical applications of pulmonary function tests. *Anaesthesia*, **18**, 355.

39 HYATT R.E. and WILCOX R.E. (1963) The pressure-flow relationships of the intrathoracic airway in man. *J. clin. Invest.* **42**, 29.

40 MCILROY M., TIERNEY D.F. and NADEL J.A. (1963) A new method for measurement of compliance and resistance of lungs and thorax. *J. appl. Physiol.* **18**, 424.

41 FERRIS B.G. jr., MEAD J. and OPIE L.H. (1964) Partitioning of respiratory flow resistance in man. *J. appl. Physiol.* **19**, 653.

42 DON H.F. and ROBSON J.G. (1965) The mechanics of the respiratory system during anesthesia. *Anesthesiology*, **26**, 168.

43 GOLD M.I. and HELRICH M. (1965) Mechanics of breathing during anesthesia. *Anesthesiology*, **26**, 751.

44 HARGREAVES M.D. (1965) Changes in respiratory resistance and compliance with posture. *Br. J. Anaesth.* **37**, 988.

45 BERGMAN N.A. (1966) Measurement of respiratory resistance in anaesthetised subjects. *J. appl. Physiol.* **21**, 1913.

46 MACINTOSH R.R., MUSHIN W.W. and EPSTEIN H.G. (1963) *Physics for the anaesthetist*, 3rd ed., p. 168. Oxford: Blackwell.

47 MACINTOSH R.R., MUSHIN W.W. and EPSTEIN H.G. (1963) *Physics for the anaesthetist*, 3rd ed., p. 97. Oxford: Blackwell.

48 BEST C.H. and TAYLOR N.B. (1966) *The physiological basis of medical practice*, 8th ed., p. 1003. Edinburgh: Livingstone.

49 KEELE C.A. and NEIL E. (1965) *Samson Wright's applied physiology*, 11th ed., p. 159. London: Oxford University Press.

50 Symposium; Physiological effects of artificial ventilation (1966) Chairman, Nunn, J.F. *Abstracts; Second European Congress of Anaesthesiology, Copenhagen* (1966) p. 86.

51 MOLGAARD H. (1915) *Fysiologisk lungekirurgi*, p. 370. Copenhagen: Gyldendal.

52 HUMPHREYS G.H., MOORE R.L., MAIER H.C. and APGAR V. (1937–38) Studies of cardiac output of anesthetized dogs during continuous and intermittent inflation of the lungs. *J. thorac. Surg.* **7**, 438.

53 HUMPHREYS G.H., MOORE R.L. and BARKLEY H. (1939) Studies of jugular, carotid, and pulmonary pressures of anesthetized dogs during positive inflation of the lungs. *J. thorac. Surg.* **8**, 553.

54 BEECHER H.K., BENNETT H.S. and BASSETT D.L. (1943) Circulatory effects of increased pressure in the airway. *Anesthesiology*, **4**, 612.

55 CARR D.T. and ESSEX H.E. (1946) Certain effects of positive pressure respiration on circulatory and respiratory systems. *Am. Heart J.* **31**, 53.

56 BARACH A.L., FENN W.O., FERRIS E.B. and SCHMIDT C.F. (1947) The physiology of pressure breathing; a brief review of its present status. *J. Aviat. Med.* **18**, 73.

57 COURNAND A., MOTLEY H.L. and WERKÖ L. (1947) Mechanism underlying cardiac output change during intermittent positive pressure breathing. *Fedn. Proc. Fedn. Am. Socs. exp. Biol.* **6**, 92.

58 PAPPER E.M. and REAVES D.P. (1947) Circulatory depression during controlled respiration—a case report. *Anesthesiology*, **8**, 407.

59 WERKÖ L. (1947) The influence of positive pressure breathing on circulation in man. *Acta. med. scand.* **128**, Suppl. 193.

60 COURNAND A., MOTLEY H.L., WERKÖ L. and RICHARDS D.W. jr. (1948) Physiological studies of effects of intermittent positive pressure breathing on cardiac output in man. *Am. J. Physiol.* **152**, 162.

61 MOTLEY H.L., COURNAND A., WERKÖ L., DRESDALE D.T., HIMMELSTEIN A. and RICHARDS D.W. jr. (1948) Intermittent positive pressure breathing; a means of administering artificial respiration in man. *J. Am. med. Ass.* **137**, 370.

62 WATROUS W.G., DAVIS F.E. and ANDERSON B.M. (1950) Manually assisted and controlled respiration; its use during inhalation anesthesia for maintenance of near-normal physiologic state. *Anesthesiology*, **11**, 538.

63 WATROUS W.G., DAVIS F.E. and ANDERSON B.M. (1950) Manually assisted and controlled respiration; its use during inhalation anesthesia for maintenance of near-normal physiologic state. *Anesthesiology*, **11**, 661.

64 WHITTENBERGER J.L. and SARNOFF S.J. (1950) Symposium on specific methods of treatment; physiologic principles in treatment of respiratory failure. *Med. Clins N. Am.* **34**, 1335.

65 EDWARDS W.S. (1951) The effects of lung inflation and epinephrine on pulmonary vascular resistance. *Am. J. Physiol.* **167**, 756.

66 PRICE H.L., BENTON D.K., ELDER J.D., LIBIEN B.H. and DRIPPS R.D. (1951) Circulatory effects of raised airway pressure during cyclopropane anesthesia in man. *J. clin. Invest.* **30**, 1243.

67 TAYLOR G. and GERBODE F. (1951) Observations on the circulatory effects of short duration positive pressure pulmonary inflation. *Surgery, St. Louis*, **30**, 56.

68 WATROUS W.G., DAVIS F.E. and ANDERSON B.M. (1951) Manually assisted and controlled respiration; its use during inhalation anesthesia for maintenance of near-normal physiologic state. *Anesthesiology*, **12**, 33.

69 BRECHER G.A. (1953) Venous return during intermittent positive-negative pressure respiration studied wiith a new catheter flowmeter. *Am. J. Physiol.* **174**, 299.

70 MALONEY J.V. jr., ELAM J.O., HANDFORD S.W., BALLA G.A., EASTWOOD D.W., BROWN E.S. and TEN PAS R.H. (1953) The importance of negative pressure phase in mechanical respirators. *J. Am. med. Ass.* **152**, 212.

71 ANKENEY J.L., HUBAY C.A., HACKETT P.R. and HINGSON R.A. (1954) The effect of positive and negative pressure respiration on unilateral pulmonary blood flow in the open chest. *Surgery Gynec. Obstet.* **98**, 600.

72 ASTRUP P., GOTZCHE H. and NEUKIRCH F. (1954) Laboratory investigations during treatment of patients with poliomyelitis and respiratory paralysis. *Br. med. J.* **1**, 780.

73 HUBAY C.A., WALTZ R.C., BRECHER G.A., PRAGLIN J. and HINGSON R.A. (1954) Circulatory dynamics of venous return during positive-negative pressure respiration. *Anesthesiology*, **15**, 445.

74 MALONEY J.V. and HANDFORD S.W. (1954) Circulatory responses to intermittent positive and alternating positive-negative pressure respirators. *J. appl. Physiol.* **6**, 453.

75 PRICE H.L., CONNER E.H. and DRIPPS R.D. (1954) Some respiratory and circulatory effects of mechanical respirators. *J. appl. Physiol.* **6**, 517.

76 HUBAY C.A., BRECHER G.A. and CLEMENT F.L. (1955) Etiological factors affecting pulmonary artery flow with controlled respiration. *Surgery, St. Louis*, **38**, 215.

77 LINDERHOLM H. (1955) *Proceedings of the Third Congress of the Scandinavian Society of Anaesthesiologists, Copenhagen*, 1954, p. 24.

78 PASK E.A. (1955) The maintenance of respiration in respiratory paralysis. *Proc. R. Soc. Med.* **48**, 239.

79 WHITTENBERGER J.L. (1955) Artificial respiration. *Physiol. Rev.* **35**, 611.

80 BERGEN F.H.V., BUCKLEY J.J., WEATHERHEAD D.S.P., SCHULTZ E.A. and GORDON J.R. (1956) A new respirator. *Anesthesiology*, **17**, 708.

81 BJÖRK V.O., ENGSTRÖM C.G., FRIBERG O., FEYCHTING H. and SWENSSON A. (1956) Ventilatory problems in thoracic anaesthesia. *J. thorac. Surg.* **31**, 117.

82 BRECHER G.A. (1956) *Venous return.* p. 100 et seq. New York: Grune and Stratton.

83 CATHCART R.T., NEALON T.F. jr., FRAIMOW W., HAMPTON L.J. and GIBBON J.H. jr. (1958). Cardiac output under general anesthesia: effect of mean endotracheal pressure. *Ann. Surg.* **148**, 488.

84 MÖRCH E.T., ENGEL R. and LIGHT G.A. (1959) Effects of pressure breathing on the peripheral circulation. *Archs Surg., Chicago*, **79**, 493.

85 NEALON T.F. jr., CATHCART R.T., FRAIMOW W., MCLAUGHLIN E.D. and GIBBON J.H. jr. (1959) The effect of mean endotracheal pressure on the cardiac output of patients undergoing intrathoracic operations. *J. thorac. Surg.* **38**, 449.

86 CATHCART R.T., FRAIMOW W., NEALON T.F. jr. and PRICE J. (1960) Effect of intermittent positive pressure breathing on the cardiac output of patients with chronic pulmonary disease. *Dis. Chest*, **37**, 222.

87 WHITTENBERGER J.L., MCGREGOR M., BERLUND E. and BORST H.G. (1960) Influence of state of inflation of lung on pulmonary vascular resistance. *J. appl. Physiol.* **15**, 878.

88 BOHME H. (1961) Der Einfluß künstlicher Beatmung auf die intrathorakalen Kreislaufabschnitte mit besonderer Berücksichtigung des Lungenkreislaufes. *Anaesthesist*, **10**, 184.

89 VIRTUE R.W., CARANNA L.J. and TAKAOKA K. (1961) The respiratory pattern and cardiac output. *Br. J. Anaesth.* **33**, 77.

90 DALY W.J., ROSS J.C. and BEHNKE R.H. (1963) The effect of changes in the pulmonary vascular bed produced by atropine, pulmonary engorgement, and positive-pressure breathing on diffusing and mechanical properties of the lung. *J. clin. Invest.* **42**, 1083.

91 DALY W.J., GIAMMONA S.T. and ROSS J.C. (1965) The pressure-volume relationship of the normal pulmonary capillary bed. *J. clin. Invest.* **44**, 1261.

92 NORDENSTRÖM B. and NORHAGEN A. (1965) Effect of respiration on venous return to the heart. *Am. J. Roentg.* **95**, 655.

93 GRENVIK Å. (1966) Respiratory, circulatory and metabolic effects of respirator treatment. *Acta anaesth. scand.* Suppl. XIX.

94 MORGAN B.C., MARTIN W.E., HORNBEIN T.F., CRAWFORD E.W. and GUNTEROTH W.G. (1966) Hemodynamic effects of intermittent positive pressure respiration. *Anesthesiology*, **27**, 584.

95 NAKHJAVAN F.K. and PALMER W.H. (1966) Influence of the respiration on venous return in pulmonary emphysema. *Circulation*, **33**, 8.

96 a. KELMAN G.R. and PRYS-ROBERTS C. (1967) Circulatory influences of artificial ventilation during nitrous oxide anaesthesia in man. I. Introduction and methods. *Br. J. Anaesth.* **39**, 523.
b. PRYS-ROBERTS C., KELMAN G.R. and GREENBAUM R. (1967). Circulatory influences of artificial ventilation during nitrous oxide anaesthesia in man. II. Results: the relative influence of mean intrathoracic pressure and arterial carbon dioxide tension. *Br. J. Anaesth.* **39**, 533.

97 WASSERMAN K., BUTLER J. and VAN KESSEL A. (1966) Factors affecting the pulmonary capillary blood flow pulse in man. *J. appl. Physiol.* **21**, 890.

98 MORGAGNI J.B. (1761) 'Epistola anatomico-medica XIX', in *De sedibus, et causis morborum per anatomen indagatis libri quinque*. Ex Typographia Remondiniana, Venetiis. (Cited by Franklin K.J. (1937). *A monograph on veins*. Springfield, Illinois: Charles C. Thomas.)

99 KLEIN L.J., SALTZMAN H.A., HEYMAN A. and SIEKER H.O. (1964) Syncope induced by the Valsalva maneuver. *Am. J. Med.* **37**, 263.

100 STONE D.J., LYON A.F. and TEIRSTEIN A.S. (1965) A reappraisal of the circulatory effects of the Valsalva maneuver. *Am. J. Med.* **39**, 923.

101 BRECHER G.A. (1956) *Venous return*, p. 71 et seq. New York: Grune and Stratton.

102 KEELE C.A. and NEIL E. (1965) *Samson Wright's applied physiology*, 11th ed., pp. 113–4. London: Oxford University Press.

103 BEST C.H. and TAYLOR N.B. (1966) *The physiological basis of medical practice*, 8th ed., p. 784. Edinburgh: Livingstone.

104 KEELE C.A. and NEIL E. (1965) *Samson Wright's applied physiology*, 11th ed., p. 139. London: Oxford University Press.

105 WOOLSEY W.C. (1912) Intratracheal insufflation anesthesia. *N.Y. St. J. Med.* **12**, 167.

106 LUKE H.C. (1913) A case of extensive subcutaneous emphysema following intratracheal anaesthesia with recovery. *Surgery Gynec. Obstet.* **16**, 204.

107 MACKLIN C.C. (1937) Pneumothorax with massive collapse from experimental local overinflation of lung substance. *Can. med. Ass. J.* **36**, 414.

108 MACKLIN C.C. (1939) Transport of air along sheaths of pulmonic blood vessels from alveoli to mediastinum; clinical implications. *Archs intern. Med.* **64**, 913.

109 ADAMS W.E. (1940) Differential pressures and reduced lung function in intrathoracic operations. *J. thorac. Surg.* **9**, 254.

110 HEIDRICK A.F., ADAMS W.E. and LIVINGSTONE H.M. (1940) Spontaneous pneumothorax following positive pressure intratracheal anesthesia: a case report. *Archs Surg., Chicago*, **41**, 61.

111 MARCOTTE R.J., PHILLIPS F.J., ADAMS W.E. and LIVINGSTONE H. (1940) Differential intrabronchial pressures and mediastinal emphysema. *J. thorac. Surg.* **9**, 346.

112 MACKLIN M.T. and MACKLIN C.C. (1944) Malignant interstitial emphysema of the lungs and mediastinum as an important occult complication in many respiratory diseases and other conditions: an interpretation of the clinical literature in the light of laboratory experiment. *Medicine, Baltimore*, **23**, 281.

113 HENRY J.P. (1945) National Research Council, Division of Medical Sciences, acting for the Committee on Medical Research and the Office of Scientific Research and Development. Committee on Aviation Medicine Report No. 463, May 30th, 1945.

114 LASSEN H.C.A. (1953) A preliminary report on the 1952 epidemic of poliomyelitis in Copenhagen, with special reference to the treatment of acute respiratory insufficiency. *Lancet*, **1**, 37.

115 ANDERSEN E.W. and IBSEN B. (1954) The anaesthetic management of patients with poliomyelitis and respiratory paralysis. *Br. med. J.* **1**, 786.

116 Hay P. (1954) Pneumothorax complicating intermittent positive-pressure respiration. *Lancet*, **2**, 1156.

117 Waltz R.C., Hubay C.A., Ankeney J.L. and Merrill J. (1954) Experimental study of pulmonary histopathology following positive and negative pressure respirations. *Surgery Gynec. Obstet.* **99**, 580.

118 Ozinsky J. and Bull A.B. (1955) Surgical emphysema as a complication of anaesthesia. *Br. med. J.* **1**, 460.

119 Dobkin A.B., Hubay C.A., Mendelsohn H.J. and Hingson R.A. (1956) Anaesthesia with controlled positive and negative pressure respiration. *Br. J. Anaesth.* **28**, 296.

120 Johnstone M. (1956) Emphysema and controlled respiration. *Anaesthesia*, **11**, 165.

121 Lawes W.E. and Harries J.R. (1956) Intermittent positive-pressure respiration: an unusual complication in an infant. *Lancet*, **1**, 783.

122 Boyd W. (1961) *A textbook of pathology*, 7th ed., p. 680. London: Kimpton.

123 Nicholas J.N. (1958) Mediastinal emphysema. *Br. J. Anaesth.* **30**, 63.

124 Gray T.C. (1959) A clinical note on the difficulties of maintaining adequate pulmonary ventilation during hypothemia, in, *Symposium on pulmonary ventilation*, ed. Harbord R.P. and Woolmer R., p. 43. Altrincham: Sherratt.

125 Thompson P.W. (1963) Anaesthetic problems associated with certain surgical procedures, in, *Thoracic anaesthesia*, ed. Mushin, W.W., p. 355. Oxford: Blackwell.

126 O'Reilly R.J. (1960) The clinical recognition of carbon dioxide intoxication. *Dis. Chest*, **37**, 185.

127 Gross N.J. and Hamilton J.D. (1963) Correlation between the physical signs of hypercapnia and the mixed venous P_{CO_2}. *Br. med. J.* **2**, 1096.

128 Millar R.A. and Marshall B.E. (1965) Acid-base changes in arterial blood associated with spontaneous and controlled ventilation during anaesthesia. *Br. J. Anaesth.* **37**, 492.

129 Geddes I.C. and Gray T.C. (1959) Hyperventilation for the maintenance of anaesthesia. *Lancet*, **2**, 4.

130 Sokoloff L. (1960) The effects of carbon dioxide on the cerebral circulation. *Anesthesiology*, **21**, 664.

131 Robinson J.S. and Gray T.C. (1961) Observations on the cerebral effects of passive hyperventilation. *Br. J. Anaesth.* **33**, 62.

132 Gotoh F., Meyer J.S. and Takagi Y. (1965) Cerebral effects of hyperventilation in man. *Archs. Neurol., Chicago*, **12**, 410.

133 Kety S.S. and Schmidt C.F. (1946) The effects of active and passive hyperventilation on cerebral blood flow, cerebral oxygen consumption, cardiac output, and blood pressure of normal young men. *J. clin. Invest.* **25**, 107.

134 Wollman H., Craighead A., Cohen P.J., Smith T.C., Chase P.E. and van der Molen, R.A. (1965) Cerebral circulation during general anesthesia and hyperventilation in man. *Anesthesiology*, **26**, 329.

135 Clutton-Brock J. (1957) The cerebral effects of overventilation. *Br. J. Anaesth.* **29**, 111.

136 Asmussen E. (1955) *Proceedings of the Third Congress of the Scandinavian Society of Anaesthesiologists, Copenhagen*, 1954. p. 22.

137 Neff W., Phillips W. and Gunn G. (1942) Anesthesia for pneumonectomy in man. *Anesthesiology*, **3**, 314.

138 Spalding J.M.K. (1955) Pressure and duration of inspiration during artificial respiration by intermittent positive pressure. *Lancet*, **1**, 1099.

139 Gordon A.S., Frye C.W. and Langston H.T. (1956) The cardiorespiratory dynamics of controlled respiration in the open and closed chest. *J. thorac. Surg.* **32**, 431.

140 ATTINGER E.O., GOLDSTEIN M.M. and SEGAL M.S. (1956) Ventilation in chronic pulmonary emphysema. *Am. Rev. Tuberc. pulm. Dis.* **74**, 211.

141 CAMPBELL E.J.M. (1959) Mechanisms of airway obstruction, in, *Symposium on pulmonary ventilation*, ed. Harbord R.P. and Woolmer R., p. 73. Altrincham: Sherratt.

142 GALLOON S. and ROSEN N. (1965) Changes in airway resistance and alveolar trapping with positive-negative ventilation. *Anaesthesia*, **20**, 429.

143 SPALDING J.M.K. and SMITH A.C. (1963) *Clinical practice and physiology of artificial respiration*, p. 63. Oxford: Blackwell.

144 ROSEN M. and HILLARD E.K. (1960) The use of suction in clinical medicine. *Br. J. Anaesth.* **32**, 486.

CHAPTER 2

Clinical Aspects of Controlled Respiration

CLINICAL CIRCUMSTANCES IN WHICH CONTROLLED RESPIRATION IS NEEDED

The commonest and most important indication for controlled respiration is respiratory insufficiency. This term is used for any condition in which either respiratory activity is completely absent, or, if present, is insufficient to maintain either adequate oxygenation or carbon-dioxide clearance. The main circumstances in which this occurs are as follows.

Respiratory insufficiency associated with anaesthesia

During anaesthesia, the deliberate production of apnoea is the common reason for controlled respiration. Originally, such a state, produced by a combination of anaesthetic overdose and hyperventilation,[1–6] was only considered really necessary during open-chest surgery. Nowadays, relaxants have made the induction of apnoea easy, and this technique is employed not only in thoracic surgery, but in a wide range of operations, particularly those in the abdomen, in which profound relaxation and the abolition of spontaneous respiration are advantageous.

Post-operatively,[7–12] respiratory insufficiency or even respiratory arrest may need controlled respiration. Prolonged or disordered action of relaxant drugs, the combined effects of circulatory and respiratory depressants, the effect of oedema of the brain and of raised intracranial pressure generally, may all produce respiratory insufficiency during this period. Indeed, apnoea is sometimes deliberately maintained for one or two days after open-heart operations in order to reduce the patient's muscle metabolism, and hence his need for oxygen.

Respiratory insufficiency in diseased states unconnected with surgery or anaesthesia

Spino-bulbar poliomyelitis,[13–28] and other neurological conditions in which respiratory activity is impaired such as polyneuritis, myelitis, etc.,[29] overdose of narcotic, hypnotic, or other drugs[30,31] and severe cases of myasthenia gravis[32,33] are important indications for controlled respiration. Tetanus is also an indication in certain circumstances;[26,34–47] the spasms are controlled by relaxants or other drugs, the consequent respiratory insufficiency needing controlled respiration.

Patients suffering from carbon-dioxide poisoning, due to respiratory disease, may be tided over a critical period.[48, 49, 50] The method is being increasingly used not only in the respiratory crises [51, 52, 53] of such diseases as chronic bronchitis, asthma, and emphysema in the adult, but also in the 'respiratory distress syndrome' of the newborn.[54–60] Beneficial effects may be obtained by treating patients with crush injuries of the chest by controlled respiration.[61–72] In these cases the paradoxical movement of the chest wall has the same significance, and is as harmful, as paradoxical movement of the lungs during open-chest surgery.[73]

Other uses of controlled respiration

(a) Neurosurgery.[74, 75, 76] Here the patient derives benefit not only from the respiratory effects of controlled respiration, but also from what would ordinarily be regarded as a side-effect. Controlled respiration lowers the intracranial pressure and reduces both the brain volume and the C.S.F. pressure. These effects are shown in figs. 2.1 and 2.2.[74] An

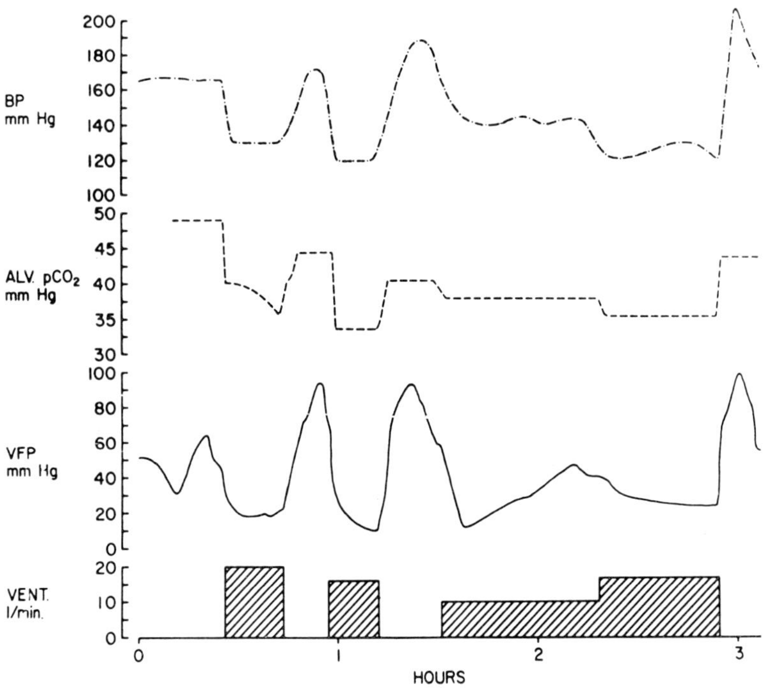

Fig. 2.1. The effect of variations in total minute-volume ventilation during I.P.P.R. on arterial blood pressure (BP), alveolar P_{CO_2} (ALV.pCO$_2$), and cerebrospinal-fluid pressure (VFP).

Courtesy of *Acta Psychiatrica et Neurologica Scandinavica*[74] and Dr N.Lundberg.

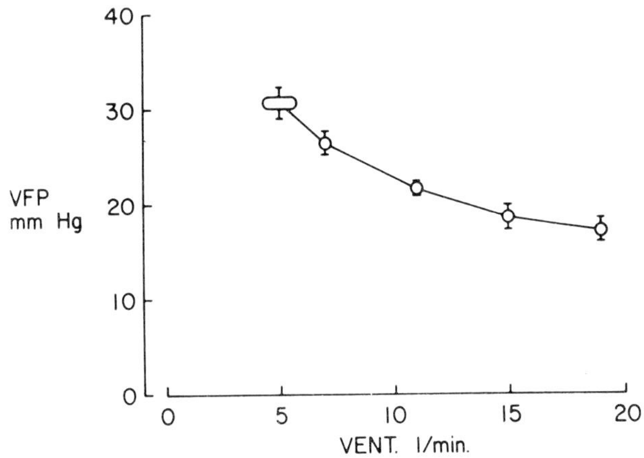

Fig 2.2. The effect of variations in total minute-volume ventilation during I.P.P.R. on cerebrospinal-fluid pressure (VFP).

Courtesy of *Acta Psychiatrica et Neurologica Scandinavica*[74] and Dr N.Lundberg.

increase in the minute-volume ventilation produces a fall in the alveolar P_{CO_2}, the systolic blood pressure and the ventricular fluid pressure. The effect on the brain itself is shown in fig. 2.3.[76] The introduction of negative pressure clearly reduces the brain volume.

(b) Induced hypotension. Controlled respiration tends to exaggerate the hypotension produced by ganglion-blocking drugs now commonly used to lower the blood pressure deliberately, when this is considered desirable during anaesthesia. This effect is due to a combination of its cardiovascular effects and hypocapnia.

(c) Pulmonary oedema.[77] Whatever the cause, this condition represents a disturbance of the balance of forces across the alveolar membrane. Controlled respiration, by its

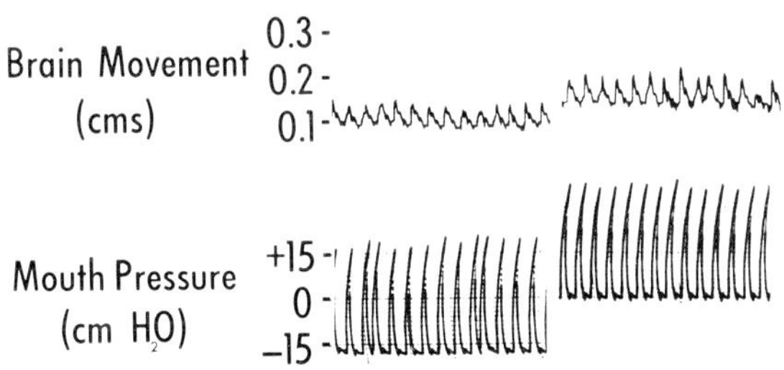

Fig. 2.3. The effect of a negative-pressure expiratory phase on the brain volume during artificial ventilation. Displacement of the 'brain movement' tracing away from the zero line reflects the increase in the brain volume which occurs when the mean pressure at the mouth is raised.

Courtesy of Dr S.Galloon.[76]

ability to increase the mean intra-alveolar pressure, increases the force tending to drive liquid back into the circulation, and to prevent further exudation into the alveoli taking place.

(d) The use of controlled respiration has from time to time been reported [78, 79, 80] for other conditions than those already mentioned.

WHEN TO START CONTROLLED RESPIRATION

Whenever it can be predicted that respiratory insufficiency will occur, controlled respiration should be instituted to forestall it. In the course of anaesthesia, it should be assumed that any dose of relaxant sufficient for abdominal relaxation, or even for intubation, will reduce the ventilation to such an extent as to make controlled respiration essential for some time at least.

The effectiveness of controlled respiration in maintaining life is so indisputable that there must be no hesitation in using it whenever signs of respiratory insufficiency appear, however mild or transient they may be.

The existence of cardiovascular disease or the possibility of aggravating cardiovascular depression should not be a deterrent to the use of controlled respiration when it is clearly indicated for the treatment or prevention of respiratory insufficiency. However, much can be done to reduce the possibility of further cardiovascular harm in these cases by careful attention to the factors already discussed in Chapter 1.

In general, the earlier that controlled respiration is started the better, particularly when excessive secretions are present. A combination of hypoxia, due to weak respiratory efforts and to obstruction by secretions, and carbon-dioxide retention may be the starting-point of a vicious circle, in which the respiratory inadequacy is still further aggravated and the whole cardiovascular system is depressed. In some instances, the very features of the disease such as the spasms of the musculature, and, in particular, of the larynx, in tetanus, are accentuated by hypoxia. Delay in initiating adequate ventilation always decreases the chances of ultimate survival and recovery.

Particularly important signs of hypoxia, though some may not be apparent in a paralysed patient, are dyspnoea, stridor, restlessness, cyanosis, the increasing use of the accessory muscles of respiration, sweating, and a rise in blood pressure and pulse rate, followed later by a fall in both.

VOLUME EXCHANGE

The tidal volume delivered by a ventilator may be inadequate for the needs of the patient. This may be the result of the incorrect setting of the ventilator, of failure to recognize the development of mechanical faults in the apparatus or of leaks between apparatus and patient, or of failure to appreciate the effect of the fresh-gas flow which, in certain circumstances, may cause the volume entering the lungs to be less than that leaving the ventilator (see p. 145). However, even when the patient's tidal volume has been estimated correctly and is entering the lungs, accumulation of secretions, or the presence of emphysema or areas of atelectasis, may interfere with proper distribution of the gas and with efficient gas exchange in the alveoli.

Poor oxygenation of the arterial blood and inadequate elimination of carbon dioxide usually occur together. However, oxygenation may be adequate while at the same time high, and possibly dangerous, levels of carbon dioxide may occur (fig. 2.4).[7, 50, 81, 82] An extreme example of this is seen when 'diffusion' respiration[83] is used during bronchoscopy; the patient, made apnoeic with relaxant, and from whom much of the blood nitrogen has been eliminated, remains oxygenated, for periods of even over half an hour, so long as the respiratory tract is kept filled with oxygen. Carbon dioxide accumulates steadily and the arterial P_{CO_2} rises at the rate of 3mmHg/min. Severe respiratory acidosis occurs, the P_{CO_2} rising to well over 100 mmHg at the end of half an hour.

Anaesthetized patients who are underventilated, but are receiving gas mixtures containing high concentrations of oxygen, may be bright pink yet have a high blood carbon-dioxide content. In the same way polio patients may easily be well oxygenated and yet suffer from carbon-dioxide accumulation.

In the absence of such factors as pulmonary shunts, atelectasis, oedema, or exudate, an alveolar oxygen tension (P_{AO_2}) of 80 mmHg (normal 100 mmHg) is sufficient to ensure an almost-normal uptake of oxygen from the lungs by the blood. However, a total minute-volume ventilation resulting in a P_{AO_2} of 80 mmHg allows the alveolar carbon-dioxide tension to rise to, say, 55 mmHg (normal 40 mmHg)—a not inconsiderable increase. Such a rise in carbon-dioxide tension would result in a blood pH as low as 7·25 (normal 7·35–7·45) if compensatory mechanisms did not operate to restore the pH towards normal.[84] Because hypoxia and hypercarbia do not necessarily occur together, they are considered separately.

Hypoxia

The danger of hypoxia needs no emphasis and its recognition is generally easy. Cyanosis is usually present, though anaemia, carboxy-haemoglobinaemia, pigmented skin, or even cosmetics, are examples of pitfalls for the unwary, since they may mask or prevent the development of cyanosis. Further, even amongst skilled observers, there may be a wide variation in the estimation of cyanosis.[85] It is therefore unsafe to assume that oxygenation is adequate simply because cyanosis is not clearly evident.

Whilst the presence of cyanosis should, in the first instance, always be assumed to be due, at least in part, to an impairment of alveolar ventilation, poor circulation in any part of the body, whether cardiac in origin or due to local causes, may also produce cyanosis. A rough and ready means of differentiation is to rub the cyanosed part briskly; if the part flushes pink, the cyanosis is circulatory in origin, while if its colour remains

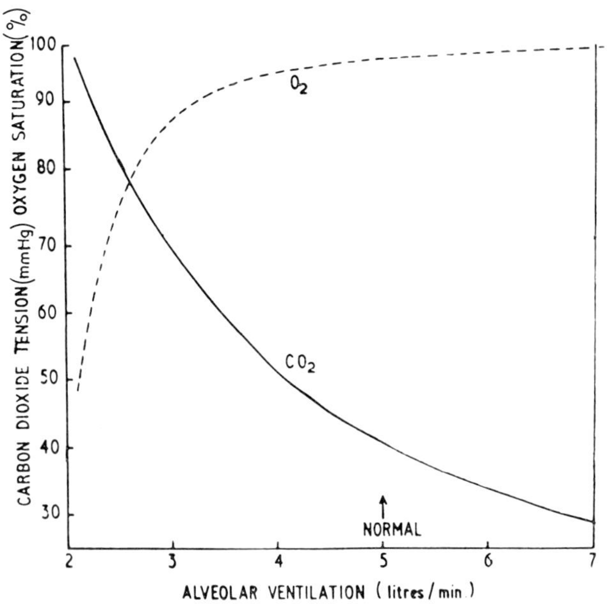

Fig. 2.4. The relation of arterial carbon-dioxide tension and oxygen saturation, to alveolar ventilation.

Courtesy of John Sherratt & Son[50] and Dr P.Hugh-Jones.

unchanged, the cyanosis is likely to be respiratory in origin. It is important to estimate with the best means available how much a cyanosed patient is suffering from a ventilation or oxygen deficiency, and how much from a cardiovascular disturbance. If this is done, not only can the correct treatment be instituted, but harm will be avoided to the occasional patient whose cardiovascular disturbance, the main cause of his cyanosis, might be aggravated by injudiciously-applied controlled ventilation.

When hypoxia develops,[86,87] compensatory circulatory changes take place which tend to maintain the supply of oxygen to the brain and the myocardium. The blood pressure and the pulse rate gradually rise. Hypoxia can be suspected if the pulse rate slows down ten or more beats per minute within ten minutes of the start of pure oxygen inhalation. However, the heart itself is second only to the nervous system in vulnerability to oxygen lack. The initial rise in blood pressure and pulse rate is followed by a rather sharp and progressive fall as the hypoxic cardiac muscle fails. The patient becomes restless. Respiration, if present, becomes shallow and periodic in character. The rate of respiration gradually increases. The accessory muscles are brought into action, movement of the alae nasi being a particularly important sign.

The early signs of hypoxia may be slight and may escape the less vigilant observer.[86] The inexperienced may interpret them as due to apprehension. The degree of suboxygenation can only be accurately determined by estimating the arterial oxygen level. This is generally done by measuring the oxygen saturation of the arterial blood, but the shape of the oxygen dissociation curve is such that the method is not particularly valuable in detecting minor degrees of suboxygenation. Cyanosis is rarely clearly visible until the oxygen saturation is below 85%, a figure which corresponds to half the normal oxygen tension. The oxygen tension of the arterial blood is now recognized as a more useful guide, though not every laboratory is equipped for this estimation. When the oxygen saturation is below, say, 80%—a level which would indicate a need for assistance with ventilation—there are invariably clinical signs of respiratory insufficiency which themselves constitute an indication for respiratory aid of some kind. Measurement of oxygen saturation in practice therefore, though valuable as a guide to the effectiveness of treatment, is usually of secondary importance in, or at any rate little more than confirmatory of, the initial clinical assessment of the need for instituting such treatment.[88]

A serious cause of impairment of oxygenation may arise during the use of 'pressure-cycled' ventilators[89] (see p. 105). Owing to changes in the compliance of the lungs and thorax brought about by such factors as secretions, changes in posture, and the use of retractors during surgery, cycling from the inspiratory to the expiratory phase may occur before an adequate volume exchange has taken place. Therefore a ventilator set to deliver an adequate volume with cycling occurring at a particular pressure, may later fail to deliver this volume though still cycling at the same pressure. Anaesthetists should be alert to this possibility. In a patient who is on controlled respiration for a prolonged period of time, regular estimations[90,91,92] of tidal and minute volumes, and of the arterial carbon-dioxide and oxygen tensions will detect this trouble early and form important guides to treatment. If both the volume exchange and the oxygen concentration of the inflating gas are adequate, the uptake of oxygen will normally be adequate. If this is not so, some other factor, such as pulmonary oedema, atelectasis, or a seriously-impaired circulation, should be suspected.

Hypercarbia

The efficient removal of metabolic carbon dioxide is essential. It has already been pointed out that this does not necessarily occur when oxygenation is adequate. In healthy people, good oxygenation, as distinct from carbon-dioxide clearance, results from a volume exchange which is not particularly critical, the term 'adequate' covering a wide range round the optimum. In the absence of venous shunts, so long as the oxygen content of the inspired mixture is sufficient—say 25% and over—serious suboxygenation is unlikely to occur except in the case of obvious underventilation or maldistribution. However, the size of the volume exchange is very important for proper carbon-dioxide clearance. In fact, the relationship between the P_{CO_2} and the alveolar ventilation is a simple inverse one (fig. 2.4); thus when the alveolar ventilation is doubled, the P_{CO_2} is halved, and vice versa. An increase of alveolar ventilation from 5 to 8 litres/min (i.e. by a factor 8/5) can be expected to lower the P_{CO_2} by a factor of 5/8, e.g. from 40 mmHg to 25 mmHg. Any estimate of the required ventilation should err on the side of overventilation rather than the reverse.

When carbon-dioxide accumulation occurs,[84, 86, 93–96] the blood pressure rises, the skin becomes hot, flushed and moist, and surgical wounds bleed freely. Salivary and bronchial secretions increase. Cerebral congestion develops and the cerebrospinal fluid pressure rises. Eventually coma supervenes. The effect of hypercarbia on the pulse varies. When of moderate extent, the heart is quickened. When the accumulation is extreme the heart muscle is depressed and conduction in the bundle of His interfered with. Ultimately, heart block and a slow ventricular rate ensue. This is usually seen in the terminal phase of asphyxia.

The estimation of carbon-dioxide accumulation or deficit should always be made by measurement of tidal and minute volumes and of the arterial P_{CO_2}. The use of the Astrup method, the Severinghaus electrode, and the rebreathing method of Taylor and Campbell have made this estimation relatively easy, and generally available.

Hyperventilation[84, 86, 90, 97–102]

Hyperventilation is probably less serious and is less readily recognized than underventilation, which is usually easily detected by the serious clinical signs of suboxygenation or carbon-dioxide accumulation.

In general, controlled respiration performed by hand tends towards hyperventilation.[86] The anaesthetist usually squeezes the bag too vigorously and too often. When performed by machine, however, with the controls set in an empiric manner, it may all too easily tend in the opposite direction. The manometer reading on the apparatus is commonly confused with the alveolar pressure and incorrect deductions from it of the tidal volume may be made (see p. 5). The effect of the fresh-gas flow in certain circumstances (see p. 145), the compression of gases in the breathing system, and the compliance of the corrugated breathing tubes (see p. 43), are all factors which tend to produce underventilation.

Hyperventilation is probably only of serious consequence if prolonged or if the patient suffers from certain underlying respiratory diseases. For example, continued over-ventilation is best avoided in subjects suffering from respiratory acidosis due to chronic bronchitis and emphysema. The institution of controlled respiration with a gas mixture of high oxygen content in these patients may not only quickly remove any hypoxic drive to respiration,[103,104] but because of the good volume exchange may also lower the blood carbon dioxide below what is probably an already high threshold value.[105,106] If such a patient is hyperventilated even for so short a time as during a surgical operation, he may well remain apnoeic and fail to breathe spontaneously at the end of the operation.

One of the possible results of gross overventilation is tetany,[100,107,108] due to the alkalosis which results from an excessive elimination of carbon dioxide. Whether tetany can be detected depends on how paralysed or how deeply anaesthetized the patient is. In the case of polio patients not too extensively paralysed the onset of tetany may sometimes give an indication of carbon-dioxide depletion.[86] It may well be that the twitching of the facial muscles or limbs of anaesthetized and curarized patients, so often taken as evidence of returning consciousness, is really tetanic in origin and evidence of hyperventilation.

Another effect of hyperventilation is cerebral vasoconstriction (see p. 17) with a fall in cerebrospinal fluid pressure and a reduction in brain size. These effects may be found of value in neurosurgical anaesthesia (see p. 34). However in patients with cerebral arteriosclerosis in whom the cerebral blood-flow may already be impaired, any further reduction in cerebral blood-flow due to hyperventilation may lead to irreversible damage. It may be that the serious personality changes sometimes leading to dementia seen in old people after operation may, at least in part, be due to this mechanism (fig. 1.12). It has been suggested, since such cerebral vasoconstriction is due to a fall in the P_{ACO_2}, that where hyperventilation is deemed necessary for full oxygenation of patients at risk, it should be accompanied by measures to prevent this fall in the P_{ACO_2}, such as the addition of a suitable proportion of carbon dioxide to the inflating-gas mixture, or by the removal of the soda-lime canister from the breathing circuit.

Hyperventilation also causes a gradual fall in the blood pressure with peripheral vasoconstriction and pallor. Some at least of the clinical signs of hyperventilation are the result of interference with cardiovascular function, described in Chapter 1. In the absence of clear clinical signs, estimation of the arterial P_{CO_2} is the only certain means of confirming suspected hyperventilation.[90]

When a patient is hyperventilated for long periods, e.g. for days, a low respiratory threshold to carbon dioxide may become established.[109] Such 'acclimatized' patients, even after spontaneous breathing has restarted, may retain a blood P_{CO_2} level as low as 25–30 mmHg. However this must clearly require a greater ventilation and therefore a greater muscular power than the maintenance of a normal arterial P_{CO_2} of 40 mmHg. It may therefore be more difficult to 'wean' from a ventilator a patient who has been overventilated for some time, than one whose arterial P_{CO_2} was kept at more normal levels.

Estimation of ventilation requirement[110]

By whatever means the ventilation requirement of a patient is calculated, the best checks on its accuracy are the repeated estimation of the arterial P_{CO_2}, oxygen saturation, and arterial P_{AO_2}. The value of these estimations for the benefit of a patient suffering from respiratory insufficiency is so great as to outweigh any possible hazards of repeated arterial puncture or the insertion of an indwelling arterial catheter. The means of performing these and other investigations are unfortunately not always readily available, especially in an emergency. In any case, these laboratory estimations do not remove the need for frequent and meticulous clinical examination of the patient's chest, as well as for radiological examination, which will go far, to detect pulmonary complications at an early stage.

Use is commonly made of tables which give the estimated total minute-volume ventilation for patients of various weights and heights, in order to maintain an arterial P_{CO_2} of about 40 mmHg. These tables are based on accumulated data, linking respiratory requirements with body surface area and hence with metabolic activity. Formulae have been established for the relationship between surface area and height and weight. Radford[111,112,113] has combined these data in a practical nomogram (fig. 2.5) from which a 'basal' tidal volume for any patient may be obtained. The total minute-volume ventilation indicated by this nomogram is claimed to maintain an arterial P_{CO_2} of 40 mmHg

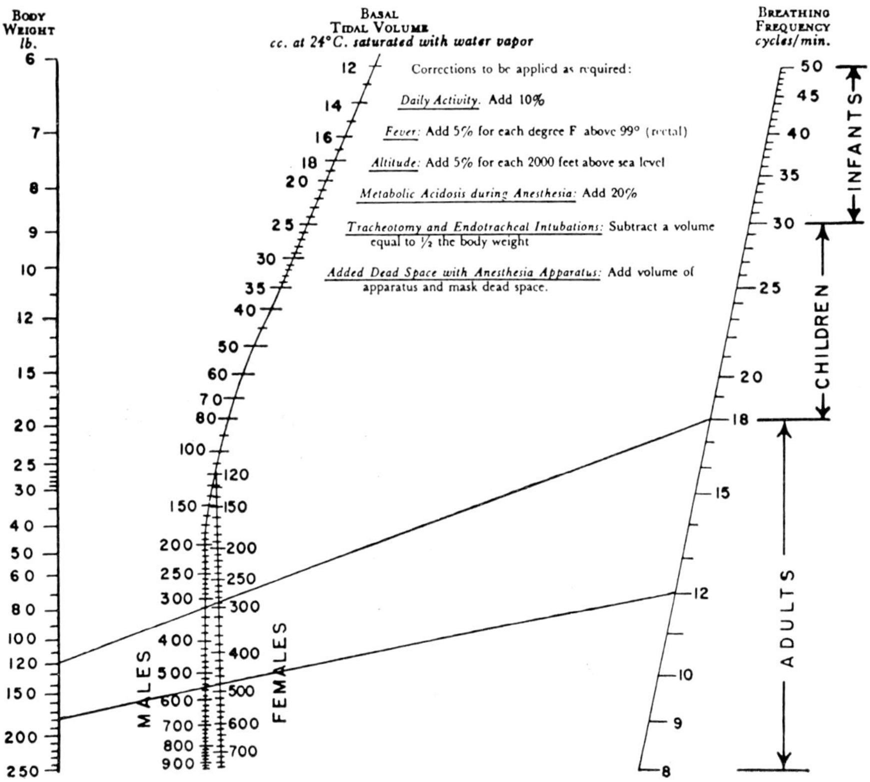

Fig. 2.5. Radford's Nomogram for predicting the optimum tidal volume from the breathing frequency, body weight, and sex of the patient. Since the original publication of this Nomogram, Radford has suggested that the correction for 'Tracheotomy and Endotracheal Intubation' should be the subtraction of a volume equal to one-quarter of the body weight rather than one-half the body weight.[113]

Courtesy of *The New England Journal of Medicine*[111] and Dr E.P.Radford.

within reasonably close limits. A tidal volume and frequency of ventilation are chosen from a range on the nomogram corresponding to the weight of the individual patient. The breathing frequency range is divided into adults, children and infants. Within each of these ranges any particular tidal volume is linked to a particular frequency, so that for a patient of any particular body weight the alveolar ventilation remains constant. The actual minute-volume ventilation resulting from the various combinations of tidal volume and frequency is larger with higher rates of ventilation; this is to take account of the variation in dead-space wastage with different ventilation frequencies. In general, the lower the ventilation frequency, the nearer the alveolar ventilation approaches the total ventilation.[114–120] The nomogram gives 'basal' tidal volume, and lists a number of corrections which must be applied. Although the Radford nomogram was widely accepted for some years, there have been reports[121,122] that the ventilation indicated by it is inadequate, particularly if the chest is open.

Another example of a nomogram for estimating ventilatory requirements is shown in fig. 2.6. This was designed by Herzog and Engström for use with the Engström ventilator. Fig. 2.7 is an adaptation of this nomogram for use for infants and children.[123] Other guides to ventilation requirements have been described.[124,125]

We have already indicated the difference which may exist between the volume leaving the ventilator and the volume entering the lungs due to the fresh-gas flow. The magnitude of the fresh-gas flow, the time during which it is in operation during the respiratory cycle, and the way in which excess gas is vented from the breathing circuit, may make the volume of gas entering the patient's lungs greater than, equal to, or less than, the volume leaving the reservoir bag. This matter is dealt with in more detail in Chapter 4.

There are two other factors which cause the tidal volume of the patient to be less than the tidal volume leaving the reservoir bag. These are the compression of the inflating gas in the breathing tubes and the airway, and the distensibility of the breathing tubes.[126] Fig. 2.8 gives some experimental figures which indicate the magnitudes of these two effects. The compressibility of the gas is in accordance with Boyle's law, and ranges from 8 ml per breath per length of breathing tube to 18·5 ml, depending on the volume of the tube, for an applied pressure of 25 cmH_2O. This is equivalent to a compliance of between 0·3 and 0·7 ml/cmH_2O. The other factor depends on the compliance of the corrugated breathing tube. The compliance of breathing tubes varies widely. We have found it to be, in a number of specimens, between 1 ml/cmH_2O and 4 ml/cmH_2O. Similar findings are shown by the figures in fig. 2.8 where the tidal volume loss may be as much as 73 ml for each tube for an applied pressure of 25 cmH_2O, i.e. a compliance of 3 ml/cmH_2O. In other words the compliance of a corrugated breathing tube together with the compressibility of the contained gas may represent a total compliance of nearly 5 ml/cmH_2O, i.e. 10% of that of the patient's total compliance. A ventilator driving 800 ml to a patient may therefore deposit as much as 80 ml in each tube at each breath, and with two corrugated tubes deliver only 640 ml to the patient. This may be a noteworthy deficiency

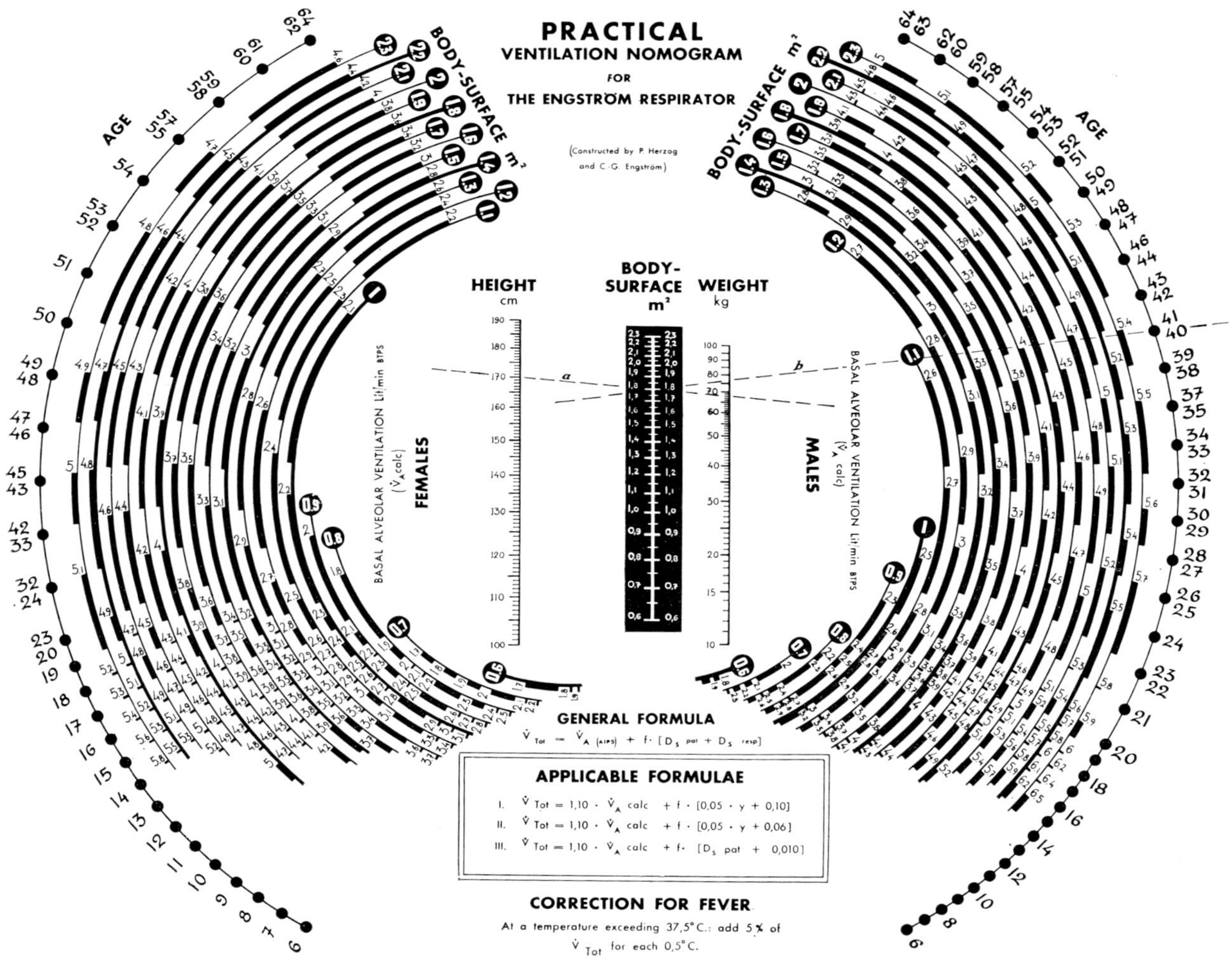

EXPLANATION

$\dot{V}_{Tot}$ — the total ventilation litre per minute to be adjusted on the respirator. Calculated on a calm patient without fever.

$\dot{V}_A$calc — the alveolar ventilation calculated by means of the nomogram litre/min. (B T P S).

f — respiration frequency per minute (adjusted on the respirator).

y — body-surface in m².

$D_s$pat — the dead space of the patient after tracheotomy, in liters, $D_s$pat = 0,05 · y (with the body-surface as a parameter).

1,10 · $\dot{V}_A$calc — includes the correction of $\dot{V}_A$calc to 24°C., and a correction for the divergents from the standard metabolic conditions.

$D_s$resp — the "functional" dead space of the respirator in liters when using different apparatus tubes: I [0,10], II [0,06], III [0,010], respectively.

APPLICATION

1) calculate y from height and weight (example line a)
2) calculate $\dot{V}_A$calc from y, age and sex (example line b)
3) place the values of $\dot{V}_A$calc and y in the formulae I, II or III, where I is to be used for standard apparatus tubes (large-size), II for micro-tubes and III when the microtubes are connected by-passing the humidifier directly to the valve-box.

EXAMPLE

Male patient: height 170 cm, weigth 68 kg, will give a body-surface of 1,8 m². At the age of 40 years, $\dot{V}_A$ calc is found to be 4,2 l/min.

To get $\dot{V}_{Tot}$ proceed as follows: The body-surface (y) was found to be 1,8 m².
Assuming the frequency (f) to have been set at 20 cycles per minute and that standard apparatus tubes are used (formula I), then $\dot{V}_{Tot}$ in liters per minute will be:
1,10 · 4,2 + 20 · [0,05 · 1,8 + 0,10]
= 8.420 lit/min.

Fig. 2.6. Ventilatory Nomogram designed by Herzog and Engström for use with the Engström ventilator.
Courtesy of P.Herzog and Dr C.G.Engström.

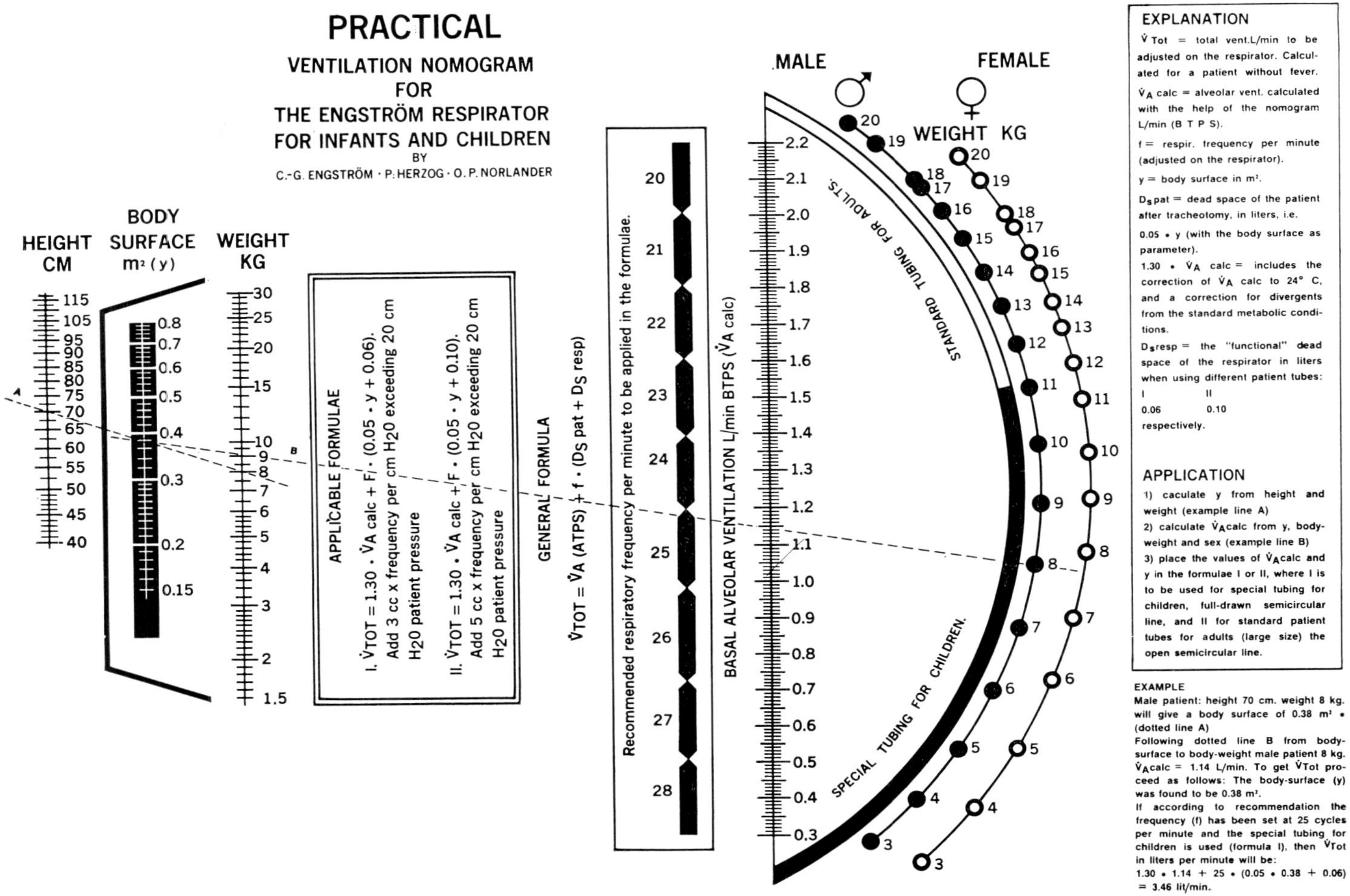

Fig. 2.7. Ventilatory Nomogram for infants and children designed by Engström, Herzog, and Norlander for use with the Engström ventilator.

Courtesy of Dr C.G.Engström and P.Herzog.

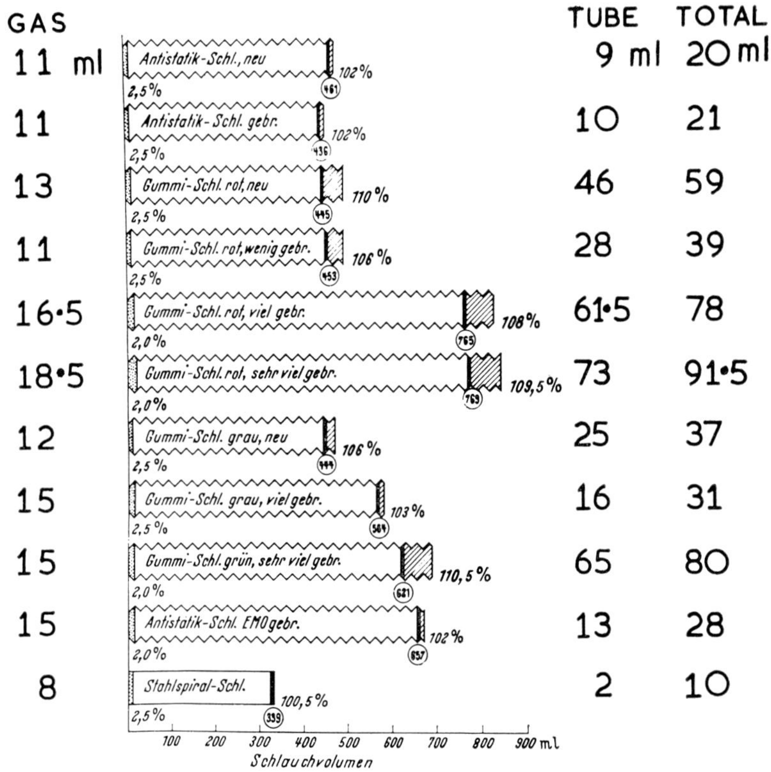

Fig. 2.8. A series of breathing tubes of varying lengths, types, and age of rubber. The pressure applied is 25 cmH_2O. The figures on the left indicate the gas lost to the patient by compression. The figures on the right indicate the volume lost to the patient by the compliance of the tube. Courtesy of *Der Anaesthesist*.[126]

if continued for any length of time, since it represents some 20% reduction in the minute volume delivered from the ventilator.

MEASUREMENT OF VENTILATION[127]

It is evident that when the tidal volume has been selected it is still necessary to ensure that this volume is in fact transferred to the patient's lungs. A common source of error is a leak between apparatus and patient. In the case of pressure-cycled ventilators, a calibrated reservoir bag is a helpful provision. An increase in the volume delivered from this bag, with the cycling pressure remaining constant, may indicate a leak rather than a greater volume going into the patient. In the case of volume-cycled ventilators, a manometer will indicate the development of a leak by showing a reduced peak pressure. It is desirable, and indeed, in cases of long-continued ventilation, essential, to incorporate some type of ventilation meter.[128] This is best placed close to the patient in the path of his expiration, so that the volume of gas measured has actually come from his lungs. Such a meter must be of a type which is not upset by the condensation of water within its mechanism. If it is, either an effective barrier to water such as a condenser humidifier must be inserted or, as an expedient, the meter must be placed in the path of the inflating gas, carefully guarding against leaks as a source of error.

As with any sensitive measuring device, regular checks should be made of the accuracy [127, 129, 130] of the calibration of the meter. In an established unit it is wise to have one robust gas meter against which at least rough checking of the more fragile meters can be made. The makers of the ventilation meters provide calibration graphs for both constant and sinusoidal flows, so that the necessary comparisons and corrections can be made.

Three small ventilation meters which are particularly useful during anaesthesia are described here.

The Wright respirometer[131]

This meter (fig. 2.9) is characterized by small size and lightness of weight. Air enters the instrument at (1) (fig. 2.10) and having passed through ten tangential slots in a cylindrical stator ring (2) escapes through the outlet (3). Within the stator ring (2) a flat two-bladed rotor (4), mounted in jewelled bearings, is turned by the passing air at a speed proportional to the air flow through the instrument and may be arrested by an 'on/off' control. A simple wheel train, similar to that in a watch, connects the rotor to the hands of the

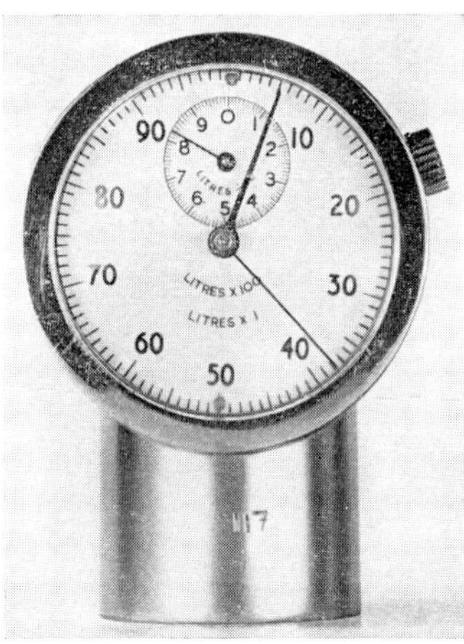

Fig. 2.9. The Wright ventilation meter.
Courtesy of British Oxygen Company Ltd.

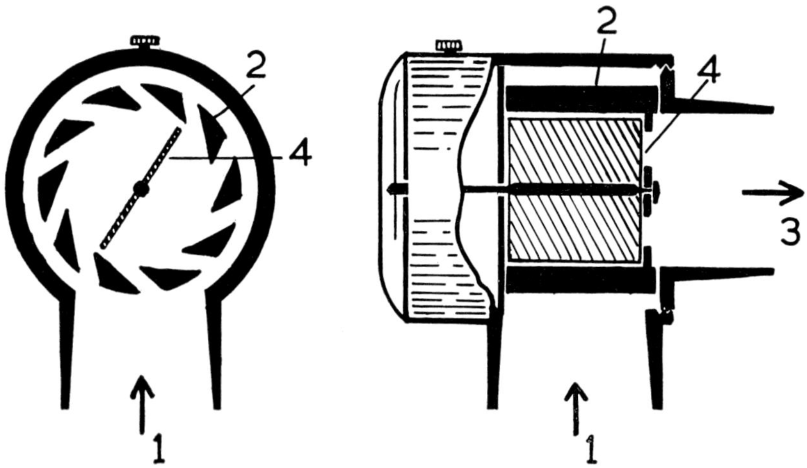

Fig. 2.10. Diagram of the Wright ventilation meter.

1. Gas inlet
2. Stator ring with ten tangential slots
3. Gas outlet
4. Two-bladed rotor running in jewelled bearings

dial. The large dial is calibrated to measure 100 litres per revolution and the smaller dial to measure 1 litre per revolution, graduated in 1/10ths of a litre. If the patient is breathing to and fro through the meter registration only occurs during one phase of each respiratory cycle. During the other phase the rotor is not turned as the air now enters the stator ring axially. A reset button returns the hands to zero when desired. A serious disadvantage of this meter, which may also be true of the others, is its fragility; if dropped on the floor—a not uncommon occurrence—expensive and prolonged repair is generally needed. The greatest care should be taken to avoid this accident.

The accuracy of this meter depends on whether the flow is steady or continuous, on the wave form and magnitude of the flow and on the gas mixture flowing through it. In general it is reasonably accurate with average conditions, but tends to over-read at high ventilations, and under-read at low ventilations.

The Bennett 'Respiratory ventilation meter' (Figs. 2.11 and 2.13)

The mechanism comprises two interlocking rotors. These are made of very light alloy and run in jewelled bearings. As the gas flow passes round the outer sides of the rotors they are both positively driven. This meter responds to flow in both directions.

A reset button is incorporated. The larger dial reads up to 1 litre and is calibrated in 25 ml units; the smaller dial reads up to 5 litres. This meter is recommended for insertion in the inspiratory pathway to avoid condensation of water within it.

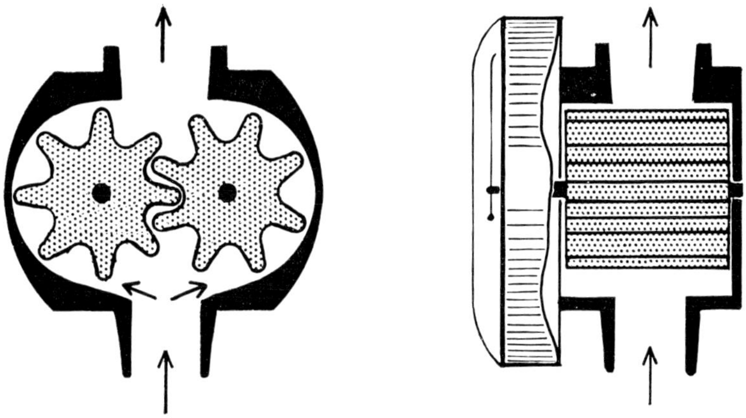

Fig. 2.11. Diagram of the Bennett ventilation meter.

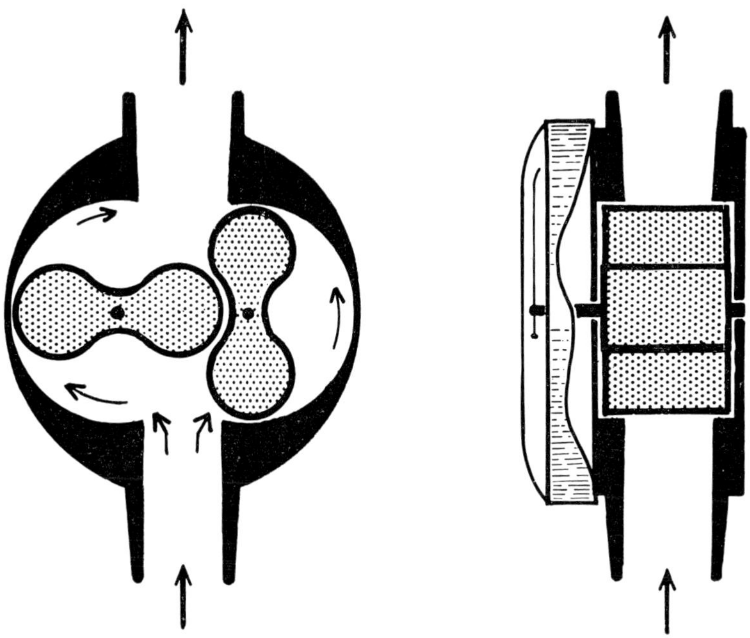

Fig. 2.12. Diagram of the Dräger 'Volumeter'.

The Drager 'Volumeter' (Figs. 2.12 and 2.13)
Two extremely light lozenge-shaped meshing rotors running in jewelled bearings are rotated positively by the passage of gases. This meter also responds to flow in both directions. The large dial reads up to 1 litre in 50 ml graduations, and the small dial up to 5 litres.

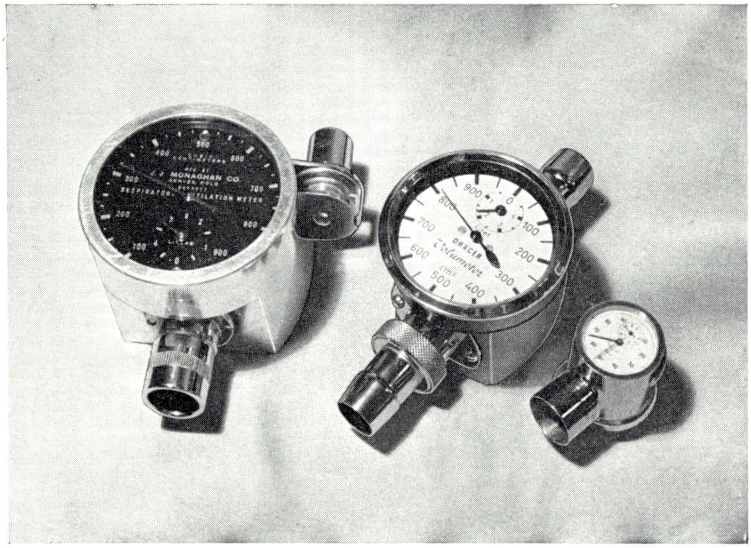

Fig. 2.13. The Bennett, Dräger, and Wright ventilation meters.
Courtesy of Department of Medical Illustration, Cardiff Royal Infirmary.

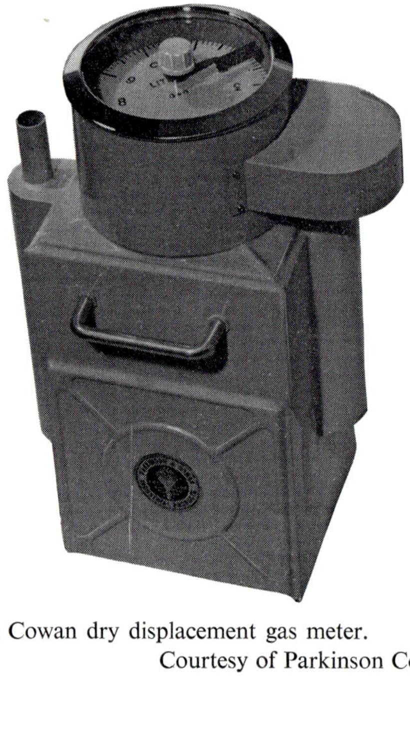

Fig. 2.14. The Parkinson Cowan dry displacement gas meter.
Courtesy of Parkinson Cowan Industrial Products.

Although the small size of the ventilation meters described above makes them particularly convenient for patients on controlled respiration, larger instruments such as the Parkinson and Cowan dry displacement gas meters[214] (fig. 2.14) give similar information and have acquired a reputation for robustness: they are now incorporated in some ventilators.

MAINTENANCE OF A CLEAR AIRWAY

We have no hesitation in asserting that any patient who is to be on controlled respiration for more than a few minutes should have an endotracheal tube inserted. This is the most effective and certain way of maintaining an adequate airway, so important in the management of these patients. Not only is the airway kept clear for the easy flow of gases, but the dead space is reduced. Secretions can be easily aspirated from the depths of the trachea and bronchi, and inflation of the stomach prevented.[132] With an inflated cuff on the tube, communication between the respiratory and alimentary tracts is virtually prevented. The cuff itself may be a source of injury because of the pressure it exerts on the tracheal mucosa. The cuff should be inflated only sufficiently to prevent leakage of gas at peak pressures of about 20–25 cmH_2O.

Such a pressure is unlikely to do more than partially compress the larger vessels in the tracheal mucosa and the chances of necrosis due to ischaemia are therefore minimized. With higher pressures this risk is very real. The pressure inside the cuff, commonly much higher, is no guide to the pressure which is applied to the mucosa. Carefully-supervised regular deflation and re-inflation still further minimizes the risk of ischaemia. The alternative to a tube through the mouth and larynx is tracheostomy. The latter has considerable advantages over the former in certain circumstances (see p. 54). Even when an endotracheal or a tracheostomy tube is in place, respiratory obstruction may still occur. Constant vigilance alone will detect and rectify this condition.

Accumulation of secretions

The average adult secretes 1,500 ml of saliva a day. Normally this is removed from the mouth by swallowing. Many times the normal rate of secretion may occur during light anaesthesia.[133] Patients who are to be anaesthetized are therefore almost invariably given atropine or a similar drug to reduce the secretion of saliva.

In other patients, particularly when the pharyngeal muscles are paralysed, accumulation of secretions may occur from a number of causes. Pooling of the saliva in the pharynx may occur through inability to swallow. The tracheo-bronchial tree itself secretes mucus and any intercurrent infection will lead to an excessive amount. Any heart failure may lead to pulmonary oedema, still further increasing the fluid in the tracheo-bronchial tree.

An adequately-inflated cuff gives a high degree of protection to the respiratory tract, but even when it is in use the accumulation of secretions in the pharynx, if allowed to occur, constitutes a danger to the patient. Deflation of the cuff may occur accidentally or deliberately for various reasons, and any accumulation of secretions above the cuff may then flood into the lower airway where it constitutes, among other things, a serious form of respiratory obstruction. The respiratory tract can theoretically be kept free of accumulated secretions by the adoption of a posture in which the mouth and pharynx are at the most dependent point. However, not only does this mean that the patient's body is in a tilt which makes nursing difficult, but experience shows this is insufficient by itself to keep the entire respiratory tract clear. It is unlikely to do more at best than keep the trachea and pharynx free of secretion. It is not a very effective means of keeping the bronchial tree clear of secretions and oedema fluid. Coughing is an important natural way of clearing the respiratory tract, but is inefficient in ill and supine patients. In particular coughing is nearly impossible in the presence of a tracheal tube, quite apart from difficulties imposed by such things as toxaemia and muscle paralysis.

Removal of secretions by suction

The important means of keeping the pharynx and tracheo-bronchial tree clear of secretions is suction. Facilities for clearing the respiratory tract by suction must be regarded as essential whenever any patient is being ventilated.

While suction may be life-saving during controlled respiration, it has dangers of its own. The tip of the catheter may be traumatic and scrape the tracheal and bronchial mucosa,[134] leading at times to what may be severe haemorrhage. Perforation of the tracheal mucosa with the occurrence of surgical mediastinal emphysema is a possibility. Gross mediastinal surgical emphysema has followed small traumata to the respiratory tract mucosa. The size of the suction catheter must be such that there is plenty of room between it and the trachea or the wall of the endotracheal tube for the passage of air from the outside.[135] If the size of the suction catheter approximates to that of the trachea or of the endotracheal tube, the large negative pressure produced in the lungs by the suction may result in gross atelectasis and dilatation of the heart.[136] A practice to be condemned, even more, is the connexion of suction direct to the endotracheal tube. Short of immediate death from acute hypoxia and heart failure, suction improperly applied in this way may lead to pulmonary oedema, by upsetting for too long a period of time, or too frequently, the delicate equilibrium of forces across the alveolar epithelium. In cases of long duration the times at which the respiratory tract should be sucked, should not be left to the judgement of an attendant. The respiratory tract should be regularly sucked clear every half-hour, whatever the condition of the patient. If between these intervals evidence of accumulated secretions appears, further suction should be carried out. As the condition of the patient improves, and infection is kept in check, so the periods for routine suction may gradually be lengthened.

Needless to say any instruments introduced into the respiratory tract of a patient should be sterile, and a full aseptic ritual should be practised by anyone using them. The tracheostomy should be regarded as though it were an open wound of the respiratory tract through which infection can easily be introduced. In particular, a fresh sterile suction catheter should be used on each occasion that suction is employed and no one should approach the patient without a mask. It is probable that infection is as important a factor in leading to muco-purulent aggregations as imperfect humidification of the inhaled gases.

Drying of secretions

The normal mechanism for moistening the inspired air is its passage through the nasal fossae and pharynx. Inspired air is usually 98% saturated at body temperature at the carina. With an endotracheal tube in place this normal mechanism is by-passed and air arrives in the lower part of the trachea drier than it does normally.[137]

A difficulty which is liable to occur as a result of this, combined with depression of ciliary activity, when controlled respiration is maintained for more than an hour or two, is the thickening of mucus into tenacious plugs or even its drying into crusts. These plugs and crusts may cause gross obstruction to respiration if within the trachea, or atelectasis if within the bronchi. For this reason, in prolonged controlled respiration the inspired air should always be effectively humidified.

A number of methods[138–144] are now available for this purpose. In the simplest, water is either instilled directly into the respiratory tract by syringe or drip, or added by bubbling the gases through water. In more sophisticated methods the gases are passed over water kept hot by means of a thermostatically-controlled electric heater. With these latter instruments provision must be made for preventing too much cooling and condensation of the water between the humidifier and the patient. An over-riding heater cut-out operated by a temperature sensor near the mouth guards against scalding of the patient in the event of such accidents as a thermostat failure in the water heater. Another method of moistening the gases is by adding water in the form of fine droplets or aerosol. This can be done by breaking up the water by a high-velocity gas flow. In another method the water is broken up by being thrown off a spinning disc, while in the most recently developed instrument it is broken up by high frequency (ultrasonic) vibrations. The quantity of water carried by gases containing a modern aerosol in which the droplets are very minute (2–5 μ) is considerably greater than that which can possibly be carried in the form of a vapour. Care must therefore be taken when using aerosols that the intake of water over long periods of time is not so excessive as to disturb the patient's water balance.[145] Water vapour will be carried with the gases to all parts of the respiratory tract. The depth to which droplets penetrate depends on their size. It is also possible to prevent excessive loss of water from the respiratory tract by interposing a condenser humidifier close to the patient. By this means 75% or more of the expired water vapour is returned to the patient on inspiration.

Obstruction in the endotracheal tube[146–152]

The presence of an endotracheal tube does not in itself constitute a guarantee of a clear airway. The tube may become obstructed from a wide variety of causes and the anaesthetist should always be on the alert to this possibility. Kinking, obstruction by inflated cuffs, and foreign bodies in the lumen are but a few examples. Special tubes[153,154] are available which mitigate some of these risks. A tube may also be passed inadvertently into a bronchus, especially in children.

ORAL TUBE[155–159] VERSUS TRACHEOSTOMY TUBE[160–175]

An endotracheal tube passed through the mouth or the nose is almost invariably used during anaesthesia when respiration is controlled. In other circumstances an endotracheal tube is valuable as an emergency measure for the rapid relief of certain forms of respiratory obstruction and to enable controlled respiration to be initiated. As a short-term procedure this is perfectly satisfactory. Indeed, we have treated a number of patients with various forms of respiratory insufficiency with controlled respiration with an endotracheal tube in place for up to three weeks without complications. However, in general, an endotracheal tube should be regarded as a satisfactory way of providing an airway in adults for up to 48 hours. Beyond this time the risk of complications such as sub-glottic stenosis increases.

If it is anticipated that the respiratory insufficiency will last for longer than this time, a tracheostomy is preferable, though, in the case of infants,[176–179] having regard to the difficulties associated with tracheostomy, prolonged intubation with specially-designed tubes has proved to be the best choice. The presence of a tube between the cords is traumatic,[180–195] and, with infection, may give rise to sub-glottic oedema and to such later complications as scarring and granulomata leading to stenosis.

A tracheostomy prevents these complications although not free from complications of its own.[196–200] The respiratory tract itself is more easily kept clear by suction through the tracheostomy tube. Furthermore, the patient, even with the tracheostomy tube in place, sooner or later regains the activity of his vocal cords which can therefore react to the presence of any foreign matter. He also becomes able to swallow his saliva. Until these natural mechanisms return, suction keeps the pharynx clear.

It can be said, therefore, that the objectives in performing a tracheostomy are to facilitate the removal of secretions from the respiratory tract by suction, to isolate the tracheo-bronchial tree from the oropharynx and the alimentary canal without injuring the larynx, and to increase alveolar ventilation by reducing the anatomical dead space. It must be pointed out however that both in the case of an endotracheal tube inserted through the larynx and a tracheostomy tube, the isolation of the respiratory tract from the alimentary canal depends largely on the cuff of the tube. Not only should the cuff of either sort of tube be carefully inspected for leaks or deterioration of its wall before the tube is inserted, but its proper functioning should be watched carefully throughout the treatment of the patient. The inflated cuff is essential for the prevention of entry of foreign material into the respiratory tract; it is not essential, although it is undoubtedly preferable, for the proper ventilation of the lungs so long as any leakage of gas around it can be compensated for by the ventilator.

The tracheostomy tube should be specially designed for its purpose. A shortened endotracheal tube is unsatisfactory because the length of the cuff is such that it may easily come to lie at the bifurcation of the trachea and occlude one or both main bronchi. A shortened endobronchial tube may serve temporarily, but the cuff here is on the small side, for it was designed for a tract of narrower diameter than the trachea. Several useful specially-designed tracheostomy tubes[201–210] with inflatable cuffs are now available.

FEEDING AND FLUID BALANCE

All food by mouth, liquid or solid, must be prohibited in patients who cannot swallow. Even when they can, nothing must be given by mouth so long as there is an endotracheal tube through the larynx. There is every likelihood of fluid collecting above the inflated cuff and finding its way into the lungs when the cuff is later deflated. A stomach tube offers a simple and effective solution. Feeding should be carried out through this until the patient can swallow a test spoonful of sterile water without it finding its way into the trachea.[211] Some go further and recommend that if the paralysis is likely to be of some duration, a gastrostomy is indicated.[114]

In a patient, on controlled respiration for more than a day, it is essential that the fluid and electrolyte balance be maintained. Any losses or deficiency should be made good. The most vital element is an adequate intake of water, and at least 2 to 3 litres a day are required. The accurate and careful charting of fluid balance should be started at the earliest moment, regard being paid to the importance of vomiting and sweating as sources of fluid loss. Nutrition becomes a problem only when treatment lasts more than a couple of days. Owing to the lower metabolism in such cases, an initial daily intake of about 1,500 calories is generally adequate. This is gradually increased to up to 3,000 calories a day.

OTHER COMPLICATIONS

Patients who are on controlled respiration apart from anaesthesia, are generally very ill. Many are either comatose or else extensively paralysed. The prolonged immobility, the inability to cough or swallow, the ever-present hazard of aspiration of food and secretions, make for a high incidence of serious complications particularly in the lungs. Daily careful clinical examination with particular scrutiny of the chest is essential, and the observations should be correlated with spirometric, blood gas and pH estimations. These, together with frequent X-ray examinations, will not only check the correctness of the ventilation but will detect chest complications such as atelectasis at their start.[212] Chemotherapy and antibiotics, combined with expert physiotherapy, frequent suction, and changes of posture, will preclude or overcome many, if not all, of these complications. Expert nursing care and physiotherapy are vital. Such complications as urinary tract sepsis through careless catheterization or the development of bed sores may be tragic events, best avoided. No less than the nurse's other contributions is the maintenance of the patient's morale and cheerfulness through what may be a prolonged illness.

It is vital that such patients should be removed, at the very earliest moment, to centres where all the facilities of modern scientific medicine are available, if the best results are to be obtained.

It is not the intention of the authors that the account given here should be the sole guide to the clinical care of patients suffering from respiratory insufficiency of long duration. Those who are called upon to undertake the treatment of such a patient, should consult the many papers and books[212,213] which have been written on this subject, for more detailed guidance on particular aspects.

REFERENCES

1 Guedel A.E. and Treweek D.N. (1934) Ether apnoeas. *Curr. Res. Anesth. Analg.* **13**, 263.

2 Waters R.M. (1936) Carbon dioxide absorption from anaesthetic atmospheres. *Proc. R. Soc. Med.* **30**, 11.

3 Guedel A.E. (1940) Cyclopropane anesthesia. *Anesthesiology*, **1**, 13.

4 Nosworthy M.D. (1941) Anaesthesia in chest surgery, with special reference to controlled respiration and cyclopropane. *Proc. R. Soc. Med.* **34**, 479.

5 Neff W., Phillips W. and Gunn G. (1942) Anesthesia for pneumonectomy in man. *Anesthesiology*, **3**, 314.

6 Waters R.M. (1945) Cyclopropane—a personal evaluation. *Surgery, St. Louis*, **18**, 26.

7 Björk V.O. and Engström C.G. (1955) The treatment of ventilatory insufficiency after pulmonary resection with tracheostomy and prolonged artificial ventilation. *J. thorac. Surg.* **30**, 356.

8 Robson J.G. (1958) Postoperative treatment with artificial respiration of two thoracic surgical patients. *Can. Anaesth. Soc. J.* **5**, 25.

9 Rudy N.E. and Crepeau J. (1958) Role of intermittent positive-pressure breathing post-operatively. *J. Am. med. Ass.* **167**, 1093.

10 Becker A., Barak S., Braun E. and Myers M.P. (1960) The treatment of post-operative pulmonary atelectasis with intermittent positive pressure breathing. *Surgery Gynec. Obstet.* **111**, 517.

11 SANGER P.W., ROBICSEK F., TAYLOR F.H., STAM R.E., REES T.T. and CHARLOTTE, N.C. (1960) Acute post-operative cardiorespiratory insufficiency: treatment by curarization and artificial breathing. *J. Am. med. Ass.* **172**, 695.

12 MACRAE W.R. and MASSON A.H.B. (1964) Assisted ventilation in the post-bypass period. *Br. J. Anaesth.* **36**, 711.

13 LASSEN H.C.A. (1953) A preliminary report on the 1952 epidemic of poliomyelitis in Copenhagen with special reference to the treatment of acute respiratory insufficiency. *Lancet*, **1**, 37.

14 MACRAE J., MCKENDRICK G.D.W., CLAREMONT J.M., SEFTON E.M. and WALLEY R.V. (1953) The Clevedon positive-pressure respirator. *Lancet*, **2**, 971.

15 Report (1953) Respiratory paralysis in poliomyelitis. *Br. med. J.* **1**, 1216.

16 IBSEN B. (1954) The anaesthetist's viewpoint on the treatment of respiratory complications in poliomyelitis during the epidemic in Copenhagen, 1952. *Proc. R. Soc. Med.* **47**, 72.

17 MARCHAND J.F. (1954) Care of respiratory paralysis from poliomyelitis. *J. Am. med. Ass.* **155**, 1297.

18 O'BRIEN W.A., SCOTT A.E., CROSBY R.C. and SIMPSON W.E. (1954) The anesthesiologist, the poliomyelitis team, and the respirator. *J. Am. med. Ass.* **156**, 27.

19 SMITH A.C., SPALDING J.M.K. and RUSSELL W.R. (1954) Artificial respiration by intermittent positive pressure in poliomyelitis and other diseases. *Lancet*, **1**, 939.

20 WISLICKI L. (1954) Positive-pressure inflation in respiratory paralysis of poliomyelitis. *Br. med. J.* **2**, 672.

21 AFFELDT J.E., COLLIER C.R., CRANE M.G. and FARR A.F. (1955) Ventilatory aspects of poliomyelitis. *Curr. Res. Anesth. Analg.* **34**, 41.

22 Annotation (1955) Artificial respiration by intermittent positive pressure. *Lancet*, **2**, 79.

23 BOWER A.G. (1955) Principles of diagnosis and treatment of acute poliomyelitis. *Curr. Res. Anesth. Analg.* **34**, 35.

24 HARRIES J.R. and LAWES W.E. (1955) Intermittent positive-pressure respiration in bulbo-spinal poliomyelitis; use of the Radcliffe respiration pump. *Br. med. J.* **1**, 448.

25 RUSSELL W.R. (1955) Respiratory insufficiency in poliomyelitis and other diseases. *Br. med. J.* **1**, 98.

26 WISLICKI L. (1955) Positive pressure respiration in infectious diseases. *Br. J. Anaesth.* **27**, 303.

27 KELLEHER W.H., MEDLOCK J.M. and POWELL D.G.B. (1956) Maintenance of respiratory function in poliomyelitis and other neuromuscular disorders. *Lancet*, **2**, 68.

28 LASSEN H.C.A. (1956) *Management of life-threatening poliomyelitis*. Edinburgh: Livingstone.

29 JAMES J.L. and PARK H.W.J. (1961) Respiratory failure due to polymyositis treated by I.P.P.R. *Lancet*, **2**, 1281.

30 Leading article (1956) Treatment of barbiturate poisoning. *Br. med. J.* **2**, 1107.

31 FREIER S., NEAL B.W., NISBET H.I.A., REES G.J. and WILSON F. (1957) Salicylate intoxication treated with intermittent positive-pressure respiration. *Br. med. J.* **1**, 1333.

32 GRIFFIN S.G., NATTRASS F.J. and PASK E.A. (1956) Thymectomy during respiratory failure in a case of myopathy with myasthenia gravis. *Lancet*, **2**, 704.

33 HEAD J. (1964) Respiratory failure after thymectomy for myasthenia gravis. *Ann. Surg.* **160**, 123.

34 FORRESTER A.T.T. (1954) Treatment of tetanus with succinylcholine. *Br. med. J.* **2**, 342.

35 HONEY G.E., DWYER B.E., SMITH A.C. and SPALDING J.M.K. (1954) Tetanus treated with tubocurarine and intermittent positive-pressure respiration. *Br. med. J.* **2**, 442.

36 LASSEN H.C.A., BJØRNEBOE M., IBSEN B. and NEUKIRCH F. (1954) Treatment of tetanus with curarization, general anaesthesia, and intratracheal positive pressure ventilation. *Lancet*, **2**, 1040.

37 SHACKLETON P. (1954) The treatment of tetanus; role of the anaesthetist. *Lancet*, **2**, 155.

38 WOOLMER R. (1954) Tetanus. *Br. med. J.* **2**, 702.

39 Annotation (1955) Treatment of tetanus. *Lancet*, **2**, 236.

40 GUSTERSON F.R. (1955) Treatment of tetanus. *Anaesthesia*, **10**, 300.

41 ABLETT J.J.L. (1956) Tetanus and the anaesthetist. A review of the symptomatology and the recent advances in treatment. *Br. J. Anaesth.* **28**, 258.

42 ANDREWS J.D.B., MARCUS A. and MUIRHEAD K.M. (1956) A fatal case of tetanus treated by suxamethonium chloride, tracheotomy, and intermittent positive pressure respiration. *Lancet*, **2**, 652.

43 SMITH A.C., HILL E.E. and HOPSON J.A. (1956) Treatment of severe tetanus with d-tubocurarine chloride and intermittent positive pressure respiration. *Lancet*, **2**, 550.

44 GLOSSOP M.W. and LOW M.D.W. (1957) Some observations on severe tetanus treated by paralysis and I.P.P.R. *Br. J. Anaesth.* **29**, 326.

45 POWELL K.J., BRIMBLECOMBE F.S.W. and STONEMAN M.E.R. (1958) Treatment of severe tetanus by curarisation and intermittent positive-pressure respiration. *Lancet*, **1**, 713.

46 WALTON W.J. (1961) Tetanus and I.P.P.R.: a partial paralysis regime. *Br. J. Anaesth.* **33**, 589.

47 ADAMS E.B., HOLLOWAY R., THOMBIRAN A.K. and DESAI S.D. (1966) Usefulness of intermittent positive pressure. *Lancet*, **2**, 1176.

48 BJØRNEBOE M., IBSEN B., ASTRUP P., EVERBERG G., HARVALD B., SØTTRUP T., THAYSEN E.H. and THORSHAUGE CHR. (1955) Active ventilation in treatment of respiratory acidosis in chronic diseases of the lungs. *Lancet*, **2**, 901.

49 HUGH-JONES P. (1958) Oligopnoea. *Proc. R. Soc. Med.* **51**, 104.

50 HUGH-JONES P. (1959) Management of pulmonary ventilation in emphysematous subjects in the state of carbon-dioxide narcosis, in, *Symposium on pulmonary ventilation*, ed. Harbord R.P. and Woolmer R., p. 55, Altrincham: Sherratt.

51 BENVENISTE D., BUCHMANN G., FOG C.V.M. and WULFF H.L.G. (1960) Positive-pressure ventilation in children with severe laryngotracheobronchitis. *Acta anaesth. scand.* Suppl. VI, 12.

52 MISURACA L. (1966) Mechanical ventilation in status asthmaticus. *New Engl. J. Med.* **275**, 318.

53 AMBIAVAGAR M., JONES E.S. and ROBERTS D.V. (1967) Intermittent positive pressure ventilation in severe asthma. *Anaesthesia*, **22**, 134.

54 DELIVORIA-PAPADOPOULOS M., LEVISON H. and SWYER P.R. (1965) Intermittent positive pressure respiration as a treatment in severe respiratory distress syndrome. *Archs Dis. Childh.* **40**, 474.

55 Leading article (1965) Respirator treatment in hyaline-membrane disease. *Lancet*, **2**, 1227.

56 GLOVER W.J. (1965) Mechanical ventilation in respiratory insufficiency in infants. *Proc. R. Soc. Med.* **58**, 902.

57 REID D.H.S. and TUNSTALL M.E. (1965) Treatment of respiratory distress syndrome of the newborn with nasotracheal intubation and intermittent positive pressure respiration. *Lancet*, **1**, 1196.

58 THOMAS D.V., FLETCHER G., SUNSHINE P., SCHAFER I.A. and KLAUS M.H. (1965) Prolonged respirator use in newborn pulmonary insufficiency. *J. Am. med. Ass.* **193**, 183.

59 REID D.H.S. and TUNSTALL M.E. (1966) The respiratory distress syndrome of the newborn. A method of treatment using prolonged nasotracheal intubation and intermittent positive pressure respiration. *Anaesthesia*, **21**, 72.

60 REID D.H.S., TUNSTALL M.E. and MITCHELL R.G. (1967) A controlled trial of artificial respiration in the respiratory distress syndrome of the newborn. *Lancet*, **1**, 532.

61 MÖRCH E.T., AVERY E.E. and BENSON D.W. (1955) Problems in pulmonary physiology and pathology. *Surg. Forum*, **6**, 270.

62 AVERY E.E., MÖRCH E.T. and BENSON D.W. (1956) Critically crushed chests. *J. thorac. Surg.* **32**, 291.

63 AVERY E.E., HEAD J.R., HUDSON T.R. and BENNETT R.J. (1957) The treatment of crushing injuries to the chest (methods old and new). *Am. J. Surg.* **93**, 540.

64 BOYLE A.K., GALLIE J.R. and MURRAY D.B. (1957) Crush injury of the chest. A report on two cases. *Anaesthesia*, **12**, 453.

65 THORNTON A. (1958) Crush injury of the chest. *Anaesthesia*, **13**, 99.

66 CLARKSON W.B. and ROBINSON J.S. (1962) Deliberate hyperventilation in the treatment of a crush injury of the chest. *Br. J. Anaesth.* **34**, 471.

67 GARDEN J. and MACKENZIE A.I. (1963) The stove-in chest: Another approach to treatment. *Br. J. Anaesth.* **35**, 731.

68 HUNTER A.R. (1964) Artificial ventilation of the lungs in combined head and chest injury. *Lancet*, **2**, 279.

69 WHITWAM J.G. and NORMAN J. (1964) Hypoxaemia after crush injury of the chest. *Br. med. J.* **1**, 349.

70 REID J.M. and BAIRD W.L.M. (1965) Crushed chest injury: some physiological disturbances and their correction. *Br. med. J.* **2**, 1105.

71 AMBIAVAGAR M., ROBINSON J.S., MORRISON I.M. and JONES E.S. (1966) Intermittent positive pressure ventilation in the treatment of severe crushing injuries of the chest. *Thorax*, **21**, 359.

72 BRYANT L.R. (1967) Mechanical respirators—their use and application in lung trauma. *J. Am. med. Ass.* **199**, 149.

73 MUSHIN W.W. and RENDELL-BAKER L. (1953) *Principles of thoracic anaesthesia*, p. 6. Oxford: Blackwell.

74 LUNDBERG N., KJALLQUIST A. and BIEN C. (1959) Reduction of increased intracranial pressure by hyperventilation. A therapeutic aid in neurological surgery. *Acta psychiat. scand.* **34** (Suppl. 139), 1.

75 MARRUBINI M.B., ROSSANDA M. and TRETOLA L. (1964) The role of artificial hyperventilation in the control of brain tension during neurosurgical operations. *Br. J. Anaesth.* **36**, 415.

76 GALLOON S. (1967) Personal communication.

77 MILLER W.F. and SPROULE B.J. (1959) Studies on the role of intermittent inspiratory positive pressure oxygen breathing (IPPB/I: O_2) in the treatment of pulmonary edema. *Dis. Chest*, **35**, 469.

78 REDDING J., VOIGT G.C. and SAFAR P. (1960) Drowning treated with intermittent positive pressure breathing. *J. appl. Physiol.* **15**, 849.

79 ABRAHAMSEN A.M. and NITTERHAUGE S. (1966) Extreme obesity with respiratory failure necessitating artificial respiration. *Acta med. scand.* **180**, 113.

80 GALLOON S. and CHAKRAVARTY K. (1967) Fat embolism treated with intermittent positive pressure ventilation. Report of three cases. *Br. J. Anaesth.* **39**, 71.

81 ASMUSSEN E. (1959) *Proceedings of the Third Congress of the Scandinavian Society of Anaesthesiologists, Copenhagen*, 1954, p. 22.

82 SCURR C.F. (1956) Controlled respiration: standardization of ventilation. *Br. J. Anaesth.* **28**, 23.

83 ROTH L.W., WHITEHEAD R.W. and DRAPER W.B. (1947) Studies on diffusion respiration. II. Survival of the dog following a prolonged period of respiratory arrest. *Anesthesiology*, **8**, 294.

84 WHITTENBERGER J.L. and SARNOFF S.G. (1950) Symposium on specific methods of treatment: physiologic principles in treatment of respiratory failure. *Med. Clins N. Amer.* **34**, 1335.

85 COMROE J.H. and BOTELHO S. (1947) Unreliability of cyanosis in recognition of arterial anoxemia. *Am. J. med. Sci.* **214**, 1.

86 LASSEN H.C.A. (1956) *Management of life-threatening poliomyelitis*, p. 40. London: Livingstone.
87 KEELE C.A. and NEIL E. (1965) *Samson Wright's applied physiology*, 11th ed., p. 196. London: Oxford University Press.
88 LASSEN H.C.A. (1956) *Management of life-threatening poliomyleitis*, p. 119. London: Livingstone.
89 ELAM J.O., KERR J.H. and JANNEY C.D. (1958) Performance of ventilators. Effect of changes in lung-thorax compliance. *Anesthesiology*, **19**, 56.
90 ASTRUP P., GØTZCHE H. and NEUKIRCH F. (1954) Laboratory investigations during treatment of patients with poliomyelitis and respiratory paralysis. *Br. med. J.* **1**, 780.
91 The poliomyelitis epidemic in Stockholm, 1953. ed. Ström J. (1956) *Acta med. scand.* **154**, Suppl. 316.
92 WALLEY R.V. (1957) Control of artificial respiration in poliomyelitis patients with paralysis of swallowing. *Lancet*, **2**, 1143.
93 KEELE C.A. and NEIL E. (1965) *Samson Wright's applied physiology*, 11th ed., pp. 124, 130–1. London: Oxford University Press.
94 SCURR C.F. (1954) Carbon dioxide retention simulating curarization. *Br. med. J.* **1**, 565.
95 BOURNE W. (1956) The effects of excess carbon dioxide (hypercapnia) during anaesthesia; (a review). *Curr. Res. Anesth. Analg.* **35**, 274.
96 PASK E.A. (1955) Committee on deaths associated with anaesthesia. Review of cases where post-operative care was inadequate to meet the circumstances which arose. *Anaesthesia*, **10**, 4.
97 SEEVERS M.H., STORMONT R.T., HATHAWAY H.R. and WATERS R.M. (1939) Respiratory alkalosis during anaesthesia. An experimental study in man. *J. Am. med. Ass.* **113**, 2131.
98 KETY S.S. and SCHMIDT C.F. (1946) The effects of active and passive hyperventilation on cerebral blood flow, cerebral oxygen consumption, cardiac output, and blood pressure of normal young men. *J. clin. Invest.* **25**, 107.
99 BOURDILLON R.B., DAVIES-JONES E., STOTT F.D. and TAYLOR L.M. (1950) Respiratory studies in paralytic poliomyelitis. *Br. med. J.* **2**, 539.
100 KEELE C.A. and NEIL E. (1965) *Samson Wright's applied physiology*, 11th ed., pp. 185–6. London: Oxford University Press.
101 BROWN E.B., jr. (1953) Physiological effects of hyperventilation. *Physiol. Rev.* **33**, 445.
102 ROLLASON W.N. and PARKES J. (1957) Anaesthesia, hyperventilation and the peripheral blood. *Anaesthesia*, **12**, 61.
103 DONALD K.W. (1953) Acute respiratory insufficiency. *Lancet*, **1**, 495.
104 AULD W. (1956) Emphysema and controlled respiration. *Anaesthesia*, **11**, 263.
105 SPURRELL W.R. (1955) Carbon dioxide. *Proc. R. Soc. Med.* **48**, 231.
106 MUSHIN W.W. (1955) Carbon dioxide. *Proc. R. Soc. Med.* **48**, 238.
107 BEST C.H. and TAYLOR N.B. (1966) *The physiological basis of medical practice*, 8th ed., p. 1586.
108 KEELE C.A. and NEIL E. (1965) *Samson Wright's applied physiology*, 11th ed., pp. 186, 478. London: Oxford University Press.
109 BROWN E.B., CAMPBELL G.S., JOHNSON M.N., HEMMINGWAY A. and VISSCHER M.B. (1948) Changes in response to inhalation of CO_2 before and after 24 hours of hyperventilation in man. *J. appl. Physiol.* **1**, 333.
110 PONTOPPIDAN H., HEDLEY-WHYTE J., BENDIXEN H.H., LAVER M.B. and RADFORD E.P., jr. (1965) Ventilation and oxygen requirements during prolonged artificial ventilation in patients with respiratory failure. *New Engl. J. Med.* **273**, 401.
111 RADFORD E.P., jr., FERRIS B.G., jr. and KRIETE B.C. (1954) Clinical use of nomogram to estimate proper ventilation during artificial respiration. *New Engl. J. Med.* **251**, 877.
112 RADFORD E.P. (1955) Ventilation standards for use in artificial respiration. *J. appl. Physiol.* **7**, 451.

113 RADFORD E.P. (1958) Personal communication.

114 WOOLMER R. (1956) The management of respiratory insufficiency. *Anaesthesia*, **11**, 281.

115 DOBKIN A.B. (1958) Regulation of controlled respiration: recent concepts important to the anaesthetist. *Br. J. Anaesth.* **30**, 282.

116 WATSON W.E. (1962) Observation on physiological dead space during intermittent positive pressure respiration. *Br. J. Anaesth.* **34**, 502.

117 COOPER E.A. (1965) Physiological deadspace under general anaesthesia and IPPR. *Br. J. Anaesth.* **37**, 555.

118 FAIRLEY H.B. and BLENKARN G.D. (1966) Effect on pulmonary gas exchange of variations in inspiratory flow rate during intermittent positive pressure ventilation. *Br. J. Anaesth.* **38**, 320.

119 COOPER E.A. (1967) Physiological deadspace in passive ventilation (1—outline of a study). *Anaesthesia*, **22**, 90.

120 COOPER E.A. (1967) Physiological deadspace in passive ventilation (2—relationship with tidal volume, frequency, age and minor upsets of respiratory health). *Anaesthesia*, **22**, 199.

121 NUNN J.F. (1960) Ventilation nomograms during anaesthesia. *Anaesthesia*, **15**, 65.

122 GAIN E.A. (1963) The adequacy of the Radford nomogram during anaesthesia. *Can. Anaesth. Soc. J.* **10**, 491.

123 ENGSTRÖM C.G., HERZOG P., NORLANDER O.P. and SWENSSON S.A. (1962) Ventilation nomogram for the newborn and small children to be used with the Engström respirator. *Acta anaesth. scand.* **6**, 175.

124 DERY R. (1963) A simple method of calculating ventilatory requirements in children. *Can. Anaesth. Soc. J.* **10**, 164.

125 KENNY S. (1967) The Adelaide ventilation guide. *Br. J. Anaesth.* **39**, 2.

126 KRONSCHWITZ H. (1959) Über das „Mitatmen“ von Atemschläuchen—ein experimenteller Beitrag. *Anaesthesist*, **8**, 180.

127 Discussion on measuring pulmonary ventilation (1959) in, *Symposium on pulmonary ventilation*, ed. Harbord R.P. and Woolmer R., p. 87. Altrincham: Sherratt.

128 SCURR C.F. (1956) Controlled respiration: standardization of ventilation. *Br. J. Anaesth.* **28**, 23.

129 BYLES P.H. (1960) Observations on some continuously-acting spirometers. *Br. J. Anaesth.* **32**, 470.

130 NUNN J.F. and EZI-ASHI T.I. (1962) The accuracy of the respirometer and ventigrator. *Br. J. Anaesth.* **34**, 422.

131 WRIGHT B.M. (1955) A respiratory anemometer. *J. Physiol., Lond.* **127**, 25.

132 MUSHIN W.W. and MORTON H.J.V. (1958) Resuscitation. *Br. med. J.* **1**, 215.

133 ROBBINS B.H. (1935) Effect of various anesthetics on salivary secretion. *J. Pharmacol. exp. Ther.* **54**, 426.

134 Morbidity conference. (1956) A complication of intrabronchial suction. *Br. J. Anaesth.* **28**, 236.

135 HILLARD E.K. and THOMPSON P.W. (1963) Instruments used in thoracic anaesthesia, in, *Thoracic anaesthesia*, ed. Mushin W.W., p. 297. Oxford: Blackwell.

136 ROSEN M. and HILLARD E.K. (1960) The use of suction in clinical medicine. *Br. J. Anaesth.* **32**, 486.

137 Leading article (1956) Humidification. *Lancet*, **2**, 344.

138 MARSHALL J. and SPALDING J.M.K. (1953) Humidification in positive-pressure respiration for bulbospinal paralysis. *Lancet*, **2**, 1022.

139 WALLEY R.V. (1956) Humidifier for use with tracheotomy and positive-pressure respiration. *Lancet*, **1**, 781.

140 SPALDING J.M.K. (1956) Humidifier for patients breathing spontaneously. *Lancet*, **2**, 1140.

141 Arnold G.T. and Tovell R.M. (1956) The production of fog as a therapeutic agent. *Anesthesiology*, **17**, 400.

142 Mapleson W.W., Morgan J.G. and Hillard E.K. (1963) Assessment of condenser-humidifiers with special reference to a multiple-gauze model. *Br. med. J.* **1**, 300.

143 Marshall M. (1964) Micro-pump for continuous instillation of saline after tracheostomy. *Lancet*, **2**, 186.

144 Freedman B.J. (1967) Is the Woulfe bottle an efficient humidifier? *Br. med. J.* **3**, 277.

145 Sykes M.K. (1967) Personal communication.

146 'Medico-legal' (1953) Choked by faulty Magill tube. *Br. med. J.* **2**, 1383.

147 Ballantine R.I.W. and Jackson I. (1954) Anaesthesia for neurosurgical operations. *Anaesthesia*, **9**, 4.

148 Burns T.H.S. (1956) A danger from flexometallic endotracheal tubes. *Br. med. J.* **1**, 439.

149 Haselhuhn D.H. (1958) Occlusion of endotracheal tube with foreign body. *Anesthesiology*, **19**, 561.

150 Donnenfield R.S. and Bishop H.F. (1959) Obstruction to airway associated with endotracheal tube. *N.Y. St. J. Med.* **59**, 2618.

151 Jenkins A.V. (1959) Unexpected hazard of anaesthesia. *Lancet*, **1**, 761.

152 Mackintosh R.R., Mushin W.W. and Epstein H.G. (1963) *Physics for the anaesthetist*, 3rd ed., p. 176. Oxford: Blackwell.

153 Alsop A.F. (1955) Non-kinking endotracheal tubes. *Anaesthesia*, **10**, 401.

154 Tunstall M.E. (1966) A useful neonatal tracheal tube for anaesthesia. *Anaesthesia*, **21**, 108.

155 Foregger R. (1946) Use of endotracheal tube in therapy of post-traumatic pulmonary secretions. *Anesthesiology*, **7**, 285.

156 Briggs B.D. (1950) Prolonged endotracheal intubation. *Anesthesiology*, **11**, 129.

157 Urry A.G. (1951) The prolonged use of endotracheal tubes: case reports. *Anesthesiology*, **12**, 662.

158 Schroth R. (1957) Vorteile und Gefahren der langdauernden orotrachealen Intubation im Hinblick auf die bisher geübte Tracheotomie. *Anaesthesist*, **6**, 309.

159 Leading article (1967) Prolonged endotracheal intubation. *Br. med. J.* **1**, 321.

160 Nelson-Jones A. and Williams R.H.H. (1945) Tracheotomy in bulbar poliomyelitis. *Lancet*, **1**, 561.

161 Priest R.E., Boies L.R. and Goltz N.F. (1947) Tracheotomy in bulbar poliomyelitis. *Ann. Otol., St. Louis*, **56**, 250.

162 Galloway T.C. and Seifert M.H. (1949) Bulbar poliomyelitis. *J. Am. med. Ass.* **141**, 1.

163 Christie A.B. and Esplen J.R. (1953) Poliomyelitis in Denmark. *Lancet*, **1**, 492.

164 Davis H.S., Kretchmer H.E. and Bryce-Smith R. (1953) Advantages and complications of tracheostomy. *J. Am. med. Ass.* **153**, 1156.

165 Galloway W.H. and Wilson H.B. (1955) Tetanus in childhood. *Anaesthesia*, **10**, 303.

166 Pitman R.G. and Wilson F. (1955) Tracheotomy in acute respiratory embarrassment. *Lancet*, **2**, 523.

167 Walford A.S.H. (1955) Discussion on the modern indications for tracheotomy. *Proc. R. Soc. Med.* **48**, 947.

168 Andrew J. (1956) Tracheostomy, and management of the unconscious patient. *Br. med. J.* **2**, 328.

169 Lassen H.C.A. (1956) *Management of life-threatening poliomyelitis*, p. 44. Edinburgh: Livingstone.

170 Kretchmer H.E. and Davis H.S. (1957) The current attitude to tracheotomy. *Anesth. Anal. curr. Res.* **36**, 67.

171 NELSON T.G., PEDIGO H.K. and BOWERS W.F. (1957) Use of tracheotomy in association with artificial and controlled respiration. *Anesthesiology*, **18**, 77.

172 CAWTHORNE T. (1959) Tracheostomy today. *Proc. R. Soc. Med.* **52**, 403.

173 WATTS J.M. (1963) Tracheostomy in modern practice. *Br. J. Surg.* **50**, 954.

174 NEVILLE W.E., SPINAZZOLA A., SCICCHITANO L.P. and LANGSTON H.D. (1964) Tracheostomy and assisted ventilation—use in respiratory insufficiency in the post surgical patient. *Archs Surg., Chicago*, **89**, 149.

175 CLARKE D.B. (1965) Tracheostomy in a thoracic surgical unit. *Thorax*, **20**, 87.

176 ABERDEEN E. (1965) Tracheostomy and tracheostomy care in infants. *Proc. R. Soc. Med.* **58**, 900.

177 ALLEN T.H. and STEVEN I.M. (1965) Prolonged endotracheal intubation in infants and children. *Br. J. Anaesth.* **37**, 566.

178 MCDONALD I.H. and STOCKS J.G. (1965) Prolonged nasotracheal intubation. A review of its development in a paediatric hospital. *Br. J. Anaesth.* **37**, 161.

179 REES G.J. and OWEN-THOMAS J.B. (1966) A technique of pulmonary ventilation with a naso-tracheal tube. *Br. J. Anaesth.* **38**, 901.

180 DONNELLY W.A., GROSSMAN A.A. and GREM F.M. (1948) Local sequelae of endotracheal anesthesia as observed by examination of one hundred patients. *Anesthesiology*, **9**, 490.

181 MOULDEN G.A. and WYNNE R.L. (1951) Post-anaesthetic granuloma of the larynx. *Br. J. Anaesth.* **23**, 92.

182 JACKSON C. (1953) Contact ulcer, granuloma and other laryngeal complications of endo-tracheal anesthesia. *Anesthesiology*, **14**, 425.

183 KAMSLER P.M. (1953) Laryngeal granuloma following endotracheal intubation. *Curr. Res. Anesth. Analg.* **32**, 51.

184 YOUNG N. and STEWART S. (1953) Laryngeal lesions following endotracheal anaesthesia: a report of twelve adult cases. *Br. J. Anaesth.* **25**, 32.

185 MALONEY W.H. (1954) Laryngeal complications of endotracheal anesthesia. *Laryngoscope, St. Louis*, **61**, 861.

186 STOUT R.J. and THOMAS C. (1954) A fatal case of post-operative obstructive tracheitis. *Br. J. Anaesth.* **26**, 35.

187 HAINES A.M. and POWELL K.J. (1955) Acute sub-glottic oedema of the larynx as a sequel to endotracheal anaesthesia. *Br. J. Anaesth.* **27**, 257.

188 CARRUTHERS H.C. and GRAVES H.B. (1956) The complications of endotracheal anaesthesia. *Can. Anaesth. Soc. J.* **3**, 244.

189 Annotation (1957) Laryngeal granuloma after intubation. *Lancet*, **1**, 415.

190 EPSTEIN S.S. and WINSTON P. (1957) Intubation granuloma. *J. Laryng.* **71**, 37.

191 HAMELBERG W., WELCH C.M., SIDDALL J. and JACOBY J. (1958) Complications of endotracheal intubation. *J. Am. med. Ass.* **168**, 1959.

192 WOLFSON B. (1958) Minor laryngeal sequelae of endotracheal intubation. *Br. J. Anaesth.* **30**, 326.

193 CAMPKIN V. (1959) Post-intubation ulcer of larynx. *Br. J. Anaesth.* **31**, 561.

194 FIELDS J.A. (1959) Injuries and sequelae associated with endotracheal anesthesia. *Laryngoscope, St. Louis*, **69**, 509.

195 SNOW J.C., HARANO, M. and BALOGH K. (1966) Postintubation granuloma of the larynx. *Anesth. Anal. curr. Res.* **45**, 425.

196 PEARCE D.J. and WALSH R.S. (1961) Respiratory obstruction due to tracheal granuloma after tracheostomy. *Lancet*, **2**, 135.

197 YARINGTON C.T. and FRAZER J.P. (1965) Complications of tracheostomy. *Archs Surg., Chicago.*, **91**, 653.

198 McClelland R.M.A. (1965) Complications of tracheostomy. *Br. med. J.* **2**, 567.

199 Lunding M. (1964) The tracheotomy tube and postoperative tracheotomy complications. *Acta anaesth. scand.* **8**, 181.

200 Lloyd J.W. and McClelland R.M.A. (1964) Tracheal dilatation. *Lancet*, **1**, 83.

201 Spalding J.M.K. and Smith A.C. (1956) A new tracheotomy tube. *Lancet*, **2**, 1247.

202 Bullough J. (1957) Tracheostomy tube and connections for patients having intermittent positive-pressure respiration. *Lancet*, **2**, 372.

203 Wilson F. (1958) Modified tracheotomy tube. *Lancet*, **1**, 569.

204 Loeb W.J. (1959) Respirator tracheotomy tube. *J. Am. med. Ass.* **169**, 1326.

205 Salt R.H., Parkhouse J. and Simpson B.R. (1960) Improved material for Radcliffe tracheostomy tube. *Lancet*, **2**, 407.

206 Gilston A. (1961) Modification of the Negus tracheotomy tube and a tracheotomy T-piece. *Lancet*, **1**, 1326.

207 Thompson P.W. (1961) A tracheostomy tube. *Br. med. J.* **2**, 1353.

208 Bain J.A. and Spoerel W.E. (1964) Observation on the use of cuffed tracheostomy tubes (especially in the James tube). *Can. Anaesth. Soc. J.* **6**, 598.

209 Bradfield W. (1964) Disposable tracheostomy tube. *Lancet*, **1**, 416.

210 Glossop M.W. (1966) A cuffed tracheotomy tube. *Lancet*, **1**, 187.

211 Smith A.C. (1955) Discussion on the modern indications for tracheostomy. *Proc. R. Soc. Med.* **48**, 952.

212 Lassen H.C.A. (1956) *Management of life-threatening poliomyelitis*, p. 39. Edinburgh: Livingstone.

213 Spalding J.M.K. and Crampton-Smith A. (1963) *Clinical practice and physiology of artificial respiration*. Oxford: Blackwell.

214 Adams A.P., Vickers M.D.A., Munroe J.P. and Parker C.W. (1967) Dry displacement gas meters. *Br. J. Anaesth.* **39**, 174.

CHAPTER 3

Physical Aspects of Automatic Ventilators: Basic Principles

The anaesthetist's primary concern with automatic ventilators is to use them in the way that is best for his patients as judged from a physiological or clinical point of view. The relationship between physiological changes in the patient and the physical effects produced in the lungs by a ventilator has been considered in the previous chapters. In later chapters the mechanical design of ventilators is considered. In this chapter attention is turned to the relationship between the physical effects produced in the lungs and the mechanical design of the ventilator. This has been a subject of study by many investigators[1–18] but usually in relation to a limited number of ventilators or to a limited range of aspects. Here a more comprehensive analysis is attempted which should be of value in making a rational choice of a ventilator to suit any particular circumstances.[19]

The physical effects in the lungs are changes of volume and pressure with time; the mechanical elements of ventilators are bags, springs, pumps, valves, and so on. It is not easy to relate the physical effects in the lungs directly to the mechanical design of the ventilator. Therefore the idea of the 'functional specification' of a ventilator, as distinct from its mechanical specification, is introduced as an essential intermediate step.

The first stage of the argument in this chapter is concerned with the relationship between the mechanical specification of a ventilator and its functional specification. The meaning and significance of the term 'functional specification' may not be fully appreciated until after the following pages have been studied; but briefly it can be defined as a statement of how the ventilator works in pneumatic terms, that is, in terms of the variations with time of flow, volume, and pressure of gas which the ventilator produces within itself. The second stage of the argument is concerned with the way in which this functional specification, in combination with the pneumatic characteristics of the patient (the compliance and resistance of the respiratory tract) determine the waveforms of flow, volume, and pressure in the lungs.

In considering the mode of operation of any ventilator it is necessary to distinguish four functions. Firstly and most obviously, the ventilator must inflate the patient's lungs. Also, and equally obviously, the ventilator must deflate the lungs or allow passive expiration. In addition, but less obviously, the ventilator must have some means by which it 'decides' when to stop the process of inflation and start the process of expiration, and some other means by which it 'decides' when to stop the process of expiration and start the process of inflation. In some ventilators it is possible to distinguish four separate mechanisms each of which serves one of these functions. In others one mechanism may serve two or more functions. But always the four functions must be provided for. Therefore the functional specification must be split into four parts:

1 The inspiratory phase.
2 The change-over from the inspiratory phase to the expiratory phase.
3 The expiratory phase.
4 The change-over from the expiratory phase to the inspiratory phase.

THE INSPIRATORY PHASE

The study of this, the first element of the respiratory cycle, is commenced with a detailed examination of just one of the mechanisms used in automatic ventilators to bring about inflation of the lungs. This serves to demonstrate, firstly, the way in which the pneumatic characteristics of a ventilator, which comprise its functional specification, are determined by its mechanical construction and, secondly, the way in which, in turn, the waveforms of flow, volume, and pressure in the lungs are dependent on the functional specification. Subsequently other mechanisms and functional specifications are considered more briefly. A number of simplifying assumptions are made initially so that a clear exposition may be developed of the principal features of the situation. Some of the ways in which these basic features are modified, by the differences between reality and assumption, are mentioned later.

During the inspiratory phase the primary function of a ventilator is simply to drive gas into the patient's lungs. Therefore the ventilator must incorporate, or be supplied with, some source of compressed gas. One such source, to be found in a number of ventilators (e.g. the East-Radcliffe and the Manley), comprises a concertina bag with a weight on top (fig. 3.1). The downward force exerted by the weight on the cross-sectional area of the bag produces a certain force per unit area, i.e. a certain pressure, within the bag. This is clearly so if the outlet from the bag is blocked; but equally, if the outlet is opened and gas flows out of the bag, the weight still exerts the same downward force and the cross-sectional area remains the same so that the pressure within the bag remains the same. That is to say, so long as the bag has not completely collapsed, the pressure within it is constant no matter whether there is a flow from it or not and no matter what the magnitude of the flow.

Suppose such a weighted bag forms part of an automatic ventilator and is connected to the patient's lungs. Then the inspiratory phase will be initiated by the opening of the

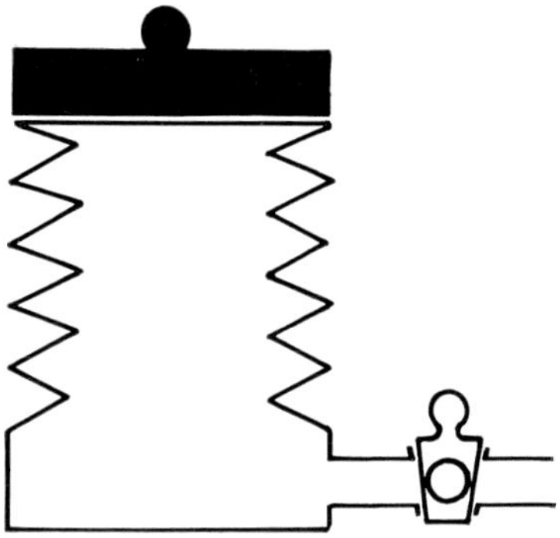

Fig. 3.1. A weighted concertina bag. An example of a constant-pressure generator.

tap in the outlet of the bag. At first the pressure in the alveoli is atmospheric, so that the whole of the positive pressure in the concertina bag is available for driving gas through the resistance of the pathway from the bag to the alveoli. The result is that the flow into the lungs is at first relatively high. However, as gas enters the lungs the pressure in the alveoli increases, so that the pressure difference between the bag and the alveoli decreases, and the flow declines from its initial high level (fig. 3.2). As inflation proceeds the alveolar pressure gradually approaches the constant pressure in the bag, while the flow gradually approaches zero.

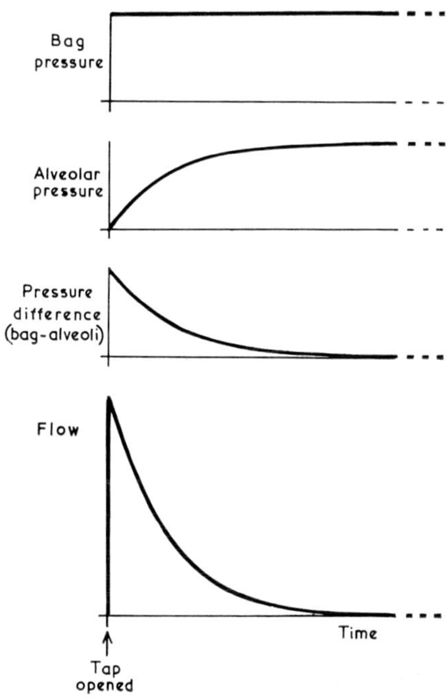

Fig 3.2. Theoretical curves, showing the variation with time of alveolar pressure and of flow when the weighted bag in fig. 3.1 is connected to a patient's lungs.

The exact nature of these approaches is discussed in detail below. For the moment, the important feature to note is that the pressure in the bag remains constant throughout the process, while the flow into the lungs varies greatly. The pressure is determined entirely by characteristics of the ventilator (the weight on the bag and the cross-sectional area of the bag) and is quite uninfluenced by the lung characteristics of the patient. On the other hand the flow is not determined by the ventilator; it is simply a product of the effect of the constant pressure in the bag on the patient's lungs and therefore changes with any change in lung characteristics. Therefore the ventilator may be said to 'generate' a constant pressure while the flow into the lungs is determined by the effect of the generated pressure on the patient's lungs. The functional specification of this mechanism is that it is a *constant-pressure generator*.

In practice, the functioning of a weighted bag is a little more complex than indicated here because, superimposed on the basic 'constant-pressure generating' process, there are some second-order effects arising from the inertia of the weight and the elasticity of the walls of the bag (see p. 94).

Another mechanism which operates more nearly as a constant-pressure generator is a reducing valve or pressure regulator. The reducing valves on anaesthetic machines deliver gas at a pressure which is usually somewhere between 5 and 60 lb/in^2 and therefore cannot be connected directly to the patient's lungs. However there exist devices, which can conveniently be called second-stage reducing valves, which, when supplied with gas at a pressure of a few pounds per square inch, will deliver that gas at a pressure of only some tens of centimetres of water. These may take the form of a relatively sophisticated piece of precision engineering, as in the Bennett ventilators, or a simple 'home-made' device, as in the 'Newcastle II' ventilator. In both cases the basic mechanism of operation is as follows.

When the outlet is blocked and the high-pressure supply is connected to the input, the pressure in the outlet rises only to some critical level at which the inflow of gas is cut off. When the outlet is opened, so that gas flows out of the valve, a very slight fall in pressure at the outlet restores the inflow of gas. Therefore, the pressure at the outlet of the valve is held constant, no matter whether there is a flow from the valve or not, and no matter how large the flow (at least within certain limits). In other words, the second-stage reducing valve operates as a constant-pressure generator: when it forms part of a ventilator and is connected to a patient the pressure is held constant at a level which is entirely determined by the design of the valve and is quite uninfluenced by the lung characteristics of the patient. On the other hand the flow is not determined by the ventilator; it is a product of the effect of the constant pressure, delivered by the valve, on the patient's lungs.

In any form of constant-pressure generator the flow may vary in a number of ways. Firstly, in a single inflation it varies with time: the flow starts high and then declines as the pressure in the alveoli of the lungs rises towards the generated pressure (fig. 3.2). Secondly, the pattern of flow varies from one inflation to another in a single patient if there are changes in the compliance or airway resistance of the lungs. This process is considered in more detail below. Finally, the pattern of flow varies from one patient to another, again in a manner dependent upon lung characteristics. But in all these instances the pressure remains constant—at the level generated by the ventilator.

This preliminary study reveals one of the advantages of making a functional analysis of a ventilator: three very different mechanisms (the weighted bag and two different forms of second-stage reducing valve) have been shown to have the same pneumatic characteristics, that is, the same functional specification. This illustrates the way in which the functional analysis of ventilators reveals that the number of basic modes of operation is less than the number of mechanical devices found in different ventilators. In addition the functional specification of a ventilator permits ready prediction of the waveforms of flow, volume, and pressure that will be developed in the lungs in various circumstances. These waveforms will now be considered in detail.

Waveforms of flow, volume, and pressure produced by a constant-pressure generator when the generated pressure is low

Waveforms for fixed lung characteristics ('standard conditions')

The factors which determine the waveforms of flow, volume, and pressure are the pneumatic characteristics of the ventilator and the pneumatic characteristics of the patient: these are the generated pressure of the ventilator, the compliance and resistance of the patient, and any compliance or resistance of the ventilator. For this study it is assumed that the patient can be adequately represented by a single compliance at the end of a single resistance and that there is some resistance within the ventilator but no compliance. To help make the explanation clear numerical values will be assumed for all the factors as follows.

Compliance, $C = 0{\cdot}05$ litre/cmH_2O.
Airway resistance*, from 'mouth' to alveoli (including endotracheal tube and connector), $R_A = 6$ cmH_2O/(litre/sec).

These values of compliance and resistance will be referred to as the 'standard conditions'.

Internal resistance of the ventilator, from the point where the pressure is generated to the 'mouth', $R_V = 2$ cmH_2O/(litre/sec).
Generated pressure, $P_G = 12$ cmH_2O.

The values chosen for C and R_A are plausible for an intubated anaesthetized patient, while the value for R_V is about the minimum likely to be found in any ventilator.

* For simplicity this is taken to include the resistance to flow of the tissues of the lung and chest wall.

The waveforms of flow, volume, and pressure which occur in these circumstances are drawn in fig. 3.3. They can be deduced by the following argument in which, as elsewhere in this book, pressures are expressed as differences from atmospheric pressure, and lung volumes are expressed as differences from the volume present when the alveolar pressure is zero. At the start of the inspiratory phase the generated pressure is applied to the system. Initially there is no pressure in the lungs (assuming that they have expired freely to atmosphere in the previous expiratory phase) so the whole of the 12 cmH_2O of generated pressure is dropped across the sum of the internal resistance of the ventilator

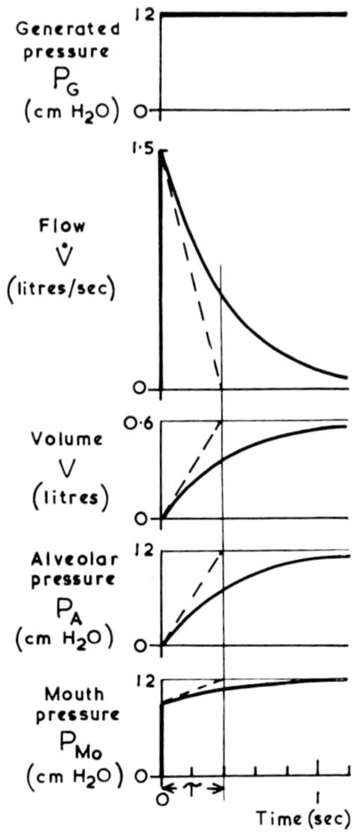

Fig. 3.3. Theoretical curves showing the variation with time during inflation of flow, volume, and pressure when a ventilator, generating a low, constant pressure and having a low internal resistance, is connected to a patient with 'standard' lung characteristics.
Generated pressure : 12 cmH_2O.
Internal resistance of ventilator : 2 cmH_2O/(litre/sec).
Airway resistance of patient : 6 cmH_2O/(litre/sec).
Compliance of patient : 0·05 litre/cmH_2O.
τ is the time constant of the exponential changes.

and the airway resistance: $2+6=8$ cmH_2O/(litre/sec). Therefore the initial flow is $12/8=1{\cdot}5$ litres/sec. If this flow were maintained the volume in the lungs would rise by 0·15 litre in 1/10 sec. Since the compliance of the lungs is 0·05 litre/cmH_2O this volume rise would be accompanied by an alveolar pressure rise of 0·15 litre divided by 0·05 litre/cmH_2O = 3 cmH_2O, in 1/10 sec. However, as the pressure in the alveoli increases, the difference between the generated pressure and the alveolar pressure decreases. It is this pressure difference, across the combined airway and ventilator resistance, which drives gas into the lungs. Therefore, as the pressure difference decreases, so the flow decreases. Consequently the rate at which the volume in the lungs increases becomes less; also the rate at which the pressure in the alveoli increases becomes less. Therefore, at the end of 1/10 sec the alveolar pressure is in fact something less than the 3 cmH_2O calculated above. However, the alveolar pressure does go on increasing, and the closer it approaches the generated pressure the smaller the flow becomes, the slower the rise of alveolar pressure becomes, and therefore the slower is the rate of decline in flow. In fact the alveolar pressure progressively approaches the generated pressure, and the flow progressively approaches zero, but neither quite reaches its equilibrium value in any finite time. Similarly, the volume in the lungs approaches a limiting value: when the pressure in the alveoli finally becomes equal to the generated pressure, the volume in the alveoli is given by the product of the compliance, 0·05 litre/cmH_2O, and the generated pressure, 12 cmH_2O, namely 0·6 litre.

The exact nature of these approaches to the equilibrium values can be deduced if the problem is considered in general terms instead of in the specific terms of the numerical example just given. In general terms, the volume added to the lungs up to any given moment during inflation is equal to the compliance C multiplied by the alveolar pressure at that moment P_A:

$$\text{volume at any moment} = CP_A. \tag{1}$$

The volume in the lungs when equilibrium has been achieved, that is when the alveolar pressure P_A has risen to equal the generated pressure P_G, is given by:

$$\text{volume at equilibrium} = CP_G. \tag{2}$$

Therefore the volume which still remains to be added at any moment is the difference between these two:

$$\text{volume remaining to be added at any moment} = C(P_G - P_A). \tag{3}$$

The flow rate of gas into the lungs is equal to the pressure difference between bag and alveoli ($P_G - P_A$) divided by the total resistance between these points R:

$$\text{flow} = \frac{P_G - P_A}{R}. \tag{4}$$

But if gas flows into the lungs at a certain rate, then the volume in the lungs (and therefore the volume remaining to be added to the lungs) changes at the same rate. That is:

$$\text{flow} = \text{rate of change of 'volume to be added'} \tag{5}$$

or, substituting for 'flow' and 'volume to be added' from equations (4) and (3),

$$\frac{P_G - P_A}{R} = \text{rate of change of } C(P_G - P_A), \tag{6}$$

or, since C and R are constants,

$$(P_G - P_A) = CR \times \text{rate of change of } (P_G - P_A). \tag{7}$$

That is to say that the rate of change of the pressure difference between bag and alveoli is proportional to the pressure difference itself. A relationship such as this, in which the rate of change of some variable is proportional to the magnitude of that variable, is the fundamental characteristic of an exponential change.[20] Therefore the pressure difference between bag and alveoli declines exponentially. Since the flow is proportional to this pressure difference, flow also declines exponentially. Similarly the alveolar pressure approaches the generated pressure exponentially and the volume approaches its limiting value exponentially.

To say that a variable changes exponentially is to give a precise definition of the general shape of the curve (see below). The particular shape of a given exponential curve is defined by two parameters which are constant for the given curve. The first is the 'magnitude constant' which defines the magnitude of the variable at zero time, e.g. the initial flow or the initial difference between alveolar and generated pressure. The second parameter is the 'time constant'. In general this expresses how drawn out the curve is in the time dimension. In particular it is the constant in the equation relating the variable to its rate of change. Thus in equation (7) above, which relates the variable $(P_G - P_A)$ to the rate of change of $(P_G - P_A)$, the time constant for the exponential change of $(P_G - P_A)$ is CR. Furthermore, the time constant is the time in which the exponential change would be completed if the rate of change were maintained at its initial level instead of decreasing. It is possible to deduce this also from equation (7) but perhaps the most convincing way of demonstrating these two properties of the time constant is to return to the numerical example.

In the example compliance is given as:

$$C = 0{\cdot}05 \text{ litre/cmH}_2\text{O} = 0{\cdot}05 \, \frac{\text{litre}}{\text{cmH}_2\text{O}};$$

and total resistance (the sum of airway and ventilator resistance) by:

$$R = 8 \text{ cmH}_2\text{O/(litre/sec)} = 8 \, \frac{\text{cmH}_2\text{O.sec}}{\text{litre}}.$$

Therefore:

$$CR = 0{\cdot}05 \times 8 \, \frac{\text{litre.cmH}_2\text{O.sec}}{\text{cmH}_2\text{O.litre}},$$

$$= 0{\cdot}4 \text{ sec.}$$

Thus the product of compliance and resistance is indeed a time. In addition, it was calculated above that, at the initial flow rate, the alveolar pressure would rise by 3

cmH_2O in each 0·1 sec. Therefore in the time constant of 0·4 sec the alveolar pressure would rise by $3 \times 0{\cdot}4/0{\cdot}1 = 12$ cmH_2O, which would indeed complete the change since 12 cmH_2O is the generated pressure.

Similarly it may be shown that all the exponential changes in fig. 3.3 have a time constant, *CR*, equal to 0·4 sec, although they all have different magnitude-constants. This is indicated by the broken lines in the figure which represent continuations of the initial rate of change of each variable: in every case, no matter where it starts, the broken line always reaches the equilibrium level in one time constant, usually represented by the Greek letter τ (tau) and, in this example, equal to 0·4 sec.

In fact, of course, the initial rate of change is not maintained but progressively decreases. The mode of decrease, as for all exponentials, is such that in one time constant the change is not complete, but only about 2/3 complete, or 1/3 incomplete. At the end of two time constants it is about 1/3 of 1/3 = 1/9 incomplete. At the end of three time constants it is about 1/3 of 1/3 of 1/3 = 1/27 incomplete. To be more precise, the fraction of change incomplete at the end of one time constant is not exactly 1/3 but 1/e where e is the base of natural logarithms and is equal to 2·718. Now 1/2·718 = 37%. Therefore, at the end of one time constant, the change is 37% incomplete and 63% complete. At the end of two time constants it is 37% of 37% = 13·5% incomplete and 86·5% complete. At the end of three time constants it is 5% incomplete and 95% complete. These results are summarized and extended in Table 3.1. With the aid of this table, supplemented by more detailed tables for intermediate values, it is possible to plot the changes of flow, volume, and pressure precisely and this is how fig. 3.3 was constructed.

Table 3.1. Progress of an exponential change

Number of time constants	Extent to which change is incomplete (%)	Extent to which change is complete (%)
0	100	0
1	37	63
2	13·5	86·5
3	5·0	95·0
4	1·8	98·2
5	0·7	99·3
6	0·25	99·75

Fig. 3.3 also shows the waveform of pressure at the mouth because this is of considerable interest later. It can be deduced as follows. The resistance between the alveoli and the mouth, $R_A = 6$ cmH_2O/(litre/sec), is three-quarters of the total resistance between the alveoli and the point in the ventilator at which the constant pressure is generated: $R_A + R_V = 8$ cmH_2O/(litre/sec). Since the same flow of gas passes through both resistances the pressure at the mouth P_{Mo} must always be three-quarters of the way from the alveolar

pressure to the generated pressure. Initially the alveolar pressure is zero. The generated pressure is always 12 cmH_2O. Therefore, at the start of the phase, the mouth pressure jumps from 0 to 9 cmH_2O. It then approaches the generated pressure in such a way that it always exceeds the alveolar pressure by three-quarters of the difference between the alveolar pressure and the generated pressure. This also is an exponential approach.

It is of considerable importance to note that the time constant is the product of the patient's compliance and the *total* resistance (airway plus ventilator resistance). In the example chosen this led to a time constant of 0·4 sec so that inflation was 95% complete in $3 \times 0{\cdot}4 = 1{\cdot}2$ sec. This is consistent with the conclusion of Spalding[17] that an inspiratory phase longer than 1·5 sec provides little useful increase in tidal air. However, in many ventilators which operate as constant-pressure generators, the internal resistance of the ventilator is considerably greater than the 2 cmH_2O/(litre/sec) assumed here. Therefore the time constant is longer and a substantial inspiratory flow may continue for well over 1·5 sec if the phase is not previously terminated.

The effect of changes of lung characteristics

It was remarked above that changes of compliance and airway resistance, either within one patient or from one patient to another, would result in changes of flow pattern but not of the generated pressure. These changes will now be examined. Two situations will be considered: in the first the compliance is halved ($C' = 0{\cdot}025$ litre/cmH_2O) but the resistance is unchanged; in the second the compliance is unchanged but the *total* resistance is doubled ($R' = 16$ cmH_2O/(litre/sec)). In the second situation, since the resistance within the ventilator is unchanged ($R_V = 2$ cmH_2O/(litre/sec)) the patient's airway resistance must be rather more than doubled: the normal value R_A is 6 cmH_2O/(litre/sec), but the increased value R'_A is 14 cmH_2O/(litre/sec). The waveforms which result from these changed circumstances are shown in fig. 3.4, together with those for the 'standard' conditions (from fig. 3.3) for comparison.

In all circumstances the generated pressure stays the same, steady at 12 cmH_2O throughout the inspiratory phase. For the waveforms of other variables three aspects must be considered: the initial values, the final steady values, and the speed with which these final values are approached.

When the compliance is halved, but the resistance is unchanged, the initial flow is unaltered because the same pressure difference is applied across the same resistance. Therefore the initial mouth pressure is the same (9 cmH_2O) and the initial rate of rise of volume is unchanged (0·15 litre in 1/10 sec). However, because of the halved compliance, relating volume to alveolar pressure, the initial rate of rise of alveolar pressure is doubled: now it is 0·15 litre divided by 0·025 litre/cmH_2O = 6 cmH_2O in 1/10 sec instead of 3 cmH_2O in 1/10 sec. So far as the final steady conditions are concerned, the flow must eventually fall to zero and the alveolar pressure and mouth pressure must approach the generated pressure, as before. However, the final steady level for the volume curve is halved: it is equal to the product of the generated pressure and the halved compliance (12 $cmH_2O \times 0{\cdot}25$ litre/$cmH_2O = 0{\cdot}3$ litre). The approach to the final steady conditions is still exponential but the time constant is halved:

$$C'R = 0{\cdot}025 \text{ litre/cmH}_2\text{O} \times 8 \text{ cmH}_2\text{O/(litre/sec)} = 0{\cdot}2 \text{ sec, instead of } 0{\cdot}4 \text{ sec.}$$

The most obvious way in which this is manifested is the more rapid decline of flow towards zero and the more rapid approach of alveolar pressure towards the generated pressure. In the standard conditions the changes became 95% complete in the 1·2 sec (3 time constants) drawn in fig. 3.4. Now, with the halved compliance and halved time constant, three time constants last only 0·6 sec and the changes are 95% complete in only half the time they were before. However, in the figure, the inflation process has been

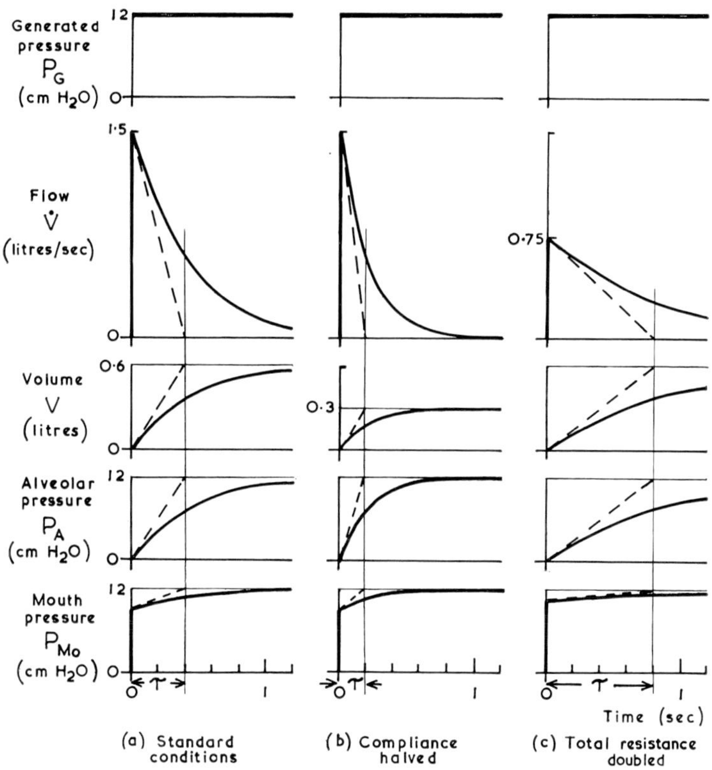

Fig. 3.4. Theoretical waveforms for inflation by a low-constant-pressure generator as in fig. 3.3:

(a) when connected to a patient with 'standard' lung characteristics, as in fig. 3.3,
(b) when the patient's compliance is halved,
(c) when the total resistance (patient plus ventilator) is doubled.

followed for 1·2 sec as before. This period of time now represents six time constants instead of only three. In the additional three time constants the degree of completeness of the changes increases from 95% to 99·75% (Table 3.1). It is still true that the time constant is the time in which the changes would be complete if the initial rate of change were maintained; for instance, the initial rate of change of alveolar pressure has just been calculated to be 6 cmH_2O in 1/10 sec which would indeed amount to 12 cmH_2O in the 0·2 sec of one time constant. This is indicated by the broken lines in fig. 3.4b all of which reach the limiting value of the corresponding variable in one time constant, τ, now equal to 0·2 sec.

When the total resistance is doubled, but the compliance is unaltered, the initial flow is halved (12 cmH_2O divided by 16 cmH_2O/(litre/sec) = 0·75 litre/sec). Therefore the initial rate of rise of volume is halved (0·075 litre in 1/10 sec). Since the compliance is unaltered the relationship between volume and alveolar pressure is the same as in the 'standard' conditions and therefore the initial rate of rise of alveolar pressure is also halved (0·075 litre divided by 0·05 litre/cmH_2O = 1·5 cmH_2O in 1/10 sec). The airway resistance, from mouth to alveoli is now 14 cmH_2O/(litre/sec) out of a total resistance of 16 cmH_2O/(litre/sec); therefore the mouth pressure rises initially to 14/16 = 7/8 of the generated pressure, that is, to 10·5 cmH_2O. As to the final steady levels: flow again declines to zero, alveolar and mouth pressures again approach the generated pressure, and the level approached by the volume curve is once more the same as under the standard conditions, since the same compliance eventually comes into equilibrium with the same generated pressure (0·05 litre/cmH_2O × 12 cmH_2O = 0·6 litre). However, the approach to these final steady levels is now much slower than before: it is still exponential but doubling the total resistance has doubled the time constant:

$$CR' = 0{\cdot}05 \text{ litre/cmH}_2\text{O} \times 16 \text{ cmH}_2\text{O/(litre/sec)} = 0{\cdot}8 \text{ sec.}$$

Therefore the period of 1·2 sec drawn in fig. 3.4 represents only $1\frac{1}{2}$ time constants in which the changes are only 78% complete. The inspiratory time would have to be extended to 2·4 sec in order to make it equal to three time constants and hence to allow the changes to become 95% complete as under the standard conditions in fig. 3.4a. However, in fig. 3.4c, if the initial rates of change were maintained, the changes would still just be complete in one time constant, τ, now equal to 0·8 sec, as shown by the broken lines.

A number of useful conclusions can be drawn from fig. 3.4 concerning the response of the waveforms produced by a constant-pressure generator to changes of lung characteristics. Thus, when the compliance is halved, the flow declines much more rapidly but from the same initial value. As a corollary of this the tidal volume is reduced although any given percentage of the ultimate maximum tidal volume is reached sooner because of the reduced time constant. When the total resistance is doubled the initial flow is halved but also the decline becomes slower so that, if the inspiratory phase is lengthened sufficiently,

out the inflation; therefore the flow into the lungs is also constant. The remaining waveforms (fig. 3.6) can now readily be derived.

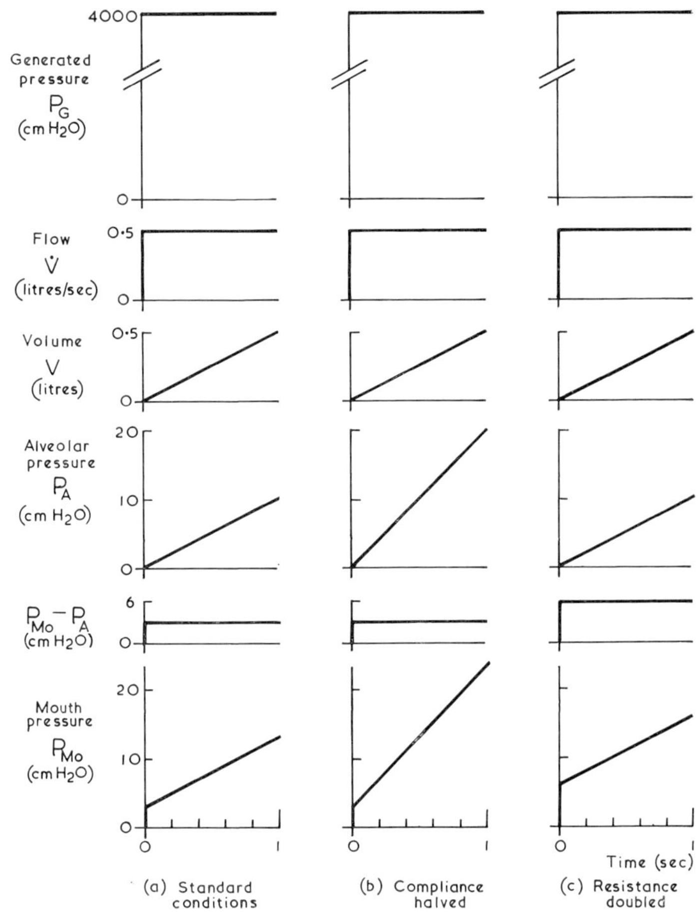

Fig. 3.6. Theoretical waveforms for inflation by a ventilator generating a very high constant pressure and having a very high internal resistance. As the waveforms show, and as is argued in the text, such a ventilator can more helpfully be regarded as a constant-flow generator.

(a) Ventilator connected to a patient with 'standard' lung characteristics.
(b) Patient's compliance halved.
(c) Patient's airway resistance doubled.

For all three sets of waveforms the characteristics are as follows.

Generated pressure : 4000 cmH_2O.
Internal resistance of ventilator : 8000 cmH_2O/(litre/sec).
Equivalent generated flow : 0·5 litre/sec.
'Standard' airway resistance of patient : 6 cmH_2O/(litre/sec).
'Standard' compliance of patient : 0·05 litre/cmH_2O.

The constant flow results in a constant rate of increase of volume of 0·5 litre/sec so that 0·5 litre is delivered in 1 sec. Similarly the alveolar pressure increases at a constant rate of 0·5 litre/sec divided by 0·05 litre/cmH_2O = 10 cmH_2O/sec and therefore reaches a value of 10 cmH_2O at the end of 1 sec. In this example it is helpful to calculate and plot, as in fig. 3.6, the pressure difference between the mouth and the alveoli, $P_{Mo} - P_A$. This is the pressure drop across the airway resistance of 6 cmH_2O/(litre/sec). At a flow of 0·5 litre/sec this amounts to 3 cmH_2O. Since the flow is constant this pressure difference also is constant throughout the inflation. The mouth pressure can now be determined as the sum of the alveolar pressure and the difference between mouth and alveolar pressures $P_{Mo} = P_A + (P_{Mo} - P_A)$: initially the mouth pressure rises suddenly to 3 cmH_2O and then increases steadily to reach 13 cmH_2O at 1 sec.

An alternative way of viewing the situation is to regard it as the first, very small, part of an exponential change. This is legitimate because, if sufficient time were allowed and various practical limitations ignored, such as the mechanical strength of the patient's lungs and of the anaesthetic circuit, the lungs would eventually inflate to a pressure of 4000 cmH_2O and the flow would finally decay to zero. In fact, the initial flow is 0·5 litre/sec for a pressure difference of 4000 cmH_2O, so that the total resistance must be 8000 cmH_2O/(litre/sec). Therefore, if inflation is to be regarded as part of an exponential process, the time constant of the exponential is

$$0{\cdot}05 \text{ litre/cmH}_2\text{O} \times 8000 \text{ cmH}_2\text{O/(litre/sec)} = 400 \text{ sec.}$$

Therefore, in the hypothetical situation proposed, it would take nearly 7 min for inflation to 4000 cmH_2O to become even 63% complete. In the practical situation, in which the inflation process is stopped after 1 sec, the inspiratory time is only 1/400th of a time constant in which time the change is 1/400th part complete; and 1/400th part of an exponential curve is, to all intents and purposes, a straight line. In other words, flow is constant throughout inflation and the rates of increase of volume and pressure are also constant.

To complete the argument it is now necessary to consider what happens when there are changes of lung characteristics. When the compliance is halved, if the original tidal volume is still to be delivered the alveolar pressure must rise to 0·5 litre divided by 0·025 litre/cmH_2O = 20 cmH_2O. Therefore the pressure drop across the total resistance will fall from 4000 cmH_2O to 3980 cmH_2O: that is, the flow will still be constant throughout inflation at 0·5 litre/sec and the tidal volume of 0·5 litre will still be delivered in 1 sec. Alveolar pressure still rises steadily, but at twice the rate obtaining under the standard conditions. The mouth pressure shows the same initial step, as before, because there is the same flow through the same airway resistance, but thereafter the mouth pressure rises at the same, doubled, rate as the alveolar pressure.

When the airway resistance is doubled to 12 cmH_2O/(litre/sec) this makes a negligible difference to the total resistance of 8000 cmH_2O/(litre/sec) so that the flow is unaltered.

Therefore, again the increase of lung volume is unaltered and, on this occasion, the increase of alveolar pressure also is the same as under the standard conditions, 10 cmH_2O in 1 sec. In fact the only changes from the standard conditions are that the pressure drop from mouth to alveoli across the doubled airway resistance is doubled, to 6 cmH_2O, and therefore the initial step in the mouth-pressure waveform is also doubled. Thereafter mouth pressure increases at the same rate as the alveolar pressure and at the same rate as under the standard conditions, 10 cmH_2O/sec.

Comparison of the waveforms produced by constant-pressure generators of different magnitudes of generated pressure: the idea of the constant-flow generator

If figs. 3.4, 3.5, and 3.6 are compared the following conclusions can be drawn about constant-pressure generators.

When the generated pressure is low (12 cmH_2O in fig. 3.4) it is clear that the generated-pressure waveform is the only one which is uninfluenced by changes of lung characteristics. The mouth-pressure waveform is not very different from the generated-pressure waveform because there is little resistance between the points at which the two pressures occur. Therefore, the mouth-pressure waveform varies little with changes of lung characteristics. On the other hand, the flow waveform varies markedly when the lung characteristics are changed.

When the generated pressure is very high indeed (4000 cmH_2O in fig. 3.6) the situation is quite different. Then the flow waveform is just as constant, and just as much uninfluenced by changes of lung characteristics, as is the waveform of generated pressure. On the other hand the mouth-pressure waveform is radically altered by changes of lung characteristics and bears no resemblance in either shape or magnitude to the generated-pressure waveform. The reasons for the constancy of the flow are twofold. Firstly, the internal resistance of the ventilator is so huge in relation to any likely airway resistance of the patient that changes of airway resistance have no appreciable effect on the total resistance. Secondly, the generated pressure at one end of this total resistance is so very large in relation to any pressure likely to develop in the alveoli that changes of compliance have no appreciable effect upon the pressure difference across the total resistance. Therefore, with no change of total resistance and no change of pressure difference there can be no change of flow.

By analogy with the definition of a constant-pressure generator, a *constant-flow generator* can be defined as a system in which the flow into the patient is held constant at a level which is determined by the ventilator and is quite uninfluenced by the lung characteristics of the patient. With a constant-flow generator the pressure waveforms, at the mouth and in the alveoli, are determined by the effect of the constant generated flow on the patient's lungs and hence vary with lung characteristics. Clearly, it is permissible to refer to the system of fig. 3.6 as a constant-flow generator. Indeed, it is not merely permissible but also positively helpful to do so. This is so because the waveforms can more readily be deduced if the ventilator is regarded as generating a constant flow of 0·5 litre/sec throughout the inspiratory phase rather than as generating a constant pressure of 4000 cmH_2O and having an internal resistance of 8000 cmH_2O/(litre/sec). Furthermore, if the nature of the mechanism inside the ventilator were unknown, examination of the other waveforms (a flow which is constant throughout the phase at a level which is independent of lung characteristics, and a mouth pressure which varies very markedly with lung characteristics) would undoubtedly lead to the conclusion that the ventilator was generating a constant flow no matter how this was achieved.

If a low pressure in series with a low resistance is to be regarded as a constant-pressure generator, and a very high pressure in series with a very high resistance is to be regarded as a constant-flow generator, then, at some intermediate point, there must be a transition from one to the other. It is pertinent to enquire where this transition occurs. In fig. 3.5 the generated pressure is 40 cmH_2O and the ventilator resistance 60 cmH_2O/(litre/sec). Should this be regarded as a constant-pressure generator or as a constant-flow generator? Certainly the flow is not constant throughout the phase and certainly the flow waveform does vary somewhat with lung characteristics. However, the mouth-pressure waveform varies much more, so that, if the nature of the mechanism inside the ventilator were unknown and a judgement had to be based on waveforms at the patient, it might seem more sensible to regard the ventilator as approximating to a constant-flow generator than to a constant-pressure generator. Indeed, if it were regarded as generating a flow of 0·5 litre/sec in all circumstances, the waveforms calculated for volume, alveolar pressure, and mouth pressure would be those of fig. 3.6 which, it can be seen, are not very different from those of fig. 3.5; therefore little error would result. However, it is important to stress that this is so only within the range of variation of lung characteristics used in constructing the figures. If the ventilator of fig. 3.5 were connected to a patient with a very low compliance, say 0·01 litre/cmH_2O, then it would be necessary to wait for almost complete equilibrium between alveolar pressure and generated pressure even to obtain a tidal volume which approached 0·4 litre (40 $cmH_2O \times$ 0·01 litre/cmH_2O). In this situation the flow would fall nearly to zero by the end of the phase while the mouth pressure would be close to the generated pressure. Therefore the system could no longer be regarded as approximating to a constant-flow generator and could only be understood in terms of its fundamental, pressure-generating, action.

In summary it may be said that, if the mechanism in a ventilator fundamentally controls a pressure at a constant level, then the waveforms can always be reliably deduced if the ventilator is regarded as a constant-pressure generator with some internal resistance. However, if the generated pressure is much higher than the highest pressure likely to be produced in the alveoli, it will usually be easier to deduce the waveforms, at least approximately, if the ventilator is regarded as approximating to a constant-flow generator. The point at which such an approximation becomes unacceptable clearly depends on the circumstances. However, as a working rule, it is suggested that the approximation will be very good if the generated pressure is more than ten times the highest alveolar pressure. It will however still be acceptable for many purposes if, as in fig. 3.5, the generated pressure is twice the highest alveolar pressure. It follows from this that a particular ventilator may be satisfactorily approximated to a constant-flow generator when delivering a given tidal volume to a given patient and yet the approximation may become unacceptable if the tidal volume is increased or if the ventilator is connected to a patient with a lower compliance.

Mechanical forms of constant-flow generator and constant-pressure generator

So far the weighted bag, the second-stage reducing valve, and the first-stage reducing valve plus needle valve have been considered. It has been shown that fundamentally these all operate as constant-pressure generators but that, when the generated pressure and internal resistance are high enough, these systems behave as constant-flow generators. Now various other devices for producing inflation will be considered and it is convenient to begin with a group which behave as constant-flow generators in their own right.

Positive-displacement pumps

Positive-displacement pumps are pumps which displace a definite volume of gas at each stroke. They draw in a fixed volume of gas and then expel the whole of it, virtually no matter what the resultant pressure. They can therefore be used as compressors and are often referred to as such. Commonly the volume displaced is small (of the order of a few millilitres) and the frequency is high (several strokes or revolutions per second) so that there is an almost continuous flow of gas. If the intake is at atmospheric pressure the mass, or quantity, of gas displaced per stroke is fixed; if the pump is driven by a constant-speed motor, such as an electric induction motor, the frequency is fixed; therefore the volume flow rate of the emergent gas (after it has expanded to atmospheric pressure) is fixed, no matter how high (within limits) the pressure at the outlet of the pump. If such a positive-displacement pump is used to inflate a patient it therefore operates as a constant-flow generator: the flow of gas into the patient's lungs is held constant throughout the inspiratory phase at a level which is determined by the ventilator and is uninfluenced by the patient's lung characteristics. The waveforms of fig. 3.6 (apart from the generated pressure waveform) are applicable. This system is found in the 'Fazakerley' ventilator and the Blease 'Pulmoflator', although in the Blease the fundamental, constant-flow-generating action is considerably modified by various factors. These are considered in detail in the full account of the Blease 'Pulmoflator' but one factor is of sufficient general importance to merit consideration here.

To permit variation of the flow rate at which the lungs are inflated a control is provided in the Blease 'Pulmoflator' which introduces a variable leak to atmosphere. Thus, when this control is open, only part of the constant flow, generated by the positive-displacement pump, goes to the patient and part escapes through the leak; from the point of view of the pump the leak is 'in parallel' with the patient; from the point of view of the patient the leak is 'in parallel' with the pump. Whatever the point of view, the fraction of the total flow from the pump which goes to the patient is not constant throughout the phase: as inflation proceeds the mouth pressure rises and therefore the pressure drop across the leak rises. Consequently the flow through the leak increases and the flow into the patient decreases. Since the way in which the mouth pressure increases depends on the patient's lung characteristics, the way in which the flow into the lungs decreases also depends on lung characteristics. Therefore, once a leak is introduced in parallel with a positive-displacement pump (or any other constant-flow generator) the system no longer operates as a constant-flow generator. However, it can be shown that a constant-flow generator with a leak in parallel behaves very similarly to a constant-pressure generator with an internal resistance in series. As the size of the leak increases so the equivalent generated pressure decreases, as also does the magnitude of the equivalent series resistance.

It can readily be appreciated that there is a maximum pressure which can be developed by a constant-flow generator with a leak: the maximum is the pressure at which the whole of the constant-flow is blown to waste through the leak. This maximum pressure is the equivalent generated pressure. If the leak is very small, the equivalent generated pressure and the equivalent internal resistance are very high and the system still makes a good approximation to a constant-flow generator; the waveforms produced will not be very different in character from those in fig. 3.6. If the leak is large, the equivalent generated pressure is small and the equivalent internal resistance is reduced, so that the device may need to be considered as a constant-pressure generator; the waveforms produced will be more like those in fig. 3.5 or even fig. 3.4.

Injectors

Many ventilators make use of an injector during the inspiratory phase. Gas at high pressure, usually 45 to 75 lb/in^2, is supplied to the jet of the injector (see fig. 3.7). The

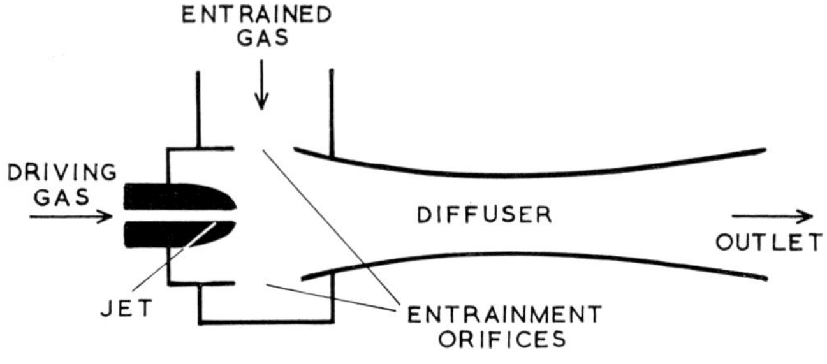

Fig. 3.7. An injector: a device which is equivalent to a constant-pressure generator with an internal resistance.

resultant high-velocity flow from the jet entrains air or other gas through the entrainment orifices and the total flow, emerging from the diffusor of the injector, inflates the patient's lungs. The performance cannot be rigorously deduced but it can perhaps be appreciated that, as the pressure at the mouth, and hence the pressure at the outlet of the injector, builds up during inflation, so the flow rate of gas which is entrained, and hence the total flow into the lungs, is reduced. Therefore an injector does not operate as a perfect constant-flow generator. Its actual mode of operation can be deduced if its characteristics are determined experimentally. The characteristics of an injector can be determined by gradually occluding the outlet and observing the way in which the emergent flow and the pressure at the outlet vary.

With no obstruction to the outlet the pressure there is atmospheric (zero) and the flow is at a maximum for the given driving pressure. As the outlet is gradually occluded the outlet pressure gradually rises and the emergent flow gradually declines. When the outlet is completely occluded the emergent flow must be zero, with the driving-gas flow being forced out through the entrainment orifices. The outlet pressure is then at a maximum.

From such an experiment it is possible to plot a graph such as that shown in fig. 3.8 for a hypothetical injector. This graph shows that when there is no obstruction of the outlet (zero outlet pressure) the emergent flow is 40 litres/min; but as the pressure at the

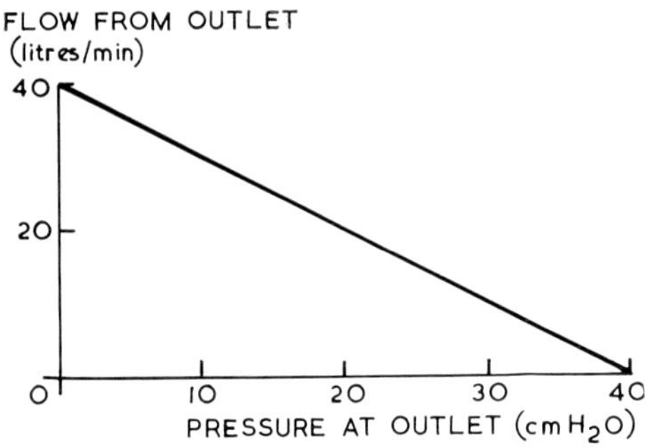

Fig. 3.8. Flow-pressure characteristic of a hypothetical injector which, with a particular driving pressure, is equivalent to a constant pressure of 40 cmH_2O in series with a resistance of 60 cmH_2O/(litre/sec).

outlet increases the flow steadily decreases, reaching zero at a pressure of 40 cmH_2O. This is precisely the same relationship between flow and pressure that would be observed at the outlet of the ventilator which produced the waveforms shown in fig. 3.5. That ventilator comprised a source of constant pressure (40 cmH_2O) and an internal resistance of 60 cmH_2O/(litre/sec). Thus, if the pressure at the outlet of that ventilator were zero (atmospheric), the whole of the generated pressure would be dropped across the internal ventilator resistance to produce a flow of 40 cmH_2O divided by 60 cmH_2O/(litre/sec) which equals 2/3 litre/sec or 40 litres/min. Further, if the outlet pressure were increased, the pressure difference, and therefore the flow, would decrease until, at an outlet pressure of 40 cmH_2O, the flow would reach zero—exactly as in fig. 3.8. Therefore the hypothetical injector whose characteristics are plotted in fig. 3.8 is precisely equivalent to a constant-pressure generator in series with a resistance. This is at least broadly true for all injectors. The equivalent constant pressure is always very much less than that of the driving gas and does not actually exist at any point in the injector. Nevertheless, the equivalent pressure, together with the equivalent resistance, accurately defines the equivalent pneumatic characteristics of the injector. Thus, suppose an injector with the characteristics shown in fig. 3.8 were substituted for the ventilator assumed in deducing the waveforms of fig. 3.5. The real constant pressure and real resistance of that ventilator were identical with the equivalent pressure and resistance of the injector. Therefore the injector would produce exactly the same waveforms as in fig. 3.5.

There is also experimental evidence of the validity of these equivalent characteristics. In the Aga 'Spiropulsator' there is one setting of the inlet pressure to the injector at which the charactistic of the injector is very similar to the hypothetical one shown in fig. 3.8, and it so happens that a setting close to this was used for making the experimental recordings on the 'Spiropulsator'. If the experimental waveforms in the inspiratory phase in fig. 10.6* are compared with the theoretical ones in fig. 3.5 then, allowing for differences of scale, they will be seen to be very similar.

With other injectors, and with other inlet pressures to the 'Spiropulsator' injector, different flow-pressure characteristics are obtained; but all those that we have recorded can be closely represented by an equivalent constant pressure and series resistance. In many cases ('Cyclator', Dräger 'Poliomat', Ohio (Monaghan) 300, and also the Aga 'Spiropulsator' at high inlet pressures) the equivalent generated pressure is as high as 100 to 200 cmH_2O, although always very much less than the inlet pressure, and the series resistance is usually from 100 up to as much as 600 cmH_2O/(litre/sec).† Therefore, remembering the criterion established above (see p. 84) these injectors will make good approximations to constant-flow generators. This can be appreciated from the flow-pressure characteristics which are shown in the accounts of the individual ventilators: the flow falls off only slowly as the pressure at the outlet increases. On the other hand, in the Bird Mark 8 ventilator, especially at low inlet pressures, (that is at low settings of the 'flowrate' control) the flow falls off much more steeply with increase of pressure (fig. 29.5). This indicates that the generated pressure and series resistance are both quite low, even down to 17 cmH_2O and 19 cmH_2O/(litre/sec) at the setting used for the recordings of fig. 29.8. Under these conditions the system must be considered as a low-constant-pressure generator.

Blowers

A number of ventilators use as their primary motive source some sort of blower. In these, a system of rotating vanes or fan blades drives gas forward. (The domestic vacuum

* If the form of this figure is not immediately understandable the reader should refer to p. 179 where the way in which the experimental recordings were obtained is described in detail.

† Unlike most real resistances in ventilators, these equivalent resistances are usually almost perfectly linear. For a brief note on the different effects of linear and non-linear resistances see p. 134.

cleaners used in several of the early ventilators come in this category.) It can perhaps readily be visualized that with a blower there will be a certain flow when the pressure at the outlet is zero but that, unlike the positive-displacement pump, as the pressure increases so the flow is dammed back, until at some limiting pressure the flow falls to zero. From this it seems likely that a blower, like an injector, can be regarded as equivalent to a constant-pressure generator with an internal resistance. Measurements have been made on only one such system, the blower in the Air-Shields 'Respirator', and the flow-pressure characteristics (fig. 14.3) confirm this equivalence. This blower, with the 'flow' control at maximum, is approximately equivalent to a generated pressure of 80 cmH_2O in series with a resistance of 110 cmH_2O/(litre/sec). At this setting, therefore, it makes a good approximation to a constant-flow generator. However, in some blowers the equivalent generated pressure may be lower and these may therefore need to be treated as low-constant-pressure generators.

Pressure transformers

In a number of ventilators the patient is inflated from a concertina bag which is mechanically linked to a piston in a cylinder. The cylinder is supplied with gas at high pressure (15 lb/in^2 upwards). A simple form is illustrated in fig. 3.9. During the inspiratory phase a high pressure P acting on the small area a of the piston produces a force

$$F = P \times a. \tag{8}$$

This force, acting on the large area A of the concertina bag produces a small pressure

$$p = F/A. \tag{9}$$

Substituting for F from equation (8) gives

$$p = P \times a/A, \tag{10}$$

or

$$p/P = a/A. \tag{11}$$

That is, the ratio of 'output' (p) and 'input' (P) pressures is constant and equal to the ratio of input to output areas. Thus the system operates in a manner analogous to that of the electrical transformer and is therefore referred to here as a 'pressure transformer'.

If the input pressure comes directly from a good reducing valve it will be constant throughout the inspiratory phase despite fluctuations in the flow drawn from the valve. Therefore, according to the theory just given, the output pressure will also be constant and the device will operate as a constant-pressure generator. The magnitude of the generated pressure depends on the dimensions of the transformer and on the input pressure but may well be high enough, as in the 'R.P.R.' ventilator, for the device to approximate to a flow generator.

In several ventilators the piston and cylinder are not directly connected to the reducing valve; instead an adjustable resistance is interposed to provide some control of the speed of inflation. Because of this resistance the input pressure to the piston varies with flow. However, it can be shown that this system is equivalent to a precisely-constant output pressure in the concertina bag with a resistance at the outlet.

A factor which may complicate the functioning of the system is that some of the force produced by the action of the input pressure on the piston may be used, not in developing output pressure, but in overcoming other forces. In the 'Jefferson' it has to overcome the heavy weight in the base of the concertina bag but this factor alone merely reduces the magnitude of the generated pressure; it is still a constant generated pressure. Other factors may alter the form of the generated pressure but these are discussed more fully elsewhere (see p. 94 and the account of the 'R.P.R.' ventilator).

The mechanical forms of the Allbritten, 'Jefferson', and U.S. Army ventilators closely match that shown in fig. 3.9 but other pressure transformers differ considerably.

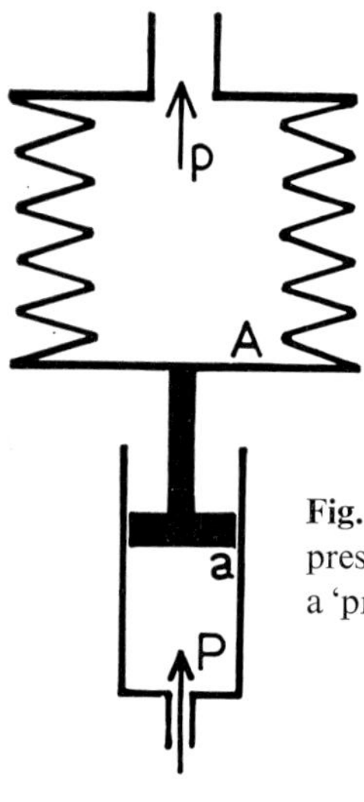

Fig. 3.9. A concertina bag driven by high-pressure gas applied to a piston in a cylinder : a 'pressure transformer'.

p, P = pressures.
a, A = cross-sectional areas.
$p/P = a/A$.

Thus, in the Stephenson and 'R.P.R.' ventilators two pistons in parallel act downwards on the concertina bag. In the Emerson gas-operated ventilator the concertina bag is replaced by a second, large bore, piston and cylinder. In the Mortimer the input 'pressure' is about half an atmosphere of vacuum and the piston and cylinder are replaced by a close-fitting paddle rotating within a semi-cylindrical space. The angular movement of the paddle, acting through a lever system, produces a smaller angular movement of the end plate of a concertina bag.

Non-constant-flow generators

There are a number of ventilators in which a concertina bag or a piston in a cylinder is driven through a simple mechanical linkage by a constant-speed electric motor. With such an arrangement the pattern of movement of the bag or piston, with respect to time, is uninfluenced by the build-up of pressure within the bag or cylinder. Therefore the pattern of flow out of the bag will not be influenced by pressure and hence will be independent of the lung characteristics of the patient to whom the ventilator is connected. On the other hand, the pattern of pressure in the bag will depend upon the effect of the flow on the patient's lungs and so will be very much influenced by changes of lung characteristics. Such a ventilator must therefore be regarded as a flow generator.

In these ventilators the pattern of flow, although the same in every inspiratory phase, is rarely constant throughout the phase. In principle the pattern of flow can have almost any shape imaginable, but in practice the flow usually starts at some low level, builds up to a maximum, and then declines again towards the end of the phase. However, whatever the pattern of flow may be, the essential characteristic is that the pattern is always the same, no matter what the lung characteristics. This is illustrated in fig. 3.10 for a pattern of flow which corresponds to a half cycle of a sine wave. (Of the curves which rise to a peak and fall again the sine wave is the simplest from the mathematical point of view, and is a tolerable approximation to many of the flow patterns which occur in practice.) The duration of the half cycle in fig. 3.10 is 1 sec and its amplitude (the peak flow half-way through the 1 sec) is such as to deliver a tidal volume of 0·5 litre in the half cycle. Thus the ventilation produced by this sine-wave-flow generator is similar to that produced by the other ventilators considered above (figs. 3.4, 3.5, 3.6). The first column of curves in fig. 3.10 shows the waveforms, deduced theoretically, which result when this pattern of flow is delivered to a patient with our 'standard' lung characteristics. The subsequent columns show the waveforms that result when the compliance is halved and when the airway resistance is doubled. It can clearly be seen that the flow, though not constant throughout the phase, follows exactly the same pattern whatever the lung characteristics, although the patterns of alveolar and mouth pressures are very much influenced by changes of lung characteristics.

In some ventilators the waveform of generated flow is close to the half cycle of a sine wave shown in fig. 3.10 (the Starling Pump and Emerson electrically-operated ventilator). In others, although the compression of the reservoir bag follows a half cycle of a sine wave quite closely, the patient is connected to the bag for only part of this half cycle (Aika, Cape-Waine). In some ventilators the performance may be modified by a blow-off valve (Aika, Beaver Mark III) or a leak (Engström). In the case of the Engström the modification is so great that its behaviour is completely altered (see below).

In one ventilator the patient is connected to the reservoir bag almost throughout its compression stroke, but the pattern of compression deviates appreciably from a sine wave: the peak flow comes later than half-way through the cycle (Lundia). In two others

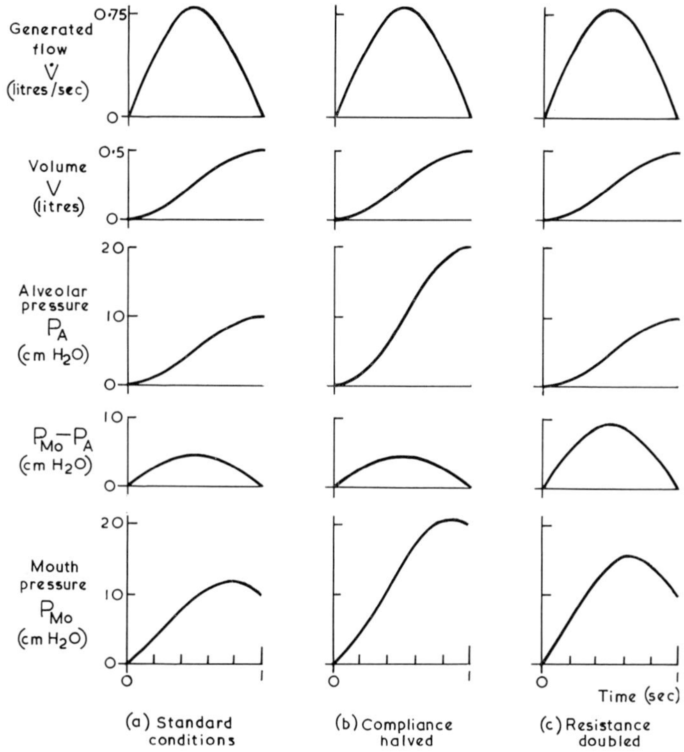

Fig. 3.10. Theoretical waveforms for inflation by a ventilator generating a half cycle of a sine wave of flow:

(a) when connected to a patient with 'standard' lung characteristics,
(b) when the patient's compliance is halved,
(c) when the patient's airway resistance is doubled.

For all three sets of waveforms the characteristics are as follows.

Peak flow : 0·79 litre/sec.
Duration of half cycle : 1 sec.
'Standard' airway resistance of patient : 6 cmH_2O/(litre/sec).
'Standard' compliance of patient : 0·05 litre/cmH_2O.

a variety of waveforms can be obtained at will by the choice of different cams ('Adelaide', Clutton-Brock).

Non-constant-pressure generators

By analogy with a non-constant-flow generator it is possible to have a non-constant-pressure generator. In such a system a waveform of pressure is generated which, though not constant throughout the inspiratory phase, is the same shape in every respiratory cycle despite changes in lung characteristics. One way in which this arises is from the combination of a non-constant-flow generator with a leak. It was mentioned above (see p. 85) that a constant-flow generator with a leak was equivalent to a constant-pressure generator. Similarly, a non-constant-flow generator with a leak behaves as a non-constant-pressure generator.

This situation exists in the Engström ventilators. During the inspiratory phase a piston in a cylinder is driven through a mechanical linkage by a constant-speed electric motor so that it expels gas according to a flow pattern which corresponds to the first one-third of a cycle of a sine wave. It does this irrespective of the pressure built up in the cylinder. However, in this one-third of a cycle, the total volume displaced is 5 litres and the peak flow (at a respiratory frequency of 20/min) is 6·6 litres/sec. Necessarily, most of this flow must be blown to waste and this is done through an orifice the size of which is adjusted to give a pattern of pressure drop of suitable amplitude for inflating the patient. Since the pattern of total flow is constant, any change in the flow into the patient, comparing one respiratory cycle with another, must be accompanied by an equal and opposite change in the flow through the orifice. However, the flow into the patient is always much less than the flow through the orifice, so that any change in the former flow results in only a small percentage change in the latter. Therefore the pattern of pressure drop across the orifice is substantially the same whatever the lung characteristics. In other words the system approximates closely to a non-constant-pressure generator and the pattern of flow into the lungs varies with changes of lung characteristics. In the first one-third of a cycle of a sine wave the flow increases for most of the time and therefore so also does the pressure-drop. Therefore the Engström ventilators can usefully be described as increasing-pressure generators. This is consistent with Norlander's[12] 'increasing force generator' since his 'force' presumably acts on a constant area, and therefore is associated with a proportionately increasing pressure. The details of the action of this ventilator are complicated by a number of other factors of which a full account is given in Chapter 52.

A mechanism which operates directly as a non-constant-pressure generator is a concertina bag compressed by a spring as in the 'Barnet' and the Howells ventilators. As the bag empties the spring relaxes, the force exerted on the bag decreases, and the pressure within it decreases. Thus it is possible to plot a graph of pressure in the bag against volume in the bag, as has been done in fig. 23.4 for the prototype of the 'Barnet' Mark III and fig. 57.4 for the Howells. The pressure in the bag, at any given bag volume, is entirely determined by the characteristics of the ventilator—primarily the force exerted by the spring at any given position of the bag, divided by the cross-sectional area of the bag. This pressure is not affected by the flow out of the bag and therefore is quite uninfluenced by the lung characteristics of the patient. On the other hand the pattern of flow out of the bag into the patient's lungs is not directly determined by the ventilator but is a product of the effect of the pattern of pressure within the bag on the patient's lungs. The flow pattern therefore does vary with lung characteristics.

Therefore this system would appear to be a pressure generator and, specifically, might be called a 'decreasing-pressure generator'. However, it should be noted that the pattern of pressure is fixed in relation to the volume in the bag and not in relation to time. Therefore a spring-loaded bag is not strictly a non-constant-pressure generator if the term 'pressure generator' is restricted to mean a device which keeps the pattern of pressure fixed in relation to time. For a precise way of expressing the behaviour of spring-loaded bags, or other systems in which the pressure is fixed in relation to volume, it is necessary to treat them as 'discharging compliances' (see p. 98). However, for many purposes the 'decreasing-pressure-generating' point of view is sufficiently accurate and is particularly useful in understanding the differences between such systems and true constant-pressure generators.

Having established the mode of action of a spring-loaded concertina bag it is opportune to look again at those ventilators in which a concertina bag is compressed by a constant force produced either by a weight or by the action of a pressure transformer. In the previous accounts of these mechanisms the elasticity of the bag wall was ignored. If this is taken into account it can be appreciated that, when the bag is extended, the elasticity supplements the external force but, when the bag approaches full compression, the elasticity opposes the external force. Therefore the pressure within the bag is not simply equal to the external force divided by the cross-sectional area; instead it ranges from rather more than this, when the bag is full, to rather less, as the bag empties. Thus the system can be regarded either as a decreasing-pressure generator or as a discharging compliance just like the spring-loaded bag. Furthermore, in the spring-loaded bag, the fall in pressure as the bag empties must be accentuated a little by the elasticity of the bag wall. When the external force is constant (weight, or pressure transformer) the extent of the fall in pressure as the bag empties depends on the shape and material of the bag wall. In the Manley ventilator (fig. 61.4) it is quite large and represents a substantial fraction of the maximum pressure when that is set low; in the 'Vellore' (fig. 89.3) it is negligible (the kinks at the extremes of extension and compression of the bag are due to other causes discussed in the full account of the ventilator).

Another complication which arises in weighted concertina bags stems from the inertia of the weight. When gas begins to flow out of the bag at the start of the inspiratory phase some of the force exerted by the weight is used in accelerating the weight downwards so that the pressure in the bag falls a little. Later the weight may gather enough speed to be moving faster than in accordance with the flow of gas out of the bag so that its inertia raises the pressure in the bag above what it would otherwise be. The overall result is a series of oscillations in the pressure in the bag and hence in the flow into the lungs. These oscillations are quite prominent in the recordings of the 'Vellore' (figs. 89.4 and 89.5) but almost absent in most of the recordings of the East-Radcliffe 'Positive-Negative' ventilator (figs. 47.7 and 47.8).

Another mechanism which may operate as a decreasing-pressure generator is the distended spherical reservoir bag. In a number of ventilators inflation is brought about by connecting the patient to an ordinary reservoir bag which has previously been inflated to a suitably high pressure. This system is discussed in detail below.

In all decreasing-pressure generators, if the pressure can be set high enough, and kept high throughout the inspiratory phase, the mode of operation will approximate to that of a flow generator—a decreasing-flow generator. This is well illustrated in the set of experimental waveforms obtained with the Howells ventilator in which the generated pressure ranges from about 120 to 80 cmH_2O as the bag empties: if fig. 57.5 is examined it will be seen that the pattern of flow, a slow steady decline throughout the phase, is little altered by the changes of lung characteristics but that the pattern of pressure at the mouth is markedly altered.

A pressure transformer can act as a non-constant-pressure generator if the mechanical advantage of the linkage between the 'piston' and the bag alters during the phase. This is the case in the 'Roswell Park' ventilator.

Another form of pressure generator

A system for inflation which was employed in many of the early ventilators (Bang, 'Clevedon', and several of the 'Newcastle' ventilators), and which has recently been brought back into use in the 'Minivent' and 'Autovent', is shown diagrammatically in fig. 3.11. Inflating gas enters the system from flowmeters at a constant rate at (A),

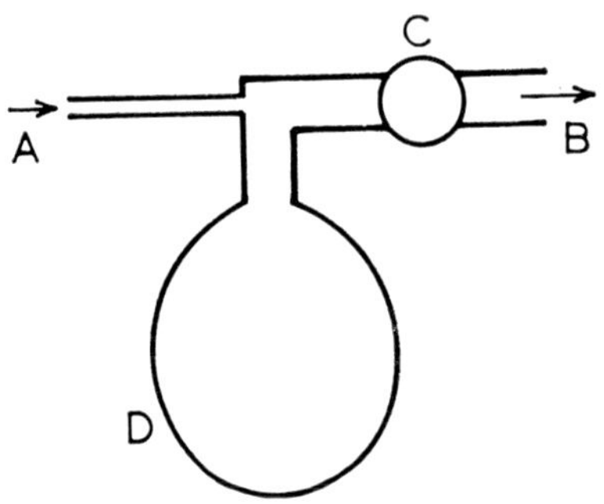

Fig. 3.11. A common supply system whose mode of operation is discussed in the text.
A. Continuous steady flow of inflating gas.
B. Connexion to patient.
C. Valve which is open for the inspiratory phase and closed for the expiratory phase.
D. Reservoir bag distended by gas under pressure.

building up pressure in the reservoir bag (D) while the tap (C) is shut. Inflation is brought about by opening the tap (C) so that gas is driven into the patient's lungs by the tension in the rubber wall of the bag. The bag therefore partly empties. During the expiratory phase the tap (C) is closed and the bag is refilled with inflating gas.

In this arrangement the pressure in the bag is due solely to the elasticity of the wall of the bag and therefore, for a given bag, varies with the volume of gas in the bag but not with the flow out of the bag. Therefore the system behaves as a pressure generator but, like the decreasing-pressure generators just discussed, the pattern of pressure is related to the volume in the bag and not to time. The pattern of generated pressure is revealed by the pressure-volume characteristic of the bag employed. This characteristic has been determined for ten 'two-litre' reservoir bags in a number of circumstances. A typical characteristic is shown in fig. 3.12. It can be seen that, as the volume increases above the two litres or so required to make the bag taut, the pressure increases fairly rapidly at first as the wall is stretched, but later, because of the physical configuration of the bag (approximately spherical) the pressure rises more slowly and eventually reaches a maximum.

It follows from the characteristics in fig. 3.12 that there are two main modes of operation. For the first mode of operation the bag is kept well inflated—always above 5 litres. Then the variation in bag volume in the course of each respiratory cycle has a negligible effect on the bag pressure. In this mode the system operates as a virtually-perfect con-

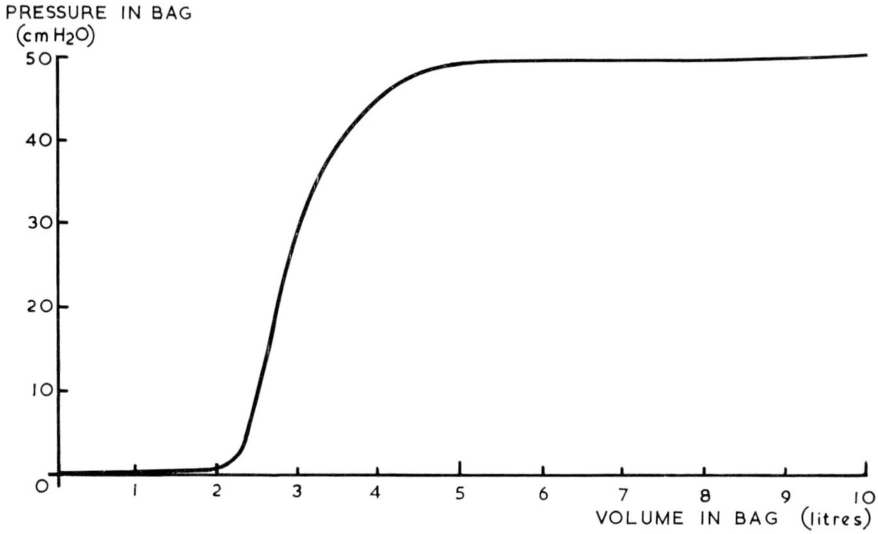

Fig. 3.12. Pressure-volume characteristic for a 'two-litre', anti-static, reservoir bag. The curve shown is for the second inflation of a new bag. The first inflation gave slightly higher pressures—a maximum of 59 cmH_2O at 5·5 litres falling to 55 cm H_2O at 10 litres. Later inflations gave results similar to that shown. In nine other bags (seven new, two old) the peak pressures in the first inflation ranged from 48 to 71 cmH_2O. In the four bags in which a second inflation was made the pressure at 5 to 6 litres was 85 to 87% of the peak pressure on the first inflation.

In all cases the steep rise of pressure to the maximum can be closely matched by that given theoretically for a spherical bag of perfectly-elastic material.[21] For higher volumes, however, the theory predicts that the pressure will gradually fall towards zero whereas experimentally it was found that the pressure stayed in the vicinity of its initial maximum up to at least 200 litres. During subsequent gradual deflation much lower pressures were obtained and the final flaccid volume was 8 litres.

stant-pressure generator. In the 'two-litre' reservoir bags studied the generated pressure was quite high, in the range 40 to 60 cmH_2O, so that in practice they would often make fair approximations to constant-flow generators. However, with other types of bag it would be possible to generate other pressures. For instance, a '30 gramme' meteorological balloon was found to exert a pressure which varied only between 9·4 and 9·6 cmH_2O for volumes between 9 and 16 litres: such a bag would form a perfect low-constant-pressure generator.

For the second mode of operation the average degree of inflation of the bag is less and therefore the variation of bag volume in the course of each respiratory cycle occurs within the steep portion of the pressure-volume characteristic. (The system must operate in this mode in the case of the 'Minivent' and 'Autovent' since the mechanism used for cycling these ventilators from the expiratory phase to the inspiratory phase depends on changes in bag pressure.) This portion of the characteristic is very similar to the pressure-volume characteristics of some of the spring-loaded or weighted concertina bags found in other ventilators. This is shown clearly in fig. 3.13 where part of the characteristic of the distended reservoir bag of fig. 3.12 has been replotted (curve b) on the scales used elsewhere in the book for plotting the pressure-volume characteristics of loaded concertina bags. Two of these characteristics are also plotted in fig. 3.13 for comparison: curve (a) is

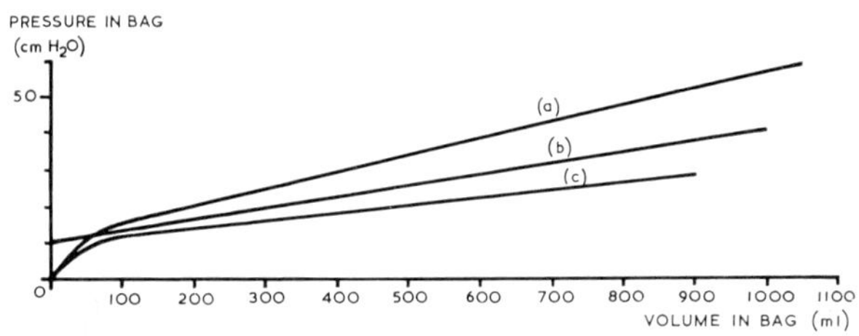

Fig. 3.13. Pressure-volume characteristics for bags in various ventilators.

(a) The spring-loaded concertina bag from the closed circuit of a prototype of the 'Barnet' Mark III.

(b) The distended reservoir bag whose full characteristic is given in fig. 3.12. (For this characteristic the 'volume in bag' axis should be read as the volume in excess of that present at a pressure of 10 cmH_2O.)

(c) The weighted concertina bag of the Manley with the weight set to minimum.

for a spring-loaded bag (prototype of the 'Barnet' Mark III); curve (c) is for a weighted bag in which the pressure is much affected by the elasticity of the bag wall (Manley). In this mode, therefore, the distended reservoir bag, like the spring-loaded concertina bag, can be regarded as a decreasing-pressure generator in which the pattern of pressure is fixed in relation to the volume in the bag but not in relation to time.

Another view of the decreasing-pressure generator: the idea of a 'discharging compliance'

The idea of a pressure generator in which the pressure decreases according to a pattern which is fixed in relation to volume but not to time is somewhat unsatisfactory, because it is not easy to deduce the resultant waveforms in a patient. An alternative way of dealing with devices with these characteristics is to regard them as 'discharging compliances'. Compliance is defined as change of volume per unit change of pressure; therefore a distended reservoir bag, or a spring-loaded or weighted concertina bag, has a compliance in just the same way that lungs have compliance. During the expiratory phase the bag is commonly inflated by a steady inflow of gas (analogous to positive-pressure inflation of the lungs of a patient) but sometimes, as in the closed circuit of the 'Barnet' Mark III, it is expanded by external means (analogous to spontaneous inspiration). Then, during the inspiratory phase, the compliance of the bag discharges into the compliance of the patient (analogous, perhaps, to mouth-to-mouth inflation). The term 'discharges' is used, by analogy with the discharge of an electrical condenser, rather than 'deflates' or 'expires', since the use of these terms might cause confusion with expiration by the patient.

The magnitude of the compliance of a bag is indicated by the slope of its pressure-volume characteristic. Since this characteristic is often curved the slope, and therefore the compliance, often varies with bag volume—just as is the case, to some extent, in the lungs. However, this is not always so, and in the spring-loaded bag of the prototype of the 'Barnet' Mark III (curve (a) in fig. 3.13) the compliance is constant over most of the range of volume.

To understand the operation of a discharging compliance it is best to consider a simple situation first. Assume that the compliance of the bag is constant. Assume also that inflating gas does not enter the system during the inspiratory phase, i.e. unlike the arrangement in fig. 3.11 but like the arrangement in the Manley and in the closed circuit of the 'Barnet' Mark III.

For a specific example assume that the lung characteristics of the patient are the same as before:

compliance of patient, $C_P = 0{\cdot}05$ litre/cmH_2O,
airway resistance, $R_A = 6$ cmH_2O/(litre/sec).

Let the compliance of the bag be given by

$C_B = 0{\cdot}02$ litre/cmH_2O,

and let there be a resistance between the bag and the patient's mouth,

$R_V = 22$ cmH_2O/(litre/sec).

Finally, let the initial pressure in the bag be 35 cmH_2O.

The resultant waveforms are shown in the left-hand column of fig. 3.14 and may be deduced as follows. At the start of the phase, assuming the alveolar pressure to be zero, the pressure difference between the bag and the alveoli is 35 cmH_2O. The total resistance between these two points is $6+22=28$ cmH_2O/(litre/sec); therefore the initial flow is

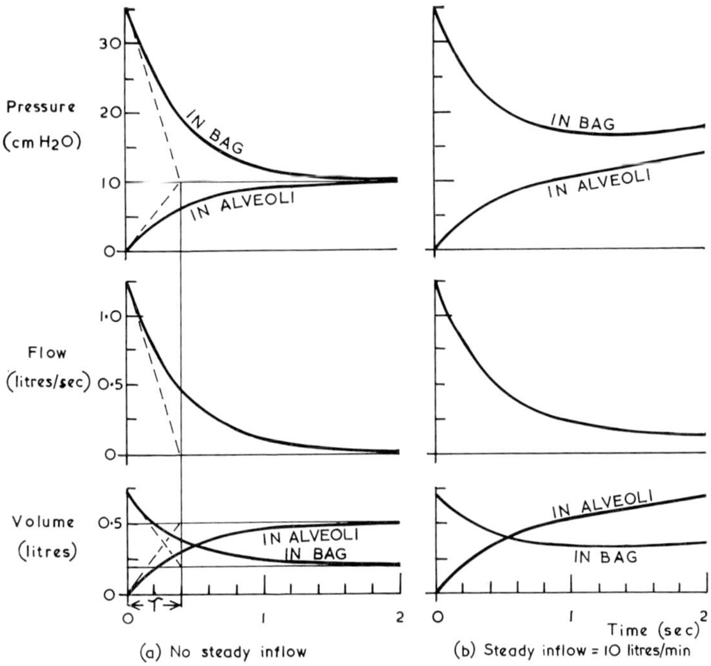

Fig. 3.14. Theoretical waveforms for inflation by a ventilator which operates as a discharging compliance connected to a patient with 'standard' lung characteristics,
(a) with no steady inflow of inflating gas,
(b) with a steady inflow of 10 litres/min.
For both sets of waveforms the characteristics are as follows.
Compliance in ventilator : 0·02 litre/cmH_2O.
Internal resistance of ventilator : 22 cmH_2O/(litre/sec).
Airway resistance of patient : 6 cmH_2O/(litre/sec).
Compliance of patient : 0·05 litre/cmH_2O.
Initial pressure in ventilator compliance : 35 cmH_2O.
τ is the time constant of the exponential changes.

$35/28=1{\cdot}25$ litres/sec. This causes the alveolar pressure to rise and the bag pressure to fall so that the pressure difference between them, and hence the flow, decreases. Eventually, if the inspiratory phase is allowed to continue long enough, a state of equilibrium is achieved in which the bag and alveolar pressures are equal and there is no flow. In this state of equilibrium the volume of gas originally in the bag,

$$0{\cdot}02 \text{ litre/cmH}_2\text{O} \times 35 \text{ cmH}_2\text{O} = 0{\cdot}7 \text{ litre},$$

is shared between the bag and the patient in proportion to their compliances: 0·5 litre is in the patient (compliance 0·05 litre/cmH_2O) and 0·2 litre is in the bag (compliance 0·02 litre/cmH_2O). Therefore the pressure in both is 10 cmH_2O. Just as with a constant-pressure generator the approach to equilibrium can be shown to be an exponential process: the flow, and the difference between the initial and equilibrium pressures in the bag and in the alveoli, all decline exponentially. The time constant of the exponential is equal to $C'R'$ where C' is the equivalent of the bag compliance C_B and the patient's compliance C_P in series and R' is the total resistance. Compliances in series add reciprocally:

$$\frac{1}{C'} = \frac{1}{C_B} + \frac{1}{C_P}.$$

Therefore,

$$\frac{1}{C'} = \frac{1}{0{\cdot}02} + \frac{1}{0{\cdot}05} = 50 + 20 = 70 \text{ cmH}_2\text{O/litre.}$$

Therefore,

$$C' = \frac{1}{70} = 0{\cdot}0143 \text{ litre/cmH}_2\text{O.}$$

This is necessarily less than either compliance on its own. The total resistance R' is 28 cmH_2O/(litre/sec), so that the time constant $C'R'$ is $0{\cdot}0143 \times 28 = 0{\cdot}4$ sec. The broken lines in fig. 3.14 indicate that if the initial rate of change of each variable were maintained the changes would be complete in one time constant, τ.

In Fig. 3.14 the process has been followed for two seconds, that is for five time constants, in which the exponential processes become 99·3% complete. Normally the inspiratory phase would be terminated much earlier but this has been avoided here to aid the comparison with the waveforms that arise when a steady flow of inflating gas enters the system (shown in the right-hand column of fig. 3.14 and discussed below).

It is now appropriate to comment on the numerical values used for fig. 3.14. The bag compliance of 0·02 litre/cmH_2O is near the lower end of the range found in practice and was chosen to bring out the differences from a constant-pressure generator. (If the bag compliance is high, the fall of pressure with fall of volume is slight, and the system is almost the same as a constant-pressure generator.) To retain the tidal volume of about 0·5 litre used in the earlier examples, this choice of bag compliance requires an initial pressure in the bag of 35 cmH_2O—similar to that used for the high-constant-pressure generator of fig. 3.5. The internal resistance of the ventilator was chosen to give the same time constant as that in the case of the low-constant-pressure generator with low internal resistance of fig. 3.4. Yet the value of resistance used, 22 cmH_2O/(litre/sec), was more akin to that of fig. 3.5, 60 cmH_2O/(litre/sec), than that of fig. 3.4, 2 cmH_2O/(litre/sec).

Thus, with a discharging compliance, if the compliance is small compared to that of the patient, the initial pressure must be high in order to deliver an adequate tidal volume.

The internal resistance may also be quite high, in which case pressure and resistance are similar to those in the high-constant-pressure generator which led to the waveforms of fig. 3.5. Yet the waveforms produced by the discharging compliance (fig. 3.14) are more like those of the low-constant-pressure generator of fig. 3.4.

The responses of the discharging compliance to changes of compliance and resistance in the patient are generally somewhere between those of a low-constant-pressure generator and those of a high-constant-pressure generator. However, these responses will not be examined here since they are often complicated by concomitant changes in the pressure to which the bag compliance is charged during the expiratory phase. The accounts of individual ventilators should be consulted for details.

A factor which will be considered here is the effect of a continuous flow of inflating gas into the system during the inspiratory phase. This is present in most of the ventilators which operate as discharging compliances. The effect of such a continuous flow into the system which has just been examined has been calculated; the resultant waveforms for a flow of 10 litres/min are plotted in the right-hand column of fig. 3.14. The explanation for these waveforms, in qualitative terms, is as follows.

The continuous inflow of inflating gas prevents the bag and alveolar pressures becoming equal and steady. If the inspiratory phase is long enough the bag pressure falls only to the point at which it is just sufficiently in excess of the rising alveolar pressure to drive the whole of the inflating-gas flow into the lungs. Thereafter, the continuing rise of alveolar pressure reduces the pressure difference between the bag and the alveoli to a level at which some of the inflating-gas flow is diverted into the bag. Therefore the bag pressure starts to rise again. The final 'steady' state is one in which the inflow is shared between the bag and the patient in proportion to their compliances. Then the pressures in both rise at the same slow rate. The difference between the two pressures is steady and just sufficient to drive through the total resistance between the bag and the alveoli that fraction of the inflating-gas flow which goes to the patient. In fig. 3.14 this 'steady' state is approached, but not quite reached, in the time for which the process is followed. Commonly the inspiratory phase will be terminated even before the bag pressure has fallen to its minimum. Indeed, in a number of ventilators, in which the change-over from the inspiratory phase to the expiratory phase occurs only when the volume or pressure in the bag has fallen to a critical level, the inspiratory phase must be terminated before this minimum pressure has been reached or the ventilator will become permanently fixed in the inspiratory phase.

Finally, it should be remembered that the concept of the discharging compliance is simply another way of viewing a pressure generator in which the pressure decreases in a manner related to volume and not to time. Therefore, if the pressure at the end of the inspiratory phase is still high, despite the decrease which has occurred during the phase, the ventilator may more usefully be regarded as approximating to a decreasing-flow generator. The way in which the Howells ventilator constitutes an example of this was discussed above (see p. 95).

THE CHANGE-OVER FROM THE INSPIRATORY PHASE TO THE EXPIRATORY PHASE

During the inspiratory phase time passes, the volume delivered to the patient builds up, the pressure in the patient increases and, often, the flow into the patient decreases. Each of these four variables, time, volume, pressure, and flow, is sensed in different ventilators and the ventilator made to change-over from the process of inflation to the process of expiration when the chosen variable has attained some predetermined critical value. The mechanism which does the sensing and performs the change-over is called the 'cycling' mechanism of which there are therefore four basic types.

1 Time-cycled, in which the change-over occurs after a preset period of time.
2 Volume-cycled, in which the change-over occurs when a preset volume has been delivered.
3 Pressure-cycled, in which the change-over occurs when a pressure, closely related to that in the lungs, reaches a preset level.
4 Flow-cycled, in which the change-over occurs when the flow falls to a preset level.

Some practical cycling mechanisms cannot be matched exclusively with just one of these basic types. These are discussed under:

5 Mixed-cycled.

Finally, there are a few cycling mechanisms which cannot be properly matched with any of the basic types. These are discussed under:

6 Other cycling mechanisms.

Time-cycling

A ventilator can be said to be time-cycled from the inspiratory phase to the expiratory phase when the change-over is brought about at a time which is determined by the action of a timing mechanism which is uninfluenced by conditions in the patient's lungs. The mechanism may be electronic (e.g. 'Barnet'), electro-mechanical (e.g. East-Radcliffe), or pneumatic (e.g. Air-Shields 'Respirator'). The essential feature, however, is that the duration of the inspiratory phase is entirely determined by the ventilator and is quite uninfluenced by the patient's lung characteristics. On the other hand, the volume delivered in this time, the pressure developed in the lungs, and the flow at the end of the phase, are all free to vary; their values at the moment of cycling will all be determined by the effect on the lungs of the flow-generating or pressure-generating mechanism which was operative during the inspiratory phase. Therefore, when the lung characteristics alter, the duration of the inspiratory phase is unaffected; but the volume, pressure, and flow at the end of the phase may all change. This is well illustrated in fig. 3.4 in which the action of a low-constant-pressure generator was followed for a period of 1.2 sec in association with each of three different sets of lung characteristics. If it is supposed that a time-cycling mechanism ended the inspiratory phase at the end of the curves drawn in fig. 3.4 it can be seen that, although the inspiratory time is always the same, the flow, volume, and alveolar pressure at the end of the phase are all substantially altered when the lung characteristics change. The mouth pressure is negligibly affected, but this is because, with the characteristics used for fig. 3.4, the mouth pressure was always close to the constant generated pressure.

Volume-cycling

The change-over from the inspiratory phase to the expiratory phase can be said to be volume-cycled when it is the volume delivered during the inspiratory phase which is determined by the ventilator while the duration of the phase, and the flow and pressure at its end, are free to vary. This can be illustrated by reference to fig. 3.15. This shows the same set of waveforms as fig. 3.5 which illustrated the first 1 sec of operation of a high-constant-pressure generator connected to lungs with different characteristics. However, in drawing fig. 3.15 it has been supposed that the pressure generator is fitted with a volume-cycling mechanism set to end the inspiratory phase when 0·4 litre has been delivered. For each set of lung characteristics this occurs when the volume trace has just reached the 0·4 litre level indicated by the dotted lines in fig. 3.15. Thus the phase does not continue for the full 1 sec drawn in fig. 3.15; instead it is cut short at times corresponding to the broken vertical lines: 0·75 sec under the standard conditions, 0·85 sec with the compliance halved, and 0·8 sec with the resistance doubled. That is, the inspiratory time varies with lung characteristics. Similarly, if the vertical lines are followed, it will be found that the flow, alveolar pressure, and mouth pressure at the end of the phase are all affected by lung characteristics. In this particular example the variation in inspiratory time is small because the high-constant-pressure generator of figs. 3.5 and 3.15 approximates to a constant-flow generator. Therefore there is not much variation in flow with lung characteristics and not much variation in the time taken to deliver the preset volume. On the other hand, if the low-constant-pressure generator of fig. 3.4 were fitted with a volume-cycling device and this were set to 0·4 litre, then when the compliance was halved the inspiratory phase would be prolonged indefinitely because, even at equilibrium, only 0·3 litre is delivered. In other words, the ventilator would become arrested in the inspiratory phase. This situation can arise in the 'Vellore' ventilator.

The physical form of almost all volume-cycling mechanisms is a piston or concertina bag, by the movement of which the patient is inflated, and the stroke of which is preset either by a mechanical drive or by means of mechanical or electrical trips. Thus it is the volume expelled from the bag or cylinder, rather than the volume which enters the lungs, which is controlled by the ventilator. It is important to realize that if any gas enters or leaves the patient circuit during the inspiratory phase there may be a discrepancy between these two volumes. This discrepancy is usually small, but in certain circumstances can be quite large. The problem is discussed in Chapter 4.

For several years now it has been possible, by means of an integrating pneumotachograph or a ventilation meter, to sense the volume entering the endotracheal tube and to use this to cycle the ventilator. However, this does not yet appear to have been attempted.

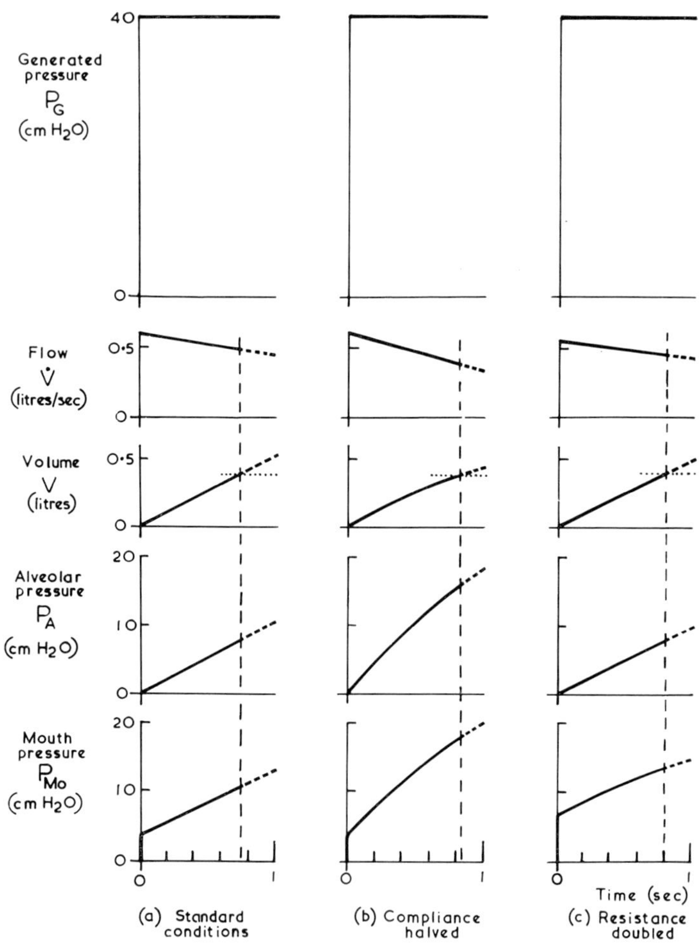

Fig. 3.15. Theoretical waveforms for inflation by a high-constant-pressure generator exactly as in fig. 3.5 but showing the effect of a volume-cycling mechanism. The dotted lines indicate the critical volume at which cycling occurs (0·4 litre). The vertical broken lines indicate the various moments at which cycling occurs and draw attention to the different flows and mouth and alveolar pressures at these moments.

The Bird Mark 17 goes one stage further, in a sense, and uses a volume-cycling mechanism which responds to the volume actually in the patient's lungs. However, the mechanism works by sensing the circumferential expansion of the chest so that its response to lung volume is indirect.

Pressure-cycling

The end of the inspiratory phase is pressure-cycled if it occurs when the pressure at the mouth, or some closely-related pressure, reaches a predetermined critical value irrespective of the time this may take, or of the volume that may have been delivered, or of the flow that may exist at the time. Therefore, with a pressure-cycled ventilator, changes of lung characteristics may alter the duration of the inspiratory phase, the volume delivered, and the flow at the end of the phase, but they will not alter the mouth pressure at the end of the phase.

This can be illustrated by reference to the waveforms of fig. 3.16. This shows the same set of waveforms as fig. 3.6, namely that for the first 1 sec of operation of a constant-flow generator. However, in drawing fig. 3.16 it has been supposed that the flow generator has been fitted with a pressure-cycling device, responding to the pressure at the mouth, and set to cycle at a pressure of 13 cmH_2O. Then, with the 'standard' lung characteristics the phase just lasts 1 sec. However, when the compliance is halved or the airway resistance doubled, the mouth pressure reaches the preset cycling pressure, shown by the dotted line, much sooner; the phase is therefore terminated after 0·5 or 0·7 sec respectively, when the volume delivered to the lungs is much smaller than under the standard conditions. In this example the flow at the end of the phase is the same in all instances since the ventilator is operating as a constant-flow generator, but note that, when the airway resistance is increased, the alveolar pressure at the end of the phase is reduced even though the mouth pressure is unaltered. This is because of the increased pressure drop across the increased airway resistance (see the graph for $P_{\mathrm{Mo}} - P_{\mathrm{A}}$ in fig. 3.16).

Pressure cycling is usually brought about by applying the mouth pressure to a diaphragm so that, as the pressure rises, the resultant force or movement is eventually sufficient to reverse a mechanical toggle (Blease 'Pulmoflator', Dräger 'Poliomat') or a magnetic 'toggle' ('Cyclator', Takaoka) or to operate electrical contacts (Air-Shields 'Pressure Breathing Assistor', 'Barnet' Mark III).

Flow-cycling

In all the Bennett ventilators described in this book the change-over from the inspiratory phase to the expiratory phase can be considered to be flow-cycled. This is because the Bennett valve, incorporated in all these ventilators, switches from the inspiratory position to the expiratory position when the flow through it to the patient has fallen to a critical

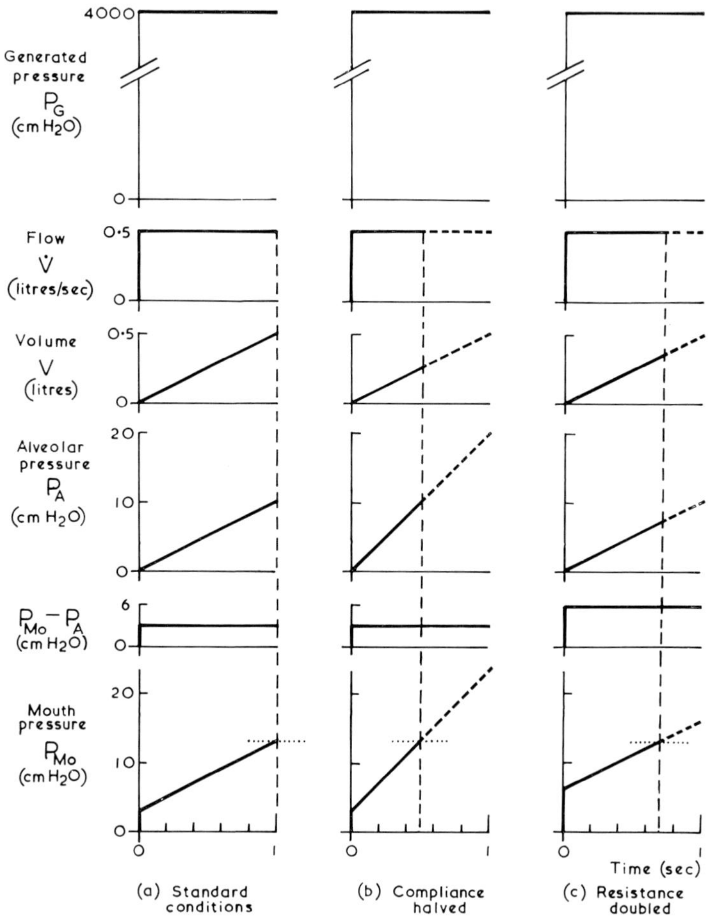

Fig. 3.16. Theoretical waveforms for inflation by a constant-flow generator exactly as in fig. 3.6 but showing the effect of a pressure-cycling mechanism. The dotted lines indicate the critical mouth pressure at which cycling occurs (13 cmH_2O). The vertical broken lines indicate the various moments at which cycling occurs.

low level (in the region of 1 to 4 litres/min) almost irrespective of the time this may take or of the volume that may have been delivered.

The 'Autovent' also is flow-cycled.

Mixed-cycling

Some ventilators cannot be allotted exclusively to any of the above classes. This may arise for a variety of reasons.

Firstly, a ventilator may have two or more different and independent cycling mechanisms. For instance, the 'Barnet' Mark III has three separate mechanisms, one for time-cycling, one for volume-cycling, and one for pressure-cycling. Any one of these may be brought into operation at any one time and the ventilator may be used in any of these three ways. In the Bennett PR-2 the flow-cycling mechanism, described in the previous section, is always operative, but a separate, time-cycling, mechanism can also be brought into play. Then the inspiratory phase ends either when the flow has fallen to the preset level or when the preset time has elapsed, whichever event occurs first. A change from one to the other would generally be indicative of a change of lung characteristics or of the development of a leak.

Secondly, a single mechanism can result in two different types of cycling. For instance, in some ventilators (e.g. Aga 'Spiropulsator', Ohio (Monaghan) 300) the patient is inflated from a concertina bag contained in a rigid pressure chamber to which compressed gas is supplied. The cycling mechanism senses the pressure in the pressure chamber. So long as the bag is moving freely this pressure is similar to that at the mouth; therefore the change-over to expiration is then pressure-cycled. However, if the concertina bag empties or reaches an adjustable stop before the critical pressure has been reached, no further volume can be expelled from the ventilator and the pressure in the pressure chamber rises rapidly to the cycling pressure. In this situation, provided the compliance of the pressure chamber is small, the change-over occurs almost immediately the bag has delivered a given volume and so may be regarded as volume-cycled. Thus, in general, the inspiratory phase ends either when a preset volume has been delivered, or when the mouth pressure has risen to a preset level, whichever event occurs first. Again a change from one to the other would probably be indicative of a leak or of a change of lung characteristics.

Thirdly, in some ventilators it may not be evident from recordings of their action what sort of cycling-mechanism is in operation. Thus, suppose fig. 3.6 represented a set of experimental recordings of the full inspiratory phase of a ventilator about whose mechanism nothing was known. Clearly the ventilator could not be pressure-cycled at the end of the inspiratory phase because the mouth pressure at that time is very much influenced by changes of lung characteristics. Also it could not be flow-cycled because the flow is constant throughout the phase and does not just attain some critical level at the end of the phase. However, all three sets of tracings end both, just as the time reaches 1 sec, and, just as the volume reaches 0·5 litre. Therefore, is the ventilator time-cycled or volume-cycled? Clearly, in a sense, it is effectively both; and this is necessarily true for any constant-flow generator (and even for a non-constant-flow generator). This is because, if a constant flow is delivered for a preset time then a preset volume is delivered irrespective of changes of lung characteristics. Equally, if a preset volume is to be delivered at a constant flow rate it will take a preset time. However, the fundamental nature of the cycling mechanism is revealed if the generated flow is altered. Then, if the change-over is fundamentally volume-cycled, as in the Bourns 'Pediatric' and the Greer and Donald ventilators, the delivered volume is unaltered but the inspiratory time is changed. On the other hand, if the change-over is fundamentally time-cycled, as in the Air-Shields 'Ventimeter' and the 'Amsterdam', the inspiratory time is unaltered but the delivered volume is changed.

Another example of a cycling-mechanism which may appear to be operating in two different ways simultaneously is the flow-cycling mechanism of the Bennett ventilators. When the lung characteristics change, the flow at the end of the inspiratory phase is unaltered. However, these ventilators operate as constant-pressure generators during at least the last part of the inspiratory phase; therefore, at the end of the phase, the predetermined flow through the preset internal resistance of the ventilator produces a preset pressure drop from the point where the pressure is generated to the mouth. Therefore changes of lung characteristics do not alter the pressure at the mouth at the end of the phase; that is, the ventilator behaves as if it were pressure-cycled as well as flow-cycled. The fundamental nature of the mechanism is revealed only when the generated pressure is altered; then the mouth pressure at the end of the phase is changed but the flow remains the same.

Fourthly, there are some ventilators which are genuinely both volume-cycled and time-cycled. These are the ventilators in which a concertina bag or a piston in a cylinder is moved through a preset stroke in a preset time by means of a constant-speed electric motor. Here again, changes in lung characteristics have no effect on delivered volume or inspiratory time; but in these ventilators both volume and time are directly controlled and one is not determined indirectly from the setting of the other and the setting of a separate flow control. Instead it is the amplitude of the flow pattern that is determined by the independent volume and time controls. This is quite well illustrated in the experimental recordings of the Lundia ventilator which is primarily a volume-cycled and time-cycled non-constant-flow generator. In fig. 60.5 it can be seen that changes of lung characteristics alter neither the tidal volume nor the inspiratory time. (The flow waveform at the start of the phase is somewhat altered because there is a component of the ventilator which, at that time, operates as a discharging compliance.) Furthermore, in fig. 60.6 it can be seen that, when the delivered volume is increased (fig. 60.6b) the inspiratory time is unaltered and it is the amplitude of the flow waveform which is increased. Similarly, when the inspiratory time is decreased (fig. 60.6c) the tidal volume is unaltered and again the flow is increased.

Finally, there are a few ventilators in which the moment of change-over cannot be related exclusively to any one of the four variables under consideration but depends on the values of two or more of them.

In the 'Minivent' the change-over occurs when a certain force has reached a critical value, but this force is made up of two components: one component can be related to the flow into the patient, the other can be related either to the pressure in a discharging compliance (and hence to the volume discharged) or else to the pressure in the lungs.

In some of the early ventilators ('Clevedon', Pires and Mentz, and Williams) and in the so-called 'pressure-cycled' mode of the 'Barnet' Mark III, the change-over occurs when the pressure in an auxiliary circuit reaches a critical level. The auxiliary circuit consists, in effect, of a small compliance, connected through a high resistance to a point in the patient circuit where the pressure is similar to that at the mouth. Thus this auxiliary circuit effectively constitutes a miniature lung which is inflated in parallel with the patient. If the patient's lung characteristics change in such a way as to cause the mouth pressure to rise more rapidly, then the pressure in the auxiliary circuit will reach the critical level in a shorter time but at a higher mouth pressure. In the Pires and Mentz and in the Williams the critical pressure is fixed. Adjustment is obtained by variation of the resistance of the 'miniature lung' thereby altering its time constant and the speed with which it responds to the rise of mouth pressure. In the 'Barnet' Mark III the resistance, and hence the time constant, is fixed but the cycling pressure is adjustable. In the 'Clevedon', both cycling pressure and resistance are adjustable.

Other cycling mechanisms

In the 'Cyclator CAV' and a few of the early ventilators (Dennis, Emerson 'Assistor', and Mörch I and II) the cycling mechanism is such that changes of lung characteristics may alter the magnitude of all four variables, time, volume, pressure, and flow, at the moment at which cycling occurs. The arrangement which gives rise to this situation is a 'bag in a bottle' ventilator (see p. 132) with a blow-off valve (see p. 145) in the patient circuit, and with the change-over occurring when a critical pressure is reached in the driving circuit outside the bag. The mode of action is discussed fully in the account of the 'Cyclator CAV'. There it is shown that the change-over occurs when a particular volume has been delivered from the ventilator but that the delivered volume includes the tidal volume which happened to be expired by the patient in the previous respiratory cycle. This expired tidal volume is not determined by the ventilator but depends upon lung characteristics.

THE EXPIRATORY PHASE

In the expiratory phase, just as in the inspiratory phase, it is possible to classify ventilators as flow or pressure generators. The choice depends on whether it is the flow pattern which is controlled by the ventilator and the pressure pattern which varies with lung characteristics, or the pressure pattern which is determined by the ventilator and the flow pattern which depends on the lung characteristics.

In discussing this phase the various types of generator are first considered from the point of view of the mechanisms from which they arise. Subsequently the waveforms produced by the more-important ones are examined.

Before proceeding, it should be noted that many ventilators do not operate in the same way throughout the expiratory phase. They may simply change from generating one pressure at the beginning of the phase to generating a different pressure later in the phase as in the Lundia; on the other hand, they may go through three or four sub-phases covering a variety of flow and pressure generators, as in the Cape-Waine.

It should also be noted that a ventilator which operates as a flow generator in the inspiratory phase may be a pressure generator in the expiratory phase, and vice versa. Indeed, whereas many ventilators can be classed as flow generators in the inspiratory phase only a few can be so regarded in the expiratory phase.

Constant-pressure generators

The commonest method of bringing about expiration is simply to connect the patient's lungs to the atmosphere. In this situation it is quite clear that, no matter how rapidly or slowly the patient's lungs may empty, the flow from them will have not the slightest effect on the atmospheric pressure. Therefore, this arrangement must be classed as a constant-pressure generator, specifically as a constant, atmospheric, pressure generator.

A number of ventilators operate as constant, negative, pressure generators as a result of mechanisms similar to those which produce constant, positive, pressure generation in the inspiratory phase. Thus, if the patient is connected to a suspended concertina bag with a weight in the bottom (e.g. Aga 'Spiropulsator', 'Cyclator CAV', and, in effect, Bennett BA-4), the constant downward force of the weight acting on the constant cross-sectional area of the bag may be expected to produce a constant, negative, pressure within the bag despite variations in flow. In fact, the elasticity of the wall produces some slight decrease in the magnitude of the negative pressure as the bag expands.

It is possible to imagine the large negative pressure of a suction machine or pipe-line being converted to a small, constant, negative pressure by a device equivalent to a second-stage reducing valve but this does not appear to have been done in practice. However, negative-pressure-limiting valves are found in a number of ventilators (e.g. 'Newcastle III' and Air-Shields 'Ventimeter') and these operate as constant, negative, pressure generators so long as gas is being drawn in through them.

In the Dräger 'Spiromat 661' and the Engström 'Narcosis' ventilators expiration can be made to occur through a spring-loaded valve to produce a small constant positive pressure during the expiratory phase.

In many ventilators the patient is connected to the entrainment orifice of an injector. Usually the jet of the injector is connected to a constant high-pressure supply so that, in just the same way as when the patient is connected to the diffuser outlet of an injector for inflation, this arrangement behaves as though it were a constant-pressure generator, negative in this case, with some series resistance. In most cases the negative pressure and the resistance are quite small; see fig. 28.3 for the Bennett PR-2 and fig.29. 5 curves (g) and (h) for the Bird Mark 8. However, in the Dräger 'Poliomat' (fig. 42.3) and the Takaoka the equivalent negative pressure and series resistance are both large enough for the mechanism to make a good approximation to a constant-flow generator. In two ventilators part of the flow which would otherwise drive the injector can be diverted, either to the entrainment port ('Amsterdam') or to the diffuser outlet (Blease 'Pulmoflator'), so that the generated pressure can be adjusted and even made positive.

Mechanisms which operated as pressure transformers during the inspiratory phase (fig. 3.9) may simply refill the bag or cylinder with fresh gas while the patient expires to atmosphere (e.g. U.S. Army, Emerson gas-operated). In other instances pressure-transformer action is applied to the patient during the expiratory phase and is usually equivalent to a constant, negative, pressure in series with a resistance. In the 'Jefferson' ventilator the high-pressure input is shut off and the piston is connected to the atmosphere so that the input pressure is zero. The driving force comes from the heavy weight in the concertina bag. Therefore the generated, negative, pressure arises directly from the downward force of the weight acting on the cross-sectional area of the bag. However the effective resistance on the patient side of the transformer arises indirectly from the actual resistance on the piston side. In the Allbritten and the Mortimer ventilators high pressure is applied to the opposite side of the piston to that used in the inspiratory phase, so that a constant, negative, pressure is generated equal to the positive pressure in the inspiratory phase; a somewhat similar arrangement is used in the Stephenson. In at least some of these pressure transformers the generated negative pressure and the series resistance must be large enough for the mechanism to make a good approximation to a flow generator.

Constant-flow generators

It has already been mentioned that an injector may approximate to a constant-flow generator if the equivalent (negative) generated pressure and equivalent series resistance are large enough. In a similar manner the actual large negative pressure generated by the Mörch I in combination with its actual large resistance must have made a similar close approximation to a flow generator.

Another mechanism which operates as a constant-flow generator is to be found in the 'Barnet', Manley and 'R.P.R.' ventilators. The constant flow of gas into one concertina bag produces a constant flow into another concertina bag to which it is mechanically linked and to which the patient is connected.

Non-constant flow and pressure generators

In the East-Radcliffe 'Positive-Negative' ventilator negative pressure is generated by the pull of a spring on a concertina bag. As the bag expands the pull of the spring decreases so that the negative pressure decreases. It does so in a manner which is entirely determined by the ventilator and is uninfluenced by the patient, so that it is indeed a non-constant-pressure generator—specifically a decreasing-pressure generator. However, the pattern of pressure is fixed in relation to bag volume and not to time. Therefore the mechanism could be regarded as a discharging compliance in the way that similar devices were so regarded in the inspiratory phase.

The 'Roswell Park' ventilator is a pressure transformer which operates as a non-constant, negative, pressure generator because of the nature of the mechanical linkage between the 'piston' and the concertina bag. Again the pattern of pressure is fixed in relation to volume and not to time.

In the Aika and Engström ventilators the jet of an injector is supplied with a half cycle of a sine wave of flow. Therefore it generates something like a half cycle of a sine wave of negative pressure. In this instance the pattern of pressure is fixed in relation to time and not to volume.

Non-constant flow generation arises, as in the inspiratory phase, when a bag, or a piston in a cylinder, is driven through a simple mechanical linkage by a constant-speed electric motor. The waveform depends on the nature of the linkage: in the Cape, Cape-Waine, and James ventilators and in the 'Respirateur MMS 104' the waveform is roughly sinusoidal; in the 'Respirateur SF4' it is probably not far from constant. In the 'Adelaide' and Clutton-Brock ventilators various waveforms can be achieved by the use of different cams.

The discharging compliance

It has already been mentioned that the spring-loaded bag of the East-Radcliffe 'Positive-Negative' ventilator can be regarded as a discharging compliance rather than as a decreasing-pressure generator. The same is true of the Van Bergen. In the latter ventilator gas is continuously pumped out of a large rigid vessel, throughout the respiratory cycle, but the patient is connected to the vessel only during the expiratory phase. Therefore, during the inspiratory phase the pressure in the vessel gradually becomes more negative: during the expiratory phase the pressure gradually becomes less negative and the flow from the patient rapidly diminishes. Therefore, both pressure and flow vary during the expiratory phase, but the waveforms are determined by the fact that one compliance, that of the patient, is discharging into another, that of the rigid vessel, which has previously been discharged to a negative pressure.

Since the pressure in the rigid vessel of the Van Bergen and in the bag of the East-Radcliffe 'Positive-Negative' ventilators rises during this process perhaps they should be referred to as charging compliances rather than discharging compliances.

Waveforms produced by a constant, atmospheric, pressure generator

The waveforms of flow, volume and pressure which result from the use of a constant, atmospheric, pressure generator can be deduced as follows. Curves for a specific example are shown in fig. 3.17.

At the start of the expiratory phase the lungs contain a certain volume of gas from the previous inflation, and this is associated with a proportionate alveolar pressure:

$$\text{volume} \propto \text{alveolar pressure.}$$

Since the generated pressure is zero, the whole of the alveolar pressure is dropped across

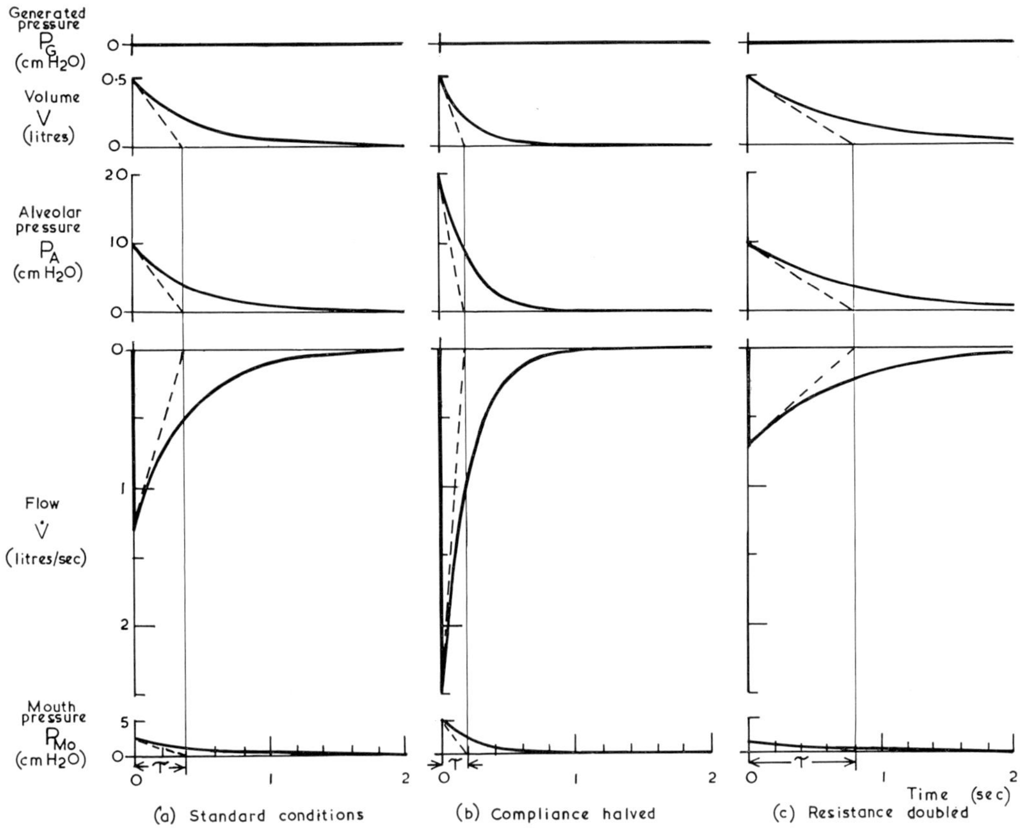

Fig. 3.17. Theoretical waveforms for the expiratory phase for a constant, atmospheric, pressure generator having a low internal resistance:

(a) when connected to a patient with 'standard' lung characteristics,

(b) when the patient's compliance is halved,

(c) when the patient's airway resistance is doubled.

For all three sets of waveforms the characteristics are as follows.

Generated pressure : 0 cmH_2O.

Internal resistance of ventilator : 2 cmH_2O/(litre/sec).

'Standard' airway resistance of patient : 6 cmH_2O/(litre/sec).

'Standard' compliance of patient : 0·05 litre/cmH_2O.

Lungs previously inflated to 0·5 litre above the volume present at zero alveolar pressure.

τ is the time constant of the exponential changes.

the combined resistance of the patient and the ventilator to produce a proportionate expiratory flow:

$$\text{alveolar pressure} \propto \text{flow}.$$

But expiratory flow is the same thing as the rate of change of volume in the lungs:

$$\text{flow} \equiv \text{rate of change of volume}.$$

Therefore the rate of change of volume is proportional to the alveolar pressure which, in turn, is proportional to the volume itself:

$$\text{rate of change of volume} \propto \text{volume}.$$

It will be recalled that proportionality between the rate of change of a variable and the magnitude of that variable is the fundamental characteristic of an exponential change. Therefore the volume in the lungs decreases exponentially. Furthermore, since alveolar pressure is proportional to volume, and flow to alveolar pressure, these also decrease exponentially. Just as with a constant-pressure generator in the inspiratory phase it can easily be shown that the time constant of all the exponential changes is CR where C is the total compliance of the patient and R is the total resistance of the system (airways plus internal resistance of the ventilator). The final steady values which the exponential processes approach can also be described in the same terms as in the inspiratory phase: the flow approaches zero, the alveolar pressure approaches the generated pressure (regarded as zero for an atmospheric-pressure generator) and the volume approaches that volume present in the lungs when they are in equilibrium with the generated pressure.

Fig. 3.17 shows the waveforms that result in a specific instance. Flow is plotted as negative since it is in the reverse direction from that in the inspiratory phase. A constant, atmospheric, pressure generator with a low internal resistance of 2 cmH_2O/(litre/sec) is assumed to be connected in turn to (a) a patient with the 'standard' lung characteristics used before, (b) a patient with halved compliance, and (c) a patient with doubled *airway* resistance. In each instance it is assumed that the patient has previously been inflated with 0·5 litre. It is immediately apparent that the waveform of generated pressure (zero throughout the phase) is the only waveform to be uninfluenced by changes of lung characteristics. Of the others, the flow waveform is the most strikingly influenced while the mouth-pressure waveform is the least affected. However the mouth pressure is not quite the same as the generated pressure because of the internal resistance of the ventilator which separates these two pressures and must be present in some degree in any ventilator. In the numerical example the internal resistance is one-quarter of the total (one-seventh when the airway resistance is doubled) so the mouth pressure is always one-quarter (or one-seventh) of the alveolar pressure.

As with a constant-pressure generator in the inspiratory phase, the exponential changes would all be complete in one time constant (τ) if their initial rates of change were maintained. This is illustrated by the broken lines in fig. 3.17. Similarly, the degree of completion of the exponential changes again increases in accordance with the number of time constants that have elapsed. Since the expiratory phase is usually allowed to continue for longer than the inspiratory phase, the changes have been followed for 2 sec in fig. 3.17. In the standard conditions this represents five time constants (each 0·4 sec) and the changes are accordingly 99·3% complete. With the compliance halved 2 sec represents 10 time constants giving an even closer approach to completion (99·995%!). With the airway resistance doubled (and the internal resistance of the ventilator unaltered) the total resistance is increased to 14 cmH_2O/(litre/sec) and the time constant to 0·7 sec; therefore 2 sec represents only 2·86 time constants in which the change is only 94·3% complete.

In the inspiratory phase, when the primary object was simply to drive gas into the lungs, 95% completion of an exponential change was regarded as virtually the same as absolute completion. In the expiratory phase, however, at least with free expiration to atmosphere, the objective is a little different and usually the anaesthetist is anxious to achieve 'complete' expiration, that is for the alveolar pressure to fall fully to atmospheric pressure before the end of the phase. In fig. 3.17 it is clear that expiration is near enough complete under the standard conditions and with the compliance halved. However, with the airway resistance doubled, there is still 0·5 cmH_2O positive pressure left in the alveoli at the end of the phase. Therefore it may be considered that an expiratory time equal to three time constants is only on the borderline of adequacy for achieving 'complete' expiration.

In drawing fig. 3.17 it was assumed that, in all instances, the lungs had previously been inflated with a tidal volume of 0·5 litre. Therefore, when the compliance was halved, the alveolar pressure was raised to 20 cmH_2O by the beginning of the phase instead of only to 10 cmH_2O. (It may be supposed either that this resulted from the action of a volume-cycling mechanism in the inspiratory phase or else that the inspiratory-phase controls were suitably adjusted when the compliance was halved.) This high alveolar pressure serves to produce a very high initial flow in this instance*, so accentuating the effect of changes of lung characteristics on the flow waveform. However, even if it were assumed, instead, that the lungs were always inflated to the same pressure then, although the peak flow would be the same as under the standard conditions, it would still decline much more rapidly because of the halved time constant.

Waveforms produced by a constant, negative, pressure generator

Negative-pressure generators commonly have larger internal resistances than atmospheric-pressure generators. For instance, injectors necessarily have some effective resistance in series with their effective generated pressure. The same is also usually true

* It is unlikely that such a high flow as 2·5 litres/sec would be achieved in practice because of the way in which resistance, instead of being constant, increases with flow, especially in expiration (see p. 134).

of pressure transformers. Even with an inverted, weighted, bag or a negative-pressure-limiting valve there is commonly some real resistance in the associated tubing and connexions although careful design could reduce this. For a specific example, therefore, (fig. 3.18) an internal resistance of 6 cmH_2O/(litre/sec) has been assumed. This is three times that assumed for the atmospheric-pressure generator of fig. 3.17 and is equal to the patient's 'standard' airway resistance. A generated pressure of −3 cmH_2O has been assumed.

From fig. 3.18 it is evident that again the generated pressure waveform is the only one to be unaffected by changes of lung characteristics. The other waveforms are affected in varying ways but are broadly similar to those for the constant, atmospheric, pressure generator. They all exhibit exponential decays but the initial and ultimate values and the time constants are usually somewhat different. The most obvious difference is that the alveolar and mouth pressures now approach a limit of −3 cmH_2O instead of 0 cmH_2O. Because of the increased ventilator resistance the time constants are increased, the initial flows are decreased, and the mouth pressure is closer to the alveolar pressure than before.

Because of the increased time constants the exponential changes are less fully completed in the 2 sec for which the waveforms have been followed. Thus for the three sets of waveforms ('standard' conditions, compliance halved, and resistance doubled) the time constants are 0·6, 0·3, and 0·9 sec respectively. Two seconds therefore represents 3·33, 6·66, and 2·22 time constants respectively in which the changes become 96·4, 99·9, and 89·2% complete respectively. Thus the approach of alveolar pressure towards −3 cmH_2O and the approach of flow to zero appears complete when the compliance is halved, but not quite so under the standard conditions and clearly not so when the airway resistance is doubled.

The assumptions made about volume are slightly different from those made in respect of fig. 3.17. In this example it is assumed that in every inspiratory phase a tidal volume of 0·5 litre is driven into the lungs irrespective of how high or low the alveolar pressure may be at the end of the previous expiratory phase. Thus, when the ventilator is first connected to the patient, the alveolar pressure at the end of the first inflation may perhaps be higher than shown in fig. 3.18. If so, the expired volume will be greater than 0·5 litre. But then, over a few cycles of respiration, the alveolar pressure at the end of each inspiratory phase will progressively diminish, until it is just sufficient under the prevailing conditions to drive out 0·5 litre in the available expiratory time. Thus a steady state is reached in which the waveforms are the same in every respiratory cycle. This is the state plotted in fig. 3.18. Now suppose that the prevailing conditions change, from the 'standard' conditions to the 'doubled airway resistance'. The alveolar pressure will again adjust itself over a few respiratory cycles until it is once more just sufficient to expel 0·5 litre in the given expiratory time. This is what is plotted in the last set of waveforms in fig. 3.18. Similar arguments apply to the derivation of the waveforms for halved compliance.

The volume trace is shown as always falling from 0·5 litre exactly to zero by the end of the phase. This is because here, as in all the experimental recordings of different

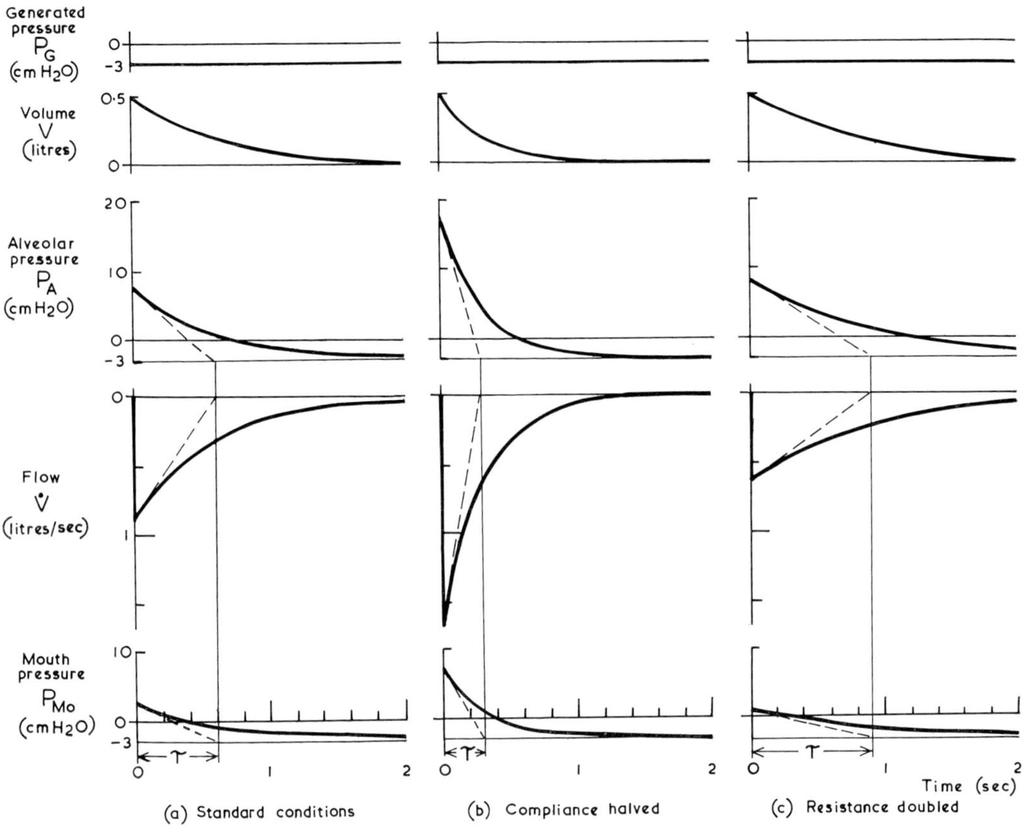

Fig. 3.18. Theoretical waveforms for the expiratory phase for a constant, negative, pressure generator having a moderate internal resistance:

(a) when connected to a patient with 'standard' lung characteristics,
(b) when the patient's compliance is halved,
(c) when the patient's airway resistance is doubled.

For all three sets of waveforms the characteristics are as follows.

Generated pressure : -3 cmH_2O.
Internal resistance of ventilator : 6 cm H_2O/(litre/sec).
'Standard' airway resistance of patient : 6 cmH_2O/(litre/sec).
'Standard' compliance of patient : 0·05 litre/cmH_2O.
Tidal volume : 0·5 litre.

τ is the time constant of the exponential changes. Volume is plotted as volume in excess of that present at the end of the two-second expiratory phase.

ventilators, volume has been measured from the working end-expiratory volume whatever that may happen to be. This arrangement has the convenience that tidal volume can be read directly from the peak of the volume trace.

Finally it should be noted that the alveolar pressure takes a substantial time to fall below atmospheric—as much as 1·5 sec when the airway resistance is doubled. It can be deduced from this that the generation of a negative pressure in the ventilator does not necessarily result in the development of negative pressure in the alveoli: if the generated negative pressure is small and is applied for only a short time, or if the total resistance is large, it is quite possible for the alveolar pressure to remain positive throughout the expiratory phase.

Waveforms produced by a constant-flow generator

For a specific example of a constant-flow generator it is assumed that the ventilator maintains a flow out of the lungs of 0·25 litre/sec irrespective of the pressures that result. Thus, in an expiratory time of 2 sec a tidal volume of 0·5 litre is expired. The resulting waveforms for the usual three sets of lung characteristics are shown in fig. 3.19.

Since the flow waveform is the one which is controlled by the ventilator it is put at the head of each set of waveforms and is exactly the same, and constant, throughout the phase, for all three sets of lung characteristics. The same constant flow in all three instances leads to the same constant rate of fall of lung volume. Therefore the three volume waveforms are the same—at least when plotted, as in fig. 3.19, in terms of volume in excess of the working end-expiratory volume. The pressure waveforms, however, are dependent on lung characteristics and therefore are not the same in the three instances. Under the standard conditions the constant flow, or rate of change of volume, produces a constant rate of change of alveolar pressure amounting to 0·25 litre/sec divided by 0·05 litre/cmH_2O = 5 cmH_2O/sec. In the 2 sec plotted in fig. 3.19 this represents a total fall of 10 cmH_2O. An initial alveolar pressure of 7 cmH_2O has been assumed so that the starting and finishing alveolar pressures are the same as with the −3 cmH_2O constant-pressure generator in fig. 3.18. When the compliance is halved the rate of fall of alveolar pressure is doubled: 0·25 litre/sec divided by 0·025 litre/cmH_2O = 10 cmH_2O/sec and the total fall in the phase is 20 cmH_2O. In drawing fig. 3.19 it has been assumed that the initial alveolar pressure is unaltered* so that the fall is from +7 to −13 cmH_2O. When the airway resistance is doubled (but the compliance is normal) the alveolar pressure again falls at 5 cmH_2O/sec from +7 to −3 cmH_2O.

To determine the mouth pressure in the various conditions it is convenient to consider the difference between mouth pressure and alveolar pressure ($P_{Mo} - P_A$). Under the standard conditions and with the compliance halved the constant flow of 0·25 litre/sec

* This assumption will not generally be fulfilled in practice; it is made here simply to emphasize the interaction between the expiratory constant-flow generator and the lung characteristics.

through the airway resistance of 6 cmH_2O/(litre/sec) produces a constant pressure difference of $6 \times 0{\cdot}25 = 1{\cdot}5$ cmH_2O. Since, in expiration, the mouth pressure is below the alveolar pressure this is shown as negative in fig. 3.19. The mouth-pressure waveform itself, therefore, is parallel to the alveolar-pressure waveform but 1·5 cmH_2O lower. When the airway resistance is doubled the pressure difference between mouth and alveoli is also doubled so that the mouth-pressure waveform runs 3 cmH_2O lower than that of alveolar pressure.

Two features of the waveforms from the expiratory constant-flow generator call for comment.

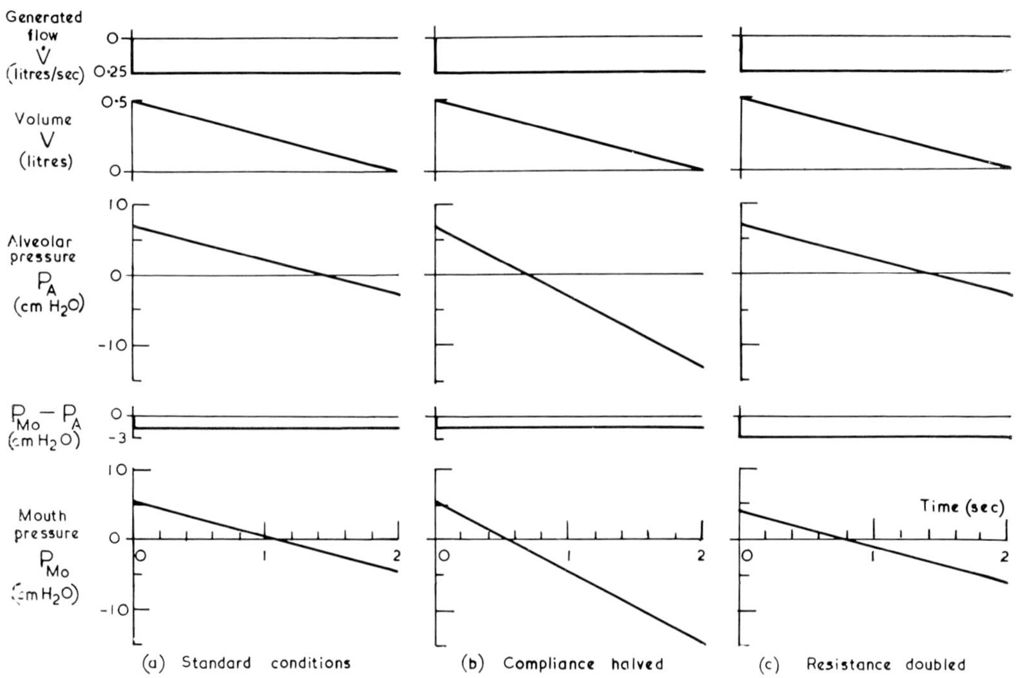

Fig. 3.19. Theoretical waveforms for the expiratory phase for a constant-flow generator:

(a) when connected to a patient with 'standard' lung characteristics,
(b) when the patient's compliance is halved,
(c) when the patient's airway resistance is doubled.

For all three sets of waveforms the characteristics are as follows.

Generated flow : 0·25 litre/sec.
'Standard' airway resistance of patient : 6 cmH_2O/(litre/sec).
'Standard' compliance of patient : 0·05 litre/cmH_2O.
Alveolar pressure at the start of the expiratory phase : 7 cmH_2O.

Volume is plotted as volume in excess of that present at the end of the two-second expiratory phase.

Firstly, if the waveforms are compared with those for a constant, atmospheric, pressure generator (fig. 3.17) it will be seen that the pressure generator gives much higher initial flows so that the alveolar pressure at first falls much more rapidly than with the constant-flow generator. In other words, the constant-flow generator is, in a sense, impeding expiration at the start of the phase. This is further revealed by the fact that the mouth pressure early in the phase is higher with the constant-flow generator than with either of the constant-pressure generators. Presumably because of this it is quite common, in ventilators which fundamentally operate as constant-flow generators in the expiratory phase, to include a one-way valve connexion to the atmosphere. Then, if free expiration to atmosphere would produce a bigger flow than that being generated, this can occur with the excess over the generated flow escaping through the one-way valve. This is discussed in more detail below.

The second feature to note in fig. 3.19 is the large negative pressure which is developed when the compliance is halved. Because a constant-flow generator, by definition, continues to pull gas out of the lungs irrespective of the resultant negative pressure, there is clearly a possibility of harmful negative pressures being developed. This may arise not only from a reduction of compliance but also from an increase in expiratory time or a failure to put enough volume into the lungs during the inspiratory phase. In practice all expiratory constant-flow generators have some means of avoiding this hazard. In the Dräger 'Poliomat' and the Takaoka ventilators a pressure-cycling mechanism (see below) reverses the ventilator to the inspiratory phase as soon as a preset negative pressure is reached. In the 'Barnet', Manley, and 'R.P.R.' ventilators, a pressure-limiting valve prevents the mouth pressure, and hence the alveolar pressure, ever going more negative than a preset amount.

Waveforms produced by a constant-flow generator with atmospheric-pressure and negative-pressure limits

It has just been shown that a ventilator which operates as a pure constant-flow generator throughout the expiratory phase may exhibit characteristics at the beginning and end of the phase which may be thought undesirable. It can readily be deduced that the same characteristics may also arise with non-constant flow generators. It is probably because of these characteristics that several ventilators have been developed which, in the expiratory phase, have mechanisms essentially the same as that shown in fig. 3.20.

Steady expansion of the concertina bag (A) (or steady movement of a piston in a cylinder) provides the basic flow-generating mechanism. However, its action is modified by the two one-way valves. The valve (B) is lightly loaded and prevents any positive pressure being developed in the bag; the valve (C) is heavily loaded and prevents the pressure in the bag becoming more negative than a preset amount.

At the start of the expiratory phase the pressure difference between the alveoli and

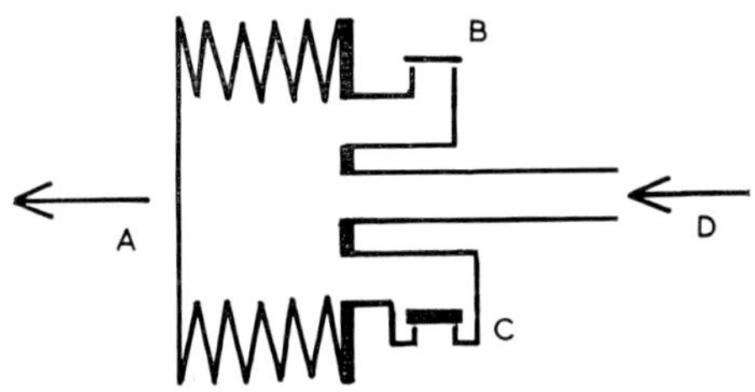

Fig. 3.20. An arrangement for the expiratory phase which operates as a flow generator with atmospheric-pressure and negative-pressure limits.
A. Concertina bag which is expanded according to a predetermined pattern—often at a constant rate.
B. Lightly-loaded one-way valve which prevents the development of any positive pressure in the bag.
C. Heavily-loaded one-way valve which prevents the development of pressures more negative than a preset amount. The loading may be adjustable.
D. Connexion from patient.

the maximum pressure that can exist in the bag (0 cmH_2O because of the valve (B)) will commonly produce a larger expiratory flow than that being generated by the concertina bag. The excess therefore escapes through the valve (B). In this part of the phase, therefore, the mechanism operates as a constant, atmospheric, pressure generator: no matter what the flow from the patient (so long as it is greater than that generated by the concertina bag) the pressure in the bag is held at atmospheric. That is, the pressure is determined by the ventilator (by the action of the valve (B)) while the flow depends on the effect of this pressure on the patient's lungs and varies with lung characteristics.

The waveforms for a specific example of a flow generator with pressure limits have been calculated and the results are shown in fig. 3.21. The generated flow chosen is constant at 0·25 litre/sec, as in fig. 3.19, with pressure limits of 0 and, as in fig. 3.18, −3 cmH_2O. The calculations are somewhat complex and so will not be described here but the principal features can readily be discerned. Thus, in the first part of the phase, it is only the bag-pressure waveform which is constant (at 0 cmH_2O) and unaltered by changes of lung characteristics. On the other hand, the flow is very variable, but always greater than the generated flow shown by the horizontal broken lines on the flow graphs.

Once the flow produced by the atmospheric-pressure-generating action has fallen to equal the flow generated by the concertina bag the valve (B) (fig. 3.20) closes. The valve (C) is also closed at this time. Therefore the bag and the patient form a closed system so that whatever flow goes into the bag must come from the patient. That is, the mechanism operates in its basic constant-flow-generating mode: the flow out of the patient is determined entirely by the ventilator (0·25 litre/sec in fig. 3.21) and is uninfluenced by the resultant pressures, subject only to the limitation that the pressure in the bag shall be between atmospheric pressure and the negative pressure which opens valve (C) (−3 cmH_2O in fig. 3.21). The pressures which in fact result are determined by the effect of the flow on the patient's lungs. The steady flow produces a steady rate of fall of alveolar

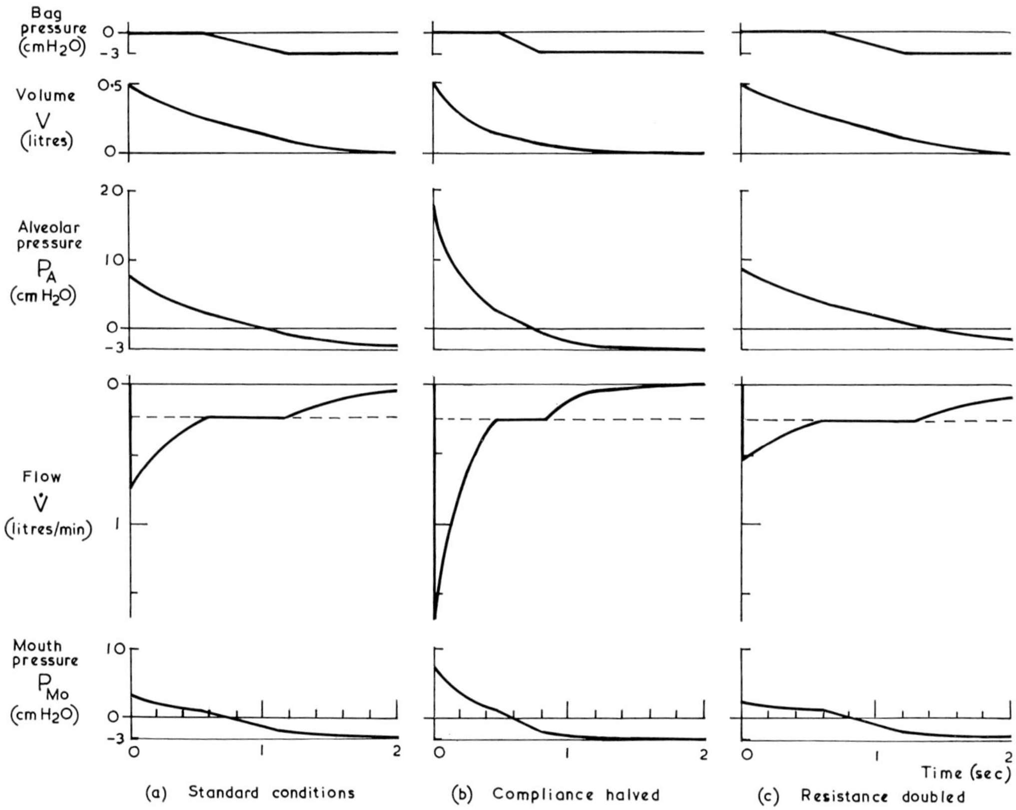

Fig. 3.21. Theoretical waveforms for the expiratory phase for a system, such as that shown in fig. 3.20, which operates as a constant-flow generator with atmospheric-pressure and negative-pressure limits:

(a) when connected to a patient with 'standard' lung characteristics,
(b) when the patient's compliance is halved,
(c) when the patient's airway resistance is doubled.

For all three sets of waveforms the characteristics are as follows.

Generated flow : 0·25 litre/sec.
Upper limit to bag pressure : 0 cmH_2O.
Lower limit to bag pressure : -3 cmH_2O.
Internal resistance of ventilator : 4 cmH_2O/(litre/sec).
'Standard' airway resistance of patient : 6 cmH_2O/(litre/sec).
'Standard' compliance of patient : 0·05 litre/cmH_2O.
Tidal volume : 0·5 litre.

Volume is plotted as volume in excess of that present at the end of the two-second expiratory phase.

pressure and a constant pressure difference between the alveoli and the bag. Therefore there is a steady fall of bag pressure from atmospheric towards the negative pressure at which the valve (C) opens.

Once the pressure in the bag has fallen to the critical level the valve (C) opens and the third part of the phase commences. There is still the same constant flow into the bag (shown by the horizontal broken line in fig. 3.21) but now part of it comes through the valve (C) and therefore only part of it from the patient. The only feature which is now fully determined by the ventilator is the pressure within the bag which is held constant at the (negative) opening pressure of the valve (C) (-3 cmH_2O in fig. 3.21) irrespective of what flow from the patient may result, subject only to the limitation that it is less than the total flow into the bag. The flow which does result is determined by the effect of the constant, negative, pressure in the bag on the lungs and varies with lung characteristics. Therefore, in this last part of the phase, the system operates as a constant, negative, pressure generator.

In real ventilators the actions are not generally quite as clear cut as described above but in the recordings of the Manley ventilator (fig. 61.5) the waveforms of the expiratory phase are recognizably similar to the theoretical waveforms in fig. 3.21. Other ventilators which more or less correspond to fig. 3.20 are the 'Barnet', Dräger 'Spiromat', 'R.P.R.', 'Respirateur SF4', and Stephenson. The accounts of the individual ventilators indicate the ways in which they deviate from the basic form. In addition the Cape and Cape-Waine ventilators, as well as the 'Respirateur MMS 104', are similar except that the concertina bag is re-expanded, not at a constant rate, but approximately according to a half cycle of a sine wave of flow.

It is worth noting that the times at which the system changes from atmospheric-pressure generation to flow generation, and from flow generation to negative-pressure generation, are not fixed in time. Thus, in fig. 3.21 the first change occurs after 0·55 sec under the standard conditions, 0·48 sec with the compliance halved and 0·6 sec with the resistance doubled. The corresponding times for the second change are 1·15, 0·78, and 1·2 sec. The times at which the changes occur depend solely on when the flow from the patient has fallen to the generated flow and when the pressure in the bag has fallen to the negative-pressure limit. As a result of this it is possible in some circumstances that one, or other, or both, of these changes will not occur during the phase. For instance, if the air-way resistance or ventilator resistance is very high, it may be that the initial flow that would result with atmospheric pressure in the bag would be less than the generated flow. In this case the atmospheric-pressure-generating 'sub phase' will be missing, and the expiratory phase will commence with the constant-flow-generating 'sub phase', with the bag pressure steadily falling towards the negative-pressure limit. Indeed, in extreme cases, the system may go straight into its negative-pressure-generating 'sub phase'. On the other hand, if a large tidal volume has been delivered in the previous inspiratory phase, and perhaps also the expiratory phase is limited to a short time, the phase may end before the bag pressure has fallen to the negative-pressure limit or even before the flow has fallen to the generated flow, in which case the third, and even also the second, 'sub phases' will not be reached.

THE CHANGE-OVER FROM THE EXPIRATORY PHASE TO THE INSPIRATORY PHASE

The change-over from the expiratory phase to the inspiratory phase, just as that from the inspiratory phase to the expiratory phase, may be:

1 Time-cycled, in which the change-over occurs after a preset period of time.
2 Volume-cycled, in which the change-over occurs when a preset volume has passed some point.
3 Pressure-cycled, in which the change-over occurs when a pressure, closely related to that in the lungs, reaches a preset level.
4 Flow-cycled, in which the change-over occurs when the flow falls to a preset level.

In addition, in this change-over, it is useful to distinguish a fifth category:

5 Patient-cycled, in which the change-over occurs when the patient makes an inspiratory effort.

There are some cycling mechanisms which cannot be matched exclusively with just one of these basic types. These are discussed under:

6 Mixed-cycled.

Finally there are a few cycling mechanisms which cannot be properly matched with any of the basic types. These are discussed under:

7 Other cycling mechanisms.

The mode of cycling at the end of the expiratory phase frequently differs from that at the end of the inspiratory phase. For instance, most of the ventilators which are pressure-cycled at the end of the inspiratory phase are time-cycled at the end of the expiratory phase.

Some ventilators operate according to a number of different modes in succession and it is possible to distinguish a number of additional cycling mechanisms between successive modes within the phase. However, in the functional analyses of the individual ventilators this has been done only where it seemed essential.

Time-cycling

A ventilator can be said to be time-cycled from the expiratory phase to the inspiratory phase when the change-over is brought about by a timing mechanism which is uninfluenced by conditions in the patient's lungs. The pressure and volume in the lungs and the flow out of them are free to vary and will be determined by the effect on the lungs of whatever flow-generating or pressure-generating mechanism has been operative during the expiratory phase. Therefore, when the lung characteristics alter, the duration of the expiratory phase is unaffected; but the volume, flow, and pressure at the end of the phase may all change. This can be seen from the waveforms of figs. 3.17, 3.18, 3.19, and 3.21 if they are regarded as sets of complete expiratory waveforms of various time-cycled ventilators in which the cycling time has been set to 2 sec: the expiratory time is always the same but the other parameters at the end of the phase are liable to vary with changes of lung characteristics. In the case of ventilators which operate as constant-pressure generators during the phase the effect of changes of lung characteristics on the final values of flow and alveolar pressure is less than in the equivalent situation in the inspiratory phase, because the expiratory phase is usually longer than the inspiratory phase and this allows the exponential changes to become more nearly complete (compare fig. 3.17 with 3.4). On the other hand, in a ventilator which operates as a time-cycled flow generator in the expiratory phase (fig. 3.19) a change of compliance can produce a change of mouth pressure at the end of the phase which is just as striking as in the equivalent case in the inspiratory phase (compare fig. 3.19 with fig. 3.6). Usually the change-over is brought about at a preset time after the start of the expiratory phase, but in the Bennett BA-4 ventilator it normally occurs at a preset time after the start of the previous inspiratory phase. Thus, in this ventilator, it is the total respiratory period which is determined by the time-cycling mechanism and not the duration of the expiratory phase.

Volume-cycling

The change-over from the expiratory phase to the inspiratory phase can be said to be volume-cycled when it is the volume moved during the phase which is determined by the ventilator while the duration of the phase, and the flow and pressure at its end, are free to vary. Most of the ventilators which are volume-cycled at the end of the expiratory phase operate, at least approximately, as flow generators during the phase. Therefore the flow at the end of the phase, and the time taken to move the preset volume, vary little or not at all with changes of lung characteristics. On the other hand the alveolar and mouth pressures may vary considerably. This can be illustrated by reference to fig. 3.19. The waveforms there can be regarded as complete expiratory waveforms from a volume-cycled (0·5 litre) constant-flow generator (0·25 litre/sec) so that, despite changes of lung characteristics, the phase always lasts 0·5/0·25 = 2 sec and the flow at the end is always 0·25 litre/sec. However, the mouth and alveolar pressures at the end of the phase are greatly modified by changes of lung characteristics.

The mechanical form which results in volume-cycling at the end of the expiratory phase is invariably a concertina bag, which forms the reservoir bag of a closed circuit and which is moved through a preset stroke, either mechanically (Clutton-Brock and James), pneumatically (Dräger 'Pulmomat' and Mörch II) or as part of a pressure transformer (Mortimer, 'Roswell Park'). Thus it is the volume drawn into the bag which is determined by the ventilator. Since there is usually a steady flow of fresh gas into the patient circuit the volume drawn out of the patient's lung is somewhat less.

Pressure-cycling

The end of the expiratory phase is pressure-cycled if it occurs when the pressure at the mouth, or some closely-related pressure, reaches some predetermined critical value, irrespective of the time this may take, or of the volume that may have come out of the lungs or of the flow that may exist at the time.

This can be illustrated by reference to fig. 3.22. This shows the same set of waveforms as fig. 3.19 which illustrated the first 2 sec of operation of a constant-flow generator connected to lungs with different characteristics. However, in drawing fig. 3.22 it has been supposed that the constant-flow generator has been fitted with a pressure-cycling

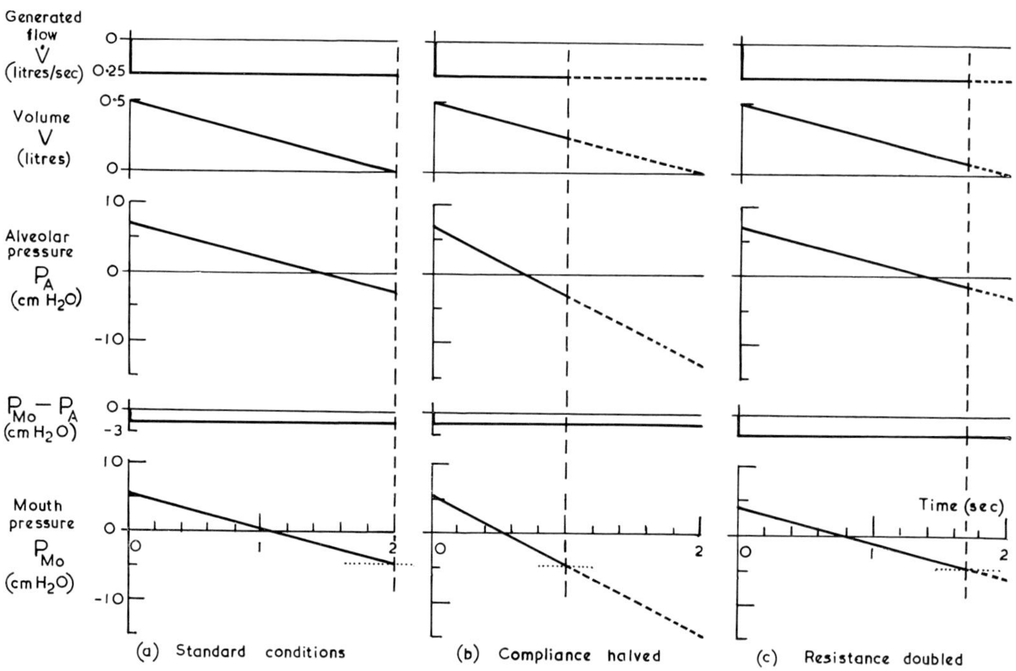

Fig. 3.22. Theoretical waveforms for the expiratory phase for a constant-flow generator exactly as in fig. 3.19 but showing the effect of a pressure-cycling mechanism. The dotted lines indicate the critical pressure at which cycling occurs ($-4{\cdot}5$ cmH_2O). The vertical broken lines indicate the various moments at which cycling occurs and draw attention to the different volumes and alveolar pressures at these moments.

mechanism set to end the expiratory phase when the mouth pressure has fallen to $-4\cdot5$ cmH$_2$O. Thus for each set of lung characteristics, cycling occurs when the sloping line representing the mouth pressure reaches the dotted line indicating the cycling pressure of $-4\cdot5$ cmH$_2$O. Under the standard conditions the expiratory phase still just lasts the full 2 sec for which the waveforms have been drawn. However, when the compliance is halved or the resistance is doubled, the cycling pressure is reached sooner and the phase ends after only 1 sec or 1·7 sec respectively, as indicated by the vertical broken lines. In these shorter times less volume comes out of the lungs and, in the case of the increased resistance, the alveolar pressure falls less.

Flow-cycling

No ventilators appear to utilize flow-cycling for the change-over from the expiratory phase to the inspiratory phase although there seems to be no physical or mechanical reason why this should not be done. Obviously flow-cycling at the end of the phase could not be combined with flow generation during the phase but only with pressure generation. In practice, however, nearly all ventilators which operate as pressure generators in the expiratory phase are time-cycled. This probably arises partly from a desire to prevent too-great changes in respiratory rhythm when lung characteristics change and partly to allow plenty of time for the alveolar pressure to fall to the generated pressure in order to achieve a low mean pressure. However, there is one situation in which it seems possible that flow-cycling at the end of the expiratory phase could be of value. This is in the patient whose airway resistance is so high that it is difficult to achieve an adequate ventilation. In these circumstances any fraction of the respiratory cycle in which there is little or no flow is being 'wasted' from the point of view of ventilation. Therefore, if the ventilator in use operates as a pressure generator in the expiratory phase, a flow-cycling mechanism could be set to end the phase as soon as the flow has fallen to some chosen suitable level. This would come near to allowing the maximum degree of emptying of the lungs which was possible, consistent with achieving the desired total ventilation.

Patient-cycling

A ventilator is patient-cycled or 'patient-triggered' when the change-over from the expiratory phase to the inspiratory phase is initiated by an attempt at inspiration by the patient. Most of the mechanisms used are constructed so that when a small negative pressure is applied to a diaphragm some electrical or pneumatic trip is operated which initiates the next inspiratory phase. In some closed-circuit ventilators if excess gas is spilt at the end of the expiratory phase (Bennett BA-4, Ohio (Monaghan) 300) the patient may have to inspire at a flow greater than the fresh-gas flow before any negative pressure can be developed at the cycling mechanism. In ventilators which operate as constant, atmospheric, pressure generators, the cycling mechanism can be set to operate at a very small negative pressure. With constant, negative, pressure generators however, the cycling mechanism must clearly be set so that it operates only when the patient's efforts produce a pressure more negative than that being generated. Alternatively, as in the 'Jefferson' ventilator, the cycling mechanism may be arranged to respond to the pressure difference across a small resistance and hence to spontaneously-produced inspiratory flow rather than to spontaneously-produced negative pressure.

Mixed-cycling

As at the end of the inspiratory phase, some ventilators can cycle according to more than one rule. For instance, almost all the patient-cycled ventilators are fitted with time-cycling mechanisms which are often set so that, if the patient does not make an inspiratory effort within a certain time, the ventilator cycles automatically to the inspiratory phase.

Those closed-circuit ventilators in which a concertina bag is expanded over a preset stroke by a constant-speed or controlled-speed electric motor (e.g. 'Adelaide', Clutton-Brock, James) can be regarded as both volume-cycled and time-cycled just as at the end of the inspiratory phase. Similarly, the combination of a pressure-cycling mechanism with an adjustable mechanical limit to the stroke of a concertina bag, as in the Dräger 'Pulmomat' and Mörch II, will again operate as volume-cycled or pressure-cycled whichever limit is reached first.

Other cycling mechanisms

Finally there are a few ventilators in which the change-over from the expiratory phase to the inspiratory phase is not related to any particular value of flow, volume, or pressure in the lungs, nor exactly to any particular time. For instance, in the 'Autovent' and 'Minivent' the change-over occurs when the pressure, and therefore the volume, in a distended reservoir bag reaches a critical level. But the pressure and volume in the bag are not related to the pressure and volume in the patient's lungs, and clearly cannot be related to the flow out of the lungs. However, it is possible to say something definite about the time at which the change-over occurs.

During each inspiratory phase a tidal volume of gas is transferred from the bag to the lungs and the bag is replenished by a steady inflow of inflating gas. Therefore the time it takes for the bag to be replenished (and regain its critical pressure and volume) is equal to the previous tidal volume divided by the inflating-gas flow and this time is the duration of the complete respiratory cycle. The inflating-gas flow is determined by the ventilator and, if the tidal volume were also so determined, the respiratory period would be determined by the ventilator. The change-over would then be time-cycled in a conventional sense—

except that, as in the Bennett BA-4, it would be the duration of the complete respiratory cycle and not that of the expiratory phase which was determined. However, in the 'Autovent' the change-over from the inspiratory phase to the expiratory phase is flow-cycled, and in the 'Minivent' it is a hybrid mixture of flow-cycled and pressure-cycled. Therefore the tidal volume is not controlled by the ventilator and consequently the change-over from the expiratory phase to the inspiratory phase is not time-cycled in the conventional sense. Therefore changes of lung characteristics can alter all four parameters, pressure, flow, volume, and time, at the end of the expiratory phase. All that can be said is that the change-over occurs at a time, after the end of the previous expiratory phase, equal to the previous tidal volume (whatever that may happen to have been) divided by the inflating-gas flow.

A similar situation can arise in the Manley ventilator. Here also the fundamental factor controlling the change-over from the expiratory phase to the inspiratory phase is that it occurs at a time, after the end of the previous expiratory phase, equal to the previous tidal volume divided by the steady inflating-gas flow. In the Manley, however, the tidal volume is normally controlled by a volume-limiting device (see p. 130) and therefore the time of the change-over is controlled by the ventilator. However, if the volume limit is not reached, perhaps because of a fall of compliance, the tidal volume is reduced and with it the duration of the respiratory cycle which then becomes dependent upon lung characteristics.

OTHER FACTORS AFFECTING THE WAVEFORMS OF FLOW, VOLUME, AND PRESSURE

Fresh-gas flow to the patient circuit

In many ventilators inflation is brought about by the compression of a bag either by a mechanical or pneumatic drive or by means of weights or springs. All these ventilators incorporate some mechanism to supply fresh gas to the patient circuit and to remove excess gas from it. In many cases the fresh gas enters continuously from a reducing valve and needle valve and hence at a constant flow rate which is often indicated by a flow-meter. In these circumstances the fresh-gas supply constitutes a small-constant-flow generator in parallel with the ventilator.

Often the effect of this is not apparent. In the inspiratory phase, if the ventilator operates primarily as a low-pressure generator, the constant-flow-generating effect of the fresh-gas flow is completely overridden. If the ventilator operates primarily as a constant-flow generator, either exactly or approximately, the fresh gas simply increases this generated flow a little. In the expiratory phase, if the ventilator has a non-rebreathing circuit the fresh-gas flow merely helps to refill the bag while expiration occurs by some other route. In a closed-circuit ventilator if the main mechanism operates as a pressure-generator, either atmospheric or moderately negative, the constant-flow-generating effect of the fresh-gas flow is overridden; if the main mechanism operates as a flow generator the fresh-gas flow slightly diminishes the net generated flow.

However, the effect does become apparent if a volume limit is reached before the end of the phase (see below) and it may have considerable repercussions on the overall action of the ventilator (see Chapter 4).

Volume limiting

In all ventilators in which the patient is inflated by the compression of a bag, or by the movement of a piston in a cylinder, the volume of gas which can be delivered from the bag or cylinder during the inspiratory phase is obviously limited to the volume in the bag or cylinder at the start of the phase. Commonly the phase ends before or as soon as this limit is reached but in some ventilators (e.g. 'Barnet', Engström, 'Jefferson', Manley) the phase may continue for a further period of time in which the lungs are held inflated. The one factor in the situation which, during this period, is entirely determined by the ventilator and uninfluenced by the patient is that there is no flow into the patient's lungs. To be consistent with the terminology already devised it is logical to call such an arrangement a 'zero-flow generator'. Admittedly the pressure in the bag may be constant after the volume limit has been reached (although there may be some drop in pressure due to stress relaxation in the lungs[22]) but the magnitude of the pressure is not fully determined by the ventilator: it depends on the effect of the previously-delivered volume on the patient's lungs and therefore changes with any change of compliance. The only factor which is fixed is the flow and this is fixed at zero.

There are two special situations in which a ventilator which has reached a volume limit will not operate as a zero-flow generator for the rest of the inspiratory phase. One of these exists where a steady flow of fresh gas into the patient circuit from a first-stage reducing valve constitutes a small-constant-flow generator in parallel with the main zero-flow generator. Then the patient continues to be inflated by the fresh-gas flow. This can occur in the Engström ventilators and is demonstrated by the small steady flow in the last part of the inspiratory phase in fig. 52.7. The second situation arises in ventilators in which the volume limit is produced by mechanically limiting the travel of the end-plate of a concertina bag before the bag has fully collapsed. Then if the pressure outside the bag continues to rise (as it does for instance in the Blease 'Pulmoflator' in the volume-limited mode) the corrugations of the concertina-bag wall may be gradually compressed, thereby driving more gas into the patient's lungs. This is illustrated by the gradual decline of flow in the last part of the inspiratory phase in fig. 30.5.

A bag can also act as a volume limit in expiration, although if a spill valve is incorporated this may allow expiration to continue after the bag has expanded to its limit.

Pressure limiting

As their name implies, pressure-limiting valves set some sort of limit to the pressure that can be developed in the circuit in which they are connected; but the precise effect depends upon their functional characteristics which can vary widely with their construction.

A well-constructed 'dead-weight' or gravity-operated valve[23] will open at a given pressure, equal to its effective weight divided by the area of its seating. So long as there is a clear path for escaping gas it will allow large flows to pass without the pressure inside the valve increasing appreciably above the opening pressure. Fig. 3.23(a) shows the pressure-flow characteristic of such a valve.

A spring-loaded valve can likewise be set to open at a given pressure, equal to the force of the spring divided by the area of the seating. However, as the flow through the valve increases, the valve disc has to be lifted further. This further compresses the spring and so increases the pressure within the valve. If the valve is so designed that quite a large movement of the disc does not greatly alter the force of the spring (as in the 'positive-pressure' valve of the 'Cyclator CAV', fig. 37.3) the pressure-flow characteristic may be something like that in fig. 3.23(b), i.e. not very different from that of the gravity-operated valve. On the other hand, in a poorly-designed valve, the pressure may increase very rapidly with flow. Then either the opening pressure is kept at a normal value, in which case very high pressures may occur at large flows, as in fig. 3.23(c); or else the pressure at the expected maximum flow is kept at a normal value and the valve first opens at a very low pressure as in fig. 3.23(d). Examples of both these types have been encountered on ventilators which are available commercially.

As gas enters a circuit incorporating a gravity-operated positive-pressure-limiting valve, the pressure rises normally until it reaches the limit set by the valve. Then gas begins to blow off through the valve and the pressure in the circuit stays constant until the end of the phase: i.e. the system becomes a constant-pressure generator. A gravity-operated negative-pressure-limiting valve operates in a similar manner. With a spring-loaded valve the pressure will not be limited to a precise value but will increase as the flow through it increases. It can be shown that such a situation is equivalent to a constant-pressure generator with some series resistance.

Many ventilators contain positive-pressure-limiting valves. Some are intended solely as safety devices in which case they normally remain closed throughout the respiratory cycle. Others are provided as a means of venting excess gas from a closed circuit. In this case they come into operation regularly towards the end of every inspiratory phase but only for a small fraction of the duration of the phase unless the fresh-gas flow is large. Pressure-limiting valves are also used to spill excess gas from a driving circuit (Allbritten, Gullberg, 'Jefferson') in which case they may be operative for the greater part of the inspiratory phase.

Several ventilators incorporate negative-pressure-limiting valves. These are mostly used to limit the negative pressure developed by a flow-generating mechanism (e.g.

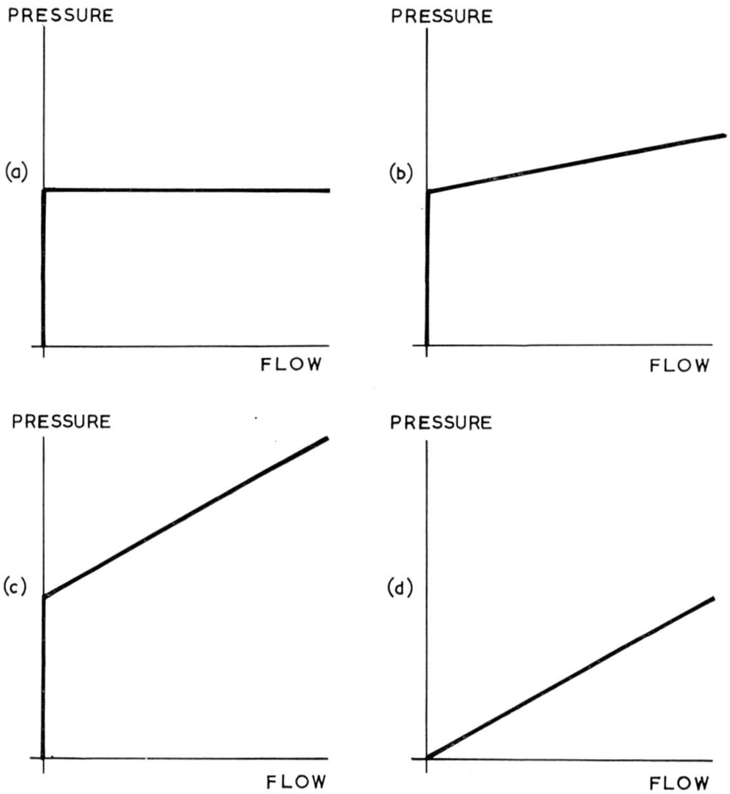

Fig. 3.23. Pressure-flow characteristics of various types of pressure-limiting valves. The graphs show the relationship between the pressure inside the valve and the flow through the valve.

(a) Gravity-operated or dead-weight valve.

(b) 'Good' spring-loaded valve.

(c) 'Bad' spring-loaded valve, set to open at the same pressure as (a).

(d) 'Bad' spring-loaded valve, set to give the same pressure as (a) at a high flow.

'Barnet', Cape-Waine, 'Jefferson', Manley). In this situation, when the valve opens the ventilator changes from flow generation to constant, negative, pressure generation as in fig. 3.21.

The 'bag in a bottle' arrangement

Many ventilators incorporate a 'bag in a bottle' arrangement. The bag is connected to the patient, at least during the inspiratory phase, and contains the gas to be delivered to the patient. It is compressed, thereby inflating the patient, by supplying compressed gas to the 'bottle' during the inspiratory phase. During the expiratory phase, the bottle is opened to the atmosphere or subjected to a negative pressure, permitting expansion of the bag and expiration by the patient. Alternatively, in a non-rebreathing circuit, the patient expires directly to the atmosphere while the bag refills with fresh gas.

The bag may be a common, rubber, anaesthetic bag, although more usually it is of concertina pattern, in which case the estimation or control of tidal volume is possible. The 'bottle' may be almost anything from a small plastic bag, as in the Bird Mark 2, to a large metal casting, as in the Blease 'Pulmoflator'.

From a functional point of view most of these differences are unimportant. So long as the bag is limp and free to expand or contract there will normally be little pressure difference between the inside and outside. One exception to this is when there is a weight in a bag of concertina pattern; this results in a nearly-constant pressure difference between the inside and outside. Therefore, apart from a possible fixed pressure difference, the flow and pressure patterns produced in the patient are, for most of the respiratory cycle, almost exactly as they would be if the lungs were connected directly to the bottle. However, the bag does impose a volume limit to inflation. In closed-circuit systems it also imposes a volume limit to expiration, unless a one-way spill valve is fitted to permit the escape of gas to the bottle when the bag becomes full. These limits may never be reached in normal operation but, if either or both of them are, they may form part of a volume-cycling mechanism, as in the Greer and Donald ventilator, or serve to convert a pressure-cycling mechanism to a volume-cycling one, as in the Dräger 'Pulmomat'. In a time-cycled ventilator the lungs are usually held inflated or deflated from the time that the limit is reached until the end of the phase. However, if there is a steady inflow of fresh gas to the patient circuit this may produce a slow, constant-flow inflation.

In comparing a 'bag in a bottle' ventilator with one in which the driving gas enters the patient's lungs directly, it must not be overlooked that, in the former, the driving gas has to compress the air in the 'bottle' as well as drive some of the contents of the bag into the lungs. This is equivalent to putting an additional 'compliance' in parallel with the patient. In most cases the effect is negligible because of the relative smallness of the 'compliance' of a rigid chamber. In the Blease 'Pulmoflator', however, with its large metal casting, and large diaphragm which also contributes to compliance, the 'compliance' of the 'bottle' has been found to be about 0·016 litre/cmH_2O, or about one-third of a typical patient compliance of 0·05 litre/cmH_2O. In these circumstances the flow into the patient's lungs is only about three-quarters of that from the compressor.

A common reason for using a 'bag in a bottle' arrangement is to allow the patient to breathe a gas mixture different from that which drives the ventilator. Voss[25] has recently shown that adequate separation can be achieved between the patient-circuit gas and the driving gas if the bag and bottle are replaced by a long, relatively-narrow tube and if an adequate fresh-gas flow is used.

CHANGES OF RESISTANCE DURING THE RESPIRATORY CYCLE

In this chapter it has been assumed that, although compliance and resistance change from patient to patient and from time to time in the same patient, at least these two parameters are constant throughout a single cycle of respiration. In fact the resistance changes appreciably in the course of each respiratory cycle. It is higher in expiration than in inspiration, especially in emphysema; it increases as lung volume decreases; and it increases as flow increases. All three of these phenomena must have some influence on the functioning of automatic ventilators, particularly in respect of the exact waveforms of flow produced by pressure generators and the exact waveforms of pressure produced by flow generators.[24] However, it is considered that the implications of these phenomena are beyond the scope of this edition. Here we seek to give a basic account which is accurate enough to explain the great majority of the functional characteristics encountered in clinical practice.

Nevertheless, in the case of constant-pressure generators, the perceptive reader will recognize certain systematic discrepancies between the waveforms deduced theoretically in this chapter and those recorded experimentally from the model lung, and reproduced in the accounts of various ventilators in the later chapters. Some brief explanation is due to him.

In the theoretical deductions in this chapter it was assumed that the pressure drop across the resistance to respiration was proportional to flow. This led to the conclusion that, with a constant-pressure generator, flow, volume, and alveolar pressure all change exponentially. In the model lung the characteristics of the resistance were such that pressure drop was almost entirely proportional to the square of flow (see p. 183). It can be shown theoretically, and the experimental recordings confirm, that this leads to flow declining nearly *linearly* with time and to volume and pressure changing parabolically.

In any practical situation, with a real patient, the pressure drop across the respiratory resistance is partly proportional to flow and partly proportional to the square of flow. Therefore the waveforms with a real patient can be expected to be intermediate between the theoretical ones given in this chapter and the experimental ones given in the accounts of individual ventilators in later chapters. It is hoped to expound these phenomena more fully elsewhere.

REFERENCES

1 Babbage E.D., Elam J.O. and Baver R.O. (1958) Mechanical ventilators. *N.Y. St. J. Med.* **58**, 2653–2657.

2 Collis J.M. (1967) Three simple ventilators: an assessment. *Anaesthesia*, **22**, 598–606.

3 Collis J.M. and Bushman J.A. (1966) An assessment of ten lung ventilators. *Wld. med. Electronics*, **4**, 134–142, 166–170, and 199–202.

4 ELAM J.O., KERR J.H. and JANNEY C.D. (1958) Performance of ventilators. Effect of changes in lung-thorax compliance. *Anesthesiology*, **19**, 56–63.

5 ELDER J.D. jr., DUNCALF D., BINDER L.S. and HARMEL M.H. (1963) An evaluation of mechanical ventilating devices. *Anesthesiology*, **24**, 95–100.

6 FAIRLEY H.B. and HUNTER D.D. (1963) Mechanical ventilators: an assessment of two new machines for use in the operating room. *Can. Anaesth. Soc. J.* **10**, 364–379.

7 FAIRLEY H.B. and HUNTER D.D. (1964) The performance of respirators used in the treatment of respiratory insufficiency. *Can. med. Ass. J.* **90**, 1397–1406.

8 GROGONO A.W. (1966) Mechanical ventilators. In Dobkin A.B. (Ed.) *Ventilators and inhalation therapy*. (International Anesthesiology Clinics Vol. 4, No. 3), p. 497–532, Boston: Little, Brown.

9 HUNTER A.R. (1966) *Essentials of artificial ventilation of the lungs*. p. 20–40. London : J. & A. Churchill.

10 HOLADAY D.A. and RATTENBORG C.C. (1962) Automatic lung ventilators. *Anesthesiology*, **23**, 493–506.

11 HOWELLS T.H. (1963) Automatic pulmonary ventilators. *Wld. med. Electronics*, **1**, 106–112.

12 NORLANDER O.P. (1964) Functional analysis of force and power of mechanical ventilators. *Acta anaesth. Scand.* **8**, 57–77.

13 RATTENBORG C.C. (1956) Basic mechanics of artificial ventilation. In Lassen H.C.A. (Ed.) *Management of life-threatening poliomyelitis*, p. 23–35. Edinburgh: E.&S. Livingstone.

14 SAKLAD M., SAKLAD E. and COX C.V. (1959) Choice of pressure-breathing apparatus—factors to consider. *Anesth. Anal. curr. Res.* **38**, 32–41.

15 SAKLAD M. and WICKLIFF D. (1967) Functional characteristics of artificial ventilators. *Anesthesiology*, **28**, 716–722.

16 SCHORER R., STOFFREGEN J. and HEISLER N. (1966) Assistierte Spontanatmung. Vergleichende Untersuchungen am Bird- und Bennett-Assistor, einschliesslich Narkose-Respiration. *Anaesthesist*, **15**, 113–116.

17 SPALDING J.M.K. (1955) Pressure and duration of inspiration during artificial respiration by intermittent positive pressure. *Lancet*, **1**, 1099–1102.

18 STOFFREGEN J. and HOHMANN G. (1958) Fehler und Gefahren bei automatischer Narkose-Beatmung. *Anaesthesist*, **7**, 311–315.

19 ROBINSON J.S. (1967) The choice of a ventilator. In Evans F.T. and Gray T.C. (Ed.) *Modern trends in anaesthesia 3—aspects of metabolism and pulmonary ventilation*, p. 190–216. London: Butterworths.

20 WATERS D.J. and MAPLESON W.W. (1964) Exponentials and the anaesthetist. *Anaesthesia*, **19**, 274–293.

21 GREEN A.E. and SHIELD R.T. (1950) Finite elastic deformation of incompressible isotropic bodies. *Proc. R. Soc. A.* 202, 407–419.

22 DON H.F. and ROBSON J.G. (1965) The mechanics of the respiratory system during anesthesia. *Anesthesiology*, **26**, 168–178.

23 SMITH W.D.A. (1962) A dead weight expiratory resistance. *Br. J. Anaesth.* **34**, 290–293.

24 RATTENBORG C.C. and HOLADAY D.A. (1966) Constant-flow inflation of the lungs. Theoretical analysis. *Acta anaesth. Scand.* Supp. **23**, 211–223.

25 VOSS T.J.V. (1967) The adaption of ventilators for anaesthesia, with particular reference to paediatric anaesthesia. *S. Afr. med. J.* **41**, 1079–1082.

CHAPTER 4

Physical Aspects of Automatic Ventilators: Some Applications of the Basic Principles

If the full functional specification of a ventilator is given in the terms discussed in the previous chapter, it is possible to deduce how it will perform in terms of the flows, volumes, and pressures which occur when it is connected to a patient with known lung characteristics. It is possible to calculate these flows, volumes, and pressures for various points in the circuit and from moment to moment throughout the respiratory cycle; but to do this completely, even for only one ventilator, would be tedious and unnecessary. It is more useful to determine the more-important features of the volume and pressure patterns in the lungs, and the way in which these patterns depend on the patient's lung characteristics.

The features to which most importance is attached to-day are as follows:

1 The total ventilation, and the tidal volume and frequency which are used to achieve it.
2 The associated maximum and minimum pressures in the lungs.

Therefore one of the main concerns of this chapter is to show how these features are determined for the various combinations of the chief types of generator and cycling mechanism. Before embarking on this, however, it is necessary to consider the problems arising from the supply of fresh gas to the patient circuit and the removal of excess gas from it.

DIFFERENCES BETWEEN THE VOLUME EXCURSION OF THE RESERVOIR BAG OF A VENTILATOR AND THE TIDAL VOLUME RECEIVED BY THE PATIENT

In any ventilator which inflates the patient by the compression of a reservoir bag it is tempting to assume that the volume discharged from the bag is the same as the tidal volume delivered to the patient. The temptation is particularly strong when the bag is of concertina pattern and is compressed past a calibrated scale. However, several factors can cause differences between these two volumes.

It has already been explained (see p. 43) how some of the volume discharged from the reservoir bag is used in compressing the gas in the patient circuit and some in distending any corrugated tubing connecting the bag to the patient. These two factors, together with the distensibility of the convolutions of the concertina bag itself, constitute the compliance of the breathing circuit of the ventilator which is inevitably inflated along with the patient. Therefore the tidal volume of the patient is less than the volume excursion of the bag by the volume absorbed in the compliance of the breathing circuit.

In practice, circuit compliance is always present to a greater or lesser degree. For the sake of simplicity in the following argument, however, it will be assumed to be zero. Therefore, whenever it is concluded below that, in any given circumstances, the tidal volume of the patient is equal to the stroke volume of the reservoir bag, it must be understood that, in practice, the tidal volume would be less than the stroke volume to the extent of the compliance loss.

Non-rebreathing circuits

In a non-rebreathing circuit the whole of the patient's expiration is discharged to atmosphere. While this is going on, that is during the expiratory phase, the bag from which the patient is subsequently inflated is refilled with fresh gas. Then, during the inspiratory phase, gas is driven from the bag to the lungs. In some ventilators fresh gas enters the bag only during the expiratory phase; in others it enters also during the inspiratory phase while the bag is being compressed.

If fresh gas can enter the reservoir bag only during the expiratory phase and not during the inspiratory phase (as for instance in the circuit shown in fig. 4.1) then, during the inspiratory phase, the bag and lungs form a closed system whose total volume is constant (assuming that there is no leak or blow off). Therefore, whatever volume is expelled from the bag during the inspiratory phase must enter the lungs and there is no discrepancy between the stroke volume of the bag and the tidal volume of the patient. The condition that fresh gas shall enter the reservoir bag only during the expiratory phase is usually met in those ventilators in which force is applied to the bag so as to suck in fresh gas from some reservoir at or near atmospheric pressure. The reservoir may in fact be the atmosphere (e.g. Air-Shields 'Respirator') or it may comprise a circuit such as that shown in fig. 4.1 (e.g. Lundia) to permit the enrichment of air with oxygen or the administration of anaesthetic gases.

In many non-rebreathing-circuit ventilators the entry of fresh gas to the reservoir bag is not confined to the expiratory phase but occurs continuously at a steady rate throughout the respiratory cycle as in fig. 4.2. In some ventilators the bag is quite free to expand during the expiratory phase (e.g. Air-Shields 'Ventimeter' and Blease 'Paediatric'), in

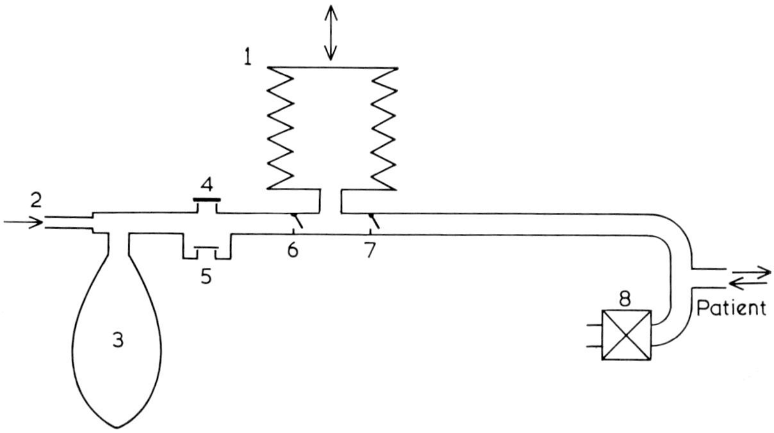

Fig. 4.1. A non-rebreathing circuit in which entry of fresh gas to the concertina reservoir bag is confined to the expiratory phase so that (apart from leaks and losses in the circuit compliance) the tidal volume of the patient is the same as the stroke volume of the bag (e.g. Dräger 'Spiromat 661', Emerson gas-operated, Lundia).

1 Concertina reservoir bag driven up and down mechanically or pneumatically.
2 Continuous inflow of fresh gas.
3 Storage bag.
4, 5, 6, 7 One-way valves.
8 Valve which is closed for inflation and open for expiration.

others the expansion occurs against the force of springs (e.g. 'Barnet' II and III) or the elasticity of the bag wall (e.g. 'Autovent' and 'Minivent'). But in all cases, so long as the fresh-gas flow is derived from a high-pressure source and needle valve, variations in the pressure inside the bag, in either the expiratory or inspiratory phase, have no effect on the fresh-gas flow which is constant throughout the respiratory cycle. In these circumstances the total volume of the system (bag plus lungs) is not constant but increases throughout the inspiratory phase. Therefore the tidal volume of the patient exceeds the stroke volume of the bag to the extent of the volume of fresh gas which enters the bag during the inspiratory phase.

Thus:

$$\text{excess of patient's tidal volume over stroke volume of bag} = \text{fresh-gas flow} \times \text{inspiratory time.} \tag{1}$$

But:

$$\begin{aligned}\text{stroke volume of bag} &= \text{volume of fresh gas entering during expiratory phase,}\\ &= \text{fresh-gas flow} \times \text{expiratory time.}\end{aligned} \tag{2}$$

Therefore, adding equations (1) and (2):

$$\begin{aligned}\text{tidal volume} &= \text{fresh-gas flow} \times (\text{inspiratory time} + \text{expiratory time}),\\ &= \text{fresh-gas flow} \times \text{respiratory period.}\end{aligned} \tag{3}$$

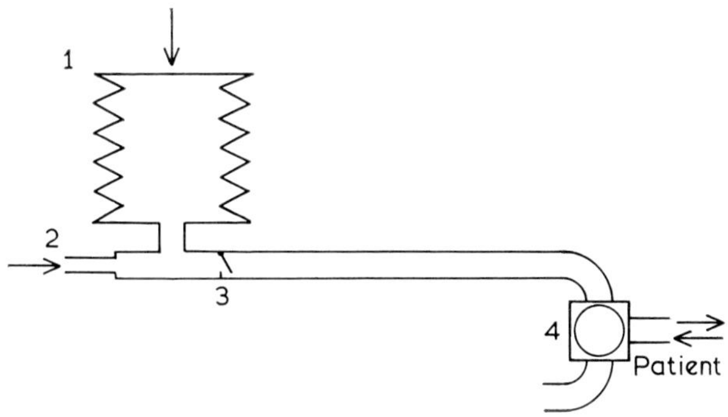

Fig. 4.2. A non-rebreathing circuit in which fresh gas enters the concertina reservoir bag continuously throughout the respiratory cycle (e.g. Blease 'Paediatric' and 'Barnet' Mark III on non-rebreathing circuit). The tidal volume of the patient exceeds the stroke volume of the bag to the extent of the volume of fresh gas which enters during the inspiratory phase. Provided that the drive is sufficient to empty the bag in every inspiratory phase such an arrangement operates as a 'minute-volume divider' (see text).

1 Concertina reservoir bag which may be spring-loaded or otherwise driven down for inflation.

2 Continuous steady inflow of fresh gas.

3 One-way valve.

4 Valve which, for the inspiratory phase, connects the patient to the bag and, for the expiratory phase, connects the patient to the atmosphere.

Two deductions may be made from this calculation. The first, which is immediately relevant, is that the difference between tidal volume and stroke volume can most clearly be expressed by dividing equation (3) by equation (2):

$$\frac{\text{tidal volume}}{\text{stroke volume}}=\frac{\text{respiratory period}}{\text{expiratory time}}. \tag{4}$$

Thus, if the inspiratory-expiratory ratio is 1 : 1 (the expiratory phase occupies $\frac{1}{2}$ the respiratory cycle) the tidal volume is twice the stroke volume; if the ratio is 1 : 2 (the expiratory phase occupies 2/3 of the respiratory cycle) the tidal volume is $3/2=1\frac{1}{2}$ times the stroke volume.

The second deduction is incidental but it is convenient to make it here. Since, from equation (3),

$$\text{tidal volume}=\text{fresh-gas flow}\times\text{respiratory period},$$

$$\text{fresh-gas flow}=\frac{\text{tidal volume}}{\text{respiratory period}},$$

$$=\text{total, minute-volume, ventilation}.$$

That is, the total ventilation is equal to the fresh-gas flow. This could, of course, have been deduced directly from the fact that, in the arrangement described, the whole of the fresh-gas flow and nothing but the fresh-gas flow goes into the patient's lungs. The important conclusion here is that the ventilator accepts the total, minute-volume, ventilation set by the fresh-gas flow and divides it up into tidal volumes. It is for this reason that such ventilators have been called 'minute-volume dividers'.[1]

The argument so far has been quite general with the one reservation that the mechanism for compressing the reservoir bag in the inspiratory phase shall be sufficiently powerful to expel from it all the fresh gas which enters it during the expiratory phase. The effect of increasing the fresh-gas flow, however, depends on the functional specification of the ventilator. If the ventilator is time-cycled in both phases (e.g. Air-Shields 'Ventimeter' and one mode of operation of the 'Barnet' Mark III) the respiratory period is fixed so that increasing the fresh-gas flow increases the tidal volume in proportion (equation 3). In addition, the expiratory time is fixed so that the ratio of tidal volume to stroke volume is fixed (equation 4). That is, both the tidal volume and the stroke volume increase in proportion to the fresh-gas flow (fig. 4.3). On the other hand, if the ventilator is volume-cycled (by the movement of the bag) in both phases (e.g. Howells, 'R.P.R.'), then the stroke volume is fixed. Therefore, increasing the fresh-gas flow decreases the expiratory time (equation 2), increases the excess of tidal volume over stroke volume (equation 1), and hence increases the tidal volume. This generally leads to some increase in the inspiratory time (fig. 4.4).

Closed circuits

In a 'closed circuit' system, with soda-lime absorption of carbon dioxide, if the fresh-gas supply is just equal to the patient's oxygen consumption the system is truly 'closed'. This neglects any uptake of anaesthetic agent. Although this is often negligible it can be considerable during induction with nitrous oxide.[2] Throughout this section, therefore, the term 'oxygen consumption' should be taken to include any anaesthetic uptake. The total volume of the system (bag plus lungs) is constant throughout the respiratory cycle. Therefore whatever volume is expelled from the bag during the inspiratory phase must enter the patient's lungs and there is no discrepancy between the stroke volume of the bag and the tidal volume of the patient.

If the fresh-gas flow exceeds the patient's oxygen consumption the excess must somehow be discharged to the atmosphere to prevent the system indefinitely overfilling. That is, the volume of fresh gas which enters the patient circuit during one respiratory cycle must be balanced by the discharge of an equal volume of gas (after allowing for oxygen consumption) during the same cycle. Three basic mechanisms have been used to achieve this balance: the spill valve, the blow-off valve, and the auxiliary circuit.

Spill valve

The essential characteristic of a spill valve is that it permits the escape of excess gas from

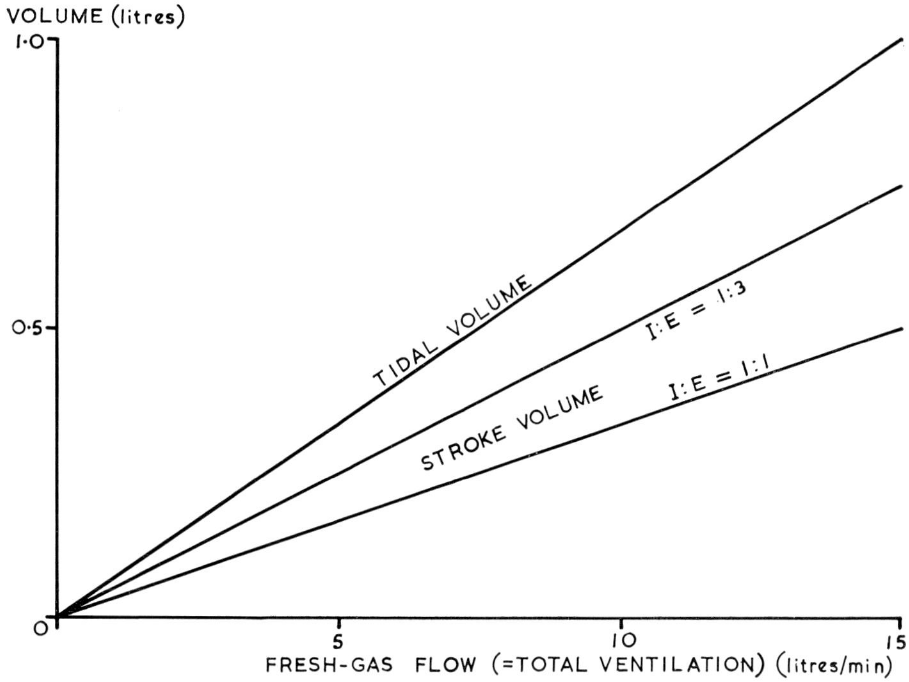

Fig. 4.3. The calculated effect of the fresh-gas flow on the tidal volume of the patient and the stroke volume of the reservoir bag for a ventilator with the following characteristics (e.g. Air-Shields 'Ventimeter' and 'Barnet' Mark III in the time-cycled, non-rebreathing mode):

Non-rebreathing circuit.

Fresh-gas flow enters the reservoir bag continuously.

Time-cycled in both phases.

Sufficient drive to empty the bag completely during the inspiratory phase.

The lines have been calculated for a respiratory frequency fixed at 15/min and an inspiratory-expiratory ratio fixed at 1 : 1 or 1 : 3.

the patient circuit during the expiratory phase, usually towards the end of the phase when the bag is fully expanded. The valve may be opened mechanically, as in the Emerson 'Controller-Assistor' and, as such, could be used on a mechanically-driven bag. In fact, however, spill valves are associated only with the 'bag in a bottle' arrangement and usually comprise just a one-way valve permitting flow of gas from bag to bottle but not in the opposite direction. With one exception they are associated only with a continuous steady inflow of fresh gas.

A typical arrangement is shown in fig. 4.5. During the inspiratory phase the entry of compressed gas to the pressure chamber maintains a higher pressure there than in the bag, thereby holding the spill valve shut and driving gas into the lungs. During the expiratory phase the weight of the bag produces a pressure difference which keeps the spill valve shut until the expansion of the bag is complete or has been arrested by an

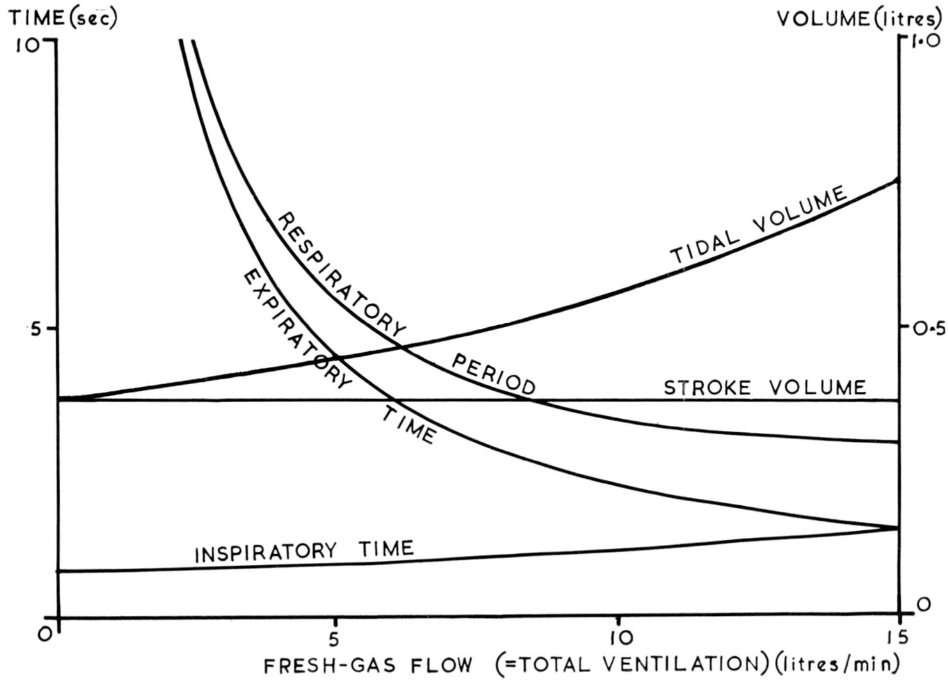

Fig. 4.4. The calculated effect of the fresh-gas flow for a ventilator with the following characteristics (e.g. Howells, 'R.P.R.'):

Non-rebreathing circuit.

Fresh-gas flow continuous.

Volume-cycled in both phases (with reference to the bag volume, not the tidal volume of the patient).

Constant-flow generator in the inspiratory phase.

The lines have been calculated for a stroke volume of the bag of 375 ml and a generated inspiratory flow of 30 litres/min (to give the same conditions as in fig. 4.3 at a fresh-gas flow of 7·5 litres/min).

adjustable stop. Then a slight rise in pressure within the bag is sufficient to open the valve and gas spills freely from the patient circuit. This spill is stopped as soon as the next inspiratory phase commences. Therefore the escape of excess gas is confined to the expiratory phase.

If also the supply of fresh gas were confined to the expiratory phase, the bag and lungs would form a closed system during the inspiratory phase, and the patient's tidal volume would be equal to the stroke volume of the bag. However, this facility is available in only one of the many ventilators with spill valves in closed circuits—the Frumin.

In all other closed-circuit ventilators with spill valves the inflow of fresh gas is continuous throughout the respiratory cycle (as in fig. 4.5) so that, as in similar circumstances with a non-rebreathing circuit (fig. 4.2), the tidal volume of the patient exceeds

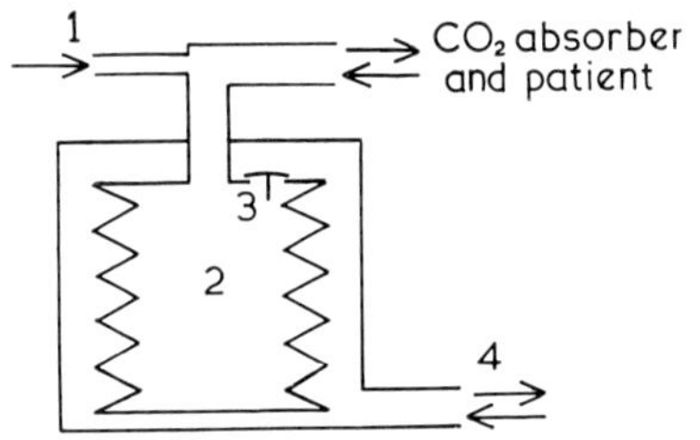

Fig. 4.5. A closed circuit in which the discharge of excess gas occurs through a spill valve at the end of the expiratory phase and fresh gas enters continuously throughout the respiratory cycle (e.g. Aga 'Spiropulsator', Bennett BA-4, Blease 'Pulmoflator' on closed circuit). The tidal volume of the patient exceeds the stroke volume of the bag to the extent of the volume of fresh gas which enters during the inspiratory phase.

1 Continuous inflow of fresh gas.
2 Concertina reservoir bag.
3 Spill valve.
4 Driving gas.

the stroke volume of the bag by the volume of fresh gas which enters during the inspiratory phase. This is equal to the fresh-gas flow multiplied by the inspiratory time. Therefore, increasing the fresh-gas flow increases the excess of tidal volume over stroke volume.

If the ventilator is volume-cycled, as it can be for instance in the Bennett BA-4 or Ohio (Monaghan) 300, or if it is volume-limited as in the Dräger 'Narkose Spiromat 650' or Blease 'Pulmoflator' on closed circuit, it is almost certainly the stroke volume of the bag which is controlled; therefore increasing the fresh-gas flow increases the tidal volume. The manner of the increase is as shown in fig. 4.6 provided that the ventilator is time-cycled at the end of the inspiratory phase as well as volume-cycled or volume-limited—as can be at least approximately the case for the four examples quoted.

On the other hand if the ventilator is pressure-cycled, as it can be for instance in the Blease 'Pulmoflator' or Ohio (Monaghan) 300, increasing the fresh-gas flow has little effect on the tidal volume and therefore the stroke volume of the bag is reduced and the manner of the decrease is as shown in fig. 4.7 except that increasing the fresh-gas flow may, in some circumstances, speed up the inflation and shorten the inspiratory time.

Since, with a spill valve, the effect of the fresh-gas flow is to make the true ventilation greater than the apparent ventilation, neglect of the correction factor is unlikely to cause the patient great harm. However such neglect might be important in the following circumstances. Suppose that, at the start of an anaesthetic, a very high fresh-gas flow was used to achieve rapid build-up of anaesthetic tension in the circuit, and that the stroke volume of the bag was set (at a low level) to give a normal tidal-volume reading on a Wright respirometer near the patient. Later, when anaesthesia was established, the fresh-gas flow might be greatly reduced. If the resultant change in the respirometer reading went unobserved and if no compensating increase were made in the setting of the stroke

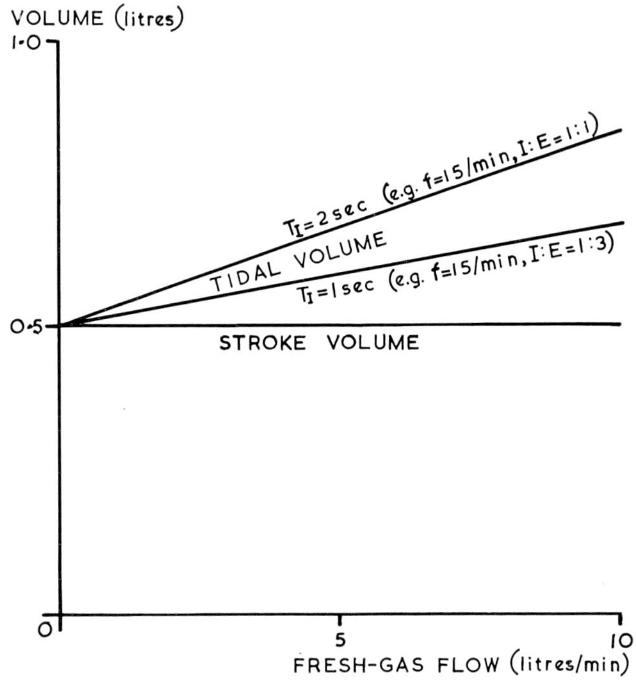

Fig. 4.6. The calculated effect of the fresh-gas flow on the tidal volume of the patient in a ventilator with the following characteristics (e.g. Dräger 'Narkose Spiromat 650' on closed circuit):

Closed circuit.
Fresh-gas flow continuous.
Spill valve.
Time-cycled at the end of the inspiratory phase and also either simultaneously volume-cycled or else volume-limited.

volume, the tidal volume would be greatly reduced and the patient might be seriously underventilated.

There is an important corollary to the use of a spill valve. At the end of every expiratory phase (in the steady state) there must be some spillage of gas. Therefore there must be at least a small pressure gradient at the end of the phase from the alveoli to the outside of the bag. Therefore, if the bag is a hanging one, and a weight in the bag is used to generate negative pressure, this negative pressure can develop only in the early part of the phase. Before the end of the phase the bag must reach a stop which supports the weight and allows the pressure within it to rise above that outside. Therefore a weighted concertina bag with a spill valve generates negative pressure only for the first part of the expiratory phase and this negative pressure can do no more than accelerate the removal of gas from the lungs. It cannot produce a negative pressure in the alveoli since the

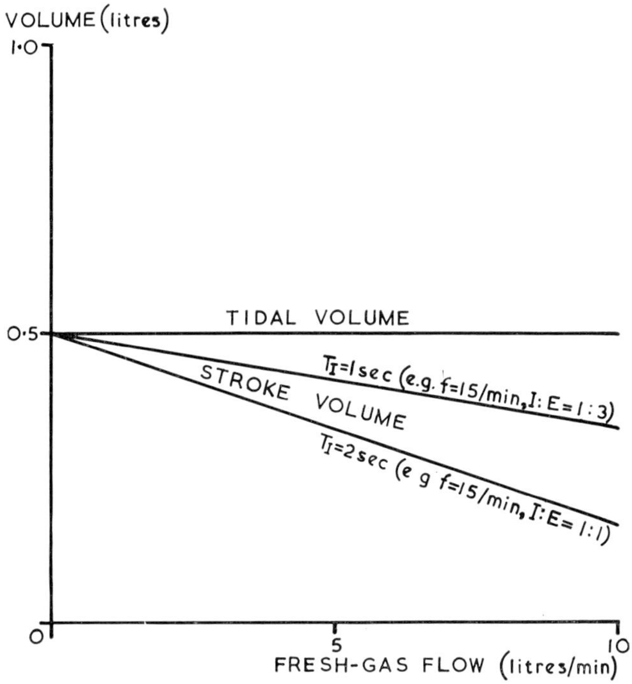

Fig. 4.7. The calculated effect of the fresh-gas flow on the stroke volume of the bag in a ventilator with the following characteristics (e.g. pressure-cycled mode of the Blease 'Pulmoflator' and the Ohio (Monaghan) 300):

Closed circuit.
Fresh-gas flow continuous.
Spill valve.
Pressure-cycled.

The lines have been calculated for a cycling pressure such that the tidal volume is 500 ml and for inspiratory times (T_I) of 1 sec and 2 sec. Increasing the fresh-gas flow may make inflation faster and shorten the inspiratory time slightly.

pressure there must be slightly positive at the end of the phase to produce the spill of excess gas. The only way in which negative pressure can be produced in the alveoli if a spill valve is used is by applying negative pressure *outside* the reservoir bag (e.g. Air-Shields 'Ventimeter', 'Jefferson'). The only way in which a weighted bag can produce negative pressure in the alveoli is by using a blow-off valve (see below) instead of a spill valve to dispose of excess gas so that the bag does not reach a stop and the weight is operative throughout the phase.

Blow-off valve

The essential characteristic of a blow-off valve is that it permits the escape of excess gas from the patient circuit when the pressure within the circuit is high, that is, towards the end of the inspiratory phase. A typical arrangement is shown in fig. 4.8. During the inspiratory phase, as the bag is compressed, gas from the bag, together with the steady inflow of fresh gas, inflates the patient's lungs until the opening pressure of the blow-off valve is reached. Then gas escapes to the atmosphere. Thus the fresh-gas flow tends to make the tidal volume of the patient greater than the stroke volume of the bag, but the

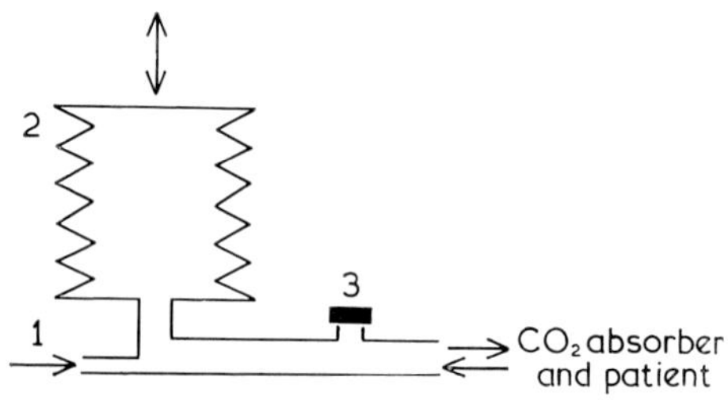

Fig. 4.8. A closed circuit in which the discharge of excess gas occurs through a blow-off valve, towards the end of the inspiratory phase, and fresh gas enters continuously, throughout the respiratory cycle (e.g. 'Cyclator CAV', Dräger 'Pulmomat'). The tidal volume of the patient is less than the stroke volume of the bag to the extent of the volume of fresh gas which enters during the expiratory phase.

1 Continuous inflow of fresh gas.
2 Concertina reservoir bag.
3 Blow-off valve.

escape through the blow-off valve more than overcomes this tendency. The functioning can be more easily understood if the expiratory phase is considered. Then pressure in the circuit is low and the blow-off valve remains shut. The bag refills only partly from the patient, and partly from the fresh-gas flow. Consequently the tidal volume of the patient is less than the stroke volume of the bag by the volume of fresh gas which enters during the phase, that is, by a volume which is equal to the fresh-gas flow multiplied by the expiratory time.

Although the above statement is generally true (apart from corrections for losses through leaks, circuit compliance, and oxygen consumption) the result of increasing the fresh-gas flow depends upon the mode of functioning of the ventilator in the expiratory phase. In certain circumstances the stroke volume remains unchanged and the tidal volume is reduced while, in others, the tidal volume remains unchanged and the stroke volume is increased. However, the general principle is maintained that increasing the fresh-gas flow diminishes the tidal volume in relation to the stroke volume. A number of specific modes of functioning will now be considered.

If the ventilator operates as a constant-flow generator in the expiratory phase it is helpful to remember that the fresh-gas flow can be considered as a supplementary constant-flow generator which, in the expiratory phase, is opposed to the main flow generator. Therefore the flow leaving the lungs (the net generated flow) is less than the main generated flow to the extent of the fresh-gas flow. If, in addition, the ventilator is time-cycled, or else volume-cycled and hence effectively time-cycled (e.g. Dräger 'Pulmomat'), increasing the fresh-gas flow, by decreasing the net generated flow, must decrease the tidal volume. If the ventilator is pressure-cycled (e.g. the Mörch I) a decreased net generated flow may have little effect on tidal volume but will take longer to lower the pressure to the cycling level and the expiratory time will therefore be increased. Therefore, in a ventilator which operates as a flow generator in the expiratory phase, no matter what the cycling mechanism at the end of the phase, increasing the fresh-gas flow leads to a decrease in ventilation. Indeed, in a constant-flow generator, if the fresh-gas flow is made equal to the main generated flow, the net generated flow becomes zero and ventilation ceases altogether. Such high fresh-gas flows (up to twice the total ventilation depending on the inspiratory-expiratory ratio) are obviously abnormal for a closed anaesthetic circuit but may be approached when the circuit is flushed to achieve a rapid change of inspired concentration of anaesthetic.

If the ventilator operates as a constant-pressure generator during the expiratory phase the steady fresh-gas flow has little direct effect on the flow from the patient. If the ventilator is time-cycled (e.g. 'Cyclator CAV') or pressure-cycled (e.g. Mörch II in one mode of operation) increasing the fresh-gas flow will have little effect on the tidal volume expired by the patient; it will merely increase the stroke volume of the bag provided that this is not limited. However, this may well lead to a prolongation of the *inspiratory* phase and hence to a reduction in frequency and total ventilation. If the ventilator is volume-cycled (as in the other mode of operation of the Mörch II) increasing the fresh-gas flow cannot alter the stroke volume of the bag and must therefore decrease the tidal volume of the patient. However, it will also increase the speed of filling of the bag and hence shorten the expiratory time. This will tend to compensate for the decreased tidal volume.

To summarize, in a closed circuit with continuous inflow of fresh gas the difference between the effects of a blow-off valve and a spill valve is as follows. With a blow-off valve the tidal volume is less than the stroke volume to an extent equal to the product of the fresh-gas flow and the expiratory time. With a spill valve the tidal volume is greater than the stroke volume to an extent equal to the product of the fresh-gas flow and the inspiratory time. In both cases the detailed effects of increasing the fresh-gas flow depend on the functional specification of the ventilator. However, for circumstances in which the

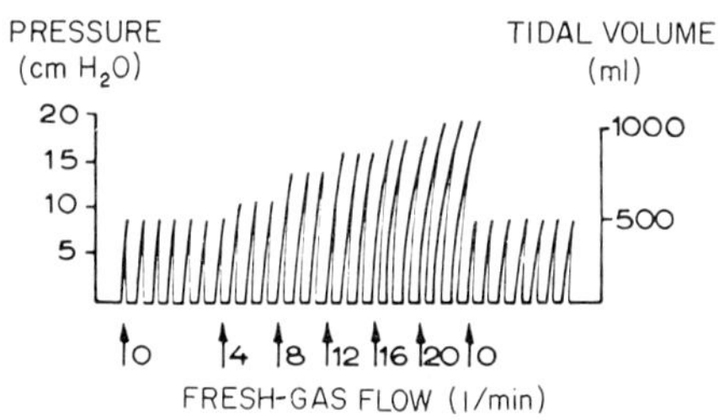

Fig. 4.9.

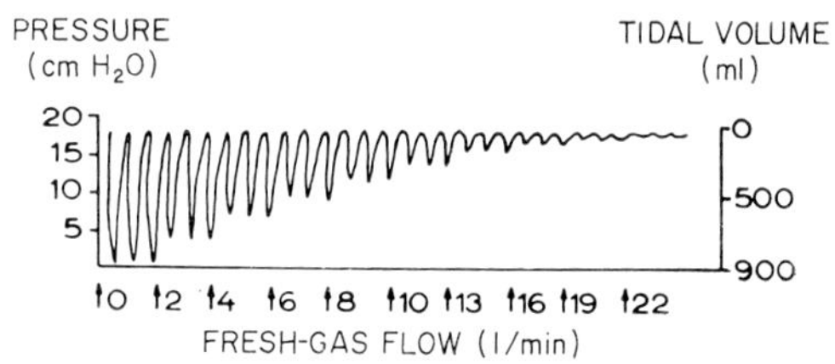

Fig. 4.10.

Fig. 4.9. Redrawn laboratory recording of the effect of increasing the fresh-gas flow in a ventilator with the following characteristics:

Closed circuit.
Fresh-gas flow enters the bag continuously.
Stroke volume of the bag constant.
Spill valve.

Fig. 4.10. As fig. 4.9 except that the ventilator is fitted with a blow-off valve.

stroke volume of the bag is held constant, the difference between the effects of a blow-off valve and a spill valve is shown vividly by the recordings of figs. 4.9 and 4.10.

Auxiliary circuit

With both the spill valve and the blow-off valve the patient expires into the same bag from which he is inflated, and it has just been shown how, with a continuous inflow of fresh gas, this leads to a discrepancy between the tidal volume of the patient and the stroke volume of the bag. In a number of the more-recently-developed ventilators this discrepancy has been avoided by using separate bags for inflation and for the collection of the patient's expiration.

A basic circuit is shown in fig. 4.11. Compression of the concertina bag (1) inflates the patient through the one-way valve (4). Meanwhile the steady inflow of fresh gas accumulates in the auxiliary storage bag (7). Therefore, during the inspiratory phase, the

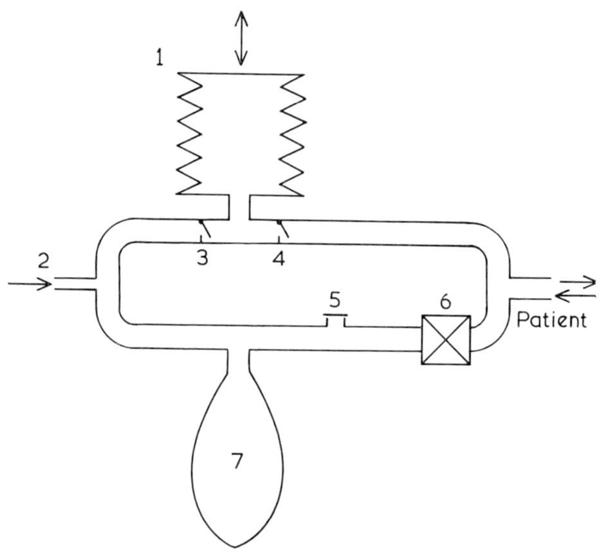

Fig. 4.11. A closed circuit in which the discharge of excess gas is carried out in an auxiliary circuit so that the tidal volume of the patient is always equal to the stroke volume of the concertina bag (apart from any losses in the compliance of the circuit).

1 Concertina bag driven up and down mechanically or pneumatically.
2 Continuous inflow of fresh gas.
3 One-way valve.
4 One-way valve.
5 Lightly-loaded one-way valve.
6 Valve which is closed during the inspiratory phase and open during the expiratory phase.
7 Storage bag.

A carbon-dioxide absorber must also be included somewhere in the circuit.

concertina bag and the lungs form a closed system whose total volume is constant so that the tidal volume of the patient is equal to the stroke volume of the bag. Therefore, alteration of the fresh-gas flow has no effect on either the tidal volume of the patient or the stroke volume of the bag. In the expiratory phase the valve (6) is open and the patient expires freely into the storage bag (7). Meanwhile the concertina bag is expanded, refilling itself from the bag (7). Usually the flow from the patient will be fast at the beginning of the phase and slow later, whereas the expansion of the concertina bag will be more-nearly steady or perhaps sine-wave throughout the phase. Therefore the bag (7) will usually become taut early in the expiratory phase and then cause excess gas to escape through the one-way valve (5). Therefore increasing the fresh-gas flow simply increases the escape of gas through the one-way valve (5). If the fresh-gas flow is very high there may also be some escape towards the end of the inspiratory phase.

The exact circuit shown in fig. 4.11 is not to be found in any ventilator at the present but the arrangements in the closed circuits of the Aika and the Engström 'Narcosis' ventilators are very similar. However, in the Engström 'Narcosis' ventilator the fresh gas enters the patient circuit on the reservoir-bag (1) side of the one-way valve (3) instead of at the position (2) shown in fig. 4.11. As a result, fresh gas flows directly to the patient during the inspiratory phase and the tidal volume exceeds the stroke volume of the reservoir bag in much the same way as in the simple circuit with spill valve (fig. 4.5). In a number of other ventilators ('Barnet' Mark III, Cape-Waine, East-Radcliffe 'Positive-Negative' PNA1) a third bag is introduced. The patient is inflated from an inspiratory concertina bag as in fig. 4.11 but expires into a second, expiratory, concertina bag which is mechanically driven to develop negative pressure. During the inspiratory phase the expiratory bag is emptied into the storage bag (7) in fig. 4.11, and during the expiratory phase the inspiratory bag refills from the storage bag. The 'Respirateur SF4' is very similar but uses pistons in cylinders instead of concertina bags.

General

The foregoing discussion has examined various particular mechanical arrangements for the supply of fresh gas and the disposal of excess gas from the patient circuit and, for each, has deduced any resultant discrepancy between the tidal volume of the patient and the stroke volume of the bag.

In general it would be possible to arrange for fresh gas to enter the reservoir bag during the inspiratory phase only, or during the expiratory phase only, or during both phases. Furthermore, each of these three cases could be combined with provision for the escape of excess gas during the inspiratory phase, or the expiratory phase, or both. Thus there are nine possible combinations of methods for the supply of fresh gas and disposal of excess gas (Table 4.1).

Any combination in which the fresh-gas inflow during the inspiratory phase is greater than the excess-gas escape during that phase results in the total volume of the bag-lungs

Table 4.1. Differences between the tidal volume of the patient (V_T) and the stroke volume of the reservoir bag (V_S) with various arrangements for the supply of fresh gas and the escape of excess gas.

		Fresh-gas Inflow		
		Inspiratory Phase Only	*Both Phases*	*Expiratory Phase Only*
Excess-gas escape	*Inspiratory Phase Only*	$V_T = V_S$ No examples	$V_T < V_S$ $(V_T = V_S - \dot{V}_F T_E)$ Closed circuit only Blow-off valve Fresh gas continuous (Fig. 4.8) e.g. 'Cyclator CAV' Dräger 'Pulmomat'	$V_T < V_S$ No current examples but see Greer and Donald CC
Excess-gas escape	*Both Phases*	$V_T > V_S$ No examples	$V_T = V_S$* No examples	$V_T < V_S$ No current examples but see Gullberg and Mörch III
Excess-gas escape	*Expiratory Phase Only*	$V_T > V_S$ No examples	$V_T > V_S$ $(V_T = V_S + \dot{V}_F T_I)$ Closed circuit Spill valve Fresh gas continuous (Fig. 4.5) e.g. Air-Shields 'Ventimeter' CC Dräger 'Narkose Spiromat 650' on CC Non-rebreathing circuit Fresh gas continuous (Fig. 4.2) e.g. Howells 'R.P.R.'	$V_T = V_S$ Closed circuit Spill valve Fresh gas stored in inspiratory phase Frumin only Closed circuit Auxiliary circuit for balancing gas volumes (Fig. 4.11) e.g. Aika CC Cape-Waine CC Non-rebreathing circuit Fresh gas sucked in from atmosphere, e.g. Lundia Non-rebreathing circuit Fresh gas shut off during inspiration 'Vellore' only Non-rebreathing circuit Fresh gas stored during inspiration (Fig. 4.1) e.g. East-Radcliffe 'Positive-Negative' Manley

V_T = Tidal volume of patient $\dot{V}_F$ = Fresh-gas flow T_E = Expiratory time
V_S = Stroke volume of bag T_I = Inspiratory time   CC = Closed circuit
* Assuming that inflow and escape both occur at a steady rate throughout the cycle.

system increasing during the phase; therefore the tidal volume received by the patient is greater than the stroke volume leaving the bag (the three cells in the bottom left-hand corner of Table 4.1). Any combination in which the fresh-gas inflow during the inspiratory phase is less than the excess-gas escape during that phase results in the total volume of the bag-lungs system decreasing during the phase; therefore the tidal volume is less than the stroke volume (the three cells in the top right-hand corner of Table 4.1). In the three remaining combinations (on the top-left to bottom-right diagonal of Table 4.1) the inflow during the inspiratory phase is equal to the escape in that phase (sometimes both are zero) so that the volume of the system is unaltered at the end of the phase and the tidal volume is equal to the stroke volume.

As can be seen from Table 4.1 many of the combinations have been used rarely or not at all. Only three are in common use and all the particular mechanical arrangements discussed above come within these three.

In one combination both the supply of fresh gas to the reservoir bag and the removal of excess gas are confined to the expiratory phase (bottom right of Table 4.1). Thus in the inspiratory phase there is no change in total volume and the tidal volume of the patient is equal to the stroke volume of the bag. This combination is found in both closed and non-rebreathing circuits. It is achieved by the mechanisms shown in figs. 4.11 and 4.1 and by others mentioned in Table 4.1.

In another combination the escape of excess gas is still confined to the expiratory phase but the supply of fresh gas enters the circuit continuously throughout the respiratory cycle (bottom centre of Table 4.1). In a closed circuit the excess gas escapes through a spill valve (fig. 4.5); in a non-rebreathing circuit it escapes through the expiratory valve (fig. 4.2). In either case the fresh-gas flow increases the total volume of the system (bag plus lungs) during the inspiratory phase so that the tidal volume is greater than the stroke volume of the bag to the extent of the volume of fresh gas which enters during the phase.

In the third combination the supply of fresh gas is again continuous but the escape of excess gas is confined to the inspiratory phase. Thus the fresh-gas flow increases the total volume of the system during the *expiratory* phase and the tidal volume is less than the stroke volume of the bag to the extent of the volume of fresh gas which enters during the expiratory phase. This combination occurs only in closed-circuit ventilators with blow-off valves (fig. 4.8).

FACTORS AFFECTING THE VENTILATION PRODUCED IN THE PATIENT AND THE ASSOCIATED MAXIMUM AND MINIMUM PRESSURES IN THE LUNGS

In a few ventilators the total minute-volume ventilation is directly controlled, but in most the required ventilation is obtained by setting the tidal volume and frequency separately. Tidal volume is related to the maximum and minimum pressures in the alveoli by the compliance. In fact, the difference between the maximum and minimum pressures is equal to the tidal volume divided by the compliance. For example:

if tidal volume	=0·5 litre,
and compliance	=0·05 litre/cmH_2O,
then the difference between maximum and minimum alveolar pressures	=0·5/0·05=10 cmH_2O.

In some cases the tidal volume is determined by the ventilator, and the difference between the minimum and maximum alveolar pressures depends on the patient's compliance. In others, it is rather the alveolar pressures that are determined by the ventilator, and the tidal volume which depends on the patient's lung characteristics. In a few cases both the pressures and the tidal volume depend on the lung characteristics, and only the timing is rigidly controlled by the ventilator. Therefore, in analysing the performance of different types of ventilator, it is convenient to vary the order in which the three factors of volume, pressure, and time are considered according to the type of ventilator.

Volume-cycled ventilators

In most volume-cycled ventilators the tidal volume delivered to the patient is determined by the ventilator characteristics. As has just been explained, the tidal volume may differ somewhat from the volume leaving the reservoir bag on account of the fresh-gas supply, but the difference is largely determined by the ventilator and so may be regarded as included in the ventilator characteristics.

Those volume-cycled ventilators which are also flow generators (e.g. Cape-Waine, Emerson electrically-operated, Lundia) are also time-cycled: the pattern of flow is determined by the ventilator, and therefore the time taken to deliver the volume at which cycling occurs is similarly determined. In much the same way these ventilators are invariably either effectively or actually time-cycled at the end of the expiratory phase as well. Therefore, the duration of the respiratory cycle, and hence the frequency, is determined by the ventilator. Consequently, the total ventilation is determined by the ventilator and is independent of the patient's lung characteristics. The only circumstances in which the ventilation received by the patient can change, without alteration of the ventilator controls, is if a leak develops in the patient circuit.

Those volume-cycled ventilators which are also pressure generators are not effectively time-cycled: when the patient's compliance decreases, or his airway resistance increases, the pressure generator takes longer to deliver the required volume against the increased impedance. There is, therefore, a reduction in respiratory frequency and hence in ventilation. In most ventilators in this category (e.g. Aga 'Spiropulsator', Ohio (Monaghan) 300) the generated pressure is high enough for them to approximate to flow generators (see p. 84) so that the effect of changes of compliance and resistance on the inspiratory time are usually small. In the 'Vellore' ventilator, however, the generated pressure can be set very low if desired and then a fall in compliance considerably prolongs the inspiratory phase. Indeed, it may even result in the generated pressure being inadequate to drive a sufficient volume into the patient to produce cycling, so that the ventilator becomes arrested in the inspiratory phase.

In all volume-cycled ventilators the difference between the maximum and minimum alveolar pressures is equal to the tidal volume divided by the compliance, as explained above. However, this does not determine the absolute value of either the maximum pressure, at the end of the inspiratory phase, or the minimum pressure, at the end of the expiratory phase. One of these must therefore be at least roughly controlled by an independent mechanism: otherwise, any slight difference between the inspiratory and expiratory tidal volumes would lead to progressive inflation or deflation and hence result in a gradual drift of the maximum and minimum pressures in the lungs, from one respiratory cycle to the next, until the lungs were either grossly over-inflated or else collapsed.

In a non-rebreathing circuit it is usually the pressure at the end of the expiratory phase which is controlled, by the patient expiring directly to atmosphere or to a negative pressure. In a closed circuit a spill valve controls the pressure at the end of the expiratory phase in a similar way, by connecting the patient to the atmosphere or to some negative pressure for a period at the end of the expiratory phase. If a blow-off valve is used instead of a spill valve, it is the pressure at the end of the inspiratory phase which is controlled. It should be noted that, if the blow-off valve is set at too high a pressure, the pressure at the end of the expiratory phase may still be positive. On the other hand if it is set too low, an excessive negative pressure may occur at the end of the expiratory phase. In any case, these pressures will change with changes in compliance.

Pressure-cycled ventilators

In a ventilator which is pressure-cycled at the end of either the inspiratory or the expiratory phase, the pressure at the cycling mechanism at the moment of cycling is precisely and solely determined by the ventilator. However, the pressure in the alveoli, which is the relevant one for the determination of tidal volume, differs from the cycling pressure. This is because, even at the moment of cycling, there is some flow, into or out of the lungs, which results in a pressure difference across the airway resistance between the cycling mechanism and the alveoli. Even with a normal airway resistance and a moderate flow this pressure difference can amount to 30 per cent of the maximum alveolar pressure; in an extreme case the alveolar pressure could easily be less than half the cycling pressure.

It is clear, therefore, that the tidal volume is greatly affected by changes in resistance as well as compliance. However, if the ventilator is a flow generator there will be a compensating change in the duration of the phase: roughly speaking, if the compliance is halved, half the volume will enter the lungs in half the time to produce the same cycling pressure. This compensation is slight in a ventilator which is pressure-cycled only at the end of a short inspiratory phase and time-cycled at the end of a relatively-long expiratory phase. On the other hand, in one which is a pressure-cycled flow generator in both phases, as is approximately the case in the Dräger 'Poliomat' and the Takaoka, the compensation can be complete: when the compliance is halved, not only will half the volume enter the lungs in half the time, but also it will take only half the time for this volume to come out. Therefore, in the time that used to be occupied by one respiratory cycle, there will now be two cycles, each of half the tidal volume. Therefore, the total ventilation remains unchanged, although the alveolar ventilation is decreased because the patient's dead space then forms a greater fraction of the tidal volume.[3]

If a leak develops in the patient circuit, cycling will still occur only when the cycling pressure is reached, assuming that the leak is not so large that this pressure cannot be reached. Therefore, the patient's tidal volume will not be much affected, but the generator will have to supply a greater volume of gas before cycling occurs. Consequently, with a high-pressure generator with high series resistance, or with a flow generator, the phase will be prolonged, the frequency reduced, and the ventilation decreased.

Time-cycled ventilators

A time-cycled flow generator, such as the Air-Shields 'Ventimeter' or the 'Amsterdam', is effectively volume-cycled since it supplies a fixed pattern of flow for a fixed time. Therefore the tidal volume is determined by the ventilator and is uninfluenced by the patient. If, as is invariably the case, the ventilator is time-cycled at the end of the expiratory phase as well as at the end of the inspiratory phase, the frequency is fixed and the total ventilation is uninfluenced by changes in the patient's lung characteristics. It will, however, be reduced if any leaks develop.

In time-cycled constant-pressure generators the performance depends considerably upon the type of pressure generator. If the ventilator resistance is small and the phase lasts for at least a second then, in most patients, the alveolar pressure becomes almost equal to the generated pressure by the end of the phase as in fig. 3.4. In these circumstances, therefore, the generated pressure must be relatively small. This is the type of performance to be expected of those ventilators in which the pressure is generated by a weighted concertina bag or a second-stage reducing valve, and in which adjustment of peak alveolar pressure is achieved by adjusting the weight, as in the East-Radcliffe and the East-Freeman, or by adjusting the setting of the reducing valve, as in the Bennett PR-2 and Frumin. The tidal volume then depends on the generated pressure and compliance. Further, if the airway resistance becomes very high, the full generated pressure may not be attained in the alveoli by the end of the phase. Therefore the ventilation is highly dependent upon the patient's lung characteristics. On the other hand, if a leak develops, more gas will flow from the pressure generator to compensate, and the ventilation will be little altered; except that, where inflation occurs from a bag, the volume limit set by its capacity may be reached before the end of the phase.

On the other hand, if the generated pressure is much greater than that required in the alveoli, and the ventilator resistance is much greater than the normal airway resistance, then the system becomes more like a flow generator. Therefore, if it is time-cycled in both phases, the ventilation will be nearly independent of the lung characteristics but greatly influenced by leaks. This mode of operation arises in the Air-Shields 'Respirator' from the blower characteristics.

Volume-limited ventilators

A volume-limited ventilator behaves like a volume-cycled one so far as the control of tidal volume is concerned, provided that the volume limit is determined by the characteristics of the ventilator. If, in addition, the ventilator is cycled by the pressure surrounding the volume-limiting bag cycling usually occurs immediately after the volume limit is reached, and the ventilator becomes effectively volume-cycled as explained on p. 107. This is the case for the Aga 'Spiropulsator', Dräger 'Pulmomat' and Ohio (Monaghan) 300 but not for the Blease 'Pulmoflator' for various reasons which are explained in the full account of that ventilator. If, instead, the ventilator is time-cycled then, when the volume limit is reached, the lungs are held inflated until the end of the phase (e.g. 'Barnet' Mark III on closed circuit, Dräger 'Spiromat 661' and 'Narkose Spiromat 650' on non-rebreathing circuit, Engström with no fresh-gas flow, and Manley). If the ventilator is time-cycled in both phases, as these ventilators are, the total ventilation will be uninfluenced by changes in the patient's lung characteristics—so long as the volume limit is reached in each inspiratory phase. The ventilation will, however, be reduced by any leak that may develop.

Pressure-limited ventilators

If a pressure limit comes into operation before the end of a phase then, no matter what type of generator the system may have been operating as up to that moment, it immediately becomes a constant-pressure generator although, if the pressure-limiting valve does not have 'ideal' characteristics, the pressure generator will have considerable internal resistance (see p. 131). If the valve does have ideal characteristics then, by the time it opens, the alveolar pressure has already approached the limiting pressure; therefore, in the remainder of the phase, the approach usually becomes very close. Thus an 'ideal' pressure-limiting valve has a fairly-close control over the alveolar pressure at the end of the phase in which it operates. If, in the other phase, there is no direct control of pressure, then either volume-cycling or volume-limiting must occur, as for example, in the Dräger 'Pulmomat' and the Mortimer ventilator, and in the 'Jefferson' ventilator with the volume-limited mode of operation. The pressure-limiting valve then serves merely to vent excess gas and to exercise a control over the general level of pressures in the lungs. On the other hand, if the pressure in the other phase is controlled—either by another pressure-limiting valve, as in the 'Jefferson' ventilator with the pressure-limited mode of operation; or by pressure-cycling, as in the Mörch I; or by the alveolar pressure becoming equal to the pressure from a pressure generator, as in the 'Cyclator CAV'—then the tidal volume depends on the difference between the two extremes of pressure and on the patient's lung characteristics.

If a positive-pressure-limiting valve is incorporated in the patient circuit of a 'bag in a bottle' ventilator to vent excess gas, and the ventilator is cycled by the pressure outside the bag, as, for example, in the 'Cyclator CAV', Dräger 'Pulmomat' and Mörch I, then it is the pressure set by the limiting valve and not the cycling pressure which controls the peak alveolar pressure. This is because the pressure-limiting valve must be set to open at less than the cycling pressure. Once it opens, the bag finishes emptying through the valve and then the pressure surrounding the bag, but not that inside it, quickly builds up to the cycling pressure. If the pressure-limiting valve is set to open at more than the cycling pressure, no excess gas can escape from the bag. Fresh gas, however continues to enter the bag which ultimately becomes permanently distended, and the lungs are then more or less held inflated at the pressure set by the limiting valve.

VENTILATORS IN WHICH THE TOTAL MINUTE-VOLUME VENTILATION IS DIRECTLY CONTROLLED

In a number of ventilators the total ventilation can be set directly, rather than by setting tidal volume and frequency separately. This ventilation is then maintained despite any changes in lung characteristics—at least within certain limits. The ventilation is, however, reduced if any leaks develop.

The arrangement which most commonly leads to this mode of operation is the non-rebreathing circuit shown in fig. 4.2 and discussed above. Fresh gas enters the circuit continuously at a fixed flow and eventually escapes intermittently through the expiratory port—but only after it has first been compressed into the lungs. Therefore the total minute-volume ventilation of the patient is equal to the fresh-gas flow and can be set by, and read from, a flowmeter or flowmeters in the fresh-gas supply line.

In some ventilators (Air-Shields 'Ventimeter' and 'Jefferson' on non-rebreathing circuit, and the Blease 'Paediatric') a separate driving mechanism provides the power for compressing the reservoir bag; then the requirement arises (see p. 139) that this drive shall be sufficient to empty the reservoir bag in each inspiratory phase. In other ventilators the fresh gas itself provides the power indirectly by inflating the reservoir bag against the force of springs ('Barnet' Marks II and III and Howells), of pneumatic pressure ('R.P.R.') or of the elasticity of the bag wall ('Autovent' and 'Minivent').

Many of these ventilators are, or can be, time-cycled in both phases, in which case the cycling-time controls are used to set the frequency. Then, in effect, the ventilator carries out the necessary arithmetic, of dividing the total minute-volume ventilation by the frequency, to determine the tidal volume. As mentioned above, ventilators of this type have been called 'minute-volume dividers'.[1]

In other ventilators (Howells, 'R.P.R.', and one mode of the 'Barnet' Mark III) both phases are volume-cycled, with reference to the concertina bag, so that the stroke volume of the bag is fixed. In this case the tidal volume of the patient is greater than the stroke volume of the bag (see p. 139). However, providing the ventilator operates as a flow generator or high-pressure generator during the inspiratory phase, as is the case for the three ventilators mentioned, the tidal volume is negligibly affected by changes of lung characteristics. Therefore in these ventilators the preset total minute-volume ventilation is divided by the preset tidal volume to determine the frequency.

In the 'Autovent' and 'Minivent' the tidal volume depends on the patient's lung characteristics but the frequency is still determined by dividing the tidal volume, whatever it may be, into the preset total ventilation.

The Engström ventilators can also be considered to be minute-volume dividers. This is clearly the case when the 'dosing valve' is closed and all the gas which enters the patient's lungs comes through the fresh-gas flowmeters. However, even when the dosing valve is open, providing the ventilator has been properly adjusted, the total ventilation is set by the sum of the litres/minute readings of the 'dosing valve' and the flowmeters. The frequency is set by another control and the ventilator 'works out' the appropriate tidal volume which is uninfluenced by the lung characteristics. The Engström 'Narcosis' ventilator seems to be unique in that it is intended to be operated as a minute-volume divider even on closed circuit.

SUMMARY OF THE EFFECTS OF CHANGES IN LUNG CHARACTERISTICS AND OF THE DEVELOPMENT OF LEAKS

From the foregoing study of the various types of ventilator a general rule emerges. Those ventilators which maintain a constant ventilation, irrespective of changes in lung characteristics, suffer a decrease in ventilation if any leak develops; on the other hand, the ventilation produced by those which can compensate for leaks is highly dependent upon lung characteristics.

The only exception to this rule occurs in the case of those closed-circuit ventilators with the following characteristics (e.g. Dräger 'Pulmomat', James):

Volume-cycled or time-cycled in both phases.
Flow generator or high-pressure generator in both phases.
Excess gas vented through a blow-off valve.

In these circumstances the tidal volume and frequency are fixed, or very nearly so, and therefore a ventilation is produced which is completely or substantially independent of the patient's lung characteristics. According to the general rule, therefore, the ventilation is decreased if any leaks develop. However, if the fresh-gas flow is larger than the patient's oxygen consumption, a volume of gas is normally expelled through the blow-off valve in each respiratory cycle. If now a leak gradually develops, it will progressively take over the function of the blow-off valve as a means of venting the excess gas. So long as the volume lost through the leak in each respiratory cycle is no more than that normally lost through the blow-off valve, then the patient's total ventilation will remain unchanged.

Finally, it is appropriate to mention the 'Autoanestheton' which can compensate equally well both for changes in lung characteristics and for leaks: a servo-mechanism adjusts the pressure supplied from a constant-pressure generator in each inspiratory phase in such a way as to maintain constant the end-expiratory carbon-dioxide concentration.

REFERENCES

1 WILSON A.B. Kinnier (1961) Discussion on patient-triggered ventilators. *Proc. R. Soc. Med.* **54**, 798.

2 MAPLESON W.W. (1963) An electric analogue for uptake and exchange of inert gases and other agents. *J. appl. Physiol.* **18**, 197–204.

3 COOPER E.A. (1967) Physiological deadspace in passive ventilation. *Anaesthesia*, **22**, 90–100 and 199–219.

CHAPTER 5

The Control of Automatic Ventilators

Amongst the many different automatic ventilators that have been designed and constructed there is a wide variety of functional specifications and an equally-wide variety of selections of parameters over which direct control is offered—to say nothing of the variety of wording to be found on the control knobs of different ventilators, even for controls which perform identical functions. It seems, therefore, that there is a need for some systematic technique for deducing, for any given ventilator, which controls should be adjusted, and in what way, in order to achieve any desired pattern of ventilation. Furthermore, the technique should reveal the way in which the pattern may be influenced by subsequent changes of compliance and resistance and what further adjustments might then be made to the controls to restore the desired pattern as nearly as possible.

The previous chapter included an outline of the relevant factors for the main types of functional specification. Now a diagram (fig. 5.1) is offered as a basis for developing the systematic technique just suggested for determining the mode of action of the controls of any ventilator. The diagram is first explained and then its application is illustrated by a few examples. It is hoped that the reader may find it helpful in a number of ways. For instance, for over twenty of the currently-available ventilators the mode of control has been discussed in some detail (see under 'Controls' in the individual accounts); for these discussions the diagram should form a useful 'map' of the pathways of control. Secondly, if the preceding discussion of the main types of functional specification was not clearly understood, again the diagram may serve as a useful map and guide. Finally, for ventilators in which the controls are not fully analysed in this book, it is hoped that the diagram will be helpful to the reader in making his own analyses.

THE 'BUTTERFLY' DIAGRAM

Fig. 5.1 shows, in the shape of a butterfly, the relationship between most of the parameters involved in the controlled ventilation of a patient. The parameters are of two kinds. Firstly, there are the lung characteristics of the patient (enclosed by hexagons) over which the anaesthetist has little control, and certainly no close control. Secondly,

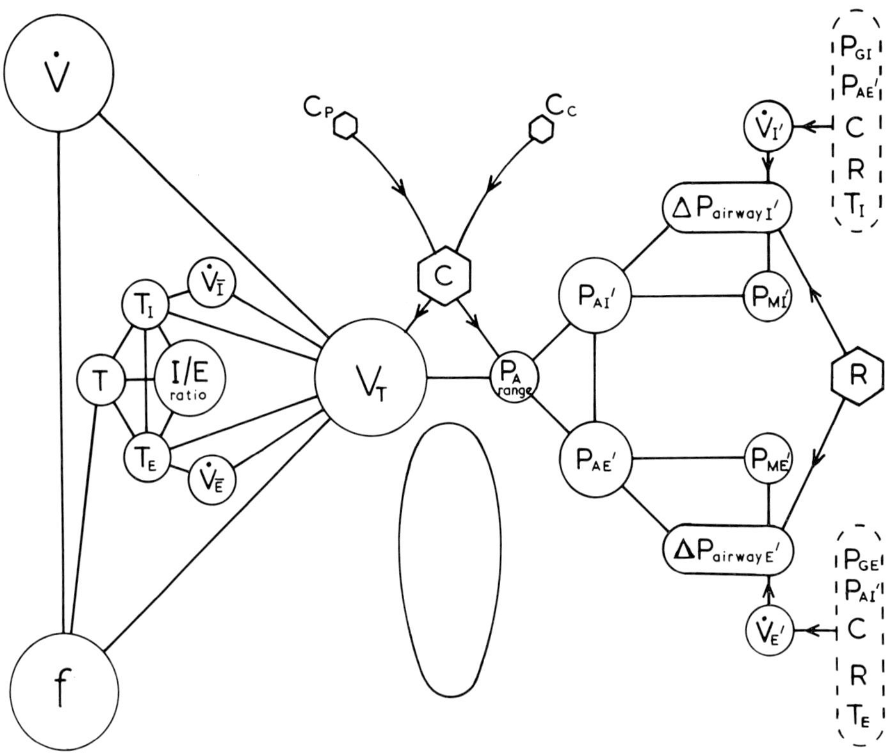

Fig. 5.1. The butterfly diagram showing the relationship between the principal parameters involved in automatic ventilation of the lungs. For full explanation see text.

C = total compliance.
C_C = chest-wall compliance.
C_P = pulmonary compliance.
f = respiratory frequency.
$P_{AI'}$ = alveolar pressure at the end of the inspiratory phase.
$P_{MI'}$ = machine pressure, which is usually similar to mouth pressure, at the end of the inspiratory phase.
$\Delta P_{airway\,I'}$ = pressure drop across the airway (from machine to alveoli) at the end of the inspiratory phase.
$P_{AE'}$, $P_{ME'}$, and $\Delta P_{airway\,E'}$ represent the corresponding pressures at the end of the expiratory phase.
$P_A$range = $P_{AI'} - P_{AE'}$.

P_{GI} = inspiratory generated pressure (if any).
P_{GE} = expiratory generated pressure (if any).
R = resistance (from machine to alveoli).
T = respiratory period.
T_I = inspiratory time.
T_E = expiratory time.
V_T = tidal volume.
$\dot{V}$ = total minute-volume ventilation.
$\dot{V}_{\bar{I}}$ = mean inspiratory flow rate.
$\dot{V}_{\bar{E}}$ = mean expiratory flow rate.
$\dot{V}_{I'}$ = flow rate at the end of the inspiratory phase.
$\dot{V}_{E'}$ = flow rate at the end of the expiratory phase.

there are those parameters (enclosed by circles) which can be controlled by the anaesthetist, usually fairly closely although often indirectly. Those which he is commonly most concerned to control are made to stand out by the use of large circles; those which he is able to control *directly* depend on the functional specification of the particular ventilator as explained below.

Where three parameters are linked together to form a triangle the three are interdependent; therefore, when any two are determined, the third is also, automatically, determined. For instance,

$$\text{total ventilation } \dot{V} = \text{tidal volume } V_{\mathrm{T}} \times \text{frequency } f.$$

Therefore the three large circles containing these parameters are linked in a triangle. Frequency f is the reciprocal of the respiratory period T so, when one is known, the other is determined. The total respiratory period T is made up of the inspiratory time T_{I} and the expiratory time T_{E}, so these three are linked in a triangle. T_{I}, T_{E} and the I/E ratio are also linked in a triangle since, if any two of these three are known, the third is determined. $\dot{V}_{\bar{\mathrm{I}}}$ is the mean inspiratory flow rate and is equal to the tidal volume V_{T} divided by the inspiratory time T_{I} although, in a time-cycled flow generator, it is T_{I} and $\dot{V}_{\bar{\mathrm{I}}}$ which are directly controlled and V_{T} which is determined indirectly as the product of the other two. Similarly, the mean expiratory flow rate $\dot{V}_{\bar{\mathrm{E}}}$ is equal to the tidal volume V_{T} divided by the expiratory time T_{E}.

This completes the left 'wing' of the 'butterfly', which is concerned with volumes, times, and flows. The right 'wing' is concerned mainly with pressures and is linked to the left 'wing' by the compliance.

Lines with arrows on them indicate that, as a general rule, influence can pass in the direction of the arrow only. Thus the pulmonary compliance C_{P} and the chest-wall compliance C_{C} together determine the total compliance C. The total compliance can influence the tidal volume V_{T} or the range of alveolar pressure P_{A}, and the last two can influence each other, but they cannot influence the compliance, except to a small and uncertain degree. Thus, if the range of alveolar pressure is determined, it and the compliance determine the tidal volume:

$$C \times (P_{\mathrm{A}}\text{range}) = V_{\mathrm{T}}.$$

Alternatively, if the tidal volume is determined, it and the compliance determine the range of alveolar pressure:

$$\frac{V_{\mathrm{T}}}{C} = P_{\mathrm{A}}\text{range}.$$

Notice, however, that it is only the *range* of alveolar pressure which is so determined and not the absolute level of either the maximum alveolar pressure which occurs at the end of the inspiratory phase, $P_{\mathrm{AI'}}$, or the minimum alveolar pressure which occurs at the end of

G

the expiratory phase, $P_{AE'}$. The range of alveolar pressure is equal to the difference between these two,

$$P_{AI'} - P_{AE'} = P_{A}\text{range},$$

so the three parameters are linked in a triangle.

Alveolar pressure can never be directly controlled whereas the pressure in the ventilator often can be, either throughout the phase by a pressure-generating mechanism, or else just at the end of a phase by a pressure-cycling mechanism. At any moment the pressure at the machine P_M is related to the alveolar pressure P_A by the pressure drop across the airway between the alveoli and the machine ΔP_{airway}:

$$P_M = P_A + \Delta P_{airway}.$$

Therefore the diagram includes two triangles, one representing the interdependence of these parameters at the end of the inspiratory phase,

$$P_{MI'} = P_{AI'} + \Delta P_{airway\ I'},$$

and the other representing it at the end of the expiratory phase,

$$P_{ME'} = P_{AE'} + \Delta P_{airway\ E'}.$$

In this last case $\Delta P_{airway\ E'}$ must be considered to be negative since the alveolar pressure is greater than the machine pressure during expiration.

The pressure drop across the airway is equal to the product of the resistance of the airway (from machine to alveoli) R and the flow rate through it. This is represented for the end of the inspiratory phase by arrowed lines from R and $\dot{V}_{I'}$ to $\Delta P_{airway\ I'}$ and for the end of the expiratory phase by arrowed lines from R and $\dot{V}_{E'}$ to $\Delta P_{airway\ E'}$.

The flow rate at the end of the inspiratory or expiratory phase is directly controlled in a ventilator which is a flow generator in the inspiratory or expiratory phase respectively. In a pressure generator the route of determination is more complex. If the inspiratory phase is considered first it will be appreciated that, in the case of a constant-pressure generator, the initial inspiratory flow will be equal to the difference between the generated pressure in inspiration P_{GI} and the initial alveolar pressure (which is the alveolar pressure at the end of expiration, $P_{AE'}$) divided by the airway resistance R:

$$\text{initial flow} = \frac{P_{GI} - P_{AE'}}{R}.$$

This flow then declines exponentially with a time constant CR for a time T_I. Therefore, in a constant-pressure generator a combination of no fewer than five factors, P_{GI}, $P_{AE'}$, C, R, and T_I, can influence the flow at the end of the inspiratory phase $\dot{V}_{I'}$. Since this is a one-way influence, and applies only to pressure generators and not to flow generators, the five parameters are enclosed by a broken line in fig. 5.1 and connected to $\dot{V}_{I'}$ by an arrowed line. In the expiratory phase similar considerations apply and the flow at the end of the expiratory phase $\dot{V}_{E'}$ is influenced by P_{GE}, $P_{AI'}$, C, R, and T_E. In expiration, however, with a constant-pressure generator, it is common for the flow to fall to zero before the end of the phase so that $\dot{V}_{E'}$ is commonly zero and $P_{AE'}$ is commonly equal to $P_{ME'}$.

Finally it should be borne in mind that, for the present purposes, the 'airway' extends from the alveoli to the ventilator and hence R includes the resistance of the endotracheal tube and connector and of the ventilator. In some ventilators, therefore, R may be markedly different in inspiration and expiration. For most purposes R should also be taken to include the tissue resistance of the lungs and chest wall.

APPLICATION OF THE BUTTERFLY DIAGRAM

The use of the butterfly diagram will be illustrated by considering three functional specifications, beginning with one in which the control of the more-important parameters is mostly indirect.

Functional Specification A

Inspiratory phase: constant-flow generator, pressure-cycled.
Expiratory phase: constant-pressure generator, time-cycled.

This specification applies to many of the earlier automatic ventilators and also to some that are in common use today—the 'Cyclator' and, in some modes of operation, the Bird Mark 7 and its variants and the Blease 'Pulmoflator'.

The first step in applying the butterfly diagram to a particular ventilator is to mark on the diagram those parameters which are directly controlled by the functional specification. This has been done by means of heavy outlines in fig. 5.2. For instance, since the ventilator is a constant-flow generator in the inspiratory phase, both the mean inspiratory flow rate $\dot{V}_{\bar{I}}$ and the flow rate at the end of inspiration $\dot{V}_{I'}$ are directly controlled. Since the ventilator is pressure-cycled at the end of the inspiratory phase, the pressure at the mouth at that time (which may be taken to be the same as the pressure at the machine) $P_{MI'}$ is directly controlled. Since the ventilator is a constant-pressure generator in the expiratory phase (P_{GE} directly controlled) the pressure at the mouth is controlled throughout the phase and therefore at the end of the phase $P_{ME'}$. Finally, since the expiratory phase is time-cycled, the expiratory time T_E is directly controlled. Compliance and resistance are, of course, determined by the patient.

At this stage it is worth noting the extent to which the total ventilation $\dot{V}$ (in many respects the most important single parameter) is separated from those parameters which are directly controlled. This emphasizes the indirectness of the control of ventilation with this functional specification. In fig. 5.2 the control pathways have been indicated by additional arrows on the lines and the logical sequence of deduction is as follows.

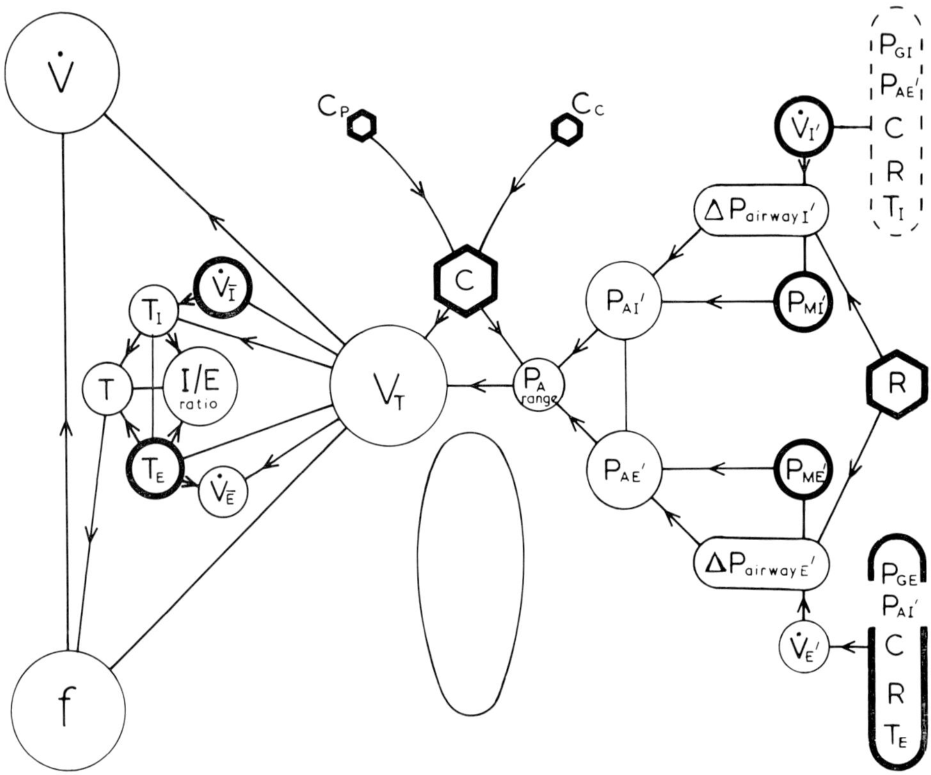

Fig. 5.2. The butterfly diagram marked for a ventilator with Functional Specification A,

inspiratory phase	:	constant-flow generator,
		pressure-cycled,
expiratory phase	:	constant-pressure generator,
		time-cycled,

(e.g. 'Cyclator', and also Bird Mark 7, and Blease 'Pulmoflator' in some modes). The parameters marked with a heavy outline are those which are directly controlled by the ventilator or determined by the lung characteristics. The remaining parameters are determined indirectly by the pathways indicated by the arrows.

Resistance R is set by the patient and $\dot{V}_{I'}$ is equal to the inspiratory generated flow. These two determine the pressure drop across the airway at the end of the inspiratory phase $\Delta P_{airway\ I'}$. This, in combination with $P_{MI'}$, which is the cycling pressure, determines $P_{AI'}$, the alveolar pressure at the end of the inspiratory phase. Commonly flow will have ceased before the end of the expiratory phase so that $\dot{V}_{E'}$ will be zero. (If not, it will be dependent upon P_{GE} and T_E which are directly controlled, C and R which are determined by the patient, and $P_{AI'}$ whose manner of determination has just been described.) If $\dot{V}_{E'}$ is zero so is $\Delta P_{airway\ E'}$. Therefore $P_{AE'}$ is equal to $P_{ME'}$; the alveolar pressure at the end of the expiratory phase is equal to the mouth pressure at the end of the phase which is the same as the expiratory generated pressure. Since $P_{AI'}$ and $P_{AE'}$ are determined, the P_A range is also determined and this, in combination with the compliance C, determines the tidal volume V_T. The inspiratory time T_I is the time taken to deliver the tidal volume at the mean inspiratory flow $\dot{V}_{\bar{I}}$, which is the inspiratory generated flow. The now-determined T_I, together with the directly-controlled T_E, determines the I/E ratio and the inspiratory period T, and hence the frequency f. Finally, V_T and f determine the total ventilation $\dot{V}$.

The above argument shows the pathways by which each parameter of ventilation is determined when a ventilator with this functional specification is connected to a patient. But the anaesthetist does not have to follow these pathways in order to make the ventilator work: the ventilator follows them automatically and delivers the ventilation which is dictated (in the manner just described) by the lung characteristics of the patient and the particular numerical values of the four elements of the functional specification. The anaesthetist becomes involved when, having connected the ventilator to the patient and switched on, he realizes that the ventilation is unsatisfactory in some way and seeks to rectify it.

Suppose he wishes to increase the tidal volume. The obvious course is to increase the cycling pressure $P_{MI'}$. $\Delta P_{airway\ I'}$ is unaltered, so $P_{AI'}$ is increased by an equal amount. Assuming that $P_{AE'}$ is unaltered there will be an equal increase in $P_A$range and so the tidal volume V_T will indeed be increased. However, various repercussions follow. Increasing V_T while leaving $\dot{V}_{\bar{I}}$ unaltered must increase T_I. This alters the I/E ratio and increases T. Therefore, the respiratory frequency f is decreased and the increase in total ventilation $\dot{V}$ is less than the increase in tidal volume. If these repercussions are to be avoided it is necessary to increase the generated flow so that $\dot{V}_{\bar{I}}$ is increased in proportion to V_T; then T_I, T, and f are unaltered. However, if the generated flow is increased, then so is the flow at the end of inspiration $\dot{V}_{I'}$. Therefore $\Delta P_{airway\ I'}$ is increased and so $P_{AI'}$ and the tidal volume are decreased and a further increase of the cycling pressure $P_{MI'}$ will be necessary to compensate.

Suppose now that the anaesthetist wishes to increase the frequency. The simplest way of doing this is to reduce the cycling time in the expiratory phase T_E. This, by means of reducing T, will increase f and hence $\dot{V}$. It will also incidentally alter the I/E ratio but perhaps the anaesthetist will not think this important enough to correct. However, it should be noted that T_E is also involved in the control of $\dot{V}_{E'}$: if the expiratory time is made too short the expiratory flow may not fall to zero by the end of the phase. If this occurs $\Delta P_{airway\ E'}$ will no longer be zero and $P_{AE'}$ will be increased: if the generated pressure in the expiratory phase was previously atmospheric the alveolar pressure will not now fall fully to atmospheric. Furthermore this will lead to a reduction in P_A range, V_T, T_I, and T unless the generated pressure can be made sufficiently negative to restore $P_{AE'}$ to its former level.

Having worked through these two instances of how deliberately to alter a parameter of ventilation, the reader can no doubt see how to use the diagram to work out the effects of a change in compliance or resistance and how to correct them as far as possible.

It is evident that, with Functional Specification A, the precise control of what are usually considered the more-important parameters of ventilation is very indirect and is complicated by interactions between controls. Therefore it is appropriate to look at other ventilators offering direct control of the more important parameters.

Functional Specification B

The Air-Shields 'Ventimeter' and 'E.G.C. Paediatric' ventilators have the following functional specification:

Inspiratory phase: constant-flow generator, time-cycled.
Expiratory phase: constant-pressure generator, time-cycled.

A diagram, suitably marked and arrowed, is shown in fig. 5.3. The control pathways are generally much shorter than for the previous example. Thus the constant inspiratory generated flow $\dot{V}_{\bar{I}}$ and inspiratory cycling time T_I determine the tidal volume V_T, while the two cycling times determine the I/E ratio and T and hence the frequency f and so, with V_T, the total ventilation $\dot{V}$. In this example the only pressures to be in any way directly controlled are expiratory ones. $P_{ME'}$ is equal to the generated pressure and, as with the first example, if $\dot{V}_{E'}$ is zero, $P_{AE'}$ is equal to $P_{ME'}$. Inspiratory pressures are dependent on the tidal volume V_T. V_T, in combination with the compliance C, determines the P_A range which, together with $P_{AE'}$, determines $P_{AI'}$. The mouth pressure at the end of the inspiratory phase $P_{MI'}$ exceeds this by the pressure drop across the airway at the time $\Delta P_{\text{airway I}'}$ which, as before, is determined by R and $\dot{V}_{I'}$.

With this functional specification the interaction of controls is considerably-less complex but their use is not entirely straightforward. Thus, increasing the generated flow, and thereby $\dot{V}_{\bar{I}}$, while leaving T_I unaltered will increase V_T and $\dot{V}$; but if the frequency f is increased without change of the I/E ratio, by decreasing T_I and T_E in the same proportion, the tidal volume V_T will be decreased and the ventilation $\dot{V}$ will remain unaltered. This may perhaps be considered to be a desirable characteristic but no doubt some would also consider it to be a little unexpected.

Similar considerations apply to the 'Amsterdam Infant Ventilator'. This has the same functional specification but the control of the inspiratory and expiratory cycling times T_I and T_E is not direct. Instead, controls are provided for the frequency f (and hence T) and for the I/E ratio so that T_I and T_E are determined indirectly. But if the frequency f is increased, the inspiratory and expiratory times T_I and T_E are decreased so that the tidal volume V_T is decreased but the ventilation $\dot{V}$ is unaltered.

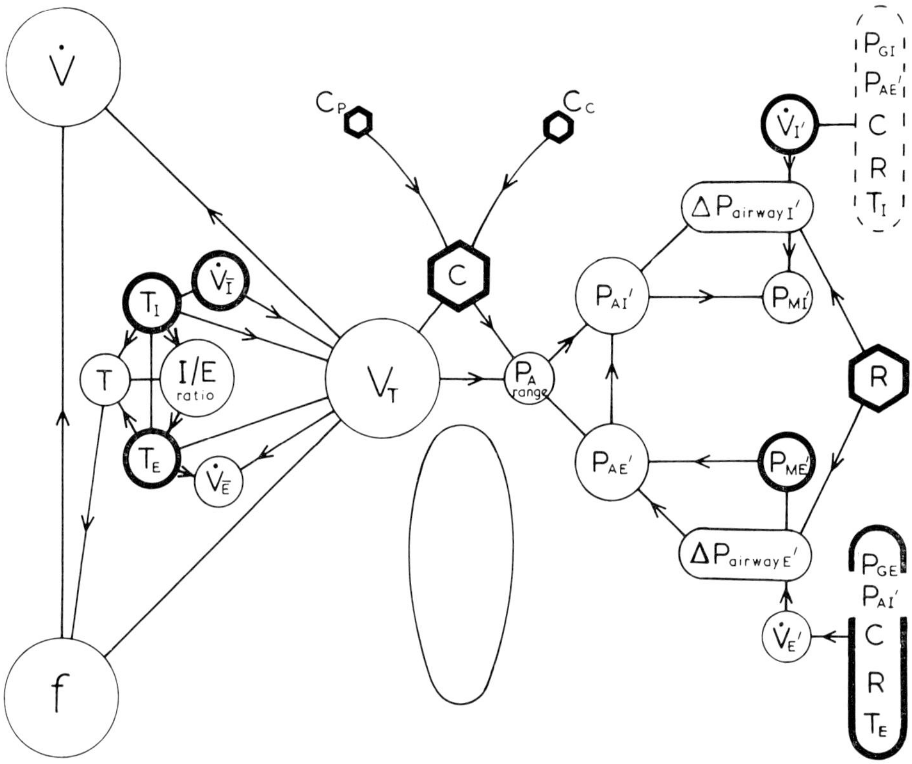

Fig. 5.3. The butterfly diagram marked (as in fig. 5.2) for a ventilator with Functional Specification B,

inspiratory phase : constant-flow generator,
time-cycled,
expiratory phase : constant-pressure generator,
time-cycled,

in which the inspiratory and expiratory times and the inspiratory generated flow are directly controlled (e.g. Air-Shields 'Ventimeter' and 'E.G.C. Paediatric').

Functional Specification C

The more-obvious arrangement of direct control of tidal volume and frequency is provided in the Cape-Waine and the Lundia ventilators. For both these ventilators the functional specification at its simplest is as follows:

Inspiratory phase: non-constant-flow generator, volume-cycled and time-cycled.
Expiratory phase: constant-pressure generator, time-cycled.

A marked and arrowed diagram is shown in fig. 5.4. As in the 'Amsterdam' the cycling times T_I and T_E are not directly controlled but are determined by the frequency f which is adjustable and the I/E ratio which in these ventilators is, at least nominally,

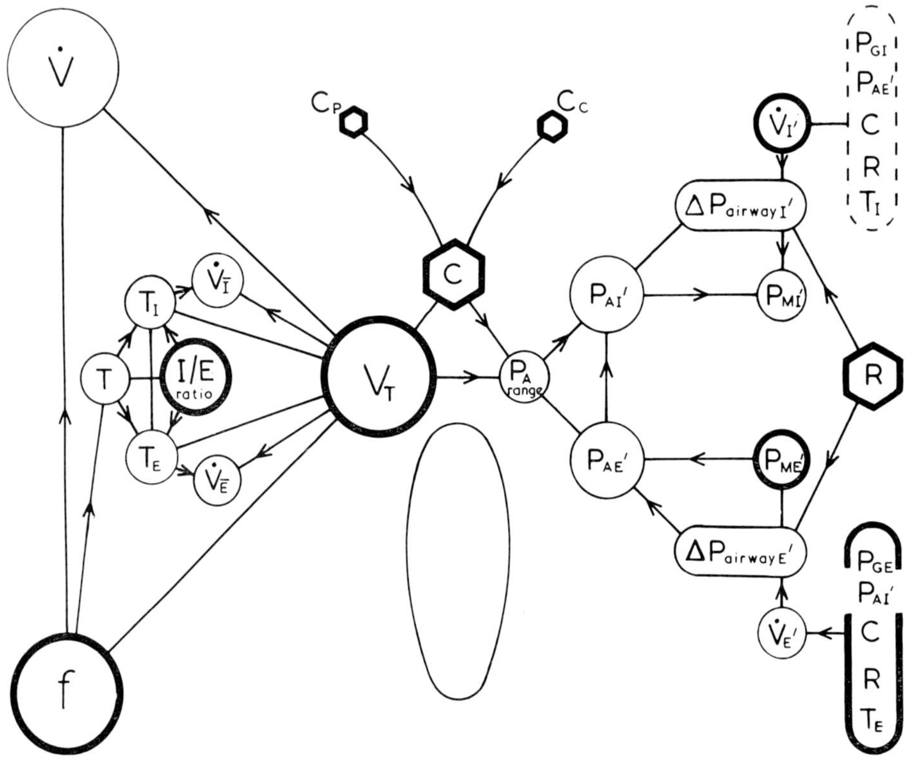

Fig. 5.4. The butterfly diagram marked (as in fig. 5.2) for a ventilator with Functional Specification C,

inspiratory phase	:	non-constant-flow generator, volume-cycled and time-cycled,
expiratory phase	:	constant-pressure generator, time-cycled,

in which, although the cycling volume is directly controlled, the inspiratory and expiratory times are determined indirectly from direct control of the frequency and from a fixed inspiratory-expiratory ratio, and the generated flow is determined indirectly from the tidal volume and the inspiratory time (e.g. Cape-Waine and Lundia ventilators at their simplest).

fixed. Therefore, increasing the frequency f decreases the inspiratory and expiratory times T_I and T_E but leaves the tidal volume V_T unaltered since this is separately regulated by the volume control. Thus the diagram reflects the fact that the inspiratory generated flow is not directly controlled but is determined indirectly from the tidal volume and inspiratory time. Pressures are determined in the same way as in Functional Specification B except that the pattern of inspiratory generated flow is such that the flow at the end of the inspiratory phase $\dot{V}_{I'}$ is always zero.

'Volume preset', 'pressure preset', and 'ventilation preset'

In the U.S.A. it is common to speak of ventilators as 'volume preset' or 'pressure preset'.

The term 'volume preset' is applied to those ventilators in which the tidal volume is controlled by the ventilator and is uninfluenced by lung characteristics. This can arise from volume-cycling or volume-limiting or because the ventilator operates as a time-cycled flow generator in one phase. Thus the control of tidal volume is either direct or at least derived from the left wing of the butterfly diagram. Control of some of the pressures in the right wing of the diagram is also derived partly from the left wing. Thus the flux of control is from left to right.

The term 'pressure preset' is applied to those ventilators in which pressures are controlled by pressure-cycling, pressure-limiting, or low-pressure generation, and the tidal volume is determined only indirectly through the compliance. In other words the flux of control in the diagram is from right to left.

Thus the terms 'volume preset' and 'pressure preset' provide a useful distinction which correlates closely with the construction of the diagram. However, it is very relevant to note that time is an important element in the diagram and to realize that total ventilation involves time as well as volume.

Therefore a ventilator which can be classed as 'volume preset' does not necessarily produce a fixed total ventilation, irrespective of lung characteristics, because the timing may alter. For instance, a volume-cycled low-pressure generator (the 'Vellore') would be classed as 'volume preset'; but, as explained in Chapter 4, an increase in resistance or decrease in compliance would reduce the mean inspiratory flow rate $\dot{V}_{\bar{I}}$ and prolong the inspiratory phase T_I so that the frequency f and the ventilation $\dot{V}$ would be reduced. On the other hand, a ventilator which is a pressure-cycled flow generator in both phases, as is approximately the case in the Dräger 'Poliomat' and Takaoka, would be classed as 'pressure preset'; yet any change in tidal volume V_T which resulted from a change in compliance or resistance would, with the constant $\dot{V}_{\bar{I}}$ and $\dot{V}_{\bar{E}}$ result in proportional changes in T_I and T_E and hence in T. Therefore there would be a precisely-compensating change in f, leaving the total ventilation $\dot{V}$ unaltered.

Thus, if the terms 'volume preset' and 'pressure preset' are to be used at all, it seems sensible to add the term 'ventilation preset'. Then a ventilator which is a pressure-cycled flow generator in both phases is 'ventilation preset' as well as 'pressure preset'; on the other hand a 'volume preset' ventilator is also 'ventilation preset' only if its timing is uninfluenced by lung characteristics.

All ventilators which operate as 'minute-volume dividers' are 'ventilation preset' although only some of them (the ones with fixed timing) are also 'volume preset'.

In the 'Autovent' and 'Minivent' both tidal volume and peak alveolar and mouth pressures are dependent upon lung characteristics although the total ventilation is preset. Therefore these ventilators, although 'ventilation preset', are neither 'volume preset' nor 'pressure preset'.

CHAPTER 6

Automatic Ventilation of Infants

Small children and neonates who require artificial ventilation present special problems. These derive from their low compliance, and the need for small tidal volumes, high respiratory frequencies, and low inspiratory flows. In general, automatic ventilators designed for adults are not able to meet these requirements in one or more respects, and, at least for the duration of surgical procedures, manual ventilation is commonly preferred. However, this is not practicable when a longer period of ventilation is needed, and it is then necessary to make use of an automatic ventilator.

Most automatic ventilators are designed for adults and trial confirms that, while some may just be satisfactory, the majority are not suitable for infants and children. A few ventilators designed specifically for this purpose and special attachments for fitting to some adult ventilators are now available. Nevertheless, an awareness of the problems involved is essential before an assessment can be made of the suitability of any ventilator, with or without modification, for paediatric use.

PHYSIOLOGICAL CRITERIA FOR VENTILATION IN INFANTS AND CHILDREN

There is general agreement about the range of normal values of ventilatory parameters in spontaneously-breathing adults and infants, although there are comparatively few reports on the latter. Typical values of these are set out in Table 6.1.

Clearly any ventilator designed or modified for artificial ventilation of infants must be capable of providing respiratory parameters which conform with those indicated in this table.

General theoretical considerations

Inspiratory flow rate

In the case of an adult, typical parameters of ventilation, taken from Table 6.1, are:

tidal volume = 500 ml,
respiratory frequency = 16 per minute.

Table 6.1

	Weight (kg)	Height (cm)	Total ventilation (litres/min)	Respiratory frequency (per min)	Tidal volume (ml)	Total compliance (ml/cmH$_2$O)	Airway resistance (cmH$_2$O/(litre/sec))
Neonate	3·2	49·4	0·64	40	16	2·5	31
1 year	9·0	71·0	1·5	30	50	10	20
8 years	25·0	125	4·0	20	200	25	6
Adult	66·0	171	8·0	16	500	50	2

Therefore, each respiratory cycle lasts $\frac{60}{16} = 3{\cdot}75$ sec.

If the inspiratory-expiratory ratio = 1 : 2,

the inspiratory phase lasts $\frac{1}{3} \times 3{\cdot}75 = 1{\cdot}25$ sec.

In order that 500 ml shall enter the lungs in 1·25 sec,

$$\text{the average inspiratory flow must} = \frac{500}{1{\cdot}25}\ \text{ml/sec}, \quad = 24\ \text{litres/min}.$$

In the case of a neonate, typical parameters of ventilation, taken from Table 6.1, are:—

tidal volume = 16 ml,
respiratory frequency = 40 per minute.

Therefore, each respiratory cycle lasts $\frac{60}{40} = 1{\cdot}5$ sec.

Assume the inspiratory-expiratory ratio to be kept at 1 : 2.
Then, the inspiratory phase lasts $\frac{1}{3} \times 1{\cdot}5 = 0{\cdot}5$ sec.

In order that 16 ml shall enter the lungs in 0·5 sec,

$$\text{the average inspiratory flow must} = \frac{16}{0{\cdot}5}\ \text{ml/sec}, \quad = 1{\cdot}9\ \text{litres/min}.$$

Pressure in the alveoli

$$\text{Compliance} = \frac{\text{tidal volume}}{\text{pressure in the alveoli}}.$$

Therefore, pressure in the alveoli at the end of the inspiratory phase.

$$= \frac{\text{tidal volume}}{\text{compliance}} = \frac{16}{2{\cdot}5}\ \text{cmH}_2\text{O} = 6{\cdot}4\ \text{cmH}_2\text{O}.$$

Pressure at the mouth

Pressure at the mouth at the end of the inspiratory phase

$$= \text{pressure in the alveoli} + \text{pressure drop across the airway.}$$

Pressure drop across the airway = inspiratory flow × airway resistance,

$$= \frac{1{\cdot}9}{60} \times 31 = 1{\cdot}0 \text{ cmH}_2\text{O}.$$

Therefore, pressure at the mouth = 6·4 + 1·0,

$$= 7{\cdot}4 \text{ cmH}_2\text{O}.$$

It is now necessary to examine the performance of various ventilators.

FLOW GENERATORS

Theoretical considerations

A flow generator whose flow rate can be adjusted to the necessary low level will function so long as its cycling mechanism can be appropriately adjusted, i.e. to 16 ml for volume cycling; to 0·5 sec for time cycling; and to 7·4 cmH_2O for pressure cycling.

If the flow is much greater than 2 litres/min then either too large a tidal volume will be delivered in the right time, or else the desired tidal volume will be delivered in too short a time, resulting in an extreme inspiratory-expiratory ratio. For instance, suppose the flow from the ventilator can be brought down to 20 litres/min; then a tidal volume of 16 ml will be delivered in 0·05 sec. At the end of this time the pressure in the lungs will be 6·4 cmH_2O as before. However, the pressure drop across the airway would now be 20/60 × 31 = 10·3 cmH_2O if the resistance were linear, and, because of turbulence, could well rise above 40 cmH_2O, in which case the pressure at the mouth at the end of the inspiratory phase would be at least 16·7 cmH_2O and could well be over 46 cmH_2O.

If such a ventilator were pressure-cycled it would have to be possible to adjust the cycling mechanism to as high a value as 46 cmH_2O. If it were time-cycled it would have to be possible to adjust the cycling mechanism to the low value of 0·05 sec. With higher flows the cycling time would have to be even shorter and the cycling pressure even greater!

If a time-cycled ventilator cannot be adjusted to the short time required, too large a tidal volume will be delivered. If a pressure-cycled mechanism cannot be adjusted to the required high level, the machine may cycle immediately flow starts, the cycling mechanism being actuated merely by the pressure difference across the airway.

Some experimental results

Some experiments have been reported[1] in which certain flow generators were connected to models of neonatal and infant lungs. In the case of the 'Aintree' ventilator, a pressure-cycled flow generator, the flow could be adjusted to the level required and the ventilator functioned for all model sizes. However, with the 'Cyclator' Mark I, another pressure-cycled flow generator, the flow was at that time fixed at about 40 litres/min by the design of the injector and the pressure of the driving gas. In the models of a 1-year old and an 8-year old child the desired ventilation could be obtained with this ventilator, but the tidal volume was delivered in a very short time. This resulted in inspiratory-expiratory ratios of 1 : 9 and 1 : 6 respectively. In the neonate model the maximum cycling pressure of 35 cmH_2O was reached before any appreciable volume exchange occurred. Recently, the 'Cyclator' Mark II has become available which, with suitable injectors and with a variable restrictor for the entrainment port, permits the adjustment of the inspiratory flow to low levels.

A Beaver II ventilator, a volume-cycled flow generator, performed adequately for the model of an 8-year old. With the smaller model lungs a serious defect was found. The Beaver valve permitted total rebreathing to occur at the low volumes required. This could be eliminated by substituting a Ruben valve but a considerable volume of gas then escaped during the inspiratory phase through the expiratory port. This was wasteful, but did not prevent ventilation of the model.

PRESSURE GENERATORS

Theoretical considerations

In a pressure generator which is pressure-cycled the performance of the ventilator depends upon the relationship between the generated pressure and the cycling pressure. If the generated pressure is much higher than the cycling pressure the inflating flow will not fall off much as inflation proceeds. The performance of such a ventilator therefore approaches that of a flow generator and the same disadvantages apply. If, on the other hand, the generated pressure is only slightly in excess of the cycling pressure, the ventilator will be as suitable for small subjects as for adults, always assuming that the cycling pressure can be set low enough.

If a constant pressure is applied to the lungs for long enough, the pressure in the alveoli will rise to equal it. Whether or not this is achieved within the allotted inspiratory time depends on the relationship between the respiratory time and the time constant of the lungs and airways. This time constant is equal to the product of compliance and resistance.

$$=0{\cdot}0025\,\frac{\text{litre}}{\text{cmH}_2\text{O}}\times 31\,\frac{\text{cmH}_2\text{O.sec}}{\text{litre}}=0{\cdot}08\text{ sec.}$$

If the duration of the inspiratory phase is 3 or more times the time constant then at the end of the phase the pressure in the alveoli will be at least 95% of the generated pressure (see Chapter 3). The inspiratory time of 0·5 sec is indeed more than 3 times the time constant of 0·08 sec; therefore the pressure in the alveoli will virtually equal the generated pressure by the end of the inspiratory phase. The pressure in the alveoli has already been determined as being 6·4 cmH_2O at the end of the inspiratory phase. The generated pressure must therefore be 6·4 cmH_2O. Table 6.2 summarizes the values to which the various parameters must be adjusted if a ventilator is to provide a normal total ventilation in a neonate. Approximate values for an adult are listed for comparison. If an adult ventilator is capable of providing the small total ventilation required by the neonate, then it will also be able to ventilate larger children.

Table 6.2

	Neonate	Adult
Total minute-volume ventilation (ml)	640	8000
Tidal volume (ml)	16	500
Frequency per minute	40	16
Inspiratory time (sec)	0·5	1·25
Inspiratory flow (litres/min)	1·9	24
Peak pressure in alveoli (cmH_2O)	6·4	10
Pressure at mouth (cmH_2O)	7·4	12

Some experimental results

Three pressure generators were reported on.[1] All of them were time-cycled, the 'Barnet' Mark II, the 'Jefferson', and the unmodified 'Pneumotron'. The last was found to behave as a time-cycled pressure generator. The timing and the generated pressure could be varied over a wide range and could be adjusted to suit even the neonate. The 'Jefferson' ventilator was found to have a fixed inspiratory time and the frequency could be adjusted by changing the length of the expiratory phase. When the ventilator was set to 40 and to 30 respirations per minute for the two smaller models, it was found that the inspiratory-expiratory ratios were 1·5 : 1 and 1 : 1 respectively. However, the generated pressure could be adjusted so that the required tidal volume was just delivered in the fixed inspiratory time. This ventilator was therefore satisfactory apart from the inspiratory-expiratory ratio. In the 'Barnet' Mark II the inspiratory and expiratory times could be adjusted to the required values, but the generated pressure could not be reduced below about 40 cmH_2O. Therefore the required tidal volume was delivered in a very short time (0·3 sec) in the neonate, but over-inflation did not occur because of the emptying of the concertina bag which contained only the tidal volume. During the rest of the inspiratory time the lungs were held inflated until the timing circuit cycled the mechanism to expiration. In the 'Barnet' Mark III the resistance to inspiratory flow can be adjusted so that inflation is just completed in the preset inspiratory time.

USING AN ADULT VENTILATOR ON A NEONATE

From the foregoing it is evident that the main reason why many adult ventilators fail to perform satisfactorily for infants is that the inspiratory flow is too high and cannot be reduced to the low level required. This carries with it the attendant dangers of over-inflation, or premature triggering of the cycling mechanism leading to under-inflation.

The general solution of these problems lies, either,

(A) in reducing the inflating flow by, either,

(1) a resistance in series with the ventilator

or (2) modification of the ventilator itself, or

(B) in disposing of excess flow by, either,

(1) a leak in the circuit

or (2) a device in parallel with the patient which absorbs the excess flow.

Naturally, whichever method is used should interfere as little as possible with the functioning of the ventilator controls. It should also neither cause rebreathing nor interfere with any patient-triggering device which may be part of the ventilator.

In the case of pressure generators any or all of these solutions can be applied. However, in the case of flow generators, by definition, the flow cannot be altered by adding external resistance; one of the other solutions therefore must be adopted or else the ventilator itself must be modified.

(A) Reduction of the inflating flow

(1) A resistance in the inspiratory path (fig. 61.)

A screw clamp can be placed on the inspiratory tubing and tightened until the inspiratory flow is reduced and the required tidal volume just delivered in the preset inspiratory time. The adjustment of the clamp is critical and difficult to get right. This approach is not practical unless a specially-designed adjustable resistor is available.

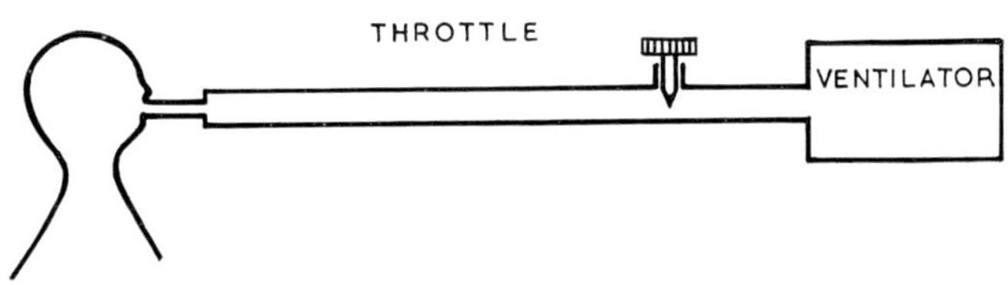

Fig. 6.1.

A period during which the pressure is held in the lungs can be avoided without the use of any external device if a more-extreme inspiratory-expiratory ratio than 1 : 2 is acceptable: the inspiratory time can be shortened until it is just sufficient for inflation to be completed and the expiratory time increased to compensate.

(2) Modification of the ventilator

This is illustrated by the introduction of the modifications already mentioned into the later Marks of the 'Barnet' and the 'Cyclator'.

(B) Disposal of excess flow

(1) A leak in the circuit (fig. 6.2)

Flow generators. If the flow from a flow-generating ventilator cannot be reduced to the required level, a leak can be introduced into the system and adjusted so as to dispose of the excess flow. The system now behaves (see p. 85) like a pressure generator with a low generated pressure which is equal to the pressure in the system when all the flow is passing through the leak. The flow into the patient is high at the beginning of the inspiratory phase, and tails off towards the end.

Perhaps fortunately, the absence of cuffs on endotracheal tubes for infants usually

Fig. 6.2.

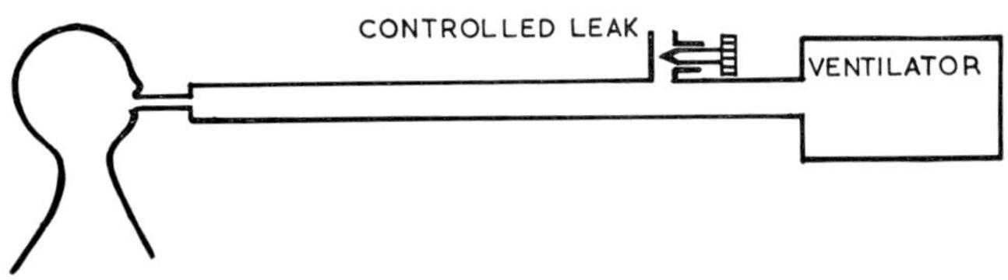

leads to a variable amount of leakage around the endotracheal tube during the inspiratory phase. Such a leak operates in the direction of making an adult ventilator perform a little better than it would do otherwise. However, the reported[1] measurements indicate that the effect is small and unlikely to make the difference between satisfactory and unsatisfactory ventilation.

In the case of the 'Cyclator' an adjustable leak can be introduced on the patient side of the inflating valve. This leak may be adjusted for each infant so that ventilation is satisfactory. The adjustment, though difficult, is quite practical and in fact the arrangement has worked well in our experience for several weeks on a child with tetanus.

The Blease 'Pulmoflator' P. 4 was reported[1] to have ventilated all the models satisfactorily. A study of its mechanism shows that it is fundamentally a flow generator in which the flow (coming from a compressor) cannot be adjusted. However, the control labelled 'length of inspiration' is in fact an adjustable leak which can be used to dispose of any excess flow. This leak happens to be in the driving circuit, and not in the patient circuit, but the effect is the same.

Pressure generators. If a pressure generator will not ventilate small subjects this is because the generated pressure is too high, and its performance approaches that of a flow generator. A controlled leak would therefore be just as effective here as in a flow generator in reducing the flow into the lungs.

With both types of ventilator the use of a leak requires a higher flow of fresh gas than the total ventilation to be delivered to the child—at least when a non-rebreathing circuit is used. It is essential therefore that care be taken to see that the supply of fresh gas is such that the proper total ventilation of the patient is maintained and that the introduction of the leak is not followed by an undesirable diminution in the ventilation.

(2) A parallel compliance and resistance (fig. 6.3)

An artificial compliance in parallel with the child's lungs can be adjusted so that the two together are equal to the compliance of an adult and will therefore accept an adult tidal volume between them. In order to ensure that the child receives its appropriate fraction of this adult tidal volume in all circumstances, it is essential that a suitable resistance be inserted in series with the artificial compliance to form a complete dummy lung.

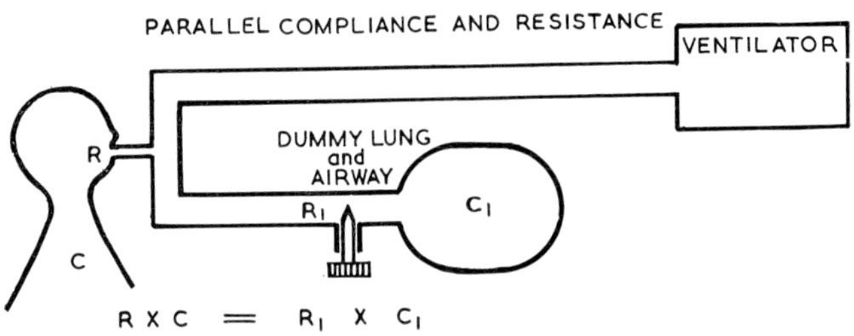

Fig. 6.3.

The product of compliance and resistance (i.e. the time constant) of the dummy lung should be equal to the product of the compliance and resistance of the child's lungs and airways. This will ensure that the inflation of the child's lung and of the dummy lung occurs simultaneously. In these circumstances the ventilator performs as though it were ventilating an adult, although at a much higher frequency and with a much shorter inspiratory period. The cycling pressure is lower and any pressure-cycling mechanism must operate at a low-enough pressure.

In principle the dummy lung should provide a general solution for all adult ventilators, since, in effect, it converts the infant into an adult, instead of seeking to convert an adult ventilator into an infant ventilator. However, one limitation is that the dummy lung interferes with the operation of many patient-triggering devices. When the infant takes a small breath this is readily drawn from the dummy lung without producing any pressure, volume, or flow, signal within the ventilator. This difficulty could be overcome by inserting a flow-sensitive trigger mechanism between the infant and the dummy lung.

CONCLUSION

It is clear that the proper ventilation of a small child does involve problems when the use of methods and equipment normally intended for ventilating adults is contemplated.

Naturally, the best solution is the use of an automatic ventilator in which the values of the various parameters approximate to those of small subjects, such as the 'Amsterdam', the 'E.G.C.', the Bourns, and the Starling, or a suitable attachment for an adult ventilator, such as the Bird 'Infant J circuit', and the Blease 'Paediatric' ventilator.

For some time to come a likely problem confronting the clinical anaesthetist is that of adapting an adult ventilator to a child. Our studies have impressed us with the primary need for a clear understanding of the physical functioning of the particular ventilator in question. Only then can the matter be taken further. No single compensatory device is universally applicable, though of the several described here the dummy lung seems most promising. There are, however, serious practical disadvantages of a bulky object near to the child's head and the still present need for the ventilator to function at high respiratory frequencies. The insertion of a resistance or of a leak in the inspiratory pathway may be suitable alternatives, but theory and our own experimental and clinical experience show that their adjustment is critical, and it is unlikely that simply-constructed devices will be more than partially satisfactory. In any case, the ultimate evidence of satisfactory ventilation must be derived from volume measurements of expiration. At the moment this cannot be done readily with the small ventilation meters on the market, like the Wright respirometer. There is clearly a need not only for specially-designed ventilators but also for ventilation-measuring equipment suitable for children. Some progress has already been made in this latter direction, and at least one satisfactory method of measuring ventilation in infants has been described.[2]

REFERENCES

1 Mushin W.W., Mapleson W.W. and Lunn J.N. (1962) Problems of automatic ventilation in infants and children. *Br. J. Anaesth.* **34**, 514.

2 Lunn J.N., Molyneux L. and Pask E.A. (1965) A device for the measurement of ventilation in young children under general anaesthesia. *Anaesthesia*, **20**, 135.

CHAPTER 7

Laboratory Testing of Automatic Ventilators

'STATIC' TESTS

It is possible to derive a certain amount of information about the functioning of a ventilator by 'static' measurements, that is, by measurements of the physical characteristics of various elements of the ventilator while it is arrested at a suitable point in its cycle of operation. Measurements of the entrainment characteristics of injectors, of the pressure-volume characteristics of weighted or spring-loaded bags, and of the pressure-flow characteristics of certain valves and breathing tubes, will usually show how closely a ventilator approximates to a flow generator or pressure generator when this is not immediately obvious from the design of the ventilator. Such tests were made on many ventilators and the results are given in graphical form in the accounts of the ventilators.

'DYNAMIC' TESTS—GENERAL

However, our main programme of testing was a 'dynamic' one in which each ventilator was connected to a model lung, the compliance and resistance of which (see below) were typical of an anaesthetized, intubated patient. Recordings were then made of the way in which flow, volume, and pressure varied with time during the respiratory cycle under a variety of conditions. The arrangement is shown schematically in fig. 7.1.

The compliance consisted of two five-gallon oil drums connected in parallel. Thus by clamping the inlet to one the compliance could readily be halved. The resistance consisted, in part, of two tubes in parallel selected so that clamping one tube doubled the resistance.

For the testing of each ventilator the compliance and resistance were first set to their 'standard' values, that is with both drums and both airway-resistance tubes in circuit. The ventilator was then connected to the model lung and switched on. The controls were adjusted to give, as nearly as possible, an arbitrary 'standard pattern' of ventilation: a tidal volume of 500 ml, at a frequency of 20 breaths/min with an inspiratory-expiratory ratio of 1 : 2. If the ventilator under test offered negative pressure in the expiratory phase this was normally used to a moderate extent. There is no special significance in the choice of pattern; it is simply one to which few anaesthetists would object strongly and one which most ventilators can be set to deliver.

When the standard pattern of ventilation was established, the flow into and out of the lung, the pressure at the 'mouth', the pressure in the 'alveoli', and the volume in the lung were recorded continuously, over a few cycles of ventilation, by means of a four-channel recording system (see below).

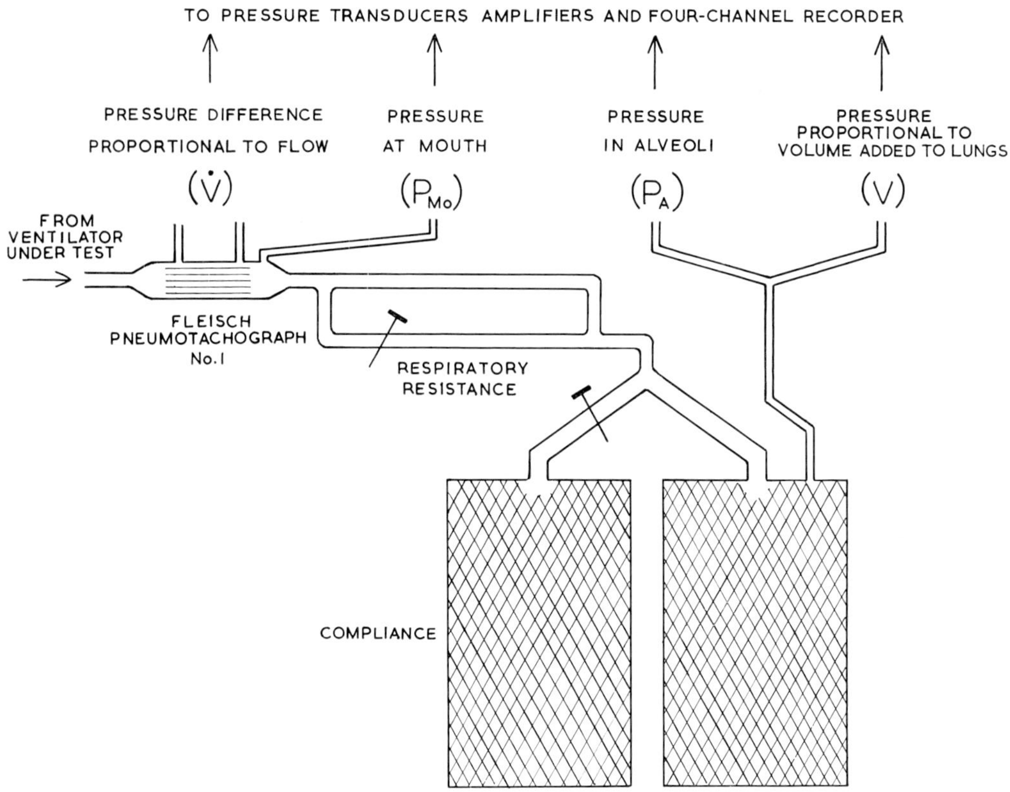

Fig. 7.1. Schematic diagram of the arrangements for the laboratory testing of automatic ventilators.

A study was then made of the effects of changing both the characteristics of the model lung and the settings of the ventilator controls. Firstly the compliance was halved, then the resistance was doubled, then each control on the ventilator was adjusted to some 'non-standard' value. After each of these changes a fresh recording of flow, pressures, and volume was made and then the parameter which had been altered was restored to its 'standard' setting before the next parameter was altered. Thus, for each recording (with one or two exceptions) only one lung characteristic or one control was at a 'non-standard' value. This technique no doubt failed to reveal certain interactions; but to have recorded the effects of all possible combinations, even of only two settings of each control and two values of each lung characteristic, would have required a prohibitively large number of recordings.

In some ventilators, after the settings of certain controls have been altered, the pattern of ventilation changes slowly and progressively over several cycles of ventilation before a new stable state is reached. All the tracings in this book were obtained only after such a stable state had been reached.

The sets of tracings reproduced in the later chapters were prepared from the original recordings by 'scissors and paste' and photography. (The 'paste' was in fact the electrostatic attraction between paper and 'Perspex' acrylic sheet[1]; the recordings were photographed on a trans-illuminated panel.[2]) Generally, there are two pages of recordings for each ventilator. The first page of recordings for the 'Cyclator' Mark II is repeated here (fig. 7.2) for convenience. Each page contains from three to six sets of tracings. Each set shows slightly more than one respiratory cycle of each of the four variables:

$\dot{V}$, flow (inspiratory flow upwards and expiratory flow downwards),
P_{Mo}, pressure at the 'mouth',
P_{A}, pressure in the 'alveoli',
V, volume added to the lungs.

The first page of recordings for each ventilator usually shows three sets of tracings. The first set on the page is for the 'standard conditions', that is with the 'standard' compliance and resistance in the model lung and with the ventilator controls set to give as nearly as possible the 'standard pattern' described above. The second set is with the compliance of the model lung halved but with no other change in the model lung or in the settings of the controls. The third set is with the resistance of the model lung doubled but with the compliance restored to 'standard' and again with no change in the controls.

This first page of recordings serves to illustrate the functional analysis of the ventilator. Thus in the 'Cyclator' (fig. 7.2) which operates as a flow generator in the inspiratory phase, the pattern of inspiratory flow can be seen to be the same in all three sets of tracings, except to the extent that the flow does not go on for so long in some sets of tracings as in others. The 'Cyclator' is a pressure generator in the expiratory phase but the pattern of mouth pressure is not quite the same in all three sets of tracings because there is some resistance between the mouth and the point where the pressure is generated; however, the pattern of flow can be seen to be markedly different in the three sets of tracings because of the three different sets of lung characteristics. Since the 'Cyclator' is pressure-cycled at the end of the inspiratory phase it can be seen that in all three sets of tracings the phase ends just as the mouth pressure reaches some critical value but that the volume delivered during the phase and its duration is very different in the three sets of tracings. Finally, since the 'Cyclator' is time-cycled in the expiratory phase, it can be seen that the duration of the expiratory phase is always the same but that the volume expired varies.

The second page of recordings shows the effect of changing the controls of the ventilator, with the model lung always adjusted to the 'standard' compliance and 'standard' resistance. The first set of tracings repeats the 'standard' set of conditions from the first page. The subsequent sets show the effect of changing the setting of each

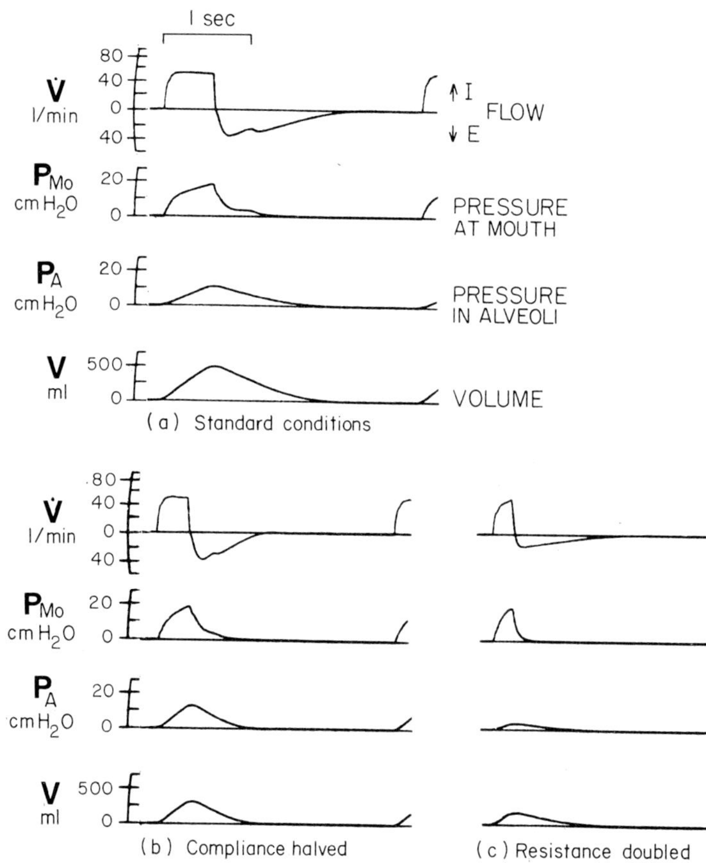

Fig. 7.2. Recordings obtained from the 'Cyclator' Mark II ventilator, when connected to the test rig of fig. 7.1, showing the effects of changes of the characteristics of the model lung. This figure is a repeat of fig. 36.5 in the full account of the 'Cyclator' Mark II.

of the ventilator controls, one at a time, up to a maximum of five. For each set of tracings all the controls, apart from the one being altered, are normally at the settings used for the 'standard conditions'. Even so, it is evident that the effect of changing the setting of a single control is often more complex than the wording on the control may suggest.

The technical details of the recording system are given below for those interested but a few matters concern the general reader.

The recorder pens wrote on curved co-ordinates so that an instantaneous change of flow or pressure, even with instantaneous response of the pen, would have produced not a straight vertical line in the recording but an arc of a circle, concave to the right. The nature of the curvature is indicated in the calibration marks in the recordings. This is of some importance when looking for simultaneity of events in two tracings in a set. For instance, if a given set of tracings is examined closely flow may appear to cross the zero line (at the change-over from the inspiratory phase to the expiratory phase) a little before the pressure at the mouth begins to fall. However, the mouth-pressure pen is then well deflected from the zero line. Therefore its tip is also slightly displaced to the right. Measurement of the distance of the points in the two tracings from the curves in their respective calibration marks will usually show that the two events are in fact simultaneous.

The deflection of the pens does not bear a strictly linear relationship to the pressure, volume, or flow represented, but the non-linearity is indicated in the calibration marks.

'DYNAMIC' TESTS—TECHNICAL DETAILS

The oil drums used were stuffed with finely-divided heat-absorbing material to ensure that the compression of the gas within them was isothermal and not adiabatic.[3] The material used was 'Brillo fine-grade' stainless-steel wool at a density of 120 g/litre. Calculation showed that this reduced the temperature change in the drums on inflation by a factor of 40. Experiment showed that the resistance to the flow of gas through the steel wool was small compared to the airway resistance used. With this arrangement the compliance of each drum was found experimentally to be 25 ml/cmH_2O.

For the resistance of the model lung, tubes and connexions were selected by a trial-and-error process so that, with both the parallel tubes open, the pressure drop across the resistance at a flow of 0·5 litre/sec was comparable to that to be expected in a normal, anaesthetized, intubated patient. However, the pressure-flow characteristic was more curved than would commonly occur with a patient and was well represented by the equation $P = 1{\cdot}2\,\dot{V} + 10{\cdot}2\,\dot{V}^2$ where P is pressure drop and $\dot{V}$ is flow. With one tube clamped the resistance was approximately doubled; the equation was $P = 2{\cdot}4\,\dot{V} + 18{\cdot}4\,\dot{V}^2$.

The connexions from the model lung to the recording system are shown diagrammatically in fig. 7.1. Flow was converted to a proportional pressure-difference by a Fleisch pneumotachograph Size 1. A recording of volume was obtained by using the model lung as its own 'pneumatic integrator'. In other words alveolar pressure, in addition to being recorded as such, was also recorded on a further channel, at different gain, as a measure of volume added to the lungs. This channel was calibrated in terms of volume. When the compliance was halved the gain of the amplifier was halved to preserve the calibration unchanged. When the alveolar pressure was not atmospheric at the end of the expiratory phase a compensating electrical bias was introduced so that the volume tracing started from zero at the beginning of each inspiratory phase.

Greer defocusing manometers[4] by Mercury Electronics were used as pressure transducers and their electrical outputs recorded on a four-channel Southern Instruments pen oscillograph. Some modifications were made to the transducers to improve their response to sudden changes of input.

Calibrations were made against a Rotameter for flow and a specially-designed water manometer[5] for pressures. This manometer was also used to calibrate the volume channel using the known compliance of the model lung. The gas used to calibrate the flow channel was always the same as that with which the model lung was inflated. Usually this was oxygen but with some ventilators it was more convenient to use air. When this was done a note is included in the captions of the recordings.

All four channels were calibrated immediately before making a set of recordings and the sensitivity was checked at the end, up to one hour later: it was always within 10% of the original value and usually within 5%. The zero was more subject to drift and therefore was checked at more-frequent intervals: the resultant errors are unlikely to have exceeded 2 litres/min, 0·5 cmH_2O, or 25 ml. For those parts of the recordings reproduced in this book, the paper speed was probably within ±3% of the indicated value.

Sudden changes of flow and of mouth pressure tended to produce oscillation in the outputs of the transducers. For the sake of providing 'clean' recordings this was eliminated by pneumatic critical damping. In the case of the flow channel the damping on the two sides of the differential-pressure transducer was very carefully matched to prevent artefacts due to sudden changes of pressure.

REFERENCES

1 MAPLESON W.W. (1965) A modern alternative to 'scissors and paste'. *Med. biol. Illust.* **15**, 195–196.

2 MARSHALL R.M. (1969) Transillumination for photography of electrostatic layouts. *Med. biol. Illust.* In press.

3 HILL D.W. and MOORE V. (1965) The action of adiabatic effects on the compliance of an artificial thorax. *Br. J. Anaesth.* **37**, 19–22.

4 GREER J.R. (1958) A sensitive defocussing photo-electric pressure transducer. *Electron. Engng.* **30**, 436–439.

5 GREER J.R. (1958) Calibrating manometer for pressure transducers. *J. scient. Instrum.* **35**, 223.

CHAPTER 8

Historical Background to Automatic Ventilation

To an onlooker in a modern operating theatre for thoracic surgery, the anaesthetic may appear to be conducted by a mechanical device whose gentle sighing supplants the patient's own breathing. The anaesthetic itself and the respiratory problems attached to it may appear relatively insignificant in this arena of surgical technical virtuosity. The anaesthetist himself may appear to be mainly concerned with fluid balance and with the correct administration of the various non-anaesthetic drugs which make the surgical procedure possible.

It is difficult to believe that until comparatively recently, the maintenance of life while the chest was open posed severe problems. At one time careful unhurried work within the thorax was impossible. No sooner would the chest be opened, than the lung would collapse, the patient's respiration would become laboured, the mediastinum would commence to 'flap' violently, and the circulation would become embarrassed; only a hurried conclusion of the operation ensured the patient's survival. This 'pneumothorax problem' had, in fact, been solved centuries before in animals. Most surgeons were well aware from physiological demonstrations and experiments dating from the time of Vesalius (1555) and Hook (1667) that life could be preserved by inflation of the lungs with bellows while an animal's thoracic wall was widely-opened.[1]

However, although the spread of aseptic, as opposed to antiseptic, surgical technique, based on the work of German bacteriologists and pioneered by the Berlin surgeon Von Bergmann (1886) and his assistant Carl Schimmelbusch, had made elective surgery within the abdomen safe from the hazard of infection for the first time, skilled surgeons like von Mikulicz, eager to extend their work into the thorax, were stopped by the 'pneumothorax problem'. To intubate a dog in the laboratory was a simple matter, but to intubate the human larynx was a problem to which at that time there was no simple answer. Some succceded like the French surgeons Tuffier and Hallion[2,3] who, in 1896, intubated a patient by touch and used their laboratory method of rhythmic artificial ventilation by means of a non-rebreathing valve attached to a cuffed endotracheal tube, to perform a successful partial resection of the lung. Although Kirstein's 'Autoscope', the first direct-vision laryngoscope, was described in 1895 in Berlin,[4] the year before

Tuffier and Hallion performed their operation in Paris, not even Kirstein envisaged the routine use of his 'Autoscope' for intubation of the larynx.

Other surgeons, like Rudolph Matas of New Orleans, also felt that only the laboratory method of artificial respiration could ensure the patient's safety during thoracic surgery.[5] In 1898[6] he used the Fell-O'Dwyer resuscitation apparatus (fig. 8.1), the metal cannula of which was passed into the larynx by touch, to perform successful resection of the chest wall. In 1902[7] Matas described his 'experimental automatic respiratory apparatus' (fig. 8.2), an improvement on the Fell O'Dwyer apparatus, though it was still used with O'Dwyer-type laryngeal cannulae which were inserted by touch. The Philadelphia surgeon Dorrance,[8] attempting to evolve in the laboratory a satisfactory method of

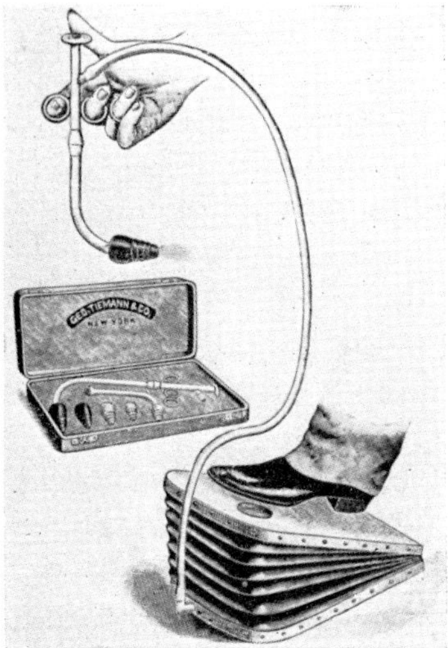

Fig. 8.1

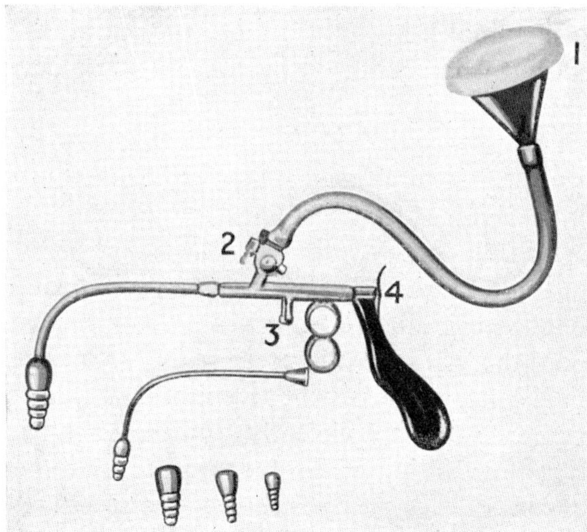

Fig. 8.2

Fig. 8.1. The Fell-O'Dwyer apparatus (c. 1888).

This apparatus was similar to the original Fell pattern but incorporated O'Dwyer's laryngeal tube which was a great improvement over the face-mask of the Fell apparatus. During inflation the operator's thumb was placed over the expiratory orifice. The interchangeable conical heads of different sizes were designed to fit securely into the larynx and prevent the escape of air during inflation.

Fig. 8.2. Matas's modification of the Fell-O'Dwyer apparatus (1900).

The device consists of an O'Dwyer pattern tube with a handle and provision for the maintenance of anaesthesia added. The anaesthetic was dripped on to the cone (1). The vapour passed, via the tap (2), into the laryngeal tube. The tap was closed during inflation and the latter would be interrupted whilst the patient inhaled air and anaesthetic vapour from the cone.

1 Anaesthetic cone (Trendelenburg pattern)
2 Tap
3 Connexion for supply of compressed air
4 Expiratory orifice—closed by thumb during inflation

'treatment of traumatic injuries of the lungs and pleura', used a Matas apparatus for rhythmic artificial respiration (fig. 8.3). He had considerable difficulty in maintaining the correct position of the laryngeal cannula and so developed the prototype of the modern

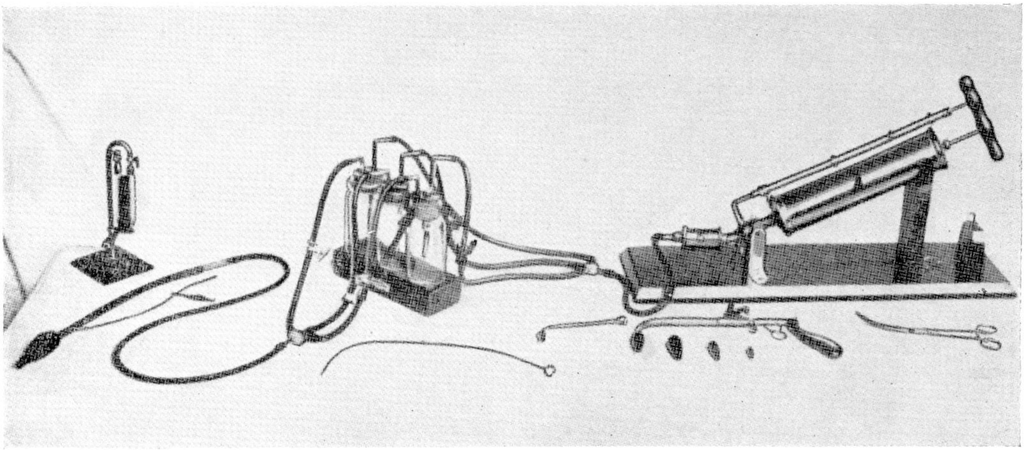

Fig. 8.3. Dorrance's outfit for anaesthesia in chest surgery (1910).
His endotracheal tube and cuff replaces the Matas cannula shown in the foreground. Behind the cannula on the right is the pump for rhythmic inflation while in the centre are the bottles for vaporizing liquid anaesthetics. Behind the endotracheal tube is the manometer for registering the intrabronchial pressure.

cuffed endotracheal tube which was inserted by touch alone through the mouth. By this means he succeeded in resuscitating several patients. The German surgeon Kuhn of Kassel, between 1900 and 1910, designed and demonstrated a whole range of flexo-metallic endotracheal tubes[9] (fig. 8.4) and anaesthetic machines.[10] He also depended upon a digital method to intubate his patients through the mouth. This cannot have appealed to his surgical colleagues for there are no accounts of other surgeons having adopted his apparatus or method.

Unfortunately, these promising attempts to evolve an anaesthetic method for thoracic surgery, based on intubation of the larynx and rhythmic inflation of the lungs, were overshadowed by the much more dramatic presentation, in 1904, by Sauerbruch,[11] from von Mikulicz's clinic in Breslau, of his negative-pressure chamber (fig. 8.5). Many European surgeons accepted Sauerbruch's assertion that the 'differential-pressure method' solved the 'pneumothorax problem' and they were relieved that it avoided the difficulty of intubating the human larynx. Many either followed Sauerbruch and constructed cumbersome differential-pressure operating chambers or adopted Brauer's[12] simpler positive-pressure anaesthetic apparatus (fig. 8.6). Sauerbruch's forceful assertion that the differential-pressure method solved the 'pneumothorax problem' and provided adequate ventilation for the patient, and the appearance of Tiegel's[13] simple positive-

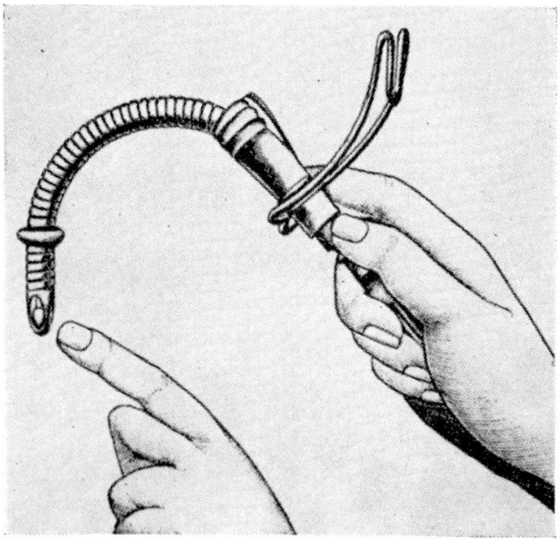

Fig. 8.4. Kuhn's endotracheal tube and introducer (1900–10).

The tube is made of flexible metal. At the tracheal end are lateral orifices so that a smooth rounded tip is obtained. Near this end is a collar which makes an air-tight fit in the larynx. At the other end of the tube is a bite block for the teeth and through this end is inserted the introducer. The wire face-loop helped to keep the tube in position.

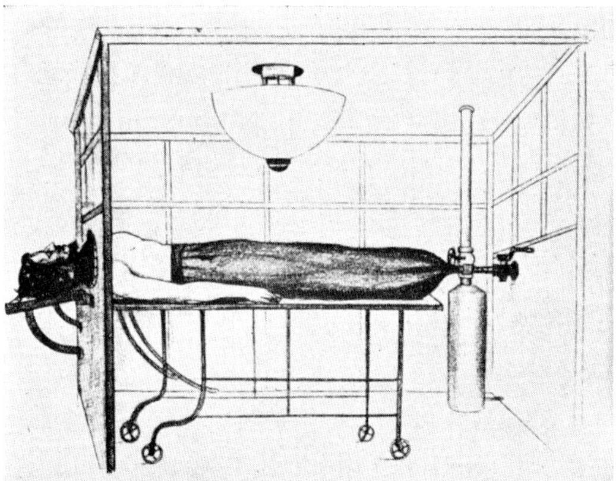

Fig. 8.5. Sauerbruch's negative-pressure operating chamber (1904).

The patient's legs and abdomen were enclosed by a cuff connected to the outside atmosphere.

pressure anaesthetic apparatus in 1908, established a method which was used by many European thoracic surgeons until the end of the 1930's.

Most American surgeons however, apart from Willy Meyer of New York, turned instead to the intratracheal insufflation method described by Meltzer and Auer[15] in 1909 as 'continuous respiration without respiratory movements' (fig. 8.7). The New York surgeon Elsberg[16] designed an insufflation anaesthetic apparatus and mastered the technique of direct laryngoscopy to ensure correct placement of the insufflation catheter. For this, Elsberg used the laryngoscopes evolved from the original Kirstein pattern by the pioneer American endoscopist Chevalier Jackson[17] of Pittsburg. Unfortunately, although Chevalier Jackson devoted his life to instructing his colleagues in the art and use of endoscopy and in 1913 wrote a paper[18] on laryngoscopy specifically for anaesthetists (fig. 8.8), very few anaesthetists or surgeons became adept in the use of the laryngoscope,

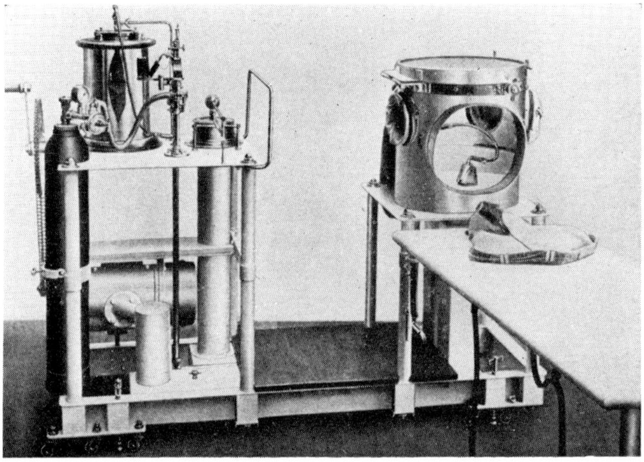

Fig. 8.6. Brauer's positive-pressure apparatus (1905).

The hand-operated compressor at the left supplied air under pressure to the cylindrical head container on the right. An airtight closure round the patient's neck was provided by the cuff lying on the operating table. Airtight cuffs on the sides of the container admitted the anaesthetist's arms. The anaesthetic was delivered separately through the mask.

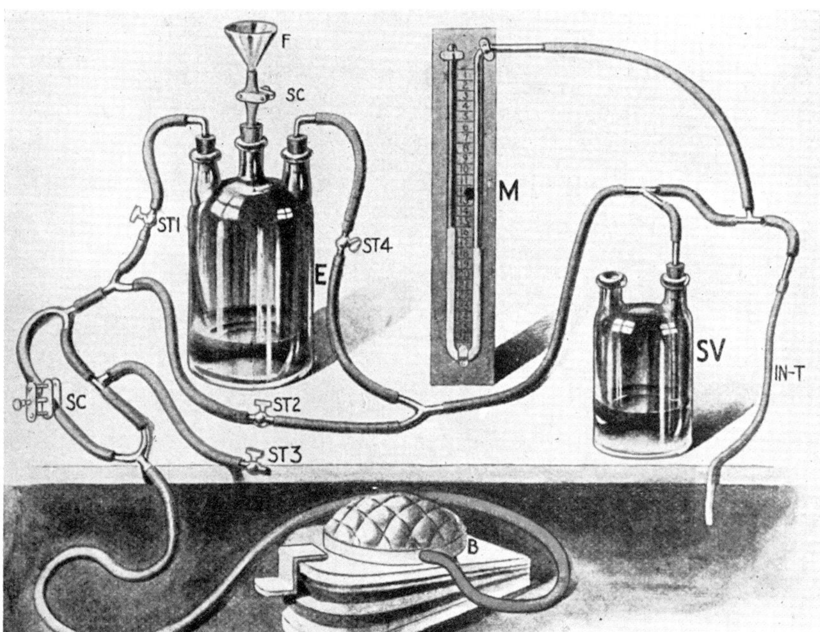

Fig. 8.7. Meltzer and Auer insufflation apparatus (1913).

A foot bellows provides a stream of air which, by means of a series of stopcocks, either passes through the ether bottle (E) or by-passes it. The air then passes to the tracheal tube (IN-T). M is a manometer. SV is a mercury blow-off safety-valve. The authors stressed the importance of tap ST3 which is used to interrupt the stream of air at regular intervals. The end of the tube SV (calibrated in mm) is lowered beneath the surface of mercury in the bottle and thus controls the pressure and acts as a safety-valve.

A 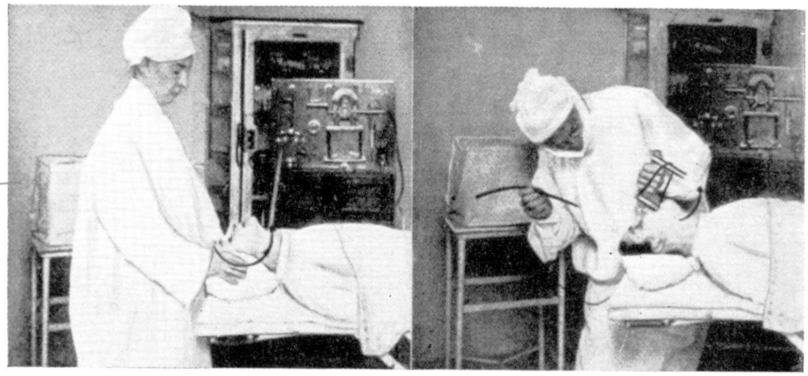 B

Fig. 8.8. Laryngoscopy for anaesthetists demonstrated by Chevalier Jackson (1913).

A. The patient's head is being placed in position for laryngoscopy. 'The pillow is removed, the head is flat on the table and the anaesthetist is beginning to force the head into the extended position. The thumbs are on the forehead and the fingers are at the side of the head. The direction of motion is shown by the dart'.

B. 'The anaesthetist is lifting with the tip of the speculum in the direction of the dart. The speculum is always held in the left hand. The right hand, of which the index has been protecting the upper lip, has now received the catheter from the nurse'.

and positive-pressure methods which did not require intubation were therefore of necessity used.

As already described, Sauerbruch's 'differential-pressure method' was widely accepted as the answer to the respiratory problems of thoracic surgery. His influence on the development of thoracic anaesthesia was described by Nissen,[19] 'Today it seems hard to believe that he rejected the method of endotracheal insufflation although this was only in small part due to an unwillingness to learn. The decisive factor lay in the organization, or rather the lack of organization, in the field of anesthesia. Sauerbruch rejected on principle the idea of setting up anesthesia as a branch in its own right, detecting in this, as he thought—quite unjustifiably—a step which would split up surgery into a number of specialized branches. His voice was sufficiently influential in the continent to hold up a development there from which, in other countries, thoracic surgery was to benefit more than any other'.

However, several investigators were fortunately not convinced. Läwen and Sievers[20] in 1910, working in Trendelenburg's department in Leipzig on the problems of pulmonary embolectomy, evolved a double-pump apparatus for artificial respiration and anaesthesia, with which they were able to maintain a patient's circulation for nine hours after respiratory arrest had occurred (figs. 8.9 and 8.10). When in 1935 Nyström and Blalock[21] commenced their work on experimental pulmonary embolectomy, they were influenced by Läwen and Sievers to employ rhythmic artificial respiration rather than the constant positive-pressure anaesthesia then in vogue for chest surgery. Unfortunately, Läwen and Sievers felt that tracheotomy cannulae[22] were essential to maintain a

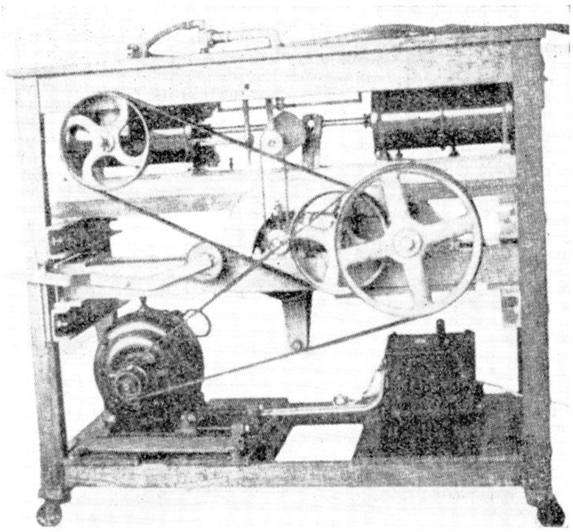

Fig. 8.9. Läwen and Sievers artificial respiration and anaesthesia apparatus (1910).
The apparatus was mounted on a table. The electric motor can be seen below the table and the inspiratory and expiratory pumps above it. The rubber tubing for connexion to the tracheotomy tube can be seen lying on the table top.

Courtesy of *Muenchener Medizinische Wochenschrift*.[20]

satisfactory airway, even though they must have been familiar with Kuhn's endotracheal tubes and his techniques of intubation.

Here was a dilemma. For success in everyday use, apparatus for artificial ventilation required intubation of the larynx, a skill possessed by only a few surgeons practising endoscopy. In 1908, when Willy Meyer[23] designed his positive-negative-pressure cabinet with his brother, an engineer, he insisted that 'what has come to be known in surgery as normal anesthesia must be applicable in the ordinary way without complication, encumbrance or hindrance and that every other consideration must be subordinated to the safe and perfect performance of anesthesia in a way which every doctor has learned and can practice'. Though he was familiar with the work of both Kuhn and Dorrance, Meyer obviously could not depend on the help of men with these advanced skills, and he had to work with whatever anaesthesia his assistants could produce. This was unfortunate, for simultaneously in New York City the experimental surgeons, Green and Janeway, evolved a series of brilliant mechanical devices which provided automatic controlled respiration throughout thoracic operations. Their first apparatus,[24] described in 1909 (fig. 8.11) was a positive-pressure headchamber which resembled Brauer's original 1904 apparatus.[12] It was, in fact, fitted with a valve which produced rhythmic fluctuation in the pressure and 'produced an artificial apnea which largely eliminated the movement of the diaphragm . . . during an operation for empyema in a child, whenever this device was utilized, the diaphragm and intercostal muscles remained at rest. This contrasted strongly with the respiratory efforts which occurred as soon as the valves were turned which permit of a change to the maintenance of the constant positive pressure. We desire to lay special stress on this point, because the absence of muscular movements during operation in the thoracic cavity contribute in an important degree to the speed and ease of operation.' A more refined model, which provided 'true artificial respiration indepen-

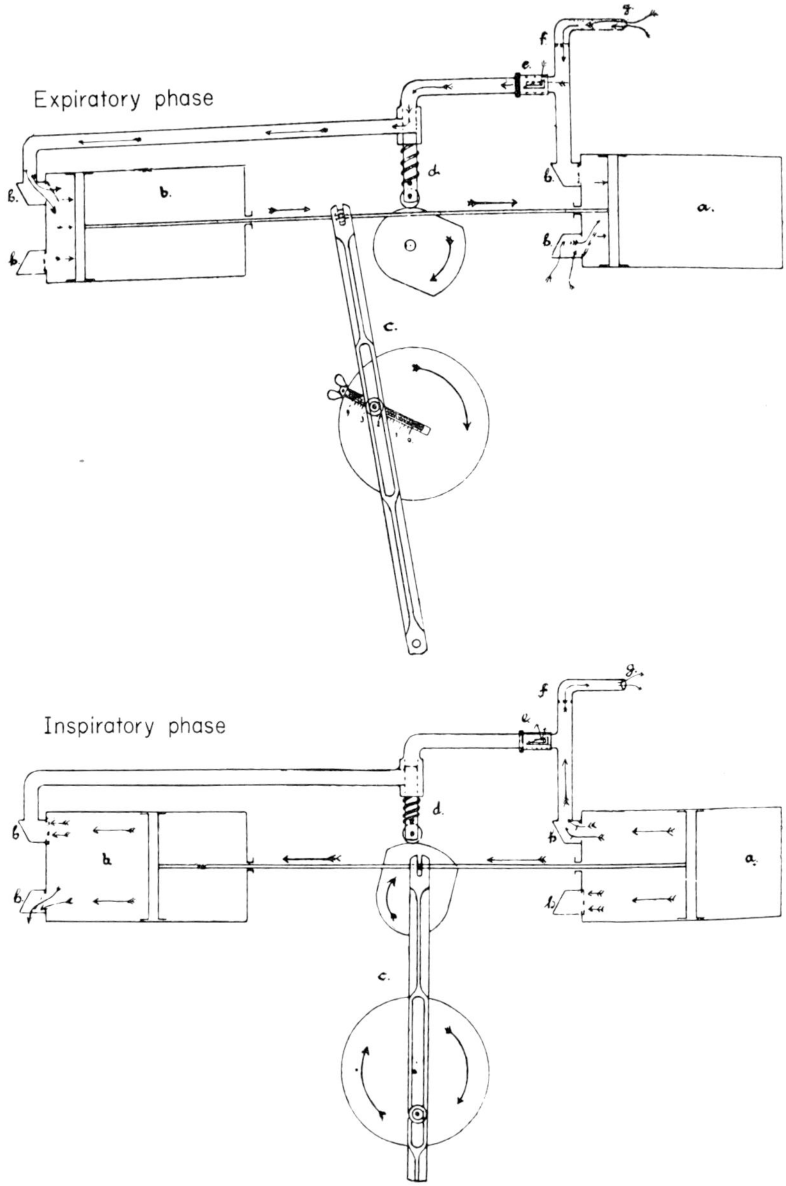

Fig. 8.10. Diagram of Läwen and Sievers positive-negative ventilator (1910).

The apparatus is operated by an electric motor which drives the variable crank (c) and the arm moving the common driving rod and the pistons (a, b) back and forth in their cylinders. The cylinder (a) supplies compressed air for inspiration and that marked (b) provides suction to assist expiration. The screw adjustment on the crank (c) permits the air delivered by the piston on inflation to be varied from one to four litres. The tidal volume can be reduced to the precise amount required by adjusting the opening of spill valve (e).

dent of the efforts of the patient' was described[25] the next year (fig. 8.12). The depth and rate of respiration and the ratio of inspiration to expiration could be varied at will. Using this apparatus, Green and Janeway 'kept a fully curarized dog alive for four hours'. Janeway[26] next accomplished the same result with an apparatus (figs. 8.13 and 8.14) which provided intermittent insufflation through a catheter in the trachea. Finally, in 1913, Janeway[27] described his automatic apparatus (fig. 8.15) which was designed to 'provide true artificial respiration synchronously with the patient's respiration; in other words, merely accentuating the patient's efforts of respiration',—in modern terminology, an assistor. This was used with nitrous oxide-oxygen mixtures and a cuffed endotracheal tube.

Unfortunately, as so often happened, once the experimental surgeons had evolved a satisfactory solution for the respiratory problems, they thenceforth concentrated exclusively upon the surgical technique. Their brilliant anaesthetic and respiratory ideas languished and withered, in the absence of skilled assistants who could adopt and develop them. Though Green[28] became a prominent thoracic surgeon and President of the American Society of Thoracic Surgeons he did not publish anything further on respiratory problems once he left Janeway's laboratory of experimental surgery at Columbia University. Janeway also left this field, in 1914, to become a pioneer of radiotherapy.[29] Similarly, Elsberg having designed the equipment and developed the clinical usefulness of Meltzer's and Auer's insufflation method, then devoted his life's efforts to the development of neurosurgery. Margaret G. Boise,[30] who was then a nurse-anesthetist at Presbyterian Hospital, New York, recalls that 'Anesthesia at that time was crude and given by the house staff who were not at all interested in the subject . . . during my time

---

Expiratory phase

Expired air from the patient is drawn into the expiratory cylinder (b). At the same time, air for inflation is drawn into the inspiratory cylinder (a) through the one-way inlet valve (k).

Inspiratory phase

Inflation has started and the cam-operated valve (d) has closed the connexion to the expiratory cylinder. Air is forced from the inspiratory cylinder to the patient. The volume reaching the patient depends upon the quantity of air permitted to escape through the spill valve (e). The expired gas in the expiratory cylinder (b) is at the same time expelled into the atmosphere. A respiratory rate of 16 breaths per minute was normally used.

Originally intended for use during the Trendelenburg pulmonary embolectomy operation, the authors felt their apparatus would be useful for resuscitation from respiratory arrest due to morphine overdose, carbon-monoxide poisoning, crush injuries of the chest, or tetanus. In tetanus, it was their intention to use curare to relax the respiratory muscles. Although the necessity for tracheotomy was a disadvantage, Läwen and Sievers felt their apparatus could be brought into service rapidly and would be easy to handle.

Courtesy of *Muenchener Medizinische Wochenschrift*.[20]

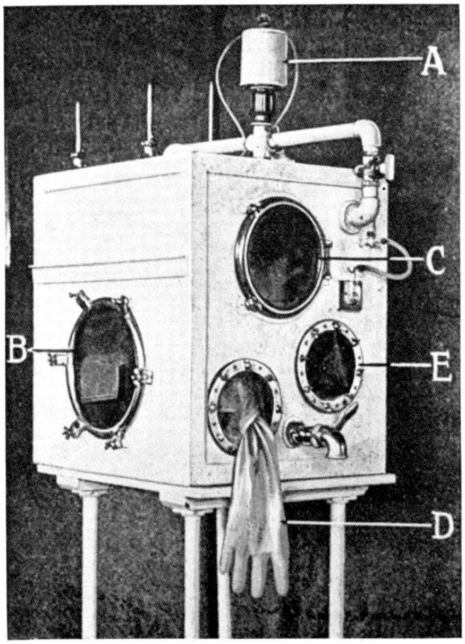

Fig. 8.11. Janeway and Green rhythmic inflation apparatus (1909).

Though similar in general appearance to Brauer's original cabinet, this one, into which the patient's head is also inserted (B), is designed to produce apnoea and practically abolish all spontaneous respiratory activity. A stream of air from a pump enters the box, thus building up a positive pressure. The valve (A), operated either by gear or cam from the electric motor, opens at regular intervals allowing the pressure inside the cabinet to drop to atmospheric. The frequency of the artificial respiration can be varied over a wide range, as can the ratio of the duration of inspiration to expiration. Port holes fitted with rubber gloves (D and E) are provided for the anaesthetist's hands and there is also a glass observation window (C).

Thus Janeway and Green accomplished in 1909 the method of anaesthesia which thirty years later was to become the standard technique for overcoming the problems incident on the widely-opened chest. Their method is identical with that now known as controlled respiration.

in New York . . . positive pressure anesthesia was invented and Doctor H.H.Janeway had his machine at Presbyterian Hospital. I learned its use but it was too cumbersome ever to be popular'. In Gwathmey's textbook on anaesthesia,[31] published in New York at this time, there was no mention of anaesthesia for thoracic surgery except by Elsberg as one indication for the insufflation method in the chapter he wrote on this method.

The First World War interrupted laboratory research and provided instead an abundance of chest injuries to be operated upon with the most rudimentary equipment. Surgeons trained in this rough school depended upon their speed to win the race against asphyxia. They returned to civilian life little interested in the 'pneumothorax problem'.

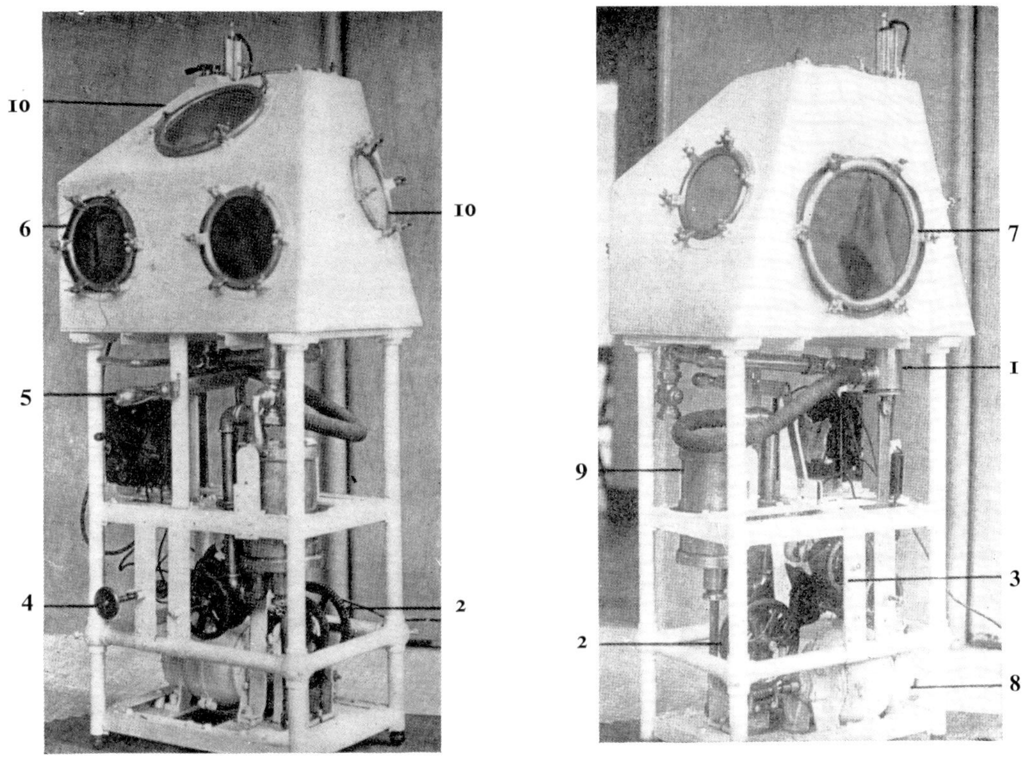

Fig. 8.12. Green and Janeway rhythmic inflation apparatus (1910).

1 Valve mechanism producing rhythmic changes in pressure
2 Speed change gears controlling valves
3 Cam
4 Frequency control
5 Lever varying ratio of inspiration to expiration
6 Gloved orifices for anaesthetist's hands
7 Head orifice with cuff
8 Motor
9 Pump
10 Windows for observation of patient

Courtesy of W.B. Saunders Company.[23]

Their post-war efforts were largely devoted to the evolution of extrapleural operations for the relief of pulmonary tuberculosis following earlier disastrous attempts at resection of such lesions. Interest in automatic ventilation was confined largely to the Fire and Police Departments in the United States and in Europe, whose rescue squads made great use of devices like the Dräger 'Pulmotor' (figs. 8.16 and 8·17).

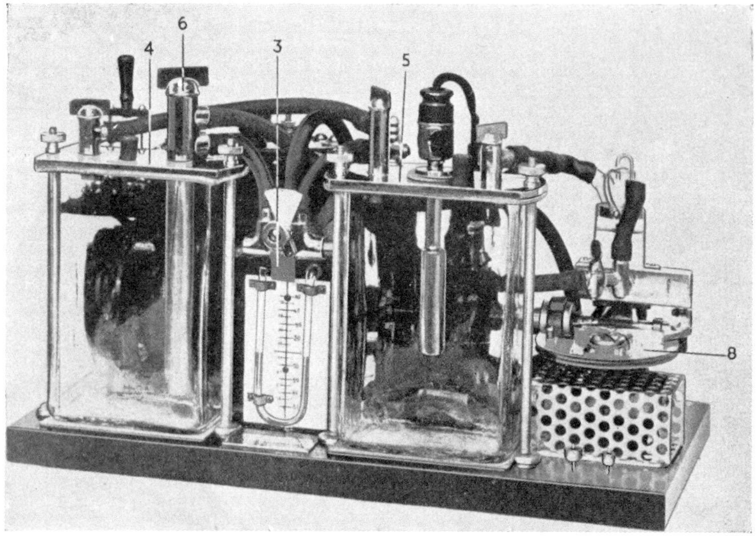

Fig. 8.13. Janeway's intermittent insufflation apparatus (1912). Front view.

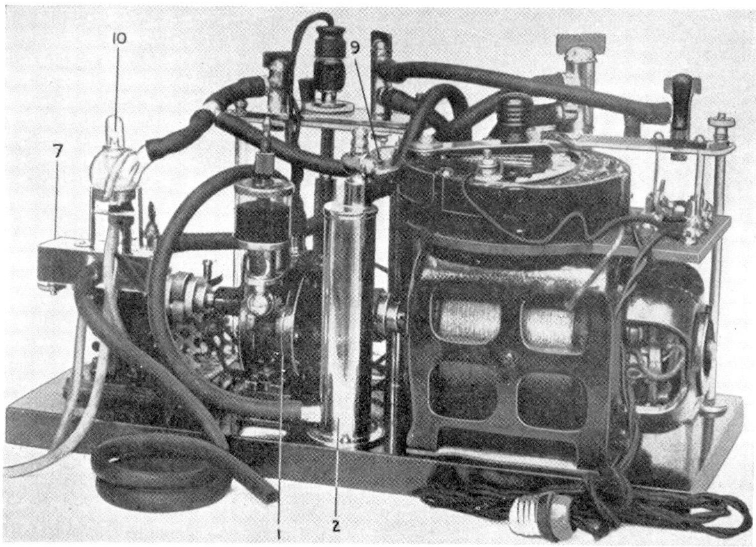

Fig. 8.14. Janeway's intermittent insufflation apparatus (1912). Rear view.

An electric motor drives a blower (1) which sends a stream of air through a filter and silencer (2). A tap (6) diverts the air either through the ether vaporizer (4) and then over the warm water in an electrically-heated jar (5) or directly through the latter. The valve (8) is opened at regular intervals by means of a cam and worm, driven by the electric motor. The air flow to the patient is thus mechanically interrupted at regular intervals, the frequency of which may be adjusted. The effect of this mechanism is to cause intermittent inflation of the patient's lungs, simulating respiration. The other function of this valve is to prevent the pressure from rising above a fixed limit.

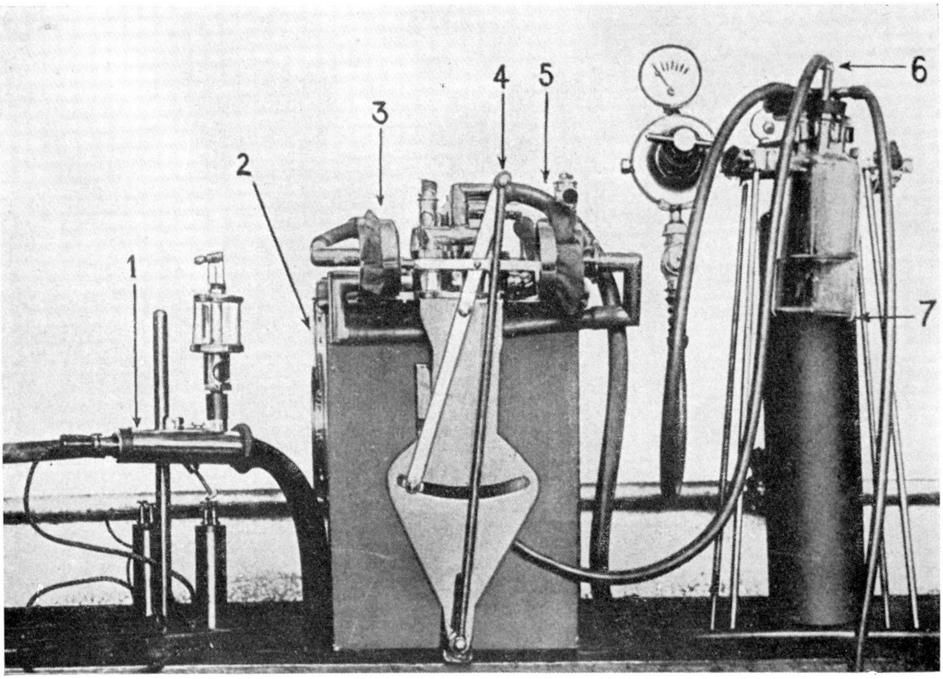

Fig 8.15. Janeway's apparatus for assisted or controlled respiration (1913).

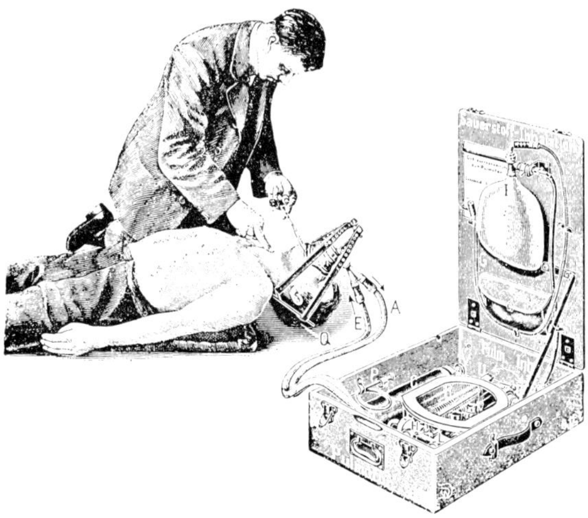

Fig. 8.16. Dräger 'Pulmotor' in use.

The operator is shown preventing inflation of the stomach by pressing on the cricoid cartilage to occlude the oesophagus. This method was recently revived by Sellick[55] to hinder regurgitation of stomach contents during intubation in emergencies. There is evidence,[56] however, that this method was used over a century earlier by obstetricians to prevent inflation of the baby's stomach during resuscitation by the mouth-to-mouth method.

Courtesy of Drägerwerk (Heinr. & Bernh. Dräger), Lubeck.

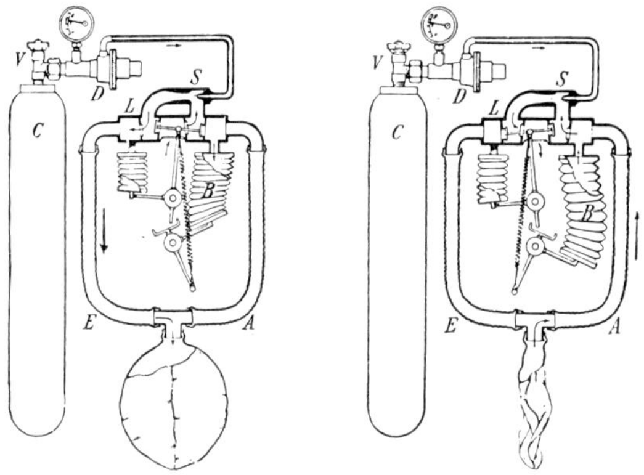

Fig. 8.17. The Dräger 'Pulmotor' (1911).

This apparatus was intended for artificial respiration for resuscitation in mines and in fires. A mixture of air and oxygen is forced into the patient's lungs at a pressure of 20 cmH_2O during the inspiratory phase. The lungs are emptied by a negative pressure of -20 cmH_2O during the expiratory phase.

The left-hand picture shows the lung (here represented by a rubber bag) being inflated. Oxygen from the cylinder passes through the injector (S) entraining air and through the open valve (L) and the breathing tube (E) to the patient's lungs. At the same time the gas mixture enters the concertina bag (B). When the pressure in the breathing tube has reached a certain level (say 20 cmH_2O) the now-distended concertina bag operates the toggle mechanism and the apparatus is now shown in the right-hand picture. When the spring-and-toggle mechanism kicks over into the expiratory position the valves are altered so that the suction produced in the injector mechanism now sucks the air out of the lungs, closes the aperture through which the gases entered the breathing tube, and instead of entraining air, now discharges the contents of the lungs through the same aperture mixed with oxygen from the cylinder.

Courtesy of Drägerwerk (Heinr. & Bernh. Dräger), Lubeck.

A notable exception was the pharmacologist Dennis E. Jackson[32,57] of Cincinnati, who repeatedly demonstrated apparatus for carbon-dioxide-absorption anaesthesia and artificial respiration to his medical colleagues (fig. 8.18). Exasperated at their slowness to benefit from laboratory experience with mechanical artificial respiration, he wrote, 'Thus it is readily obvious to anyone who possesses even a moderate familiarity with this subject that some comparatively safe and efficient means of carrying on artificial respiration should have been constantly available to all good hospitals for perhaps the last one hundred years, for 378 years ago Vesalius had fully demonstrated what artificial respiration may often accomplish in the lower animals. And in the intervening centuries these

to be varied and with this the depth of tidal exchange also. Cylinders of anaesthetic gases were fitted to the double yoke (29) and led directly into the reservoir cylinder (14). For closed-circuit anaesthesia, the pump was used merely to circulate the anaesthetic gases around the circuit and through the soda-lime. When the chest was to be opened, the machine was set to give intermittent blasts of positive pressure, so that the lungs were inflated rhythmically.

Courtesy of *Journal of Laboratory and Clinical Medicine*.[57]

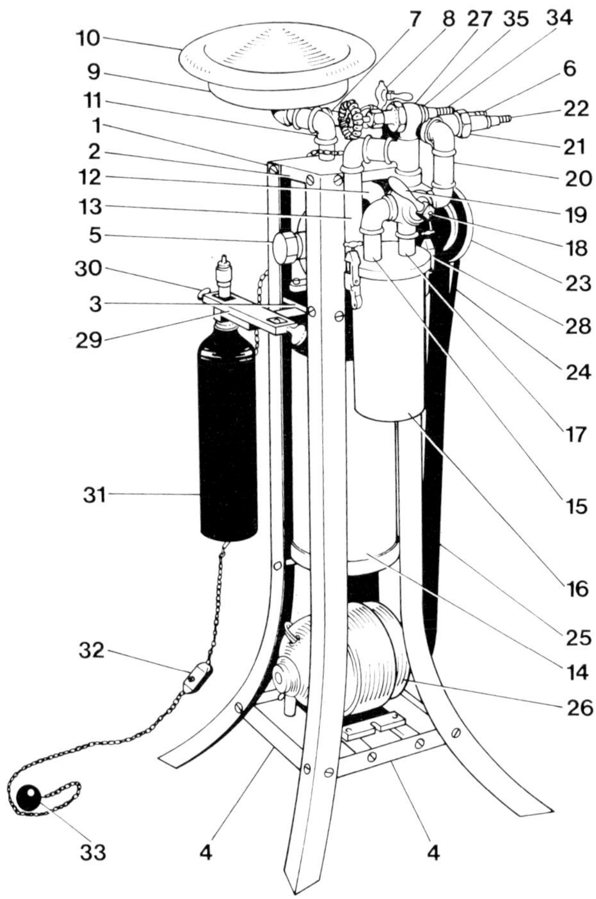

Fig. 8.18. Dennis Jackson's 'Universal artificial respiration and closed anesthesia machine' (1927).

Designed for use with laboratory animals but later used on a patient, this apparatus provided intermittent-positive-pressure inflation of the lungs. Both the respiratory frequency and the depth of respiration were variable.

An electric motor (26) drove the rotary air pump (5), by means of a belt (25). The interrupting valve (21), located just behind the outlet-tube connexion (22), was operated by a mechanism driven from the pulley (23) through the belt (24). Compressed air from the pump passed into the cylindrical container (14) and through the pipe (13) to the 4-way control valve (18). If closed-circuit anaesthesia was being employed, the air passed through (15) to the bottom of the soda-lime canister (16) where the carbon dioxide was absorbed. On leaving the canister through the tube (17), the air passed through the tubes (20) and (22) to the endotracheal tube. The tap (18) permitted the soda-lime canister to be cut out of the circuit. The air then passed directly to the tube (20) and to the patient. The expired air entered the machine through the tube connexion (6) which led into the pipe (11) and the reservoir bag (10) (for economy Jackson preferred to use a shower cap for this purpose!). The by-pass tap between the inspiratory and expiratory tubes permitted the amount of the pump's output going directly to the patient accomplishments have again been redemonstrated many thousands of times in the experimental laboratories. It would appear, however, that the interval of time required for artificial respiration in the dog to evolute into artificial respiration in man may be almost as great as that required for an animal comparable to the dog to evolute into a man. It is in the hope that this long wait may be diminished, even if ever so little, that this article is published.'

EVOLUTION OF PRESENT-DAY VENTILATORS

American and German surgeons did not return to their experiments with mechanical controlled respiration after the 1914–18 War, so that the experiments of Läwen and Sievers, and Janeway and Green did not undergo further development.

Modern ventilators can in fact be traced back[33] to the initiative of a Swedish surgeon, Giertz,[34] formerly one of Sauerbruch's assistants, who had been dissatisfied with the 'differential-pressure method'. His animal experiments showed that rhythmic inflation gave much better results, and led him to stimulate first Frenckner and then Crafoord to work on these problems. Frenckner,[35] a skilled ear, nose, and throat surgeon, evolved a series of endotracheal and endobronchial tubes and an air-driven ventilator, the 'Spiropulsator' (figs. 8.19 and 8.20). This incorporated a 'flasher' mechanism, used in automatic light buoys at sea, to control the inflation of the lungs. Crafoord,[36] then working on the technical problems of pneumonectomy, co-operated with Frenckner and the experimental engineer Anderson,[37] of the Aga Company, to develop the 'Spiropulsator'. The first commercially-available model of Crafoord and Frenckner's ventilator was announced in 1940 (figs. 8.21 and 8.22). Though Crafoord's surgical colleagues in Sweden were soon convinced of its value, and quickly included a 'Spiropulsator' in their armamentarium, Crafoord[38] found the interest of his American colleagues, at best, lukewarm, when he demonstrated this apparatus during operations on their patients. Exceptions were the experimental cardiac surgeons, Beck and Mautz,[39, 40] of Cleveland, who had already evolved their own similar apparatus in 1939.

By 1936 the work of Ralph Waters of Madison on the carbon-dioxide-absorption method[41, 42] and the use of cyclopropane[43, 44] was familiar to British anaesthetists, and these methods were in widespread use by the time war broke out. In 1941 controlled respiration with cyclopropane for thoracic surgery was described by Nosworthy[45] and the vast amount of thoracic surgery in the British Army owed its success to this solution of the 'pneumothorax problem'. Automatic apparatus for controlled respiration was at this time virtually unknown in this field.

Also during the war, in occupied Denmark, the pioneer Danish anaesthetist, Ernst Trier Mörch, familiar with Crafoord's and Gordh's method, but unable to import a 'Spiropulsator' from Sweden, commenced the design and construction of his own ventilator (fig. 8.23). When Mörch, in a paper[46] to the Royal Society of Medicine in London in 1947, enthusiastically advocated mechanical controlled respiration, he found in his audience some eager to try this new approach. Unfortunately, an early attempt to introduce the 'Spiropulsator' into British practice after World War II came to an abrupt and noisy end when cyclopropane found its way into the electrical vacuum-cleaner motor then used as a compressed-air supply. By this time, however, surgeons in many European countries no longer needed to be convinced that the abolition of spontaneous respiratory activity greatly eased their work within the chest and ensured excellent oxygenation and

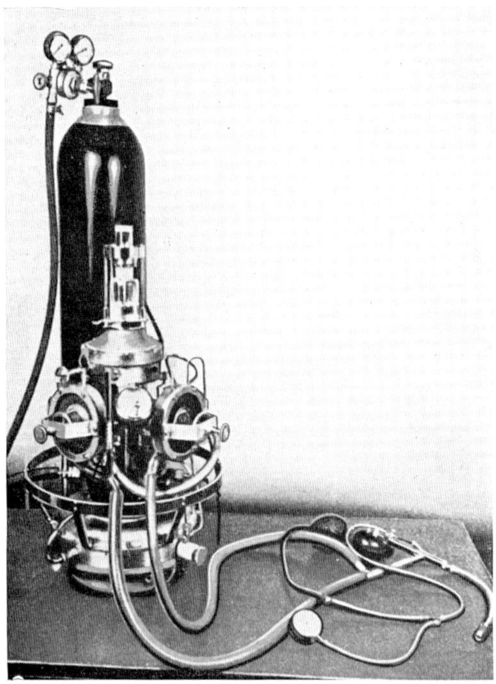

Fig. 8.19. The Frenckner 'Spiropulsator' (1934).

carbon-dioxide elimination. In Britain the ready availability of skilled anaesthetists, returning to civilian life trained to meet the needs of the armed forces, meant that, increasingly, the surgeon left these problems to his colleague. The good reception of Mörch's advocacy of ventilators was in marked contrast to that accorded to Janeway's[27] and Jackson's[32] ventilators by an earlier generation of doctors.

Pinson[47] in 1944 also devised an automatic ventilation device in which a piston pump was the main mechanism (figs. 8.24 and 8.25). He incorporated in this apparatus many refinements, the main one of which was the ability to maintain constant suction without upsetting the anaesthetic mixture containing cyclopropane by loss of gas from the circuit.

A British engineer, Blease,[48] who before the war was primarily interested in the development, building, and racing of motor cycles, became involved quite incidentally in the production of anaesthetic apparatus for a local doctor. His interest was aroused in the anaesthetic problems encountered in air-raid casualties on Merseyside during the 1939–45 War. He was stimulated by anaesthetists anxious to eliminate the drudgery of manual control of ventilation for thoracic surgery. About the end of the war the first prototype (figs. 8.26 and 8.27) of what was to become the Blease 'Pulmoflator' was used

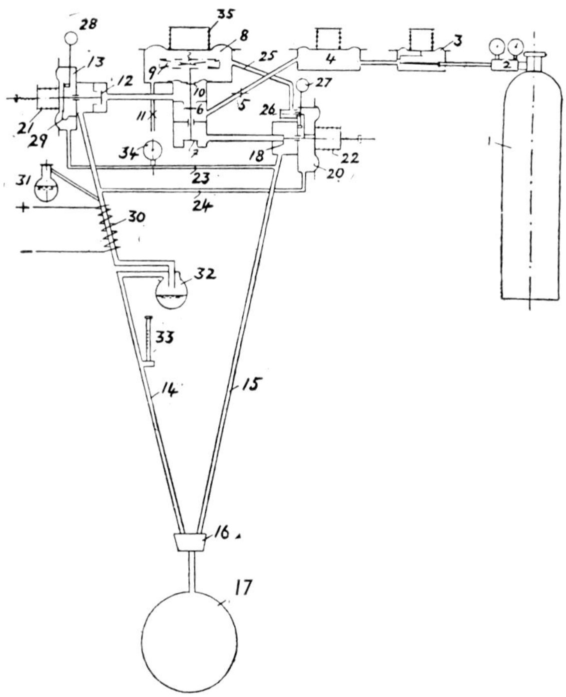

Fig. 8.20. Diagram of the Frenckner 'Spiropulsator' (1934).

Gas from the cylinder (1) passes through two reducing valves (2) and (3) and emerges at a pressure of 50 cmH_2O. The equalizer (4) acts as a reservoir, storing gas to provide a good flow on inspiration. Gas passes through tap (5), which controls the duration of inspiration, past the valves (6) and (12) and via the inspiratory tube (14) into the lungs at (17). As the pressure in the lungs rises, this is transmitted to the diaphragm chamber (13) via tubes (15) and (23). When the pressure in the circuit exceeds that exerted by the spring (21) (which controls the inspiratory pressure) valve (12) closes. The rise in pressure is also transmitted to valve chamber (20), pressing down spring (22), allowing the gas to pass via valve (18) into the 'flasher' valve chamber. Valve (7) remains closed until the pressure of gas entering the chamber via (5) (which cannot escape because valve (12) is closed) is sufficient to deflect diaphragm (9) opening the expiratory valve (7), and at the same time closing inlet valve (6). The gas in the circuit and the lungs then escapes until the pressure in both the expiratory (15) and the inspiratory tubes (14) equals the tension of the expiratory spring (22), which then closes valve (18) and expiration ends. Inspiration starts once more when sufficient gas has escaped from chamber (8) via tap (11) to enable spring (35) to overcome the tension of the 'flasher' spring, opening valve (6) and closing the expiratory valve (7). Liquid anaesthetic added from the container (31) is vaporized by the heating coil (30).

in the Wallasey Cottage Hospital. Though the reception of this prototype by some was sceptical, the convenience provided by the improved model,[49] (fig. 8.28) was especially appreciated when the introduction of curare necessitated artificial respiration throughout many other operations besides thoracic ones. Blease's efforts were followed by the

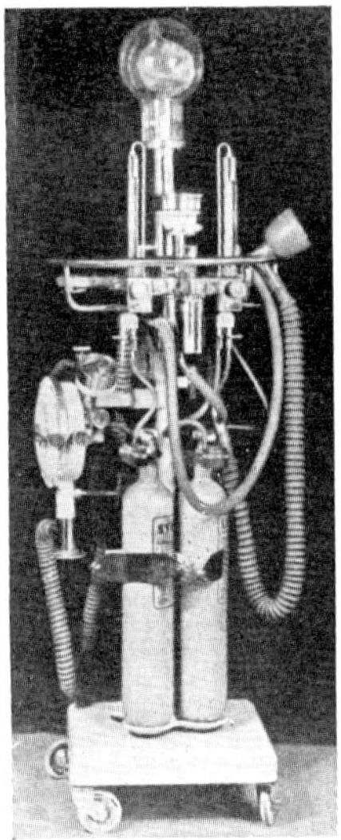

Fig. 8.21.

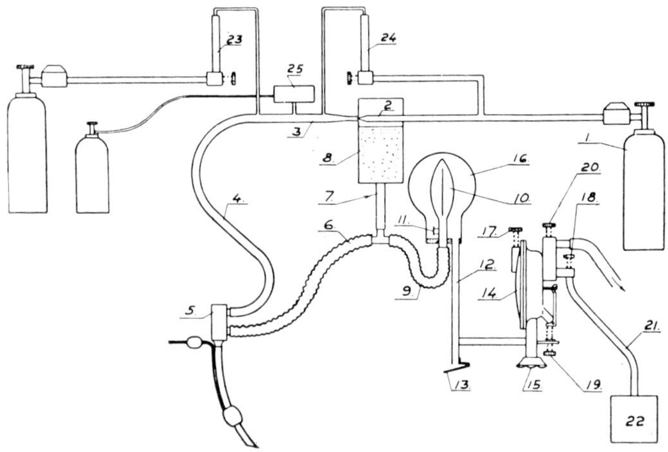

Fig. 8.22.

Fig. 8. 21. The first commercial model of the 'Spiropulsator' (1940).

This differed from the previous experimental apparatus by incorporating an absorber allowing cyclopropane to be used.

Fig. 8.22. Diagram of the 'Spiropulsator' anaesthetic apparatus.

A continuous flow of 500 ml per minute of gas from the nitrous-oxide cylinder (1) passes through the injector (2) into the pipe (3) and this creates a negative pressure in the soda-lime canister (8). This negative pressure draws gas from the rebreathing tube (6) into the absorber (8) and thus provides a circulation of gas from tube (4) into the patient's lungs and via tube (6) into the carbon-dioxide absorber. This is the principle of the Aga-Stille closed-circuit 'circle' absorber machine.

Additional nitrous oxide is added via the flowmeter (24). The flowmeters (23) and (25) control the quantities of oxygen and cyclopropane used respectively. A narrow-bore tube (4) takes the gases to the endotracheal connexion (5).

During respiration the gases pass to and fro along the tube (6) into the reservoir bag (10) which is enclosed within the glass dome (16). Any excess of gas escapes via the spring-controlled expiratory valve (11). Tube (12) connects the glass dome to the 'Spiropulsator' valve (14) which receives compressed air from the compressor (22). Valves (17) and (18) control the duration of the expiratory and inspiratory phases respectively and valves (19) and (20) the maximal and minimal pressures produced.

Valve (13) is kept open until artificial respiration is required. This permits the anaesthetic machine to be used in the normal manner. If it is closed, however, and the compressor started, the 'Spiropulsator' valve (14) produces alternating increasing and decreasing pressure in the glass chamber (16).

imaginative designs of Esplen which resulted in the appearance of the 'Aintree' ventilator in 1952 (see p. 236) and the 'Fazakerley' ventilator in 1956 (see p. 570). In the United States, unlike Britain, Scandinavia, and some other parts of Europe, the value of controlled respiration in general, to say nothing of automatic ventilation, was still

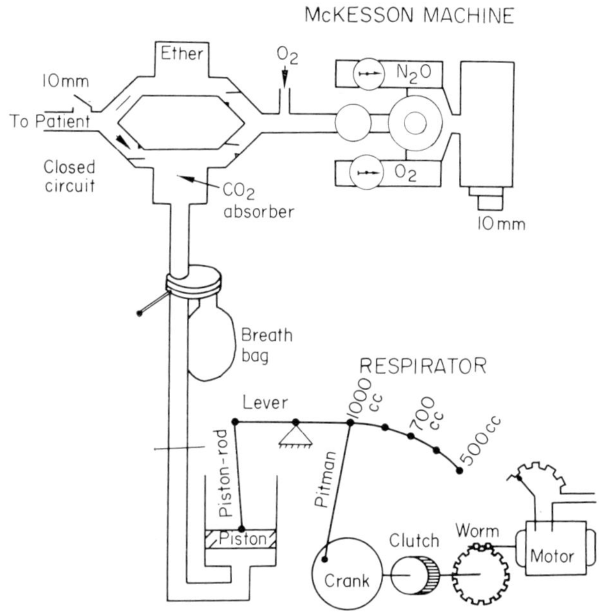

Fig. 8.23. The Mörch 'Respirator'.

In this apparatus the rhythmic inflation of the patient's chest is produced by a motor-driven piston pump. The volume of gas entering the patient's chest at each stroke can be varied by adjusting the point of attachment of the pitman to the lever. Thus each stroke of the piston delivers a certain fixed volume irrespective of the pressure within the chest. Safety-valves are obviously necessary to prevent excessive positive or negative pressures. Maximum positive pressure is controlled by the setting of the expiratory valve. The pressure control on the rebreathing bag which is kept connected to the circuit is adjusted to 10 mm Hg. The bag thus provides an additional buffer against sudden rises in pressure.

The negative pressure produced by the withdrawal action of the piston is controlled by setting the McKesson pressure dial between 'Off 'and 'O'. Should the piston produce a negative pressure of more than −3 to −5 mm Hg, fresh gases are delivered by the anaesthetic machine into the circuit.

strongly disputed even as late as the 1950's. Anesthesiologists, skilled in laboratory methods, documented the lamentably poor results obtained with the gas-oxygen-ether and 'assisted respiration' method that was then still strongly advocated. Though puzzled over the occurrence both of metabolic acidosis as well as respiratory acidosis, they were still doubtful of the value of automatically-controlled ventilation. The danger of

apparatus, not only for patients in whom a particular pattern of waveforms is desirable, but for the use of those highly-trained anaesthetists, from whom alone further knowledge and development in this field can come.

The influence of the automatic ventilator and of the respiratory unit on anaesthesia has been great. They have changed the anaesthetist, from a person who produced unconsciousness while his surgical colleague operated, into an expert physician of many parts—physiologist, physicist, biochemist, mechanic, but above all, an expert in the physiology and mechanics of respiration and in the care of patients with respiratory insufficiency whether induced by anaesthesia or not.

REFERENCES

1 MUSHIN W.W. and RENDELL-BAKER L. (1953) *The Principles of Thoracic Anaesthesia*, p. 28–30. Oxford: Blackwell.

2 TUFFIER T. and HALLION L. (1896) Intrathoracic operations with artificial respiration by insufflation. *C.R. Soc. Biol.* **48**, 951.

3 TUFFIER T. and HALLION L. (1896) On the regulation of intrabronchial pressure and anaesthesia in artificial respiration by insufflation. *C.R. Soc. Biol.* **48**, 1086.

4 MUSHIN W.W. and RENDELL-BAKER L. (1953) *The Principles of Thoracic Anaesthesia*, p. 103–141. Oxford : Blackwell.

5 MATAS R. (1899) On the management of acute traumatic pneumothorax. *Ann. Surg.* **29**, 409–434.

6 PARHAM F.W. (1899) *Thoracic Resection for Tumors*, p. 126. New Orleans.

7 MATAS R. (1902) Artificial respiration by direct intralaryngeal intubation with a new graduated air-pump, in its applications to medical and surgical practice. *Amercian Medicine*, **3**, 97–103.

8 DORRANCE G.M. (1910) Treatment of traumatic injuries of the lungs and pleura. *Surg. Gyn. Obst.* **11**, 160.

9 MUSHIN W.W. and RENDELL-BAKER L. (1953) *The Principles of Thoracic Anaesthesia*, p. 117–118. Oxford: Blackwell.

10 MUSHIN W.W. and RENDELL-BAKER L. (1953) *The Principles of Thoracic Anaesthesia*, p. 56–59. Oxford: Blackwell.

11 SAUERBRUCH F. (1904) Zur Pathologie des offenen Pneumothorax und die Grundlagen meines Verfahrens zu seiner Ausschaltung. *Mitt. Grenzgeb. Med. Chir.* **13**, 399.

12 MUSHIN W.W. and RENDELL-BAKER L. (1953) *The Principles of Thoracic Anaesthesia*, p. 51–54. Oxford: Blackwell.

13 MUSHIN W.W. and RENDELL-BAKER L. (1953) *The Principles of Thoracic Anaesthesia*, p. 60–62. Oxford: Blackwell.

14 MEYER W. (1909) Pneumectomy with the aid of differential air pressure; an experimental study. *J. Amer. med. Ass.* **53**, 1978–1987.

15 MELTZER S.J. and AUER J. (1909) Continuous respiration without respiratory movements. *J. exper. Med.* **11**, 622.

16 ELSBERG C.A. (1910) Clinical experiences with intratracheal insufflation (Meltzer) with remarks upon the value of the method for thoracic surgery. *Ann. Surg.* **52**, 23.

17 JACKSON C. (1938) *The Life of Chevalier Jackson, an autobiography*. New York: Macmillan.

18 JACKSON C. (1913) The technique of insertion of intratracheal insufflation tubes. *Surg. Gyn. Obst.* **17**, 507–509.

19 NISSEN R. (1955) Historical development of pulmonary surgery. *Amer. J. Surg.* **89**, 9.

20 LÄWEN and SIEVERS (1910) Zur praktischen Anwendung der instrumentellen künstlichen Respiration am Menschen. *Münch. med. Wchnschr*, **57**, 2221.

21 NYSTRÖM G. and BLALOCK A. (1935) Contributions to the technic of pulmonary embolectomy. *Thoracic Surg.* **5**, 169–188.

22 MUSHIN W.W. and RENDELL-BAKER L. (1953) *The Principles of Thoracic Anaesthesia*, p. 109. Oxford: Blackwell.

23 MEYER W. (1913) Anesthesia in differential pressure chambers, cabinets and other apparatus for thoracic surgery. p. 953–967 in Keen W.W. (1913) *Surgery, Its Principles and Practice*, **6**, Chap. 149. Philadelphia: Saunders.

24 JANEWAY H.H. and GREEN N.W. (1909) Experimental intrathoracic esophageal surgery. *J. Amer. med. Ass.* **53**, 1975.

25 GREEN N.W. and JANEWAY H.H. (1910) Artificial respiration and intrathoracic oesophageal surgery. *Ann. Surg.* **52**, 58–66.

26 JANEWAY H.H. (1912) An apparatus for intratracheal insufflation. *Ann. Surg.* **56**, 328–330.

27 JANEWAY H.H. (1913) Intratracheal anaesthesia. *Ann. Surg.* **58**, 927.

28 GREEN N.W. (1955) Obituary. *N.Y. State J. Med.* **55**, 1773.

29 JANEWAY H.H. (1921) Obituary and portrait. *Radium*, **16**, 82.

30 THATCHER V.S. (1953). *History of Anesthesia*, p. 84, Philadelphia: Lippincott.

31 GWATHMEY J.T. (1914) *Anesthesia.* New York: Appleton.

32 JACKSON D.E. (1930–31) The use of artificial respiration in man. Report of a case. *Cincinnati J. Med.* **11**, 515–19.

33 RENDELL-BAKER L. (1963) in Mushin, W.W. *Thoracic Anaesthesia*, p. 627. Oxford: Blackwell.

34 GIERTZ K.H. (1916–17) Studier Öfver tryckdifferensandning (rytmisk luftenblasning) vid intrathoracala operationer. *Uppsala. Lakaref.* forh. 22. Suppl., pp. 1–176. Ommexperientella lungexstirpationer. *Uppsala. Lakaref.* forh. 22. Suppl. pp. 1–109.

35 FRENCKNER P. (1943) Bronchial and tracheal catheterization. *Acta Otolaryngol.* Suppl. 20, 100.

36 CRAFOORD C. (1938) On the technique of pneumonectomy in man. *Acta chir. Scand.* Suppl. 54.

37 ANDERSON S., CRAFOORD C. and FRENCKNER P. (1940) A new and practical method of producing rhythmic ventilation during positive pressure anaesthesia: with description of apparatus. *Acta Otolaryngol.* **28**, 95–102.

38 CRAFOORD C. (1940) Pulmonary ventilation and anesthesia in major chest surgery. *J. Thorac. Surg.* **9**, 237.

39 MAUTZ F.R. (1939) Mechanical respirator as adjunct to closed system anesthesia. *Proc. Soc. exp. Biol. (N.Y.)*, **42**, 190.

40 MAUTZ F.R. (1941) Mechanism for artificial pulmonary ventilation in operating room. *J. thorac. Surg.* **10**, 544.

41 WATERS R.M. (1924) Clinical scope and utility of carbon dioxide filtration in inhalation anesthesia. *Anesth. and Analg.* **3**, 20.

42 WATERS R.M. (1936) Carbon dioxide absorption from anaesthetic atmospheres. *Proc. R. Soc. Med.* **30**, 11.

43 WATERS R.M. and SCHMIDT E.R. (1934) Cyclopropane anesthesia. *J. Amer. med. Ass.* **103**, 975–983.

44 GUEDEL A.E. and TREWEEK D.N. (1934) Ether apnoeas. *Anesth. and Analg.* **13**, 263.

45 NOSWORTHY M.D. (1941) Anaesthesia in chest surgery with special reference to controlled respiration and cyclopropane. *Proc. R. Soc. Med.*, **34**, 479.

46 MÖRCH E.T. (1947) Controlled respiration by means of special automatic machines as used in Sweden and Denmark. *Proc. R. Soc. Med.* **40**, 603.

47 PINSON K.B. and BRYCE A.G. (1944) Constant suction in thoracic surgery: Description of an anaesthetic apparatus. *Br. J. Anaesth.* **19**, 53.

48 MUSHIN W.W. and RENDELL-BAKER L. (1953) *The Principles of Thoracic Anaesthesia*, p. 97–98. Oxford: Blackwell.

49 MUSGROVE A.H. (1952) Controlled respiration in thoracic surgery. A new mechanical respirator. *Anaesthesia*, **7**, 77.

50 LASSEN H.C.A. (1956) *Management of Life-threatening Poliomyelitis.* Edinburgh: Livingstone.

51 BJÖRK V.O. and ENGSTRÖM C.G. (1955) The treatment of ventilatory insufficiency after pulmonary resection with tracheostomy and prolonged artificial ventilation. *J. Thorac. Surg.* **30**, 356.

52 MACINTOSH R.R. (1940) New use for the Both respirator. *Lancet*, **2**, 745–6.

53 MUSHIN W.W. and FAUX N. (1944) Use of the Both respirator. *Lancet*, **2**, 685–6.

54 SMITH A.C. (1963) The respiration unit, in, *The Nuffield Department of Anaesthetics Oxford 1937–1962*, p. 52. ed. Bryce-Smith R., Mitchell J.V. and Parkhouse J. Oxford: University Press.

55 SELLICK B.A. (1961) Cricoid pressure to control regurgitation of stomach contents during induction of anaesthesia. *Lancet*, **2**, 404.

56 HAIGHTON J. *Lectures on Obstetrics*, 1816. Quoted by Williams E.A. (1966) Resuscitation of the newborn. *Guy's Hospital Gazette*, **80**, 538.

57 JACKSON D.E. (1927) A universal artificial respiration and closed anesthesia machine. *J. Lab. clin. Med.* **12**, 998.

CHAPTER 9

The 'Adelaide' Ventilator

DESCRIPTION

This portable ventilator is available in several versions designed for ward or theatre use with non-rebreathing or closed circuits and in adult and infant sizes. The photograph (fig. 9.1) and the diagram (fig. 9.2) show the ventilator in the non-rebreathing circuit configuration and it is this arrangement which is described first.

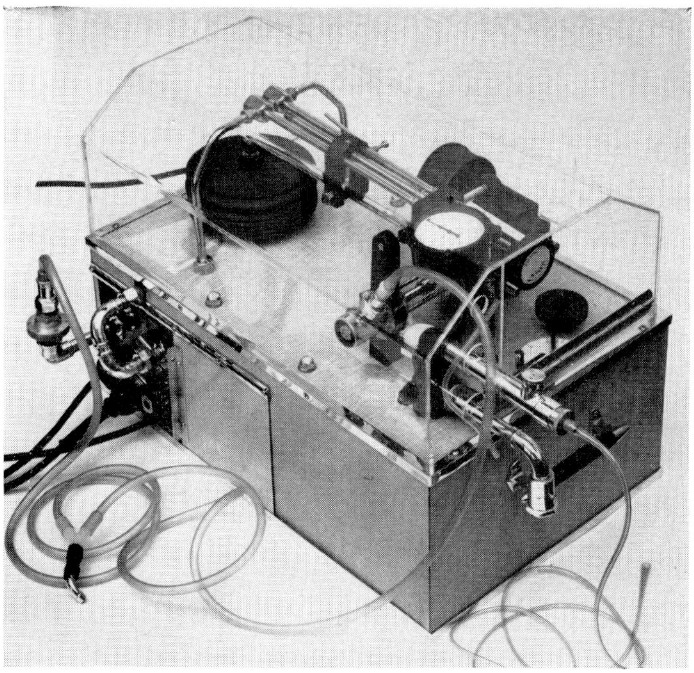

Fig 9.1. The 'Adelaide' ventilator.

Courtesy of Drs S. Kenny and M. Lewis.

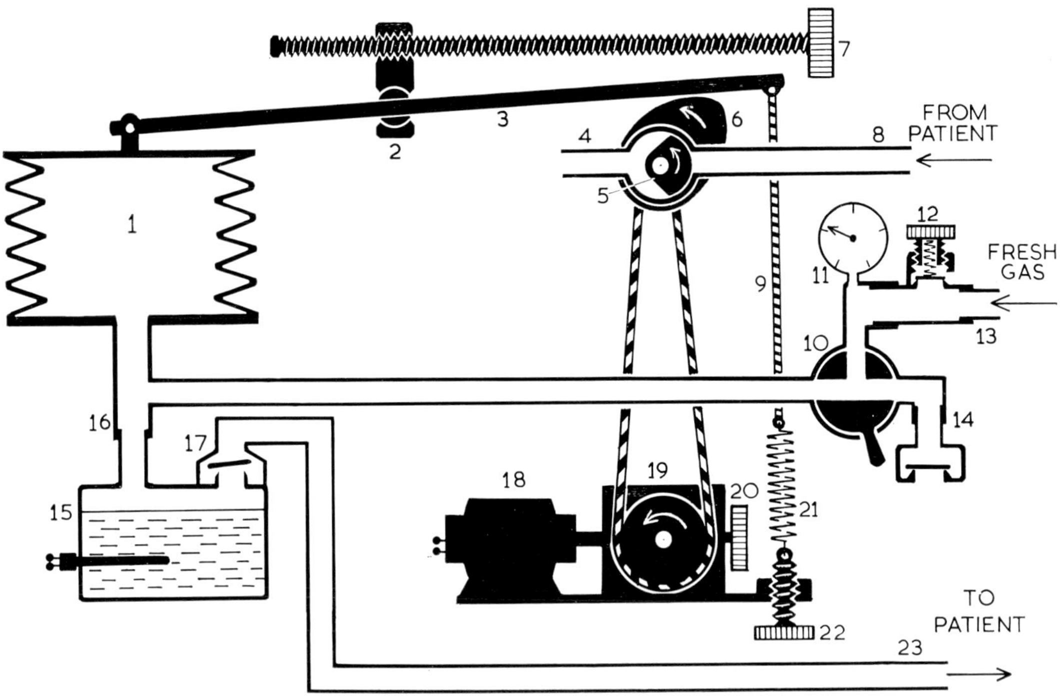

1. Concertina reservoir bag
2. Sliding pivot
3. Lever
4. Port
5. Rotary tap
6. Cam
7. 'Volume' control
8. Expiratory tube
9. String
10. Open/closed/manual tap
11. Manometer
12. Blow-off valve
13. Port
14. One-way valve
15. Heated humidifier
16. Connexion
17. One-way valve
18. a.c. mains motor
19. Gear-box
20. Speed control
21. Spring
22. Negative-pressure control
23. Inspiratory tube

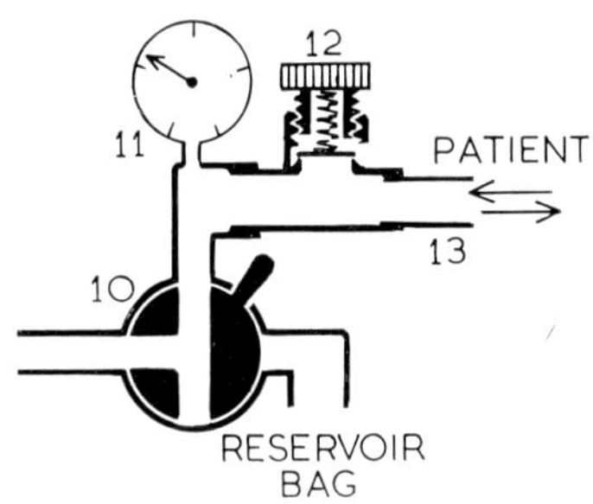

Fig. 9.2. Diagram of the 'Adelaide' ventilator.

The a.c. mains electric motor (18) (fig. 9.2) drives a variable-speed gear-box (19) which is connected by a belt-drive to a shaft which carries a rotary tap (5) and a cam (6). The lever (3) is pivoted at the fulcrum (2). One end of the lever is connected to the top-plate of the concertina reservoir bag (1) and the other is held against the cam (6) by the pull of the spring (21) on the string (9). As the cam (6) rotates, it lifts this end of the lever (3) and the concertina reservoir bag (1) is compressed. The gas within the reservoir bag (1) is forced, through the humidifier (15), the one-way valve (17), and the inspiratory tube

(23), to the patient, the tap (5) being in the closed position. The pressure developed is indicated on the manometer (11), and can be limited by the blow-off valve (12). As rotation of the driven shaft continues, the cam (6) passes its peak and the rotary tap (5) is opened. The lever (3) is drawn down by the pull of the spring (21) and the concertina bag (1) is expanded. The one-way valve (17) closes, and expired gas flows, along the expiratory tube (8), through the tap (5) and the port (4), to atmosphere. At the same time air is drawn into the reservoir bag (1) through the one-way valve (14), together with any fresh gas added at the inlet (13).

For closed-circuit operation the following changes are made (fig. 9.2 Inset). The patient is no longer connected to the ports (8 and 23) but instead only to the port (13), in place of the fresh-gas supply. The connexion is made via a closed anaesthetic circuit (either to-and-fro or circle) complete with soda-lime canister and fresh-gas inlet. The connexion (16) to the humidifier (15) is blanked off. The tap (10) is set so that the port (13), and hence the patient, is connected only to the concertina reservoir bag (1). The air-inlet valve (14) may be replaced by a reservoir bag so that, when the tap (10) is turned to its third position, the patient is connected only to this bag by means of which manual inflation via the closed circuit may be performed.

With the closed-circuit arrangement inflation occurs in the same way as with the non-rebreathing circuit except that the blow-off valve (12) must be adjusted to dispose of excess gas at the end of the inspiratory phase. However, expiration now occurs, not to atmosphere, but back into the concertina reservoir bag (1), and is therefore primarily controlled by the shape of the cam (6). If at any time during the expiratory phase this results in a faster flow rate than would be produced by free expiration to atmosphere, the pressure in the reservoir bag (1) becomes negative—provided that the spring (21) is taut enough to keep the arm (3) in contact with the cam (6). The tension of the spring (21) can be adjusted by the control (22) which can therefore set a negative-pressure limit.

In the infant version a smaller-diameter concertina bag is fitted. Alternatively, a double concertina bag may be fitted: the smaller, inner bag performs the same function as the single bag in the adult version; the larger, outer bag is used to develop negative pressure during the expiratory phase in the non-rebreathing circuit. This is achieved by connecting the port (4) to the outer bag. A one-way valve on the outer bag serves two purposes. Firstly, it allows the contents of the bag to be discharged to atmosphere during the inspiratory phase. Secondly, if free expiration produces a faster expiratory flow than the rate of expansion of the outer bag, the excess can spill through the one-way valve. After this flow falls to equal the rate of expansion of the bag, negative pressure is developed.

The control (20) allows the frequency to be varied between 12 and 60 per minute. The 'volume' control (7) determines the position of the fulcrum (2) and hence the excursion of the top-plate of the concertina bag (1), i.e. the volume delivered from the bag. This volume is indicated on a scale. In the standard ventilator the range of tidal volumes is 200–1400 ml; in the paediatric model it is 10–300 ml. The cam (6) is easily interchanged and three cams are provided, which allow three different patterns of respiratory waveform to be generated:—(*a*) a 'standard' pattern, giving 'one-third inhale, one-third exhale, one-third pause', (b) a 'maximum negative' pattern giving 'one-quarter inhale, one-quarter exhale, and one-half pause', and (c) a 'pulmonary disease' pattern, giving 'one-third inhale and two-thirds exhale'. Differently-shaped cams are used in the infant version.

FUNCTIONAL ANALYSIS

Inspiratory phase

In this phase, assuming the speed of the electric motor (18) to be constant, the ventilator operates primarily as a flow generator. The pattern of flow is, in general, not constant and is determined by the shape of the cam in use. The blow-off valve (12) can provide a pressure limit towards the end of the phase and, in the closed circuit, this limit must normally be reached in every inspiratory phase. In the closed circuit the fresh-gas flow acts as a small-constant-flow generator, supplementing the action of the main flow generator until the blow-off valve opens.

Change-over from inspiratory phase to expiratory phase

This change-over can be regarded as both volume-cycled and time-cycled. It occurs when the concertina reservoir bag completes its downstroke and commences its upstroke and (in the non-rebreathing circuit) the rotary tap (5) opens. The time at which this occurs is determined by the shape of the cam (6) and the settings of the frequency control (20), assuming that the speed of the motor is constant. The volume expelled from the bag in this time is determined by the setting of the volume control (7). However, the tidal volume of the patient falls short of this stroke volume to the extent of any volume of gas blown off through the valve (12), and exceeds this stroke volume to the extent of any steady inflow of fresh gas.

Expiratory phase

In this phase the non-rebreathing circuit of the adult version operates as a constant, atmospheric, pressure generator: the patient's expiration passes to atmosphere at the port (4).

In the closed circuit, and in the double-bag non-rebreathing circuit of the infant ventilator, the mode of operation is basically that of a flow generator. The pattern of flow is not constant and is determined by the shape of the cam (6). In the double-bag non-rebreathing circuit the one-way valve in the outer concertina bag sets an upper (atmospheric) pressure limit so that the phase may begin with a period of constant, atmospheric, pressure generation. In both the double-bag non-rebreathing and the closed circuits, the tension of the spring (21) imposes a negative-pressure limit so that there may be a period of constant, negative, pressure generation towards the end of the phase.

However, if this occurs, the arm (3) fails to follow the cam (6) and, if it has not regained contact with the cam by the end of the phase, the concertina reservoir bag (1) will not be fully expanded and the subsequent stroke volume will be correspondingly diminished.

Change-over from expiratory phase to inspiratory phase

In all circuits this change-over is time-cycled: it occurs when the concertina reservoir bag recommences its downward stroke at a time determined by the shape of the cam (6) and the setting of the frequency control (20), assuming that the speed of the motor is constant.

REFERENCES

1 KENNY S. and LEWIS M. (1960) The Adelaide respirator. *Br. J. Anaesth.* **32**, 444.

2 LEWIS M.A. (1967) A neonatal ventilator. *Br. J. Anaesth.* **39**, 448.

CHAPTER 10

The Aga 'Spiropulsator' ME–2440

DESCRIPTION

This ventilator was originally combined with the flowmeters and carbon-dioxide absorption system of the Stille anaesthetic apparatus, the whole then being known as the 'Spiropulsator' MDNC-20 (fig. 10.1). As such it was a pioneer of modern automatic ventilators and achieved a world-wide reputation for efficiency and reliability. The ventilator portion of this apparatus became available as a separate unit called the 'Vivrator'. This was essentially a closed-circuit device, but a non-rebreathing version, the 'Pulmospirator', was developed for ward use and is still available. The name 'Spiropulsator' is now applied to a slightly-modified version of the ventilator portion by itself (fig. 10.2), and this can be obtained separately for use with any anaesthetic closed circuit, or, with the Aga 'Polyvalve' inflating valve (see p. 774), in a non-rebreathing circuit.

The action of the 'Spiropulsator' (fig. 10.3) depends on a magnetic pressure-sensitive valve, called the 'Pulsator' (13–24). This was originally known as the 'flasher' because of its direct development from a similar device designed for controlling the flashing of lighthouses and marker buoys.

Compressed air or oxygen, at a pressure of 45–75 lb/in^2, enters at the inlet (27), the flow being controlled by the 'inspiratory time' control (26). During the inspiratory phase this driving gas entrains air through the injector (25). The mixture enters the 'Pulsator' through the open valve (21) and flows to the rigid plastic pressure chamber (11). The anaesthetic gas in the concertina reservoir bag (8) is forced past the diaphragm valve (7) and through the breathing tube (1).

Normally all the gas contained in the reservoir bag (8) at the start of the inspiratory phase is delivered to the patient. This volume depends on the setting of the control (12) which determines the extent to which the bag could fill during the previous expiratory phase.

When the pressure in the chamber (20) of the 'Pulsator' has risen to 35 cmH_2O the unit cycles (see below), the valve (21) is closed, and the valve (23) is opened. The mixture of driving gas and entrained air can no longer enter the 'Pulsator' and the driving gas therefore flows to atmosphere through the entrainment ports of the injector (25). Since the pressure chamber (11) is now freely connected to atmosphere through the open valve

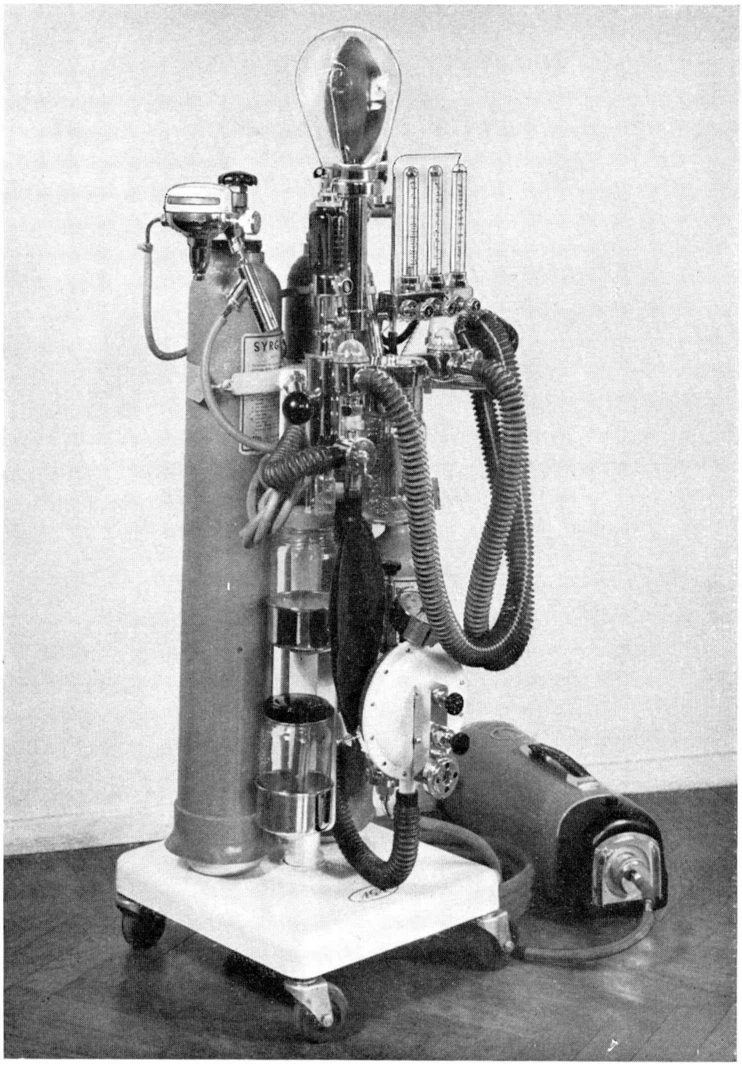

Fig. 10.1. The Aga 'Spiropulsator' MDNC–20.

Courtesy of Aga Medical Division.

(23), expired gas flows back into the concertina reservoir bag (8). This expiratory flow is assisted by the weight (10) in the base of the concertina bag. When the bag is filled, any excess gas escapes through the spill valve (9).

The mode of action of the 'Pulsator' unit is as follows. The mixture of driving gas and entrained air enters the unit at the inlet (27), at a rate controlled by the needle valve (26). The setting of this valve determines the flow rate of gas into the lungs during the inspira-

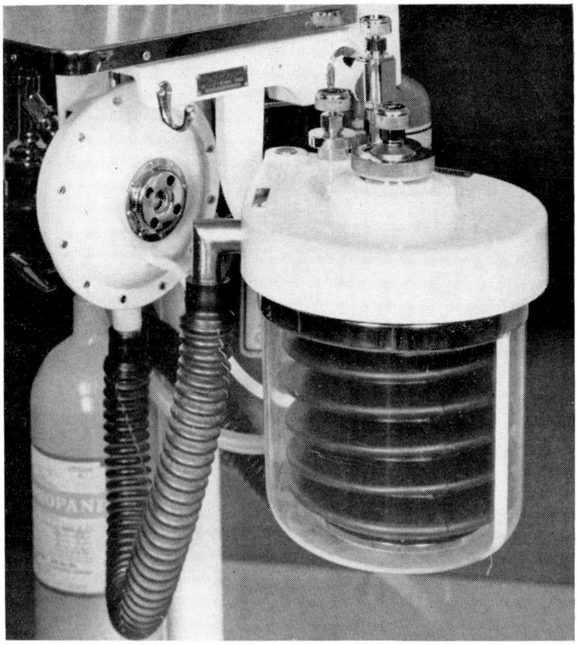

Fig. 10.2. The Aga 'Spiropulsator' ME–2440.

Courtesy of Aga Medical Division.

tory phase and, for a given tidal volume, therefore determines the inspiratory time. The driving mixture enters the chamber (20) and passes through it to the pressure chamber (11). The diaphragm (19) is connected to the rod (24) to which are attached the valves (21) and (23). This rod is held in the inspiratory position by the magnet (22), or in the expiratory position by the magnet (16). During the inspiratory phase the centre of the diaphragm cannot move until the pressure in the chamber (20) has risen to a level at which the force exerted on the diaphragm (19) is sufficient to overcome the combined effects of the spring (18) and the attraction of the magnet (22). The rod (24) now flicks over, closing the valve (21) and opening the valve (23); the inspiratory phase ends. During the inspiratory phase the one-way valve (15) allows the air in the chamber (17) to escape freely to atmosphere. At the end of the inspiratory phase the pressure in the chamber (20) falls suddenly to atmospheric. The spring (18) tends to force the diaphragm (19) back to its resting position. However, during the expiratory phase the valve (15) is closed, and therefore, until sufficient air has entered the chamber (17) by way of the pinhole in the constriction (14) and the needle valve (13) if it is open, the movement of the diaphragm (19) is impeded by the negative pressure such movement creates in the chamber (17). As air enters the chamber (17) the effective force exerted on the diaphragm increases gradually until it is sufficient to overcome the pull exerted on the rod (24) by the magnet (16).

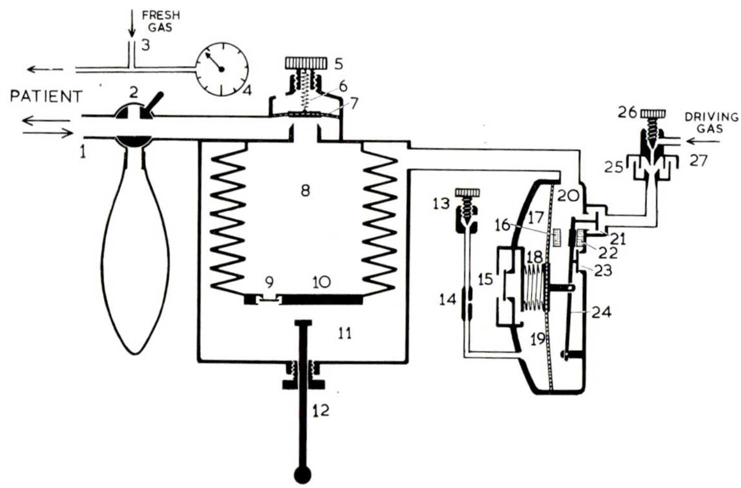

Fig. 10.3. Diagram of the Aga 'Spiropulsator' ME–2440.

1. Breathing tube
2. Manual/automatic tap
3. Fresh-gas inlet
4. Manometer
5. 'Respiratory resistance' for controlling expiratory resistance
6. Spring
7. Diaphragm
8. Concertina reservoir bag
9. Spill valve
10. Weighted base-plate
11. Rigid plastic pressure chamber
12. Stroke-volume control
13. 'Expiratory time' control
14. 'Safety device' comprising constriction and pinhole inlet
15. One-way valve
16. Magnet
17. Chamber
18. Spring
19. Diaphragm
20. Chamber
21. Inlet valve
22. Magnet
23. Exhaust valve
24. Moving rod
25. Injector
26. 'Inspiratory time' control
27. Driving-gas inlet

The rod (24) flicks over, opening the valve (21) and closing the valve (23); the expiratory phase ends. The setting of the 'expiratory time' control needle valve (13) therefore determines the duration of the expiratory phase.

The constriction in the 'safety device' (14) prevents the expiratory phase being shortened unduly, and its pinhole prevents the phase being unduly prolonged, irrespective of the setting of the needle valve (13). This ensures that the frequency cannot be set outside the range 8–40/min.

The pressure in the chamber (20) at which cycling from inspiration to expiration occurs is fixed by the characteristics of the spring (18). Normally, during the inspiratory phase, all the gas in the reservoir bag (8) is delivered to the patient before the pressure in the chamber (20) reaches the point at which cycling occurs.

During the expiratory phase the filling of the reservoir bag (8) is limited by the stop (12), which therefore acts as a tidal-volume control. Until this limit is reached the downward movement of the weight (10) in the base of the reservoir bag (8) produces a negative pressure within the bag. The pressure developed in the patient depends on the setting of the 'respiratory resistance' control (5). If this is set so that the spring (6) exerts the maximum pull on the diaphragm (7), there is no resistance to the flow of gas into or out of the concertina reservoir bag, and maximum negative pressure is developed in the patient circuit during the expiratory phase. On the other hand, if the pull on the diaphragm (7) is minimal, then the resistance of the valve is so increased that a positive pressure is maintained in the patient circuit during the expiratory phase. The use of a spring diaphragm rather than a simple throttle allows this resistance to expiration to be introduced when desired without at the same time appreciably increasing the resistance to inflation.

The tap (2) may be turned to allow manual ventilation. Fresh anaesthetic gas enters at (3). The manometer (4) indicates pressure in the patient circuit.

FUNCTIONAL ANALYSIS

This functional analysis and the 'Controls' section which follows are written on the assumption that a 'closed' patient circuit is used and that, as recommended by the manufacturers, any blow-off valve in the patient circuit is tightly closed and excess gas escapes only through the spill valve (9). Notes are appended on p. 230 on the non-rebreathing circuit and the effects of using a blow-off valve to discharge excess gas from a closed circuit. The recordings of figs. 10.6 and 10.7 were all made with a closed circuit with excess gas escaping through the spill valve.

Inspiratory phase

In this phase the 'Spiropulsator' approximates to a constant-flow generator because the characteristics of the injector (25) are such (fig. 10.4) that the flow does not fall off very much as the back pressure increases. The fall-off in flow is smaller, and therefore the approximation to constant-flow generation is closer, at high inspiratory flows than at low ones. In making the recordings of fig. 10.6 a relatively-low inspiratory flow was used and it can be seen that the flow falls off more steeply when the compliance is halved (b)

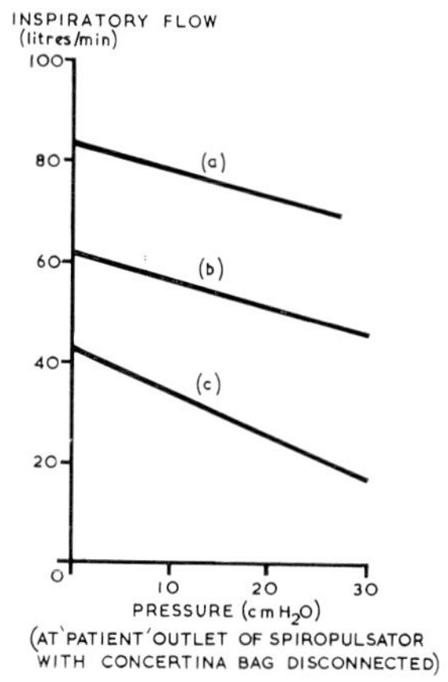

Fig. 10.4. Aga 'Spiropulsator' ME-2440. Flow-pressure characteristics of the injector for three settings of the 'inspiratory time' control:
(a) at minimum,
(b) at 1·5 turns below maximum,
(c) at 0·9 turns below maximum.
For this test the driving gas was oxygen at 60 lb/in², and flow and pressure were measured at the 'patient' outlet, (20) in fig. 10.3, of the 'Spiropulsator'.

Since, in normal operation, there is a pressure drop of about 7 cmH_2O across the wall of the reservoir bag the true flow for any given mouth pressure will be that indicated by the graph for a pressure about 7 cmH_2O greater than the given mouth pressure.

resistance between the mouth and the concertina bag, even with the 'respiratory resistance' control (5) set for minimum expiratory resistance, and also between the pressure chamber (11) and the atmosphere at exhaust valve (23). However, in fig. 10.6c, for which the airway resistance was high, it can be seen that a period of steady negative pressure at the mouth is preceded by a momentary excess of negative pressure and succeeded by a gradual decline to atmospheric pressure as the last 200 ml of gas comes out of the lungs.

Although the mouth-pressure waveforms in fig. 10.6 do not reflect the generated pressure closely the effect of changes of lung characteristics on the flow waveform can be seen clearly: halving the compliance (b) gives a higher peak expiratory flow and a more rapid decay, while doubling the airway resistance (c) leads to a lower peak flow and a slower decay.

Change-over from expiratory phase to inspiratory phase

This change-over is time-cycled. It occurs when sufficient air has leaked past the needle valve (13) and through the orifice of the 'safety device' (14) into the chamber (17) for the force on the diaphragm (19) to overcome the attraction of the magnet (16). This occurs in a time which is not affected by changes of lung characteristics as can be seen in fig. 10.6.

CONTROLS

Total ventilation

This cannot be directly controlled but is equal to the product of tidal volume and respiratory frequency.

Tidal volume

Since excess gas is spilt only during the expiratory phase, the tidal volume is equal to the stroke volume of the concertina bag plus the volume of fresh gas delivered during the inspiratory phase. So long as the 'Spiropulsator' is volume-cycled from the inspiratory phase to the expiratory phase, that is, provided the lung characteristics are not so abnormal that pressure-cycling occurs before the concertina bag is fully compressed (see the functional analysis above), the tidal volume can be directly controlled by the stroke-volume control (12). However, since the fresh-gas flow contributes to the tidal volume, increasing the fresh-gas flow (fig. 10.7f) increases the tidal volume a little.

So long as the ventilator is volume-cycled the tidal volume is not affected by changes of lung characteristics (fig. 10.6) nor by any of the other controls (fig. 10.7 except f). However, a very low compliance or a very high resistance, particularly when the stroke-volume is set high, will lead to premature pressure cycling and the tidal volume will be reduced.

When the tidal volume is deliberately increased by means of the stroke-volume control (12) the inspiratory flow is unaltered and therefore the inspiratory time is increased (fig. 10.7b). Hence the respiratory frequency is decreased and the inspiratory-expiratory ratio is changed.

Respiratory frequency and inspiratory-expiratory ratio

Neither of these parameters can be directly controlled but both are determined by the separately variable inspiratory and expiratory times.

The inspiratory time is the time taken to deliver the stroke volume of the concertina bag. It can therefore be shortened by increasing the inspiratory flow by means of turning the 'inspiratory time' control (26) in the 'minus' direction (fig. 10.7d). The inspiratory time is lengthened if the tidal volume is increased by means of the 'stroke volume' control (fig. 10.7b). The inspiratory time is not affected by any of the other controls (fig. 10.7c, e, f) and, since the ventilator is normally effectively time-cycled, it is not influenced by changes of lung characteristics (fig. 10.6). However, if a very low compliance or a very high resistance results in pressure cycling before the concertina bag has been fully compressed, then the inspiratory time is reduced.

Since the change-over at the end of the expiratory phase is time-cycled the expiratory time is directly controlled by the needle valve (13) of the 'expiratory time' control and is uninfluenced by changes of lung characteristics. The cycling mechanism, and hence the expiratory time, are uninfluenced by any other control except to a trivial extent by the 'inspiratory time' control. Moving this control in the 'minus' direction to increase the inspiratory flow increases the pressure on the inlet valve (21) during the expiratory phase and hence increases slightly the force which has to be overcome by the spring (18). Therefore a little more air has to leak into the chamber (17) behind the diaphragm (19) and this takes a little longer. However, as can be seen by comparing (d) with (a) in fig. 10.7, the effect is too small to be of clinical significance.

Thus, since the expiratory time is usually set longer than the inspiratory time, the respiratory frequency is primarily controlled by the 'expiratory time' control (13) but is also influenced by the 'inspiratory time' (26) and stroke-volume (12) controls; the inspiratory-expiratory ratio is primarily controlled by the 'inspiratory time' control but is also influenced by the 'expiratory time' and stroke-volume controls.

So long as the ventilator is effectively volume-cycled neither the respiratory frequency nor the inspiratory-expiratory ratio is appreciably influenced by changes of lung characteristics.

Inspiratory waveforms

Since this ventilator approximates to a constant-flow generator during the inspiratory phase the shape of the flow waveform cannot be varied, while the pressure waveform is determined by the interaction of the flow waveform with the lung characteristics. The amplitude of the flow waveform can be varied by means of the 'inspiratory time' control but the setting of this will normally be determined by the requirement to deliver a given tidal volume in a given inspiratory time.

Expiratory waveforms

During the expiratory phase this ventilator operates as a pressure generator and the waveform of generated pressure, though relatively complex (see the functional analysis above), cannot be adjusted. However, the resistance to expiratory flow can be adjusted by means of the 'respiratory resistance' control (5). Increasing the resistance to expiration by turning this control in the 'plus' direction (fig. 10.7e) decreases the flow at the beginning of the expiratory phase (apart from a brief initial peak) and slows down the rate at which the flow declines. The oscillation on the flow waveform under these conditions can probably be attributed to an oscillation of the diaphragm (7) engendered by the inertia of the weight (10). Since the weight generates negative pressure during the expansion of the concertina bag it is possible to introduce a certain amount of resistance by the 'respiratory resistance' control without producing a higher mean pressure than would result from the patient expiring freely to atmosphere.

Pressure limits

If the fresh-gas flow is such that the volume entering the patient circuit in one respiratory cycle is greater than the sum of the volume taken up by the patient and the volume lost through any leaks, then the excess must escape through the spill valve (9) at the end of the expiratory phase. Therefore, although negative pressure is developed inside the concertina bag (8) while its base is falling, the pressure within it must rise to atmospheric, or slightly above, before the end of the phase; that is, the base of the bag must come to rest on the adjustable stop of the stroke-volume control (12). In these circumstances the alveolar pressure can never become negative but it does normally fall to atmospheric by the end of the phase. It will fail to do so only if the airway resistance, or the expiratory resistance imposed by the 'respiratory resistance' control (5), is too high or if the expiratory time is too short. The only instance in the recordings in which the alveolar pressure did not quite fall to atmospheric is fig. 10.7e, where the 'respiratory resistance' control was set to maximum.

So long as volume-cycling occurs the peak alveolar pressure, at the end of the inspiratory phase, is determined by the fact that it must exceed the minimum at the end of the expiratory phase by an amount equal to the tidal volume divided by the compliance. If

---

Fig. 10.7. Aga 'Spiropulsator' ME–2440. Recordings showing the effects of changes in the settings of the controls, with a 'closed' patient circuit with no blow-off valve and therefore with excess gas escaping through the spill valve (9) during the expiratory phase.

(a) Standard conditions as for fig. 10.6.
(b) Stroke volume increased to produce a tidal volume of 750 ml.
(c) 'Expiratory time' decreased by 1·5 turns to produce a respiratory frequency of 30/min.
(d) 'Inspiratory time' decreased by 9 turns to minimum, that is, to give maximum inspiratory flow.
(e) 'Respiratory resistance' increased 8 turns to maximum.
(f) Fresh-gas flow increased to 4 litres/min.

pressure cycling occurs, the peak alveolar pressure is determined by the fact that it must be less than the cycling pressure by an amount equal to the sum of the pressure drop due to the weight (10) and the pressure drop across the airway and apparatus resistance due to the flow generated by the injector.

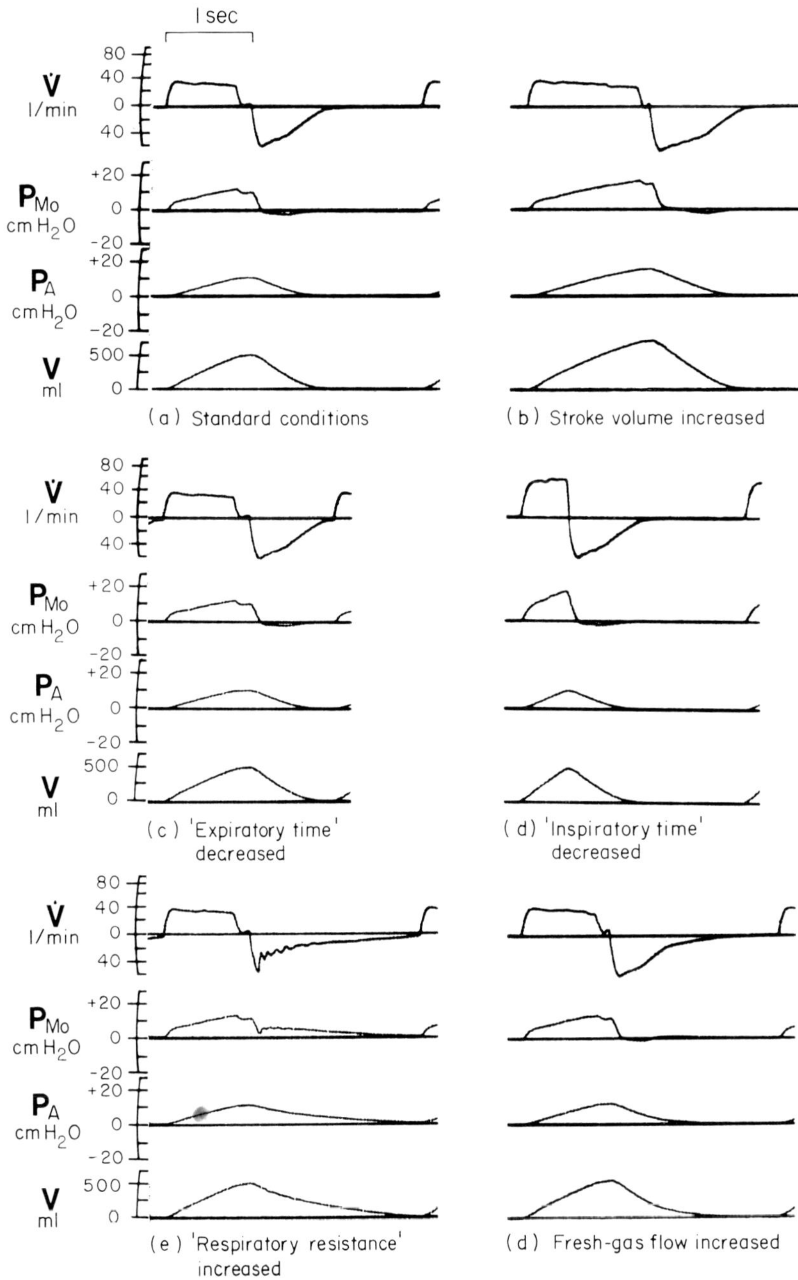

Negative pressure in the alveoli

The only way in which a negative alveolar pressure can be achieved is for the weight (10) in the concertina bag to be operative throughout the expiratory phase. This can be achieved if excess gas is discharged during the inspiratory phase, through a blow-off valve in the patient circuit, instead of during the expiratory phase, through the spill valve (9), and if, also, the stroke-volume control (12) is pulled down to its maximum position. Then, negative pressure is generated throughout the expiratory phase and therefore the alveolar pressure approaches the negative generated pressure during the phase. How closely it approaches can be regulated by the 'respiratory resistance' control (5). However, in these circumstances the ventilator is no longer volume-cycled. Instead the magnitude of the tidal volume is determined by the range of alveolar pressure multiplied by the compliance. The minimum alveolar pressure approaches the negative generated pressure in the manner described above while the peak alveolar pressure depends in a complex way on the characteristics of the expiratory valve, its setting, the inspiratory flow, and the airway resistance. Therefore, in this special mode of operation, the tidal volume, and hence the inspiratory time, inspiratory-expiratory ratio, and respiratory frequency, become dependent on lung characteristics, and tidal volume becomes dependent on the setting of the 'inspiratory time' (26) and 'respiratory resistance' (5) controls.

Non-rebreathing circuit

When an inflating valve is used, the anaesthetic circuit becomes a non-rebreathing one, and expiration occurs to atmosphere through the valve. Therefore the ventilator becomes a constant, atmospheric, pressure generator throughout the expiratory phase and the 'respiratory resistance' control becomes inoperative. Provided the Aga 'Polyvalve' is used as the inflating valve there is only one other, minor, modification to the action of the ventilator: since fresh gas enters on the atmospheric side of a one-way inlet valve (fig. 92.8, p. 775), the fresh-gas flow no longer supplements the near-flow-generating action of the injector and no longer contributes to the tidal volume. In the expiratory phase, the one-way valve permits rapid and complete refilling of the concertina reservoir bag. With other inflating valves, which do not incorporate such an inlet system, the rate of refilling of the bag in the expiratory phase is restricted to the fresh-gas flow and the action of the ventilator may be considerably modified.

CHAPTER 11

The Aika 'Respirator R–100'

DESCRIPTION

This ventilator (fig. 11.1) is designed for ward or theatre use with a closed or non-rebreathing circuit. An a.c. mains electric motor (33) (fig. 11.2) drives a gear-box (30), a crank, and a system of levers, moving the plate (15) up and down. As the plate (15) moves up the lungs are inflated from the upper concertina bag (14); as the plate moves down expiration occurs, either to atmosphere, assisted by an injector (26) driven by the compression of the lower concertina bag (16), or else into the bag (22), assisted by the expansion of the upper concertina bag (14).

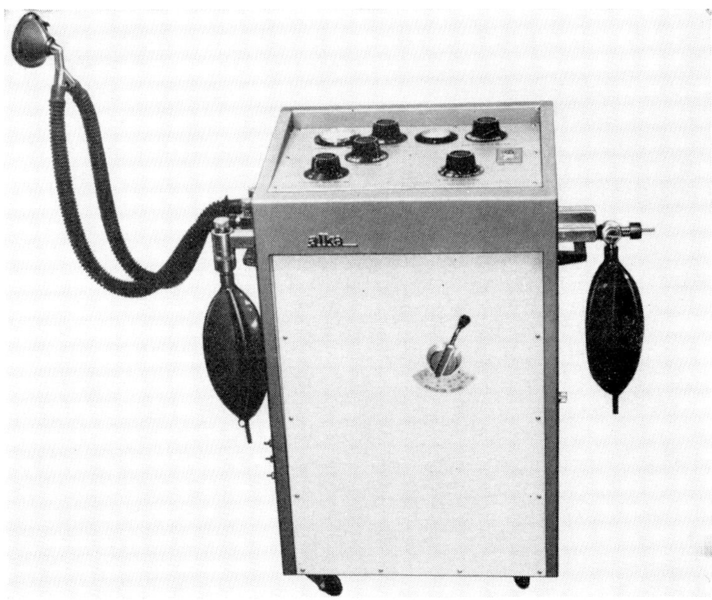

Fig. 11.1. The Aika 'Respirator R–100'.

Courtesy of Ichikawa Shiseido & Co. Ltd.

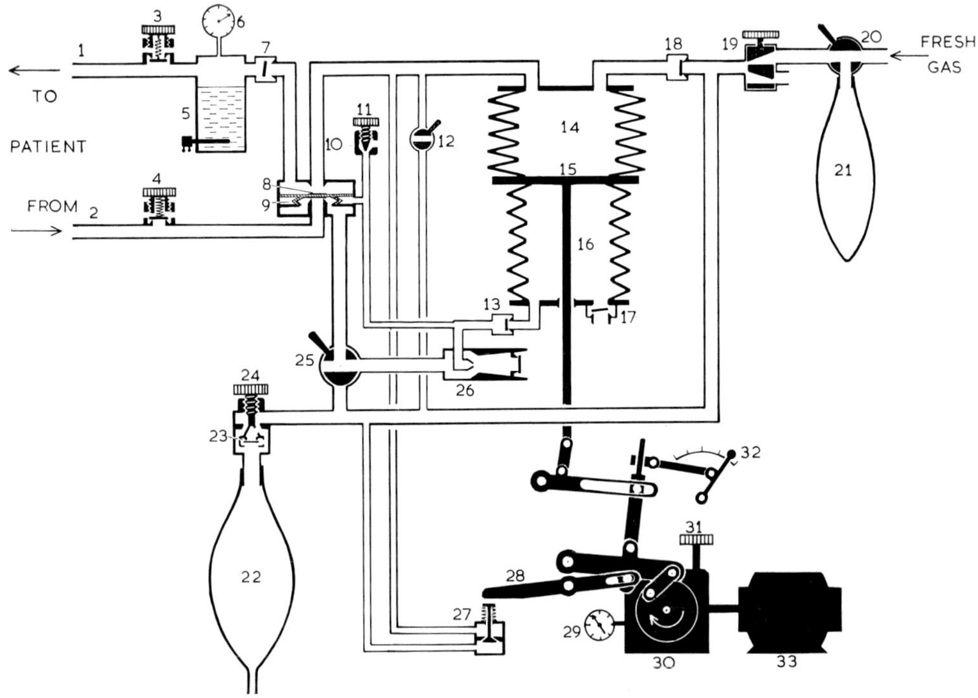

Fig. 11.2. Diagram of the Aika 'Respirator R–100'.

1. Inspiratory tube
2. Expiratory tube
3. Inlet valve
4. Positive-pressure safety-valve
5. Heated humidifier
6. Manometer
7. One-way valve
8. Diaphragm
9. Chamber
10. Tube
11. Negative-pressure control in non-rebreathing circuit
12. Manual/automatic tap
13. One-way valve
14. Concertina bag
15. Plate
16. Concertina bag
17. One-way valve
18. One-way valve
19. 'Air mixture' control
20. Fresh-gas inlet
21. Storage bag
22. Reservoir bag
23. One-way valve
24. Negative-pressure control in closed circuit
25. Closed/non-rebreathing circuit tap
26. Injector
27. Poppet valve
28. Lever
29. Tachometer
30. Gear-box
31. Frequency control
32. 'Ventilation volume' control
33. a.c. mains electric motor

When the tap (25) is in the position shown in fig. 11.2 the circuit is a non-rebreathing one. As the plate (15) moves up, the pressure within the concertina reservoir bag (14) rises, the one-way valve (18) is closed, and the diaphragm valve (8) is forced onto its lower seating, blocking the expiratory pathway. The contents of the reservoir bag (14) are now forced, through the diaphragm valve (8) and the inspiratory tube (1), to the patient. At the same time the concertina bag (16) is expanded, closing the one-way valve (13) and drawing in air through the one-way valve (17).

Shortly before the plate (15) reaches the top of its stroke the poppet valve (27) opens allowing the last of the stroke of the concertina reservoir bag (14) to be directed to the bag (22) and the pressure above the diaphragm (8) to fall. The positive pressure in the lungs causes the one-way valve (7) to close and the diaphragm (8) to move onto its upper seating so that passive expiration begins through the expiratory tube (2) and the injector (26) which is not at that time activated. Later the plate (15) commences its downward stroke so that the one-way valve (17) closes and the air driven out of the lower concertina bag (16) activates the injector (26) causing negative pressure to be developed in the expiratory tube (2). The degree of negative pressure can be adjusted, and even reduced to zero, by opening the 'negative pressure—non-rebreathing' control (11). The positive pressure which drives the injector is also applied to the small chamber (9) below the outer annulus of the diaphragm (8); this helps to ensure that the diaphragm is held against its upper seating throughout the expiratory phase.

If negative pressure is developed during the expiratory phase the pressure balance across the diaphragm (8) when the plate (15) reaches the bottom of its stroke is as follows: negative pressure is applied over the whole of the top surface except for the area of the tube (10), negative pressure is applied over the centre area of the under surface, and atmospheric pressure over the outer annulus of the under surface. Therefore the net force is upwards. Consequently, the plate (15) has to travel a little way upwards before it develops a positive pressure in the concertina reservoir bag (14) which, over the area of the tube (10), exerts enough downward force to blow the diaphragm (8) off its upper seating onto its lower seating. The next inspiratory phase then begins.

During the expiratory phase, the reservoir bag (14) is expanded and fresh gas is drawn into it through the one-way valve (18). The tap (19) may be adjusted to admit air, fresh gas supplied at the inlet (20) and stored in the bag (21), or a mixture of both.

When a closed circuit is to be used the tap (25) is turned to the 'closed' position, and the 'air-mixture' tap (19) is set to 'off' so that air is not admitted, but only fresh gas entering at the inlet (20) and stored in the bag (21). A carbon-dioxide absorber is fitted in the breathing circuit. During the expiratory phase expired gas flows, past the diaphragm valve (8), the 'non-rebreathing/closed' tap (25), and then, when expiration is passive, (that is, during at least the first part of the phase) through the one-way valve (23), into the bag (22). Later, when the concertina bag (14) begins to expand this draws gas from the bag (22). Adjustment of the 'closed-circuit negative-pressure control' (24) restricts this flow of gas from the bag (22), so that the expansion of the concertina bag (14) creates a negative pressure in the expiratory pathway and draws more gas from the lungs causing a negative pressure to develop in the alveoli.

If manual ventilation is desired the motor is switched off, the tap (12) is turned, and the bag (22) is squeezed after closing the hole in its end. The opening of the tap (12) prevents the diaphragm valve (8) being held on its lower seating at the end of the inspiratory phase by the pressure in the inspiratory pathway between the one-way valves (7) and (18). The tap (12) performs a similar function to the opening of the poppet valve

(27) in the automatic mode. Either the closed or the non-rebreathing circuit may be used during manual inflation.

The respiratory frequency may be varied between 10 and 40/min by adjusting the control (31) and is shown on the tachometer (29). The tidal-volume control (32) allows the stroke volume of the plate (15) to be varied by altering the fulcrum of the linkage between the gear-box (30) and the plate (15). In this way the tidal volume may be varied between 300 and 900 ml. The one-way valve (23) may be turned in one direction to allow the patient to inhale freely through it, or in the other direction to permit the development of negative pressure during the expiratory phase. The manometer (6) indicates the pressure in the patient circuit which is limited to any value up to 40 cmH_2O depending on the setting of the control (4). The maximum negative pressure is −15 cmH_2O. A thermostatically-controlled hot-water humidifier (5) is incorporated for use with the non-rebreathing circuit. The inspiratory-expiratory ratio is fixed at 1 : 1·5.

FUNCTIONAL ANALYSIS

Inspiratory phase

If the speed of the motor (33) is uninfluenced by the pressures in the concertina bags the ventilator operates fundamentally as a non-constant-flow generator in this phase. The pattern of flow approximates to part of a sine wave. When negative pressure is used in expiration the first part of the sine wave is distorted a little by the need to build up pressure in the concertina bag (14) before the diaphragm valve (8) opens. Since the phase ends shortly before the concertina bag (14) has completed its compression stroke the flow pattern represents something less than a half cycle of a sine wave. The positive-pressure safety-valve can be used to introduce a pressure limit before the end of the phase in which case the ventilator becomes a constant-pressure generator in the last part of the phase, but then the tidal volume of the patient is less than the volume delivered from the concertina reservoir bag (14).

Change-over from inspiratory phase to expiratory phase

This change-over is volume-cycled and time-cycled. It occurs when the poppet valve (27) is opened, releasing the pressure from the top of the diaphragm valve (8) at a particular point in the rotation of the output shaft of the gear-box (30). Therefore, if the speed of the motor (33) is constant throughout the cycle, this release occurs not only when a preset volume has been expelled from the concertina reservoir bag (14) but also in a preset time.

Expiratory phase

In the first part of this phase the ventilator operates as a constant, atmospheric, pressure generator: the patient's expiration passes to atmosphere through the injector (26) or into the bag (22) which is limp enough for the pressure inside it to be nearly atmospheric.

Subsequently, while the plate (15) is moving downwards, the ventilator operates as an approximately-sine-wave pressure generator. With the non-rebreathing circuit this arises because the lower concertina bag (16) delivers approximately a sine wave of driving flow to the injector. With the closed circuit, sine-wave pressure generation arises because the expansion of the concertina reservoir bag (14) constitutes a sine-wave-flow generator but the adjustable restriction at the head of the bag (22) constitutes a leak and a flow generator with a leak in parallel is equivalent to a pressure generator (see p. 85).

Change-over from expiratory phase to inspiratory phase

This change-over is primarily time-cycled. It occurs at the end of a short delay after the plate (15) starts to rise at a particular point in the rotation of the output shaft of the gear-box (30). The delay arises from the need to build up some positive pressure in the concertina reservoir bag (14) before the diaphragm valve (8) is displaced from its upper seating onto its lower seating. Since the positive pressure required in the bag (14) depends on the negative pressure developed in the lungs in the previous expiratory phase, the delay is slightly variable.

CHAPTER 12

The 'Aintree' Ventilator[1]

DESCRIPTION

A built-in compressor (fig. 12.1) supplies air at a pressure of 15 lb/in^2 which enters at (15) (fig. 12.2). Its flow is controlled by the needle valve (16). The compressed air passes into the chamber (10) which is closed above by the disc valve (11). This is held down by the attraction of the magnet (14) for the soft-iron disc (13). The compressed air flows into the glass pressure chamber (2) and also into the expiratory-time control chamber (19). The pressure exerted on the reservoir bag (3) forces the gas within it to the patient. When this inflating pressure has risen sufficiently, it overcomes the attraction of the magnet (14) for

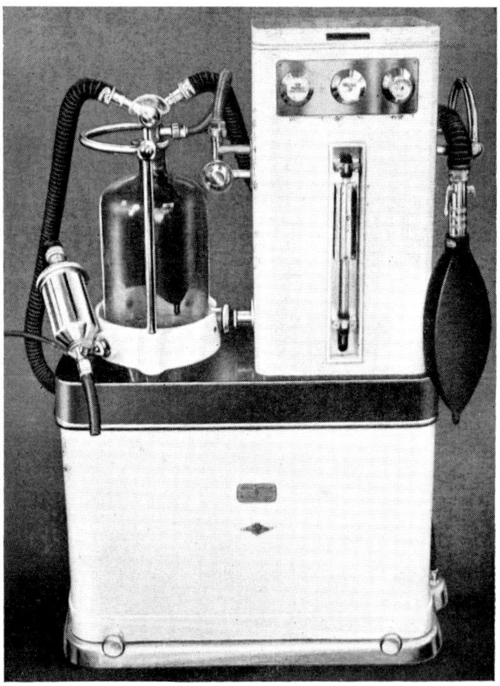

Fig. 12.1. The 'Aintree' ventilator.

Courtesy of Medical & Industrial Equipment Ltd.

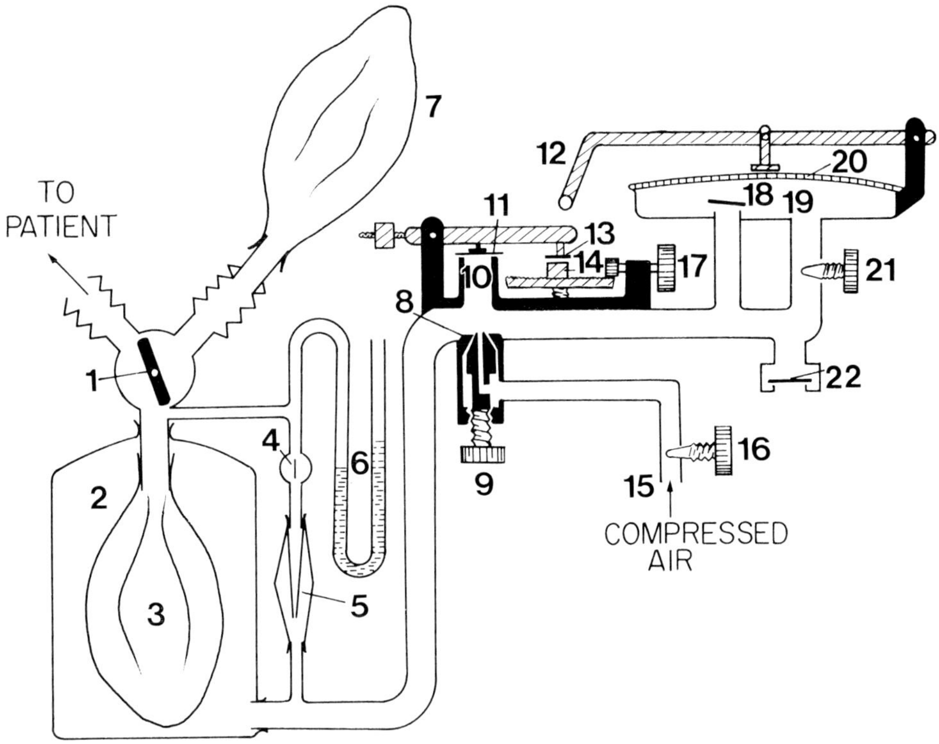

Fig. 12.2. Diagram of the 'Aintree' ventilator.

1. 'Manual/auto' control
2. Glass pressure chamber
3. Reservoir bag
4. Tap
5. Kendrick valve
6. Water manometer
7. Reservoir bag for manual ventilation
8. Injector
9. Negative-pressure control
10. Exhaust-valve chamber
11. Disc exhaust valve
12. Lever
13. Soft-iron disc
14. Magnet
15. Driving-gas inlet
16. Needle valve
17. Cycling-pressure control
18. One-way valve
19. Chamber
20. Diaphragm
21. Control for varying the expiratory time
22. Air-inlet valve

the soft-iron disc (13). The valve (11) is lifted, allowing the escape of the compressed air to the atmosphere, and expiration commences.

The flow of the compressed air through the injector (8) now produces a slight negative pressure in the pressure chamber (2), and this aids the flow of gas from the lungs. As the pressure in the chamber (2) begins to fall, the one-way valve (18) shuts, trapping the air within the chamber (19). This air slowly escapes at a rate determined by the expiratory-time control (21). The lever (12) gradually falls, pushing the arm, holding the disc (13), back within the field of the magnet (14). This snaps the exhaust valve (11) shut and so initiates another inspiratory phase. When the tap (4) is open, any excess of gas in the respiratory circuit escapes through the Kendrick valve (5) which acts as a spill valve. The tap (16) controls the flow of driving gas. The more driving gas admitted, the faster are the lungs inflated. Adjustment of the control (9) determines the negative pressure during the expiratory phase by directing the driving gas either through the injector (8) or around it. The negative pressure is limited to -5 to -7 cmH_2O by the gravity-operated inlet valve (22).

The maximum pressure during the inspiratory phase is varied by the control (17) which raises or lowers the magnet (14). If the magnet is raised closer to the metal disc (13) its effect is increased and a higher pressure must be attained before the valve (11) is lifted. A water manometer (6) indicates the pressure in the patient circuit and also acts as a safety blow-off valve. A control tap (1) allows manual inflation from the bag (7).

FUNCTIONAL ANALYSIS

Inspiratory phase

In this phase the ventilator operates as a constant-flow generator due to the constant high pressure from the compressor, applied to the resistance of the needle valve and injector. The fresh-gas supply to the patient circuit acts as a small-constant-flow generator, supplementing the main flow generator.

Change-over from inspiratory phase to expiratory phase

This change-over is pressure-cycled: the pressure in chamber (10) which produces cycling is that applied to the patient via the reservoir bag.

Expiratory phase

In this phase the ventilator operates as a constant, negative, pressure generator with substantial series resistance (due to the injector characteristics) with a limit to the negative pressure developed in the pressure chamber (2), set by the negative-pressure-limiting valve (22).

Change-over from expiratory phase to inspiratory phase

This change-over is time-cycled: the expiratory time is equal to the time in which enough air leaks out of chamber (19) for cycling to occur. This time is uninfluenced by the patient; but if the cycling pressure at the end of the inspiratory phase is raised, the volume of air which has to leak out is increased, and the expiratory phase is lengthened.

REFERENCE

1 ESPLEN J.R. (1952) A new apparatus for intermittent pulmonary inflation. *Br. J. Anaesth.* **24**, 303.

CHAPTER 13

The Air-Shields 'Pressure Breathing Assistor'

DESCRIPTION

This portable ventilator (fig. 13.1), is intended for use in the ward or at home.

Compressed air from the integral electrically-driven blower (17) (fig. 13.2) is delivered to the patient, through the solenoid-operated valve (16), the one-way valve (15), and the replaceable gauze filter (4). The chamber behind the diaphragm of the expiratory valve

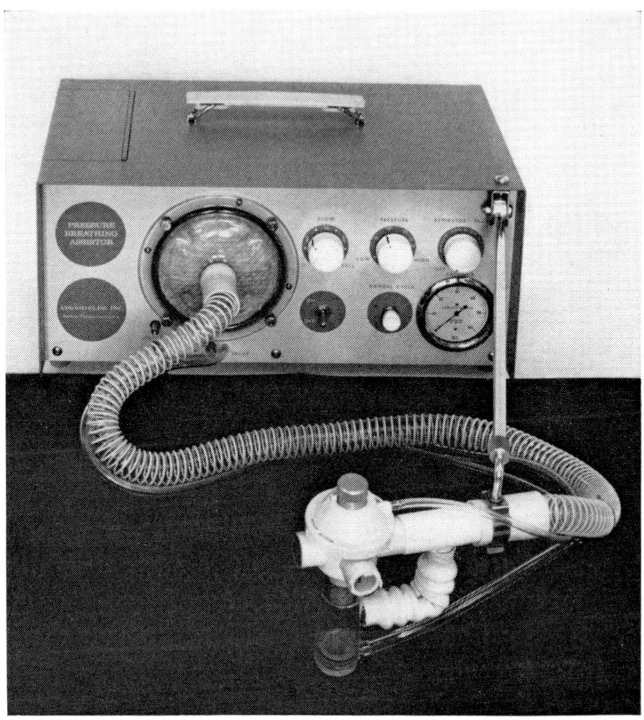

Fig. 13.1 The Air-Shields 'Pressure Breathing Assistor'.

Courtesy of Air-Shields Inc.

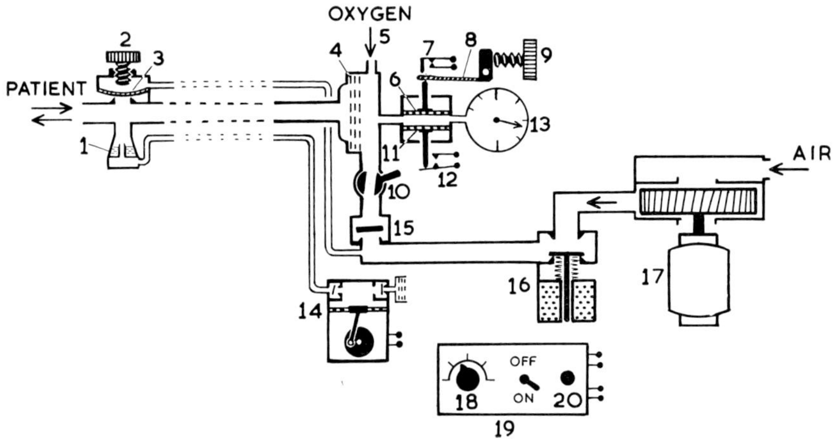

Fig. 13.2. Diagram of the Air-Shields 'Pressure Breathing Assistor'.

1. Nebulizer
2. Expiratory-resistance control
3. Expiratory valve
4. Filter
5. Oxygen inlet
6. Diaphragm
7. Microswitch for ending inspiratory phase
8. Leaf spring
9. 'Pressure' control
10. 'Flow' control
11. Diaphragm
12. Microswitch for patient-triggering of inspiration
13. Manometer
14. Diaphragm pump
15. One-way valve
16. Solenoid-operated valve
17. Electric blower
18. 'Expiratory pause' control
19. Electronic timing unit
20. 'Manual cycle' push-button

(3) is connected to the main gas pathway between the solenoid valve (16) and the one-way valve (15). So long as flow continues there is a pressure drop across the main gas pathway (15, 10, 4) and therefore the expiratory valve is held closed by the higher pressure existing in the chamber behind the diaphragm. The 'flow' control (10) allows the inspiratory flow to be restricted within the range 100 – 1 litres/min. As the pressure in the breathing tube rises during the inspiratory phase the diaphragm (6), which carries a small push-rod, is distended upwards. The microswitch (7) is in the holding circuit of the solenoid-operated valve (16) and is normally closed. When the diaphragm (6) has moved upwards sufficiently against the force exerted by the leaf spring (8), it opens the microswitch (7) and the electrical supply to the solenoid valve (16) is interrupted. The valve (16) therefore is moved by its spring into the expiratory position, and the flow of air from the blower is cut off. The chamber behind the diaphragm of the expiratory valve (3) is now connected to atmosphere through the valve (16) and pressure within the chamber falls to atmospheric. Expired gas can now escape freely to atmosphere through the expiratory valve (3). The control (2) on the expiratory-valve assembly may be adjusted to set a resistance to expiratory flow if desired. The opening of the expiratory valve (3) also allows the pressure below the diaphragm (6) to fall, and the leaf spring (8) comes away from the microswitch (7) which returns to its closed position. However, the solenoid

valve (16) remains in the expiratory position since the microswitch (7) is in its holding circuit and not its actuating circuit.

The expiratory phase continues until the next inspiratory phase is initiated. This may be done in one of three ways, patient-triggering, manual-triggering, or automatic cycling by the electronic timing unit (19). If the patient makes an inspiratory effort during the expiratory phase the negative pressure produced in the breathing tube allows the expiratory valve (3) to close and the negative pressure is then transmitted to the chamber between the two diaphragms (6) and (11). The upward movement of the diaphragm (11) allows the microswitch (12), which is normally open, to close. This completes the actuating circuit of the solenoid valve (16) which is moved to the inspiratory position. The next inspiratory phase begins, and the rise of pressure between the diaphragms (6) and (11) pushes back the lower diaphragm (11). The microswitch (12) is reopened, but the solenoid valve is kept in the inspiratory position by the holding circuit through the microswitch (7). The negative pressure required to trigger this mechanism is fixed at less than -1 cmH_2O.

The electronic timing unit (19) is in parallel with the microswitch (12) and, when switched on, automatically cycles the ventilator from expiration to inspiration if the patient fails to make an inspiratory effort within a certain time, which is determined by the setting of the 'expiratory pause' control (18).

A 'manual cycle' push-button (20), also in parallel with the microswitch (12), is provided so that a fresh inspiratory phase can be initiated at any time if desired.

The duration of the inspiratory phase depends on the time taken for the pressure below the diaphragm (6) to rise sufficiently to open the microswitch (7). The upward movement of the diaphragm (6) is opposed by the leaf spring (8), the tension of which is set by the 'pressure' control (9). The maximum inspiratory pressure is limited to 35 cmH_2O, the pressure being shown on the manometer (13).

Adjustment of the controls (9, 10, 18) allows the frequency to be varied between 6 and 60 per minute. A nebulizer (1) is an integral part of the expiratory-valve assembly. Throughout the inspiratory phase current is supplied to the small diaphragm pump (14) which drives air to the nebulizer irrespective of whether liquid is present in the container or not.

Oxygen may be added at the inlet (5).

FUNCTIONAL ANALYSIS

Inspiratory phase

In this phase the mode of operation depends on the characteristics of the blower (17). It is likely that this operates as a high-constant-pressure generator with adjustable series resistance at the 'flow' control (10).

Change-over from inspiratory phase to expiratory phase

This change-over is pressure-cycled: it occurs when the pressure below the diaphragm (6), which is similar to the pressure at the mouth, rises high enough to open the microswitch (7) against the force of the leaf spring (8).

Expiratory phase

In this phase the ventilator operates as a constant, atmospheric, pressure generator: the patient's expiration passes to atmosphere through the expiratory valve (3).

Change-over from expiratory phase to inspiratory phase

This change-over can always be patient-cycled: an inspiratory effort which reduces the pressure above the diaphragm (11) sufficiently to close the microswitch (12) will cycle the ventilator to inspiration.

If the electronic timer (19) is switched on, the change-over is patient-cycled or time-cycled whichever occurs first.

CHAPTER 14

The Air-Shields 'Respirator'

DESCRIPTION

This ventilator (fig. 14.1) is designed for ward use.

An a.c. mains electric motor (17) (fig. 14.2) drives an air blower (18) continuously. During the inspiratory phase the solenoid valve (19) is held open and air from the blower flows to the capsules of the expiratory valve (1) and the exhaust valve (12), and past the one-way valve (8) into the rigid plastic pressure chamber (10). The concertina reservoir bag (4) is compressed and its contents forced past the one-way valve (3) to the patient. A heated spinning-disc humidifier (6), driven by the electric motor (17), is incorporated in the inspiratory pathway.

After a given time, determined by the setting of the 'inspiratory time' control (21) of the electronic timing unit, the position of the valve (19) is reversed, and the pathway between the blower (18) and the pressure chamber (10) is blocked. All the air from the blower now passes to atmosphere through the outlet (16). The capsules (1) and (12) now collapse since they are in communication with the atmosphere through an outlet in the solenoid valve (19). Expired gas passes to atmosphere through the expiratory valve (1); the degree of opening of the valve may be limited by the setting of its knob thereby increasing the resistance to expiration. At the same time the concertina bag (4) is free to re-expand under the influence of the weight (9) in its base, and air is freely drawn into it through the filter (2) and the one-way valve (5), oxygen being added at the side inlet if required. The one-way valve (3) prevents any negative pressure produced in the bag (4) being transmitted to the patient. The duration of the expiratory phase depends on the setting of the 'expiratory pause' control (22) of the timing unit which determines the length of time for which the solenoid valve (19) is held closed.

The safety-valve (11) limits the positive pressure to about 50 cmH_2O. The 'flow' control (7) may be adjusted to regulate the inspiratory flow.

The inspiratory time may be varied between $\frac{1}{2}$ and 3 seconds, and the expiratory time between about $\frac{1}{2}$ and 10 seconds. The frequency is therefore variable between 5 and 60 per minute. So long as the safety-valve (11) does not open, and the bag (4) is not completely emptied, the tidal volume depends on the duration of the inspiratory phase and the flow of air blown into the pressure chamber (10). If this flow is restricted by the setting of the control (7) excess air delivered by the blower during the inspiratory phase is vented through the outlet (16). The pressure in the breathing circuit is shown in the manometer (20).

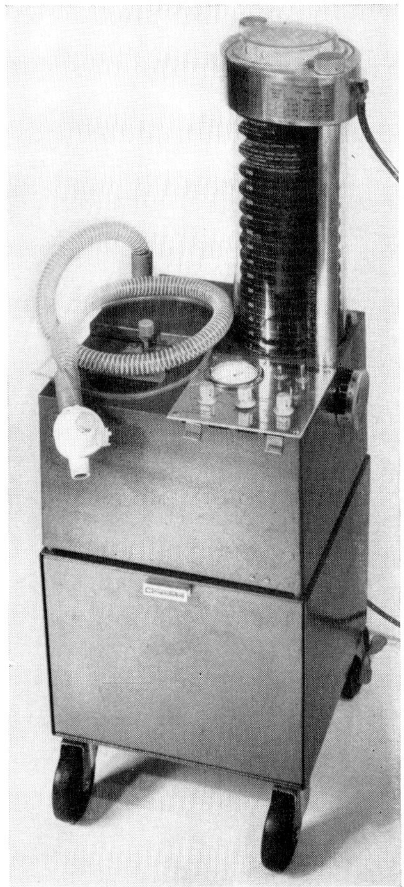

Fig. 14.1. The Air-Shields 'Respirator'.
Courtesy of Department of Medical Illustration, Cardiff Royal Infirmary.

Closure of the 'control/assist control' switch (23) activates the electrical circuit of the patient-triggering mechanism. If the patient makes an inspiratory effort during the expiratory phase, the one-way valve (1) closes and the negative pressure produced in the breathing circuit is transmitted to one side of the diaphragm (14). The diaphragm moves over, the contacts (13) are closed, and the expiratory phase is terminated by the electronic timing unit. The negative pressure required to effect this may be adjusted by the 'sensitivity' control (15).

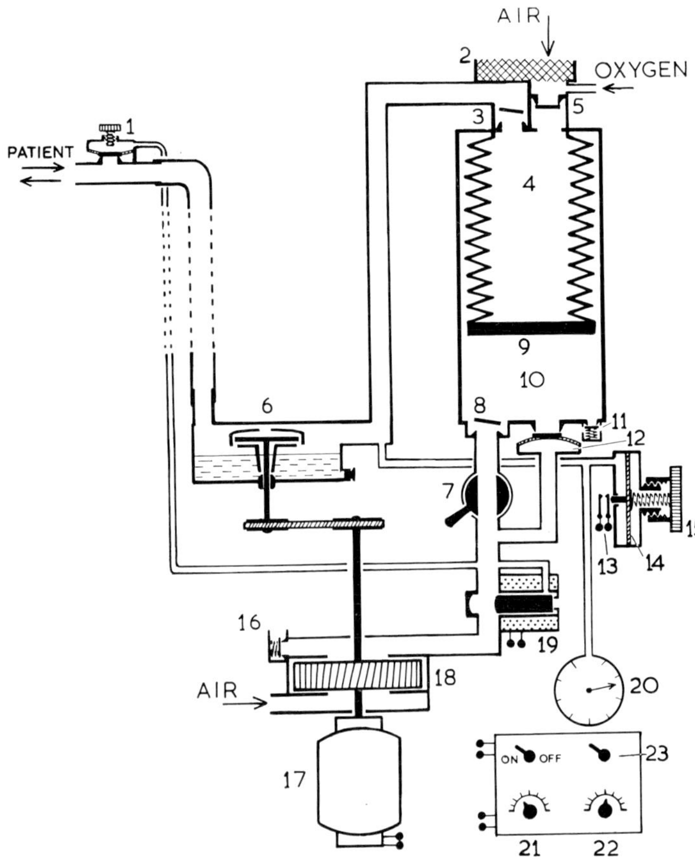

Fig. 14.2. Diagram of the Air-Shields 'Respirator'.

1. Expiratory valve
2. Air filter
3. One-way valve
4. Concertina reservoir bag
5. One-way inlet valve
6. Spinning-disc humidifier
7. Inspiratory 'flow' control
8. One-way valve
9. Weight
10. Rigid plastic pressure chamber
11. Safety-valve
12. Exhaust valve
13. Patient-trigger contacts
14. Diaphragm
15. 'Sensitivity' control
16. Outlet
17. Electric motor
18. Air blower
19. Solenoid valve
20. Manometer
21. 'Inspiratory time' control
22. 'Expiratory pause' control
23. 'Control/assist control' switch

FUNCTIONAL ANALYSIS

Inspiratory phase

The flow-pressure characteristics (fig. 14.3) of the air blower (18) with various settings of the 'flow' control (7), show that the ventilator must be regarded as fundamentally equivalent to a constant-pressure generator (about 60 to 80 cmH_2O) with a substantial series resistance, and with an overriding pressure limit of just over 50 cmH_2O. However, since the generated pressure is large compared with the range of alveolar pressure usually encountered, it is to be expected that the ventilator will normally approximate to a constant-flow generator. That this is so can be seen from the recordings of fig. 14.4 in which the inspiratory flow falls off only to a small extent during the phase and is only slightly modified by changes of lung characteristics. The mouth-pressure waveforms, on the other hand, are considerably modified by changes of lung characteristics.

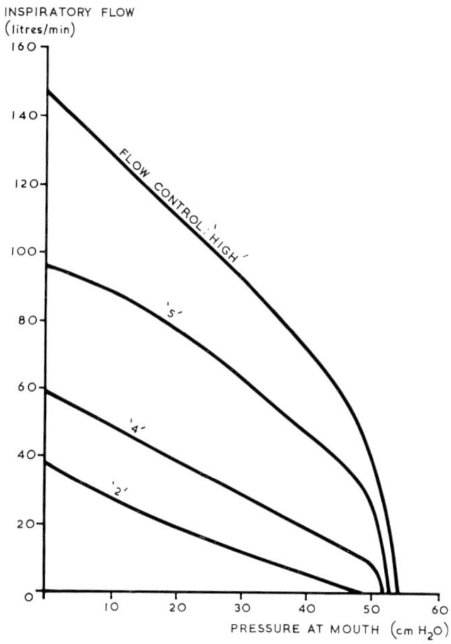

Fig. 14.3. Air-Shields 'Respirator'. Flow-pressure characteristics of the inspiratory mechanism, measured with the concertina bag *in situ*.

Change-over from inspiratory phase to expiratory phase

This change-over is time-cycled: it occurs when the solenoid valve (19) closes at a preset time after the start of the inspiratory phase determined by the electronic timing circuit. This is demonstrated in fig. 14.4 in which changes of lung characteristics are not accompanied by changes in inspiratory time.

Expiratory phase

During this phase the ventilator operates as a constant, atmospheric, pressure generator with adjustable series resistance: expiration to atmosphere occurs past the expiratory valve (1) whose maximum degree of opening can be limited by its knob.

Change-over from expiratory phase to inspiratory phase

With the switch (23) in the 'control' position this change-over is purely time-cycled: it occurs when the solenoid valve (19) opens at a preset time after the start of the expiratory phase determined by the electronic timing circuit. This is demonstrated in fig. 14.4 in which changes of lung characteristics are not accompanied by changes in expiratory time.

With the switch (23) in the 'assist/control' position the change-over is either time-

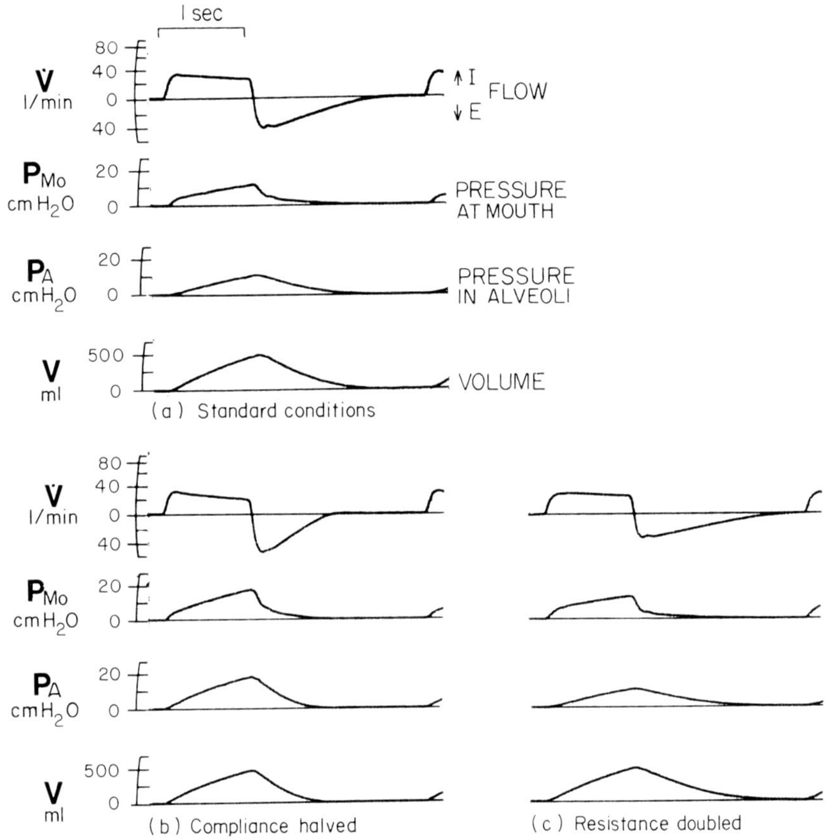

Fig. 14.4. Air-Shields 'Respirator'. Recordings showing the effects of changes of lung characteristics. Standard conditions: switch (23), in 'control' position; oxygen flow, zero; 'resistance' (to expiration), minimum; 'inspiratory time', set for an inspiratory time of 1 sec; 'expiratory pause', set for an expiratory time of 2 sec; 'flow', set for a tidal volume of 500 ml.

cycled or patient-cycled whichever event occurs first. If the patient produces enough negative pressure for the diaphragm (14) to close the electrical contacts (13) this triggers the electronic circuit to the inspiratory condition before the preset expiratory time has elapsed.

CONTROLS

Total ventilation

This cannot be directly controlled but is equal to the product of tidal volume and respiratory frequency.

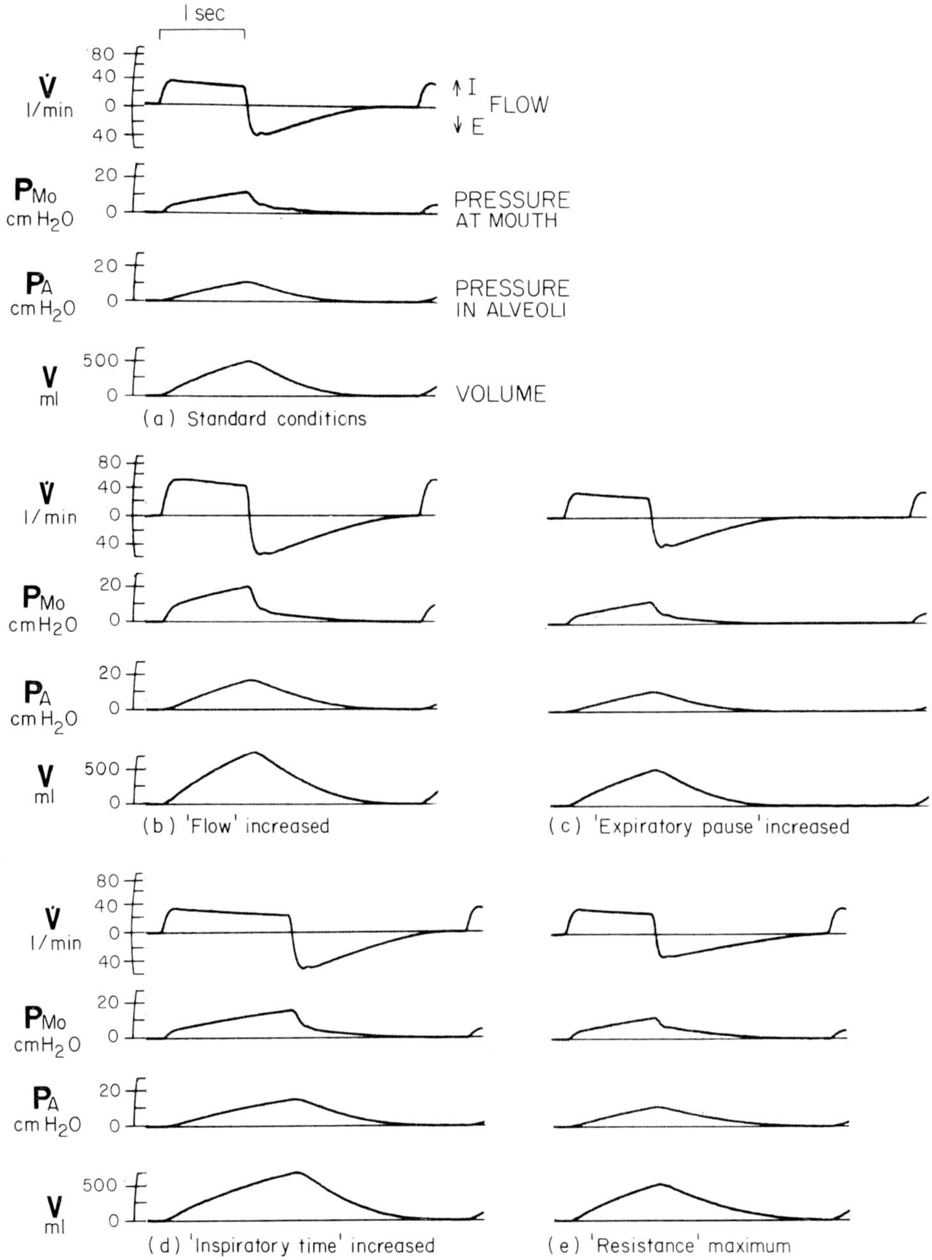

Fig. 14.5 Air-Shields 'Respirator'. Recordings showing the effects of changes in the settings of the controls.

(a) Standard conditions as in fig. 14.4.
(b) 'Flow' increased from '2·4' to '4·3' to produce a tidal volume of 750 ml.
(c) 'Expiratory pause' increased to produce an expiratory time of 3 sec.
(d) 'Inspiratory time' increased to produce an inspiratory time of 1·5 sec.
(e) 'Resistance' (to expiration) increased to maximum.

Tidal volume

This is not directly controlled but is equal to the product of mean inspiratory flow and inspiratory time. The inspiratory time is directly controlled by the electronic circuit and so is uninfluenced by lung characteristics but will normally be set in accordance with other requirements (see below). The mean inspiratory flow can be adjusted by the 'flow' control (7) and this provides the primary means of adjusting tidal volume (fig. 14.5b). However, the approximation to flow generation is only moderately close and the tidal volume is slightly diminished when the compliance is halved (fig. 14.4b) or the resistance doubled (fig. 14.4c).

Respiratory frequency and inspiratory-expiratory ratio

These are not directly controlled but both are determined by the inspiratory and expiratory times which are entirely determined by the functioning of the electronic timer and are quite uninfluenced by the patient—except when patient-triggering occurs with the switch (23) in the 'assist/control' position. The separate controls for inspiratory time (21) and expiratory time (the 'expiratory pause' control (22)) show slight interaction at short times: reducing the 'expiratory pause' setting from '2 sec' to '$\frac{1}{2}$ sec' reduces the inspiratory time, whatever it may happen to be, by about 10%; similarly, reducing the 'inspiratory time' setting from '1 sec' to '$\frac{1}{2}$ sec' reduces the expiratory time by about 10%. At longer times, however, the actions are quite independent, as is illustrated by fig. 14.5(c) and (d), and quite unaffected by other parameters, as can be seen by the other tracings in fig. 14.5 and by fig. 14.4.

When the inspiratory time is increased the tidal volume is increased. A consequence of this is that, if it is desired to increase the tidal volume and decrease the frequency while leaving the total ventilation unaltered, it will almost be sufficient just to increase the inspiratory and expiratory times in the same proportion. However, some slight increase in the setting of the flow control will be required in addition because, in the extended inspiratory time, the mouth pressure rises higher and the inspiratory flow falls slightly lower.

Inspiratory waveforms

Since the ventilator approximates to a constant-flow generator the inspiratory flow is nearly constant throughout the phase and is hardly altered by changes of lung characteristics (fig. 14.4). The magnitude of the flow can be adjusted by means of the 'flow' control (7) (fig. 14.5b) but this will normally have been set in accordance with other requirements. The waveform of flow cannot be altered.

Expiratory waveforms

Since the ventilator operates as a constant, atmospheric, pressure generator in expiration the expiratory flow rises rapidly to a peak and decays progressively to zero. The magnitude of the peak flow and the rate of decay depend on the lung characteristics but they can both be reduced by increasing the resistance (1) in series with the generated pressure (fig. 14.5e).

Pressure limits

Again, since the ventilator operates as a constant, atmospheric, pressure generator throughout the expiratory phase, the alveolar pressure falls towards that limit and in most circumstances reaches it by the end of the phase. It does so in all the tracings of fig. 14.4 and 14.5; it will fail to do so only when the total resistance to expiration is very high or when the expiratory time is very short.

CHAPTER 15

The Air-Shields 'Ventimeter Ventilator'

DESCRIPTION

This ventilator (fig. 15.1) is designed primarily for anaesthetic use with any standard circuit.

Driving gas at a pressure above 30 lb/in^2, is supplied at the inlet (32) (fig. 15.2) and flows through a sintered-bronze filter (33) to a reducing valve (26) which maintains the pressure of the driving gas at about 30 lb/in^2, this pressure being shown on the gauge (25). When the tap (27) is in the 'on' position the driving gas flows to the space beneath the diaphragm (12) and thence to the pneumatic timing unit (13–22).

During the inspiratory phase the differential diaphragms (14) in the timing unit are in their 'up' position and the valve (16) is held on its upper seating by its spring. Driving gas therefore flows, past the 'inspiratory flow' needle valve (22), through the 'bag/ventilator' tap (11), to the rigid plastic pressure chamber (1). The concertina reservoir bag (2) is compressed and the gas within it is delivered through the tube (34) to the patient. At the same time the pressure in the chamber (21) of the timing unit is holding up the differential diaphragms (18) and thus keeping open the valve (17) against the force of its spring. During the inspiratory phase gas from the chamber (21) leaks off through the 'inspiratory time' needle valve (20) and the one-way valve (19), and also through the 'expiratory pause' needle valve (13). The rate of escape from the chamber (21) depends primarily on the setting of the 'inspiratory time' control (20) but also, to some extent, on the setting of the 'expiratory pause' control (13). When the pressure has fallen sufficiently the differential diaphragms (18) return to their resting position and the valve (17) closes, thereby preventing any further escape of gas to atmosphere. Driving gas is constantly flowing past the constriction (15) but can no longer escape through the valve (17), and therefore pressure above the diaphragms (14) rises rapidly and forces them down. Driving gas then flows past the 'expiratory pause' control (13) to the chamber (21) and slowly raises the diaphragms (18) again. The downward movement of the diaphragms (14) pushes the valve (16) onto its lower seating, and the flow of driving gas to the plastic pressure chamber (1) is cut off. Driving gas can now flow through the upper seating of the valve (16) to the cylinder behind the piston (9) of the expiratory valve, thus opening the valve and releasing the pressure in the pressure chamber (1). Expired gas can now pass back freely along the tube (34) into the concertina reservoir bag (2), displacing gas from the pressure chamber past the one-way valve (5).

The expiratory phase lasts until the pressure in the chamber (21) has risen sufficiently to raise the differential diaphragms (18) and, by opening the valve (17), to allow the pressure above the diaphragms (14) to fall. The diaphragms (14) return to their resting position and the cylinder (9) of the expiratory valve is connected to atmosphere through the centre of the diaphragms (14). The expiratory valve (9) is forced into the closed position by its spring.

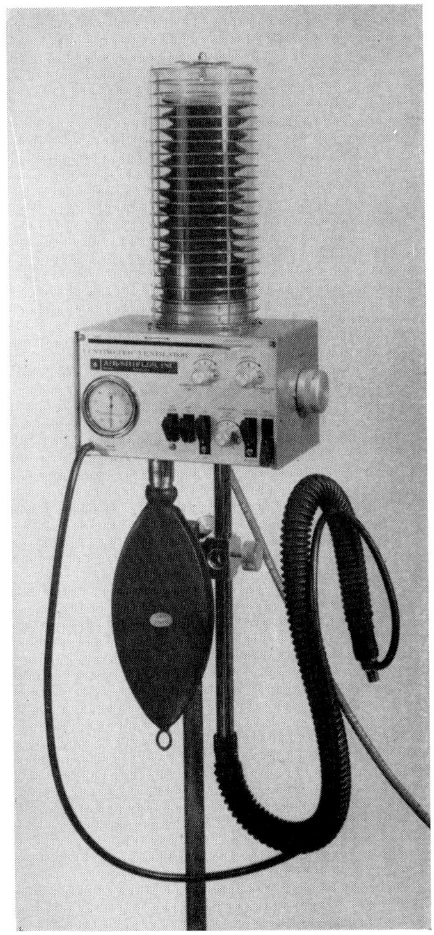

Fig. 15.1. The Air-Shields 'Ventimeter Ventilator'.
Courtesy of Department of Medical Illustration, Cardiff Royal Infirmary.

Excess gas in the breathing circuit can escape at the end of the expiratory phase past the spill valve (3). Normally the diaphragm of this valve (3) is held lightly on its seat by a small weight. During the inspiratory phase this force holding the valve (3) closed is much increased because there is a pressure difference across the reservoir bag, and because the driving-gas connexion from the needle valve (22) is directed in such a way as to exert an

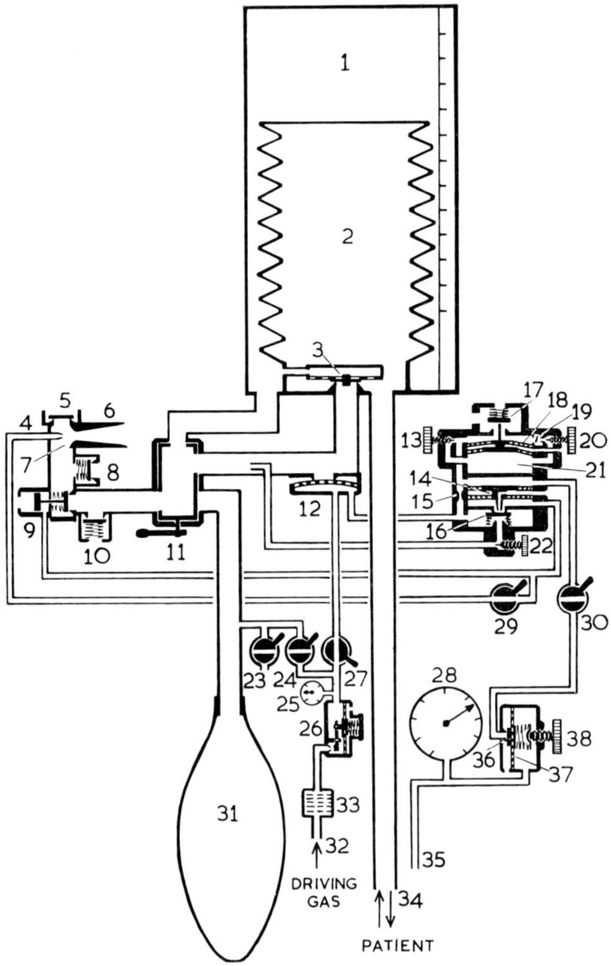

Fig. 15.2. Diagram of the Air-Shields 'Ventimeter Ventilator'.

1. Rigid plastic pressure chamber
2. Concertina reservoir bag
3. Spill valve
4. Injector
5. One-way valve
6. Diffuser tube of injector
7. Exhaust tubing
8. Negative-pressure-limiting valve
9. Cylinder and piston of expiratory valve
10. Safety-valve
11. 'Bag/ventilator' tap
12. Diaphragm valve
13. 'Expiratory pause' control
14. Differential diaphragms
15. Constriction
16. Valve
17. Valve
18. Differential diaphragms
19. One-way valve
20. 'Inspiratory time' control
21. Chamber
22. 'Inspiratory flow' control
23. 'Bag dump' tap
24. 'Bag fill' tap
25. Driving-gas pressure gauge
26. Reducing valve
27. 'On-off' tap
28. Manometer
29. 'Positive negative/positive' control
30. 'Assist control/control' control
31. Bag for manual use
32. Driving-gas inlet
33. Sintered-bronze filter
34. Breathing tube
35. Manometer and patient-triggering connexion
36. Valve
37. Diaphragm
38. 'Sensitivity' control

entrainment effect on the underside of the valve (3). During the expiratory phase the weight on the diaphragm holds the valve (3) closed until the reservoir bag (2) is fully distended and the pressure within it rises sufficiently to overcome the force exerted by the weight, whereupon excess gas spills through the open expiratory valve (9). When the driving gas is turned off, or if it should fail, the diaphragm valve (12) collapses, thereby allowing the patient to breathe spontaneously even though the expiratory valve (9) is held shut.

Negative pressure during the expiratory phase can be brought into action by opening the tap (29) which allows a supply of driving gas from the timing unit to flow to the injector (4). This functions throughout the expiratory phase, since the operation of the injector and the holding of the valve (9) in the expiratory position are synchronous.

Positive pressure is limited to 40 cmH_2O by the safety-valve (10) and the negative pressure is fixed at -4 to -5 cmH_2O by the valve (8).

The volume of the concertina reservoir bag (2) is 1500 ml. The inspiratory time is adjustable between $\frac{1}{2}$ and 3 sec, and the expiratory time between $\frac{1}{2}$ and 10 sec. The inspiratory flow is adjustable between 0 and 60 litres/min and the combination of this setting and the inspiratory time determines the tidal volume.

When the tap (30) is switched to the 'assist control' position, the ventilator may be patient-triggered. Any inspiratory effort by the patient lifts the diaphragm (37), opening the valve (36). Since the tap (30) is open, this allows the pressure above the lower differential diaphragms (14) to fall rapidly to atmospheric, and the ventilator immediately cycles to inspiration. The sensitivity of the patient-triggering diaphragm (37) can be adjusted by the control (38) in such a way that even though negative pressure is being used during the expiratory phase it responds only to an inspiratory effort.

The 'bag/ventilator' tap (11) may be turned to connect the bag (31) and the pressure chamber (1). Squeezing this bag (31) does not inflate the lungs directly but compresses the concertina reservoir bag (2). The bag (31) may be filled with driving gas by opening the spring-loaded 'bag fill' tap (24), or emptied through the 'bag dump' tap (23).

The manometer (28), which indicates pressure in the breathing circuit, is connected close to the patient through the 'airway pressure' connexion (35).

FUNCTIONAL ANALYSIS

This analysis and the 'Controls' section which follows are written mainly on the assumption that a 'closed' patient circuit is used, even though the effects of quite large fresh-gas flows are mentioned. However, where behaviour with a non-rebreathing patient circuit, incorporating an inflating valve, is substantially different this is noted briefly, but only on the assumption that the fresh-gas flow exceeds the total ventilation. If the fresh-gas flow is set to less than the ventilation which would otherwise be delivered, the ventilator operates as a minute-volume divider (see p.140). This mode of operation is included in Appendix I but is not considered further here.

Inspiratory phase

In this phase the ventilator operates as a constant-flow generator because of the very high pressure (30 lb/in^2) dropped across the very high resistance of the 'inspiratory flow' needle valve (22). This is shown by the characteristics in fig. 15.3 (curve a) in which, with the 'inspiratory flow' control (22) set at a maximum, the inspiratory flow is steady at 60 litres/min until the positive-pressure safety-valve (10) begins to open. In practice a slight deviation from pure flow generation arises from the compliance of the gas in the

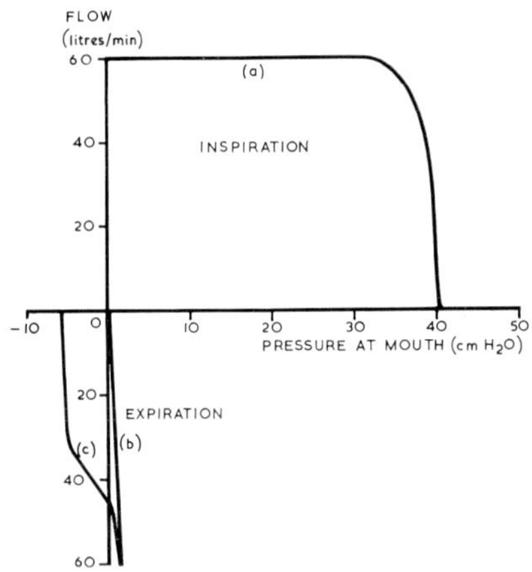

Fig. 15.3. Air-Shields 'Ventimeter Ventilator'. Flow-pressure characteristics of the inspiratory and expiratory mechanisms, measured with the concertina bag removed.
Curve (a) 'inspiratory flow' control at maximum.
Curve (b) with switch (29) (fig. 15.2) set to 'positive', i.e. with injector (4) not activated.
Curve (c) with switch (29) set to 'positive-negative'.

pressure chamber (1): a small fraction of the generated flow is used in compressing this gas and the fraction is somewhat larger when the compliance is halved because of the consequent more-rapid rise in mouth pressure and therefore in chamber pressure. Thus in fig. 15.4, when the compliance is halved (b) the flow to the patient is a little less than under the standard conditions (a) or when the resistance is doubled (c). Since the fresh-gas flow enters the patient circuit continuously and escapes only at the end of the expiratory phase it constitutes a supplementary flow generator in parallel with the main driving mechanism. If a non-rebreathing circuit with inflating valve is in use, the fresh-gas flow must be set at least equal to the desired total ventilation and therefore constitutes a substantial fraction of the total generated inspiratory flow.

If the mouth pressure rises high enough for the safety-valve to open it is clear from the characteristics in fig. 15.3 that the ventilator would then function as a constant-pressure generator for the remainder of the inspiratory phase.

Change-over from inspiratory phase to expiratory phase

This change-over is time-cycled. It occurs when sufficient gas has leaked out of chamber (21) past the needle valves (13, 20) for the pressure within the chamber to fall to a critical level (see the 'Description' above). This critical pressure is reached in a preset time which is unaffected by the pressure in the patient circuit. This is confirmed by fig. 15.4 in which changes of lung characteristics have no effect on the inspiratory time.

Since the ventilator is a flow generator in the inspiratory phase it is also effectively volume-cycled—provided the safety-valve (10) does not open. This also can be seen in

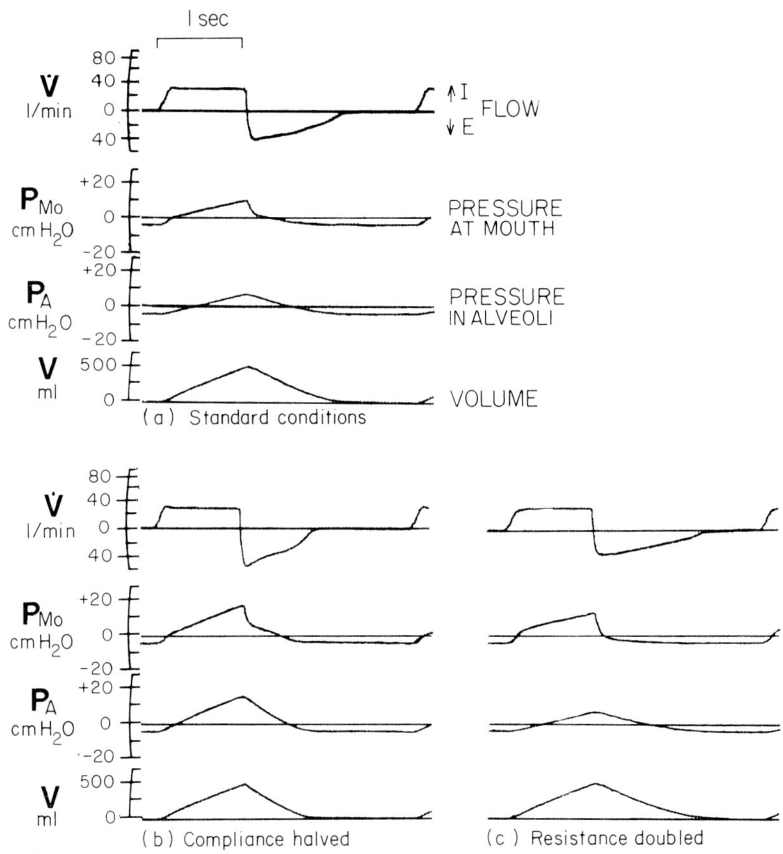

Fig. 15.4. Air-Shields 'Ventimeter Ventilator'. Recordings showing the effects of changes of lung characteristics.

Standard conditions: driving gas, oxygen at 60 lb/in²; switch (30) (fig. 15.2), in 'control' position; switch (29), in 'positive-negative' position; 'expiratory pause', set for an expiratory time of 2 sec; 'inspiratory time', set for an inspiratory time of 1 sec; 'inspiratory flow', set for a tidal volume of 500 ml; fresh-gas flow, 0·5 litre/min oxygen.

fig. 15.4: when the lung characteristics are changed (b, c) the inspiratory phase still ends as soon as the volume in the lungs has risen to the level it reached by the end of the phase under the standard conditions (a).

Expiratory phase

When the switch (29) is set to 'positive' no driving gas is supplied to the injector (4) and the ventilator operates as a constant-pressure generator with gas from the pressure chamber exhausting to atmosphere. The characteristics in fig. 15.3 show (curve b) that, when the concertina bag is removed, the apparatus is an atmospheric-pressure generator with very low series resistance: even with an expiratory flow of 60 litres/min through the ventilator the mouth pressure is only 1·5 cmH_2O. With the concertina bag in position there is a small pressure drop across the wall of the bag, rising to 1 cmH_2O as it approaches the limit of expansion and then to 2 cmH_2O when gas escapes past the spill valve (3). In practice therefore the ventilator operates as a slightly-positive-pressure generator. This has been confirmed by recordings although they are not reproduced here.

When the switch (29) is set to 'positive negative', the injector (4) is activated during the expiratory phase. It is of moderate efficiency making a tolerable approximation to a constant-flow generator. However, larger flows may come from the lungs at the start of the expiratory phase; then the excess spills through the one-way valve (5) so that the action of the injector is overridden by the atmospheric-pressure-generating action of the one-way valve (5). Later in the phase, when the flow-generating action of the injector has pulled the pressure in the exhaust tubing (7) down to about -5 cmH_2O the negative-pressure-limiting valve (8) opens and overrides the action of the injector with its own constant, negative, pressure-generating action.

The above points are illustrated by the characteristics of fig. 15.3 (curve c) although, even with the concertina bag removed, the pressure at the mouth which is plotted in fig. 15.3 is slightly above the pressure in the exhaust tube (7) because of the small expiratory resistance of the ventilator. This figure helps to show that there are potentially three parts of the expiratory phase when the injector is in use: firstly, there is constant, atmospheric, pressure generation, until the flow falls to that generated by the injector; secondly, there is near-constant-flow generation (at about 40 litres/min) until the pressure in the exhaust tubing (7) falls to the opening pressure of the limiting valve (8); and thirdly, there is constant, negative, pressure generation.

The three parts of the phase are further illustrated in the recordings of fig. 15.4 although, for these, the concertina bag was in place introducing a further small pressure difference between the mouth, where the pressure was recorded, and the exhaust tube (7), where the pressure generation occurs. The first part of the phase is clearly detectable only when the compliance has been halved (fig. 15.4b): then the initial expiratory flow is high and declines rapidly to about 40 litres/min. The second part, although it is brief, can be detected in all three sets of tracings in fig. 15.4 as a slowly-declining flow, of about 40 litres/min in all cases, while the mouth pressure falls rapidly. The third part lasts longer and can clearly be seen as a constant mouth pressure of about -4 cmH_2O, in all three sets of tracings, while the flow declines in different ways according to the nature of the lung characteristics.

If a non-rebreathing circuit is in use expiration occurs through the inflating valve which will normally act as a constant, atmospheric, pressure generator irrespective of the position of the 'positive/positive-negative' switch.

Change-over from expiratory phase to inspiratory phase

With the switch (30) closed, i.e. in the 'control' position this change-over is purely time-cycled. It occurs when sufficient gas has leaked past the 'expiratory pause' needle valve (13) for the pressure within the chamber (21) to have risen to a critical level (see the 'Description' above). This critical pressure is reached in a preset time which is unaffected by the pressure in the patient circuit. This is confirmed by fig. 15.4 in which changes of lung characteristics have no effect on the expiratory time.

With the switch (30) open, i.e. in the 'assist-control' position, the change-over is either time-cycled or patient-cycled whichever occurs first: if the patient produces enough negative pressure to lift the diaphragm (37), this will release the pressure above the diaphragm (14) before it is mediated by the attainment of the critical pressure in the chamber (21).

CONTROLS

Total ventilation

This cannot be directly controlled but is equal to the product of tidal volume and respiratory frequency.

Tidal volume

This is not directly controlled but is equal to the product of inspiratory flow and inspiratory time both of which are directly controlled and are subject to little or no change as a result of changes of lung characteristics: in fig. 15.4 it can be seen that halving the compliance or doubling the resistance does not appreciably alter the tidal volume. The inspiratory time will normally be chosen on other grounds, see below, so the 'inspiratory flow' control (22) provides the primary means of adjusting tidal volume (fig. 15.5b). However, if the inspiratory time is altered for some other reason the tidal volume will be changed. In addition, since the fresh-gas flow provides part of the generated inspiratory flow, increasing the fresh-gas flow increases the tidal volume a little (fig. 15.5f). This also results in the tidal volume exceeding the stroke volume of the concertina bag to the extent of the fresh-gas flow multiplied by the inspiratory time. The tidal volume received by the patient, however, will fall short of this to the extent of any volume absorbed in the compliance of the patient circuit.

Fig. 15.5. Air-Shields 'Ventimeter Ventilator'. Recordings showing the effects of changes in the settings of the controls.

(a) Standard conditions as in fig. 15.4.

(b) 'Inspiratory flow' increased from '11 o'clock' to '2 o'clock' to produce a tidal volume of 750 ml.

(c) 'Expiratory pause' decreased from '4 o'clock' to '1 o'clock'.

(d) 'Inspiratory time' increased from '3 o'clock' to '4.30 o'clock'.

(e) 'Positive/positive-negative' switch changed to 'positive'.

(f) Fresh-gas flow increased to 4 litres/min.

Respiratory frequency and inspiratory-expiratory ratio

These are not directly controlled but both are determined by the inspiratory and expiratory times which are entirely determined by the functioning of the pneumatic timer (13–22) and are quite uninfluenced by the patient except when patient-triggering occurs.

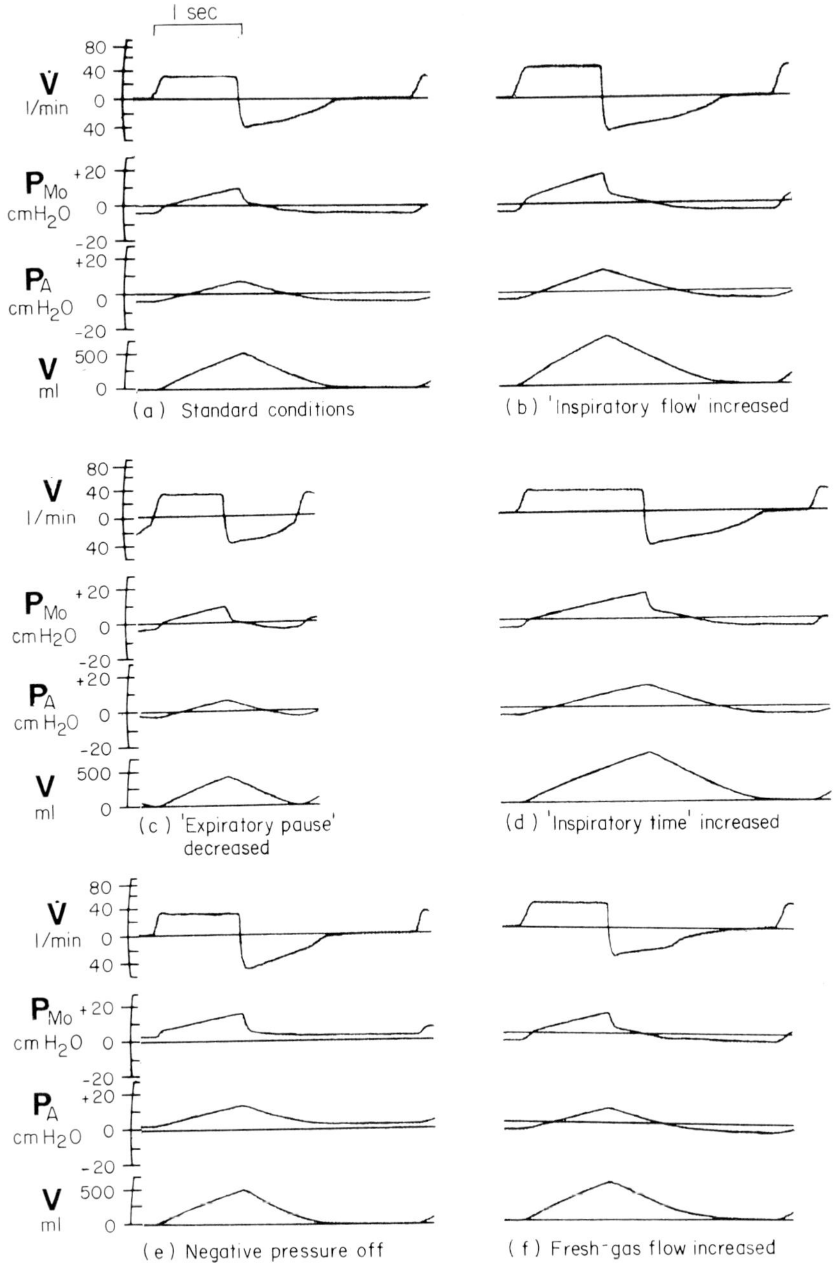

(a) Standard conditions

(b) 'Inspiratory flow' increased

(c) 'Expiratory pause' decreased

(d) 'Inspiratory time' increased

(e) Negative pressure off

(f) Fresh-gas flow increased

Separate 'inspiratory time' and 'expiratory pause' controls are provided but they interact to some extent. This arises mainly because the timing of the inspiratory phase is regulated by the leakage of gas past both the 'inspiratory time' (20) and 'expiratory pause' needle valves. Thus, if the 'expiratory pause' needle valve (13) is opened sufficiently to reduce the expiratory time below about 2 sec the inspiratory time is also decreased. This has the effect of making it impossible to produce an inspiratory time greater than the expiratory time except when the inspiratory time is at, or very near to, its maximum; even then, the inspiratory time is never more than twice the expiratory time.

This is illustrated to some extent in fig. 15.5c where the 'expiratory pause' control has been moved far enough to reduce the expiratory time from 2 sec to about 0·8 sec and this has resulted in the inspiratory time being reduced from 1 sec also to about 0·8 sec. If the expiratory time is increased from 2 sec upwards this has no effect on the inspiratory time. This is because the resistance of the 'expiratory pause' needle valve (13) is then much higher than that of the 'inspiratory time' needle valve and therefore changes in the resistance of the former have a negligible effect on the total rate of escape of gas from the chamber (21).

Changes in the setting of the 'inspiratory time' control (20) have a negligible effect on the expiratory time (fig. 15.5d) but they do, of course, alter the tidal volume in proportion. A consequence of this is that, if it is desired to, say, increase the frequency and decrease the tidal volume, while leaving the total ventilation unchanged, this can be achieved merely by adjusting the 'expiratory pause' and 'inspiratory time' controls so that both times are decreased in the same proportion; no adjustment of the 'inspiratory flow' control is required.

Inspiratory waveforms

Since the ventilator operates as a constant-flow generator throughout the inspiratory phase the inspiratory flow waveform is uninfluenced by changes of lung characteristics (fig. 15.4). The magnitude of the flow can be adjusted by means of the 'inspiratory flow' control (22) but this will normally have been set in accordance with other requirements. The waveform of flow cannot be altered.

Expiratory waveforms

The only way in which the expiratory flow waveform can be deliberately influenced is by switching the injector (4) off or on, by means of the 'positive/positive-negative' switch (29) but the choice of whether or not to use the injector will normally depend on whether or not negative pressure is required. When the injector is not in use (fig. 15.5e) the ventilator operates as a constant (slightly positive) pressure generator with low series resistance, therefore the expiratory flow starts high and declines approximately exponentially to zero in a manner dependent on lung characteristics. When the injector is in use (fig. 15.5 except (e), and fig. 15.4), the expiratory flow is controlled by the approximately flow-generating action of the injector at about 40 litres/min for a short while at or near the beginning of the phase. For the rest of the phase, however, the ventilator operates as a constant-pressure generator (nearly atmospheric at the start of the phase and negative for the last part of the phase) and the flow waveform is dependent on lung characteristics (fig. 15.4). The effect of switching off the injector in any given circumstances, as is illustrated by fig. 15.5e in comparison with fig. 15.5a, is to produce a higher peak flow (because of the higher end-inspiratory alveolar pressure) but a more rapid decay to zero flow because of the absence of the flow-generating part of the phase. In both cases, in fig. 15.5 however, most of the tidal volume has come out in half the expiratory time. On the other hand, changes of lung characteristics have an appreciable effect on the expiratory flow waveform (fig. 15.4) and influence the speed with which the tidal volume comes out.

If a non-rebreathing circuit with inflating valve is in use the ventilator operates as a constant, atmospheric, pressure generator in the expiratory phase irrespective of the setting of the 'positive/positive-negative' switch; the expiratory flow waveform, therefore depends on the lung characteristics.

Pressure limits

Since, in at least the last part of the expiratory phase, this ventilator always acts as a pressure generator with little series resistance, the alveolar pressure normally falls to the generated pressure by the end of the phase.

Thus the end-expiratory alveolar pressure is fairly firmly determined by the ventilator and is not much influenced by lung characteristics. It may be set to about $+2$ cmH_2O, with switch (29) at 'positive', or to about -4 cmH_2O, with the switch at 'positive-negative'. Starting from this end-expiratory pressure, the rest of the alveolar-pressure waveform is determined by the effects of the flow and pressure generators in the ventilator on the lungs; in particular the peak alveolar pressure at the end of the inspiratory phase exceeds the end-expiratory pressure by an amount equal to the tidal volume divided by the compliance.

Since changing the setting of the 'positive/positive-negative' switch has no effect on the inspiratory flow and not much effect on the expiratory flow (see above), it has little effect on the shape of the alveolar-pressure waveform: its main effect is simply to raise or lower the whole waveform by about 6 cmH_2O (compare (e) with (a) in fig. 15.5).

CHAPTER 16

The Allbritten Ventilator[1]

DESCRIPTION

The principle of this ventilator (fig. 16.1), the forerunner of the Jefferson, is almost identical with that of the Mortimer ventilator. Instead of compressing the reservoir bag directly, however, the windscreen-wiper arm bears on a concertina bag which, when compressed, raises the pressure in the chamber surrounding the reservoir bag.

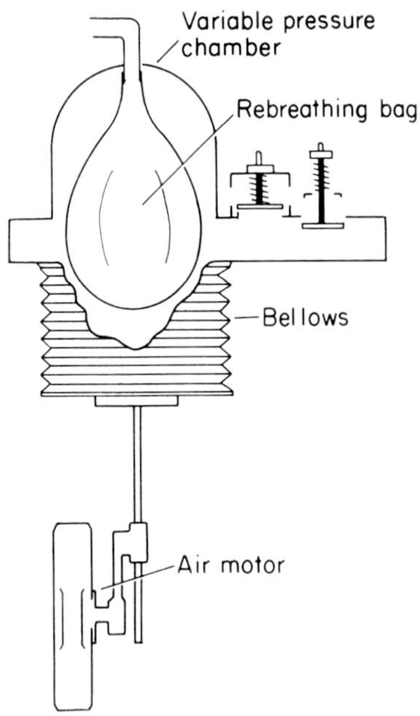

Fig. 16.1. Diagram of the Allbritten ventilator.

Courtesy of *Annals of Surgery*.[1]

FUNCTIONAL ANALYSIS

This ventilator contains a pressure transformer (see p. 89) and probably has some resistance and a constant driving pressure on the input side. Fundamentally, therefore, it is equivalent to a constant-pressure generator with a substantial series resistance between it and the patient, so that it approximates to a constant-flow generator in both phases. However, many factors complicate the action.

Inspiratory phase

Assuming that excess gas is expelled from the patient circuit by means of a blow-off valve, this must be set to open (during the inspiratory phase) at a lower pressure than the opening pressure of the positive-pressure-limiting valve in the driving circuit. Accordingly, once the blow-off valve opens, the pressure in the patient circuit, and that in the pressure chamber, are limited to the lower pressure until the reservoir bag has been completely emptied. Then the pressure in the pressure chamber rises rapidly to the opening pressure of the pressure-limiting valve in the driving circuit, and the remainder of the stroke volume of the driving concertina bag is blown to waste. Meanwhile the fresh-gas flow continues to keep the blow-off valve open so that the pressure in the patient circuit is still held constant.

Thus, so far as the patient is concerned, there are two parts to the inspiratory phase. At first the ventilator operates in its fundamental mode, approximately that of a constant-flow generator. Then, when the blow-off valve opens, the ventilator becomes a low-constant-pressure generator for the remainder of the phase. During the first part of the phase the fresh-gas supply to the patient circuit acts as a small-constant-flow generator, supplementing the main near-flow-generating action.

Change-over from inspiratory phase to expiratory phase

Fundamentally this change-over is volume-cycled: the phase ends when the driving mechanism reaches the end of its stroke and a fixed volume has been expelled from the concertina bag. However, this volume bears so little relation to the volume entering the patient's lungs that it is better to regard the change-over as time-cycled, even though the duration of the phase is slightly influenced by the patient's lung characteristics. The patient's tidal volume is governed by the setting of the blow-off valve in the patient circuit and of the negative-pressure-limiting valve in the driving circuit.

Expiratory phase

In this phase the fundamental action again approximates to that of a constant-flow generator but again this action is unmodified only for the first part of the phase. Once the pressure in the pressure chamber has become sufficiently negative to open the negative-pressure-limiting valve in the driving circuit the ventilator operates as a constant, negative, pressure generator with little series resistance. During the first part of the phase the fresh-gas supply to the patient circuit acts as a small-constant-flow generator opposing the main near-flow-generating action.

Change-over from expiratory phase to inspiratory phase

This change-over also is fundamentally volume-cycled but, like the other change-over, can more usefully be regarded as approximately time-cycled.

REFERENCE

1 Allbritten F.F., Haupt G.J. and Amadeo J.H. (1954) The change in pulmonary alveolar ventilation achieved by aiding the deflation phase of respiration during anesthesia for surgical operations. *Ann. Surg.* **140**, 569.

CHAPTER 17

The Almeida 'Pulmo-Ventilador Universal'[1]

DESCRIPTION

This ventilator (fig. 17.1), developed from an earlier, non-automatic model,[2] incorporates a variety of anaesthetic circuits any one of which may be selected by the setting of the taps (10) and (11) (fig. 17.2). It is obtainable with or without an anaesthetic apparatus. It is driven by compressed gas delivered at the inlet (22) which, when the weighted 'rhythm' valve (15) is closed, flows to the rigid plastic pressure chamber (6) and compresses the reservoir bag (5), the contents of which are forced to the patient. The driving gas is also supplied to a timing mechanism (23–33) which controls the opening and closure of the 'rhythm' valve (15).

Timing circuit

Towards the end of the inspiratory phase the timing mechanism (23–33) is in the position shown in fig. 17.2. The diaphragm (31) is in the 'down' position, and the 'rhythm' valve (15) is closed. The driving gas entering at the inlet (22) flows, past the needle valve (21) and through the drum valve (23), to the chamber (30) beneath the diaphragm (31). As the chamber (29) above the diaphragm (31) is, in this phase, connected through the drum valve (23) to atmosphere, the diaphragm (31) moves upwards fairly rapidly, at a rate determined by the setting of the needle valve (21), raising the rod (28) and compressing the spring (27). The rod (26) is pivoted and the force exerted by the spring (19) on the lever of the weighted 'rhythm' valve (15) therefore increases fairly rapidly. When this force, together with that exerted by the sliding weight (20), is sufficient to counterbalance the weight of the 'rhythm' valve (15) the pressure of the gas below it forces the valve open. The upward movement of the rod (28), which compressed the spring (27), is followed by a slower rise of the lever (25) against the resistance imposed by the dash-pot (33). The magnitude of this resistance depends on the setting of the 'frequency' control (32). When a critical position of the lever (25) is reached the click mechanism within the drum valve (23) snaps over and the flow of driving gas is now directed to the chamber (29), while the chamber (30) is connected to atmosphere. The diaphragm (31) is now fairly rapidly forced down and the rod (28) follows it, at a rate determined by the setting of the needle

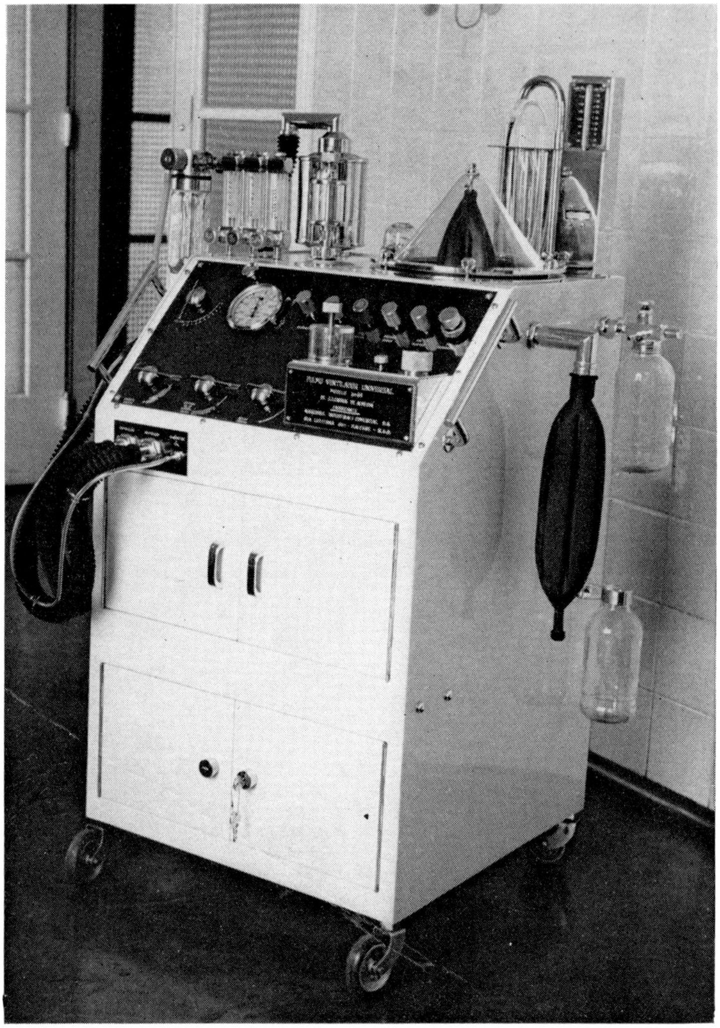

Fig. 17.1. The Almeida 'Pulmo-ventilador Universal'.

Courtesy of Dr J.J. Cabral de Almeida.

valve (21), expanding the spring (27) and pulling down the lever (25) against the resistance of the dash-pot (33). When the rod (28) has moved far enough to expand the spring (19) sufficiently, the 'rhythm' valve is closed, and the expiratory phase ends. The rate at which the 'rhythm' valve closes is fairly slow, depending on the setting of the needle valve (21), and therefore there is a progressive reduction in the escape of driving gas through the valve and a steady increase in the flow of driving gas to the plastic chamber during the first part of the inspiratory phase.

After the 'rhythm' valve (15) has closed, the tension in the spring (27) pulls down the

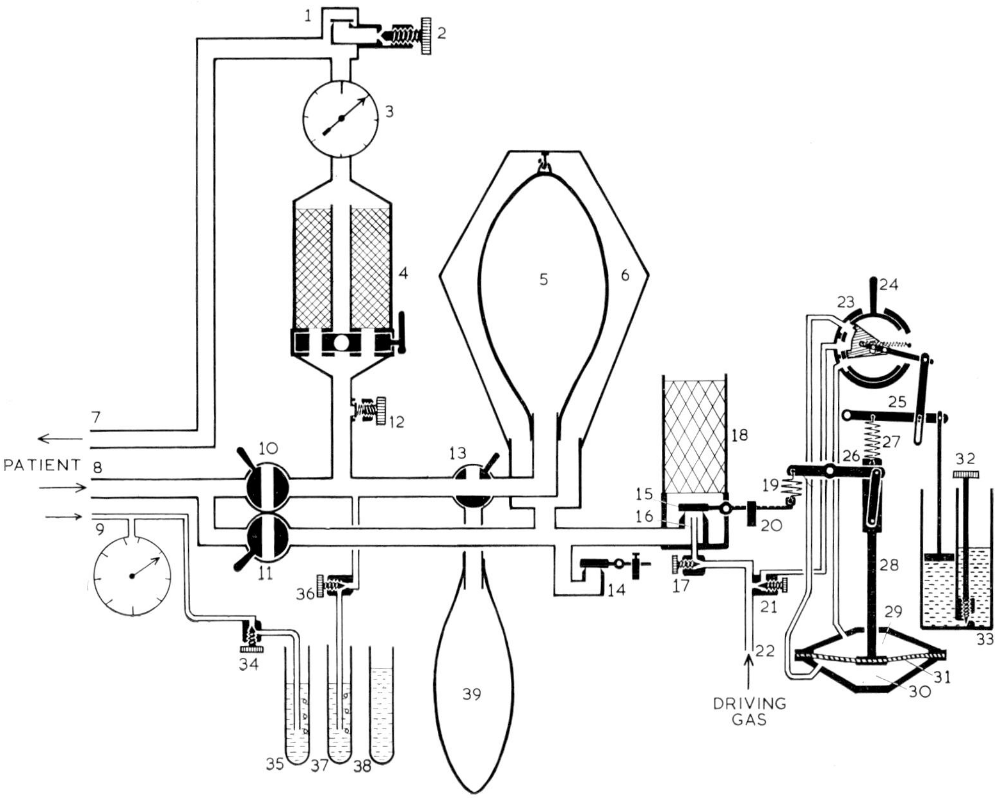

Fig. 17.2. Diagram of the Almeida 'Pulmo-ventilador Universal'.

1. One-way valve
2. Air-inlet control
3. Dräger 'Volumeter'
4. Soda-lime canister
5. Reservoir bag
6. Rigid plastic pressure chamber
7. Breathing tube
8. Breathing tube
9. Small-bore tube
10. Circuit-selection tap 'A'
11. Circuit-selection tap 'B'
12. Blow-off valve
13. 'Manual/automatic' tap
14. Safety-valve
15. 'Rhythm' valve
16. Supply tube and injector
17. Driving-gas control
18. Silencer
19. Spring
20. Sliding weight
21. Needle valve
22. Driving-gas inlet
23. Drum valve
24. Inspiratory-expiratory-ratio control lever
25. Lever
26. Pivoted rod
27. Spring
28. Rod
29. Chamber
30. Chamber
31. Diaphragm
32. 'Frequency' control
33. Dash-pot
34. Needle valve
35. Bicarbonate/bromothymol solution
36. Needle valve
37. Bicarbonate/bromothymol solution
38. Bicarbonate/bromothymol solution
39. Manual reservoir bag

connecting rod (25) against the resistance of the dash-pot (33) until the click mechanism (23) is reversed. Driving gas now flows to the chamber (30), and the chamber (29) is open to atmosphere. The diaphragm moves up, reopening the 'rhythm' valve (15), and the next expiratory phase starts.

The lever (24) allows the position of the inner drum of the valve (23) to be adjusted and thereby alters the attachment of the click spring in relation to the fulcrum of the click rod. In this way the relationship between the critical position of the click mechanism and the position of the rod (25) is changed. However, for any particular settings of the needle valve (21) and the control (32), the time taken for the diaphragm to complete a full cycle is constant, and, since the mechanical relationship between the 'rhythm' valve (15) and the rod (25) is unchanged, this adjustment of the lever (24) alters the inspiratory-expiratory ratio. Adjustment of the sliding weight (20) alters the force which must be applied to the 'rhythm' valve (15) before it is opened and hence the maximum pressure reached in the driving-gas circuit.

Breathing circuits

A 2 kg soda-lime canister (4) is fitted to the ventilator. The canister illustrated has a free central pathway which allows gas to by-pass the soda-lime when the tap in the base of the canister is turned. An alternative canister, with an external by-pass and tap, is available.

If a Y-piece with non-return valves in the inspiratory and expiratory limbs is fitted near the patient, and tap (10) is open and tap (11) is closed, the circuit becomes a closed or semi-closed circle system. Fresh gas enters the circuit on the ventilator side of the one-way valve in the inspiratory limb of the Y-piece and excess gas can spill through the spring-loaded blow-off valve (12), which also sets the maximum pressure in the breathing circuit. Depending on the amount of fresh gas entering the breathing circuit, the circuit is closed or semi-closed.

If, with the same Y-piece in place, the tap (10) is closed and the tap (11) is opened, all the expired gas escapes to atmosphere through the 'rhythm' valve (15) and the circuit is a non-rebreathing one. It should be noticed however that, unless valve (2) is admitting air due to the negative pressure produced at (16) during the expiratory phase, no air can enter the breathing circuit, and therefore the fresh-gas flow must be set equal to the desired total ventilation.

By careful adjustment of the tap (10) when a circle system is in use, or of tap (11) when the non-rebreathing or semi-closed system is in use, resistance is introduced in the expiratory pathway and a positive intrapulmonary pressure can be maintained during the expiratory phase.

With the taps (10) and (11) closed, respiratory gas can only flow along the tube (7). If a Water's soda-lime canister is placed near the patient, the circuit becomes a to-and-fro absorption system, fresh gas being added at the canister and excess gas blowing off through the valve (12). If, instead of the Water's canister, an inflating valve is included, the circuit becomes a non-rebreathing system, and the fresh-gas flow must equal the minute-volume ventilation. This system is primarily meant for use with air, which can be drawn into the circuit during the expiratory phase. The proportion of air thus drawn in depends on the setting of the valve (2) and the fresh-gas flow delivered near the patient.

The injector (16) produces a negative pressure during the expiratory phase, the limit of which depends on the driving-gas flow set by the needle valve (17). A safety-valve (14) limits the maximum positive pressure in the pressure chamber (6) to up to 100 cmH_2O.

The Dräger 'Volumeter' (3) indicates the tidal volume. The aneroid manometer (9) shows the pressure in the breathing circuit.

The 'manual/automatic' tap (13) may be turned to allow manual ventilation to be performed by squeezing the reservoir bag (39).

The respiratory gas may be sampled from near the patient and from near the reservoir bag (5) by opening the needle valves (34) and (36) respectively. The samples flow through a bicarbonate/bromothymol solution (35, 37) the colour change in which can be compared with that of a similar solution in tube (38) through which the anaesthetist has blown his own expired gas.

FUNCTIONAL ANALYSIS

Inspiratory phase

In this phase, the ventilator operates primarily as a constant-flow generator: the patient is connected to the high pressure of the compressed gas through the resistance of the needle valve (17). However, a number of factors modify the action at the beginning and end of the phase.

Firstly, the 'rhythm' valve (15) closes rather slowly and therefore some inflating flow occurs before it is fully closed. In this early part of the phase the ventilator can be regarded as an increasing-pressure generator.

Secondly, when any sort of closed anaesthetic circuit is in use, excess gas escapes through the blow-off valve (12) towards the end of the phase and therefore introduces a pressure limit which must normally be reached before the end of each inspiratory phase. Once the limit is reached the functioning changes from constant-flow generation to constant-pressure generation.

Thirdly, when a non-rebreathing anaesthetic circuit is used, the volume of gas in the reservoir bag (5) constitutes a volume limit which may be reached before the end of the phase. If it is reached, the ventilator will then operate for the remainder of the phase either as a zero-flow generator (if the only source of inflating gas is air drawn in through the control (2)) or as a small-constant-flow generator (if there is a steady inflow of fresh gas near the patient).

Change-over from inspiratory phase to expiratory phase

The change-over occurs when the balance of forces on the rhythm valve becomes such as to open it. Five forces act on this valve. Three of them are constant or preset: the weight (15) tends to close the valve, the weight (20) tends to open it, and the impact pressure of the jet of driving gas on the underside of the valve tends to open it. The other two forces vary during the respiratory cycle.

Firstly, the spring (19) tends, in the first part of the inspiratory phase, to keep the valve closed but, as the rod (28) rises, this closing force progressively diminishes and may even change to a progressively-increasing opening force. The rate at which this force changes is dependent only on the operation of the timing mechanism (21–33) and is uninfluenced by the patient's lung characteristics. Therefore, if this were the only varying force involved, the opening of the rhythm valve (15) would occur at a preset time and the change-over from the inspiratory phase to the expiratory phase would be purely time-cycled. However, there is a second varying force: the pressure in the pressure chamber (6) is added to the impact pressure on the underside of the valve and provides a progressively-increasing force tending to open the rhythm valve.

So long as the reservoir bag (5) is not collapsed, the pressure in chamber (6) is similar to the mouth pressure. Therefore, if this pressure rises more rapidly, as a result of changed lung characteristics, the rhythm valve will be opened and the change-over will occur somewhat earlier than otherwise. If the reservoir bag (5) is completely emptied during the inspiratory phase, the pressure in chamber (6) will rapidly rise to the opening pressure of the safety-valve (14). If, prior to this, the forces on the rhythm valve were already nearing a balance, the change-over would no doubt quickly follow.

In summary therefore, the change-over from the inspiratory phase to the expiratory phase is primarily time-cycled, but its occurrence may be hastened by a rapid rise in mouth pressure or by the attainment of the volume limit set by the contents of the reservoir bag (5) at the start of the inspiratory phase.

Expiratory phase

In this phase the ventilator usually operates as a constant, negative, pressure generator due to the entrainment effect of the jet of driving gas at the injector (16). The resistance of the generator may be increased by means of one of the taps (10) or (11) (depending on whether a closed or non-rebreathing circuit is in use).

However, if a non-rebreathing circuit with an inflating valve is in use, the ventilator operates as a constant, atmospheric, pressure generator: the expired gas passes to atmosphere through the expiratory port of the inflating valve.

Change-over from expiratory phase to inspiratory phase

This change-over, like the other, is actuated by the balance of forces on the rhythm valve (15). In this case, however, the only force on the underside of the valve is the impact pressure of the jet of driving gas which, for a given setting of the flow control (17), is constant. Therefore, the attainment of the balance point is dependent solely on the change of force exerted by the spring (19) and hence on the motions of the timing mechanism (21–33). Consequently the closure of the rhythm valve is time-cycled but, since its opening is somewhat influenced by pressure in the patient circuit, it is necessary to specify that the closure occurs at a preset time after the previous closure; that is, it is the duration of the complete respiratory cycle which is controlled.

The only qualification that needs to be added is to explain that the change-over from the expiratory phase to the inspiratory phase, that is, the onset of inspiratory flow, occurs some time before the complete closure of the rhythm valve. This is because the closure is a gradual process which must cause the pressure in the pressure chamber (6) to change gradually from negative to positive as the entrainment effect of the injector (16) is overcome by the pressure drop across the progressively-increasing resistance of the gradually-closing valve (15). The rate at which the pressure in chamber (6) rises, prior to the complete closure of the rhythm valve, should be substantially independent of lung characteristics; but the moment at which inspiratory flow starts is the moment at which the pressure in chamber (6) first becomes positive to the alveolar pressure, and the level to which the alveolar pressure falls during the expiratory phase is dependent on lung characteristics.

Therefore, although the change-over is primarily time-cycled (with reference to the end of the previous *expiratory* phase) its timing is slightly influenced by changes of lung characteristics.

REFERENCES

1 ALMEIDA J.J. CABRAL DE (1964) *Fisiopatologia da respiração controlada em anestesia.* Rio de Janeiro, 1964.

2 ALMEIDA J.J. CABRAL DE (1951) Nôvo método de respiração controlada mecânicamente: narcose com baro-inversão total na ventilação pelo pulmo-ventilador. *Rev. Bras. Anest.* **1**, 117.

CHAPTER 18

The 'Amsterdam Infant Ventilator'[1]

DESCRIPTION

This compact electronically-controlled ventilator (fig. 18.1) allows a preset flow of inflating gas to pass to the patient for a preset inspiratory time.

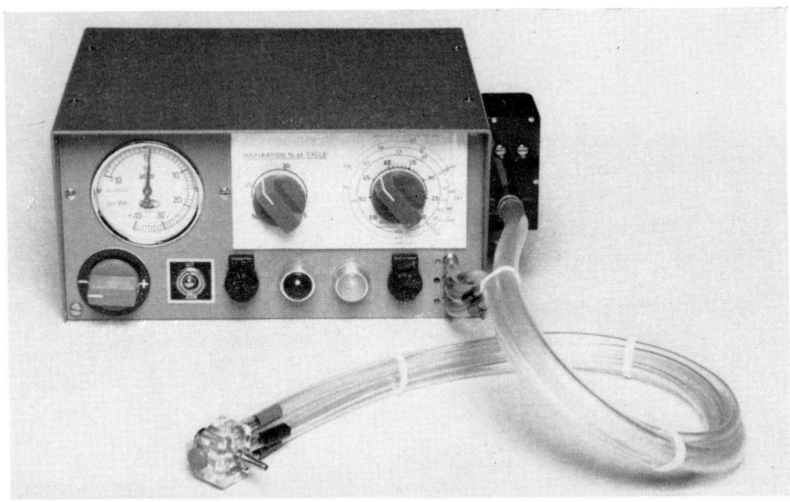

Fig. 18.1. The 'Amsterdam Infant Ventilator'.
Courtesy of G.L.Loos & Co., Amsterdam.

Compressed gas from a pipe-line, compressor, or anaesthetic apparatus, enters the ventilator continuously through the tube (11) (fig. 18.2) at a steady rate indicated by a flowmeter. During the inspiratory phase the electronic timing circuit (9) energizes the solenoid (15) and the valve (14) is held closed. Inflating gas then flows to the patient through the connector assembly (2). The pathway which it takes through the connector depends on the setting of the 'negative pressure' control (12), which determines what proportion of inflating gas flows through the tube (4) to the jet (1) of the injector in the connector, and what proportion through the tube (5) to the entrainment port in the

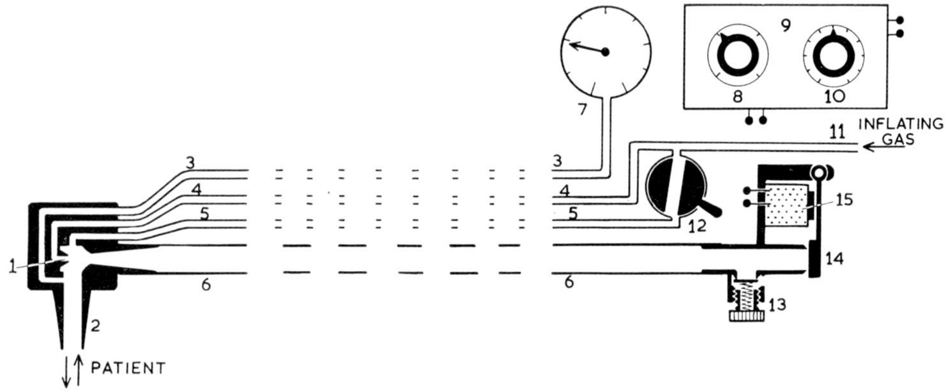

Fig. 18.2. Diagram of the 'Amsterdam Infant Ventilator'.

1. Injector
2. Endotracheal-tube connexion
3. Manometer tube
4. Supply tube to injector
5. Supply tube to airway
6. Expiratory tube
7. Manometer
8. 'Inspiration % of cycle'
9. Timing control unit
10. 'Respiratory frequency' control
11. Inflating-gas inlet
12. Negative-pressure control tap
13. Safety-valve
14. Expiratory valve
15. Solenoid

connector. The resultant pressure at the mouth is indicated by the manometer (7) and limited by the safety-valve (13) which can be adjusted from entirely closed to a few cm H_2O.

After a time set by the electronic timing circuit (9), the supply of current to the solenoid (15) is cut off and the valve (14) is free to open. The flow of gas through the jet (1) of the injector is now free to pass along the tube (6) to atmosphere, taking with it any gas entering through the tube (5) and the entrainment port of the injector and expired gas flowing from the patient. The tap (12) controls the degree of negative pressure applied at the mouth. If it is set to direct all the inflating gas through the tube (4) and the jet (1) of the injector, maximum negative pressure is developed. Adjustment of the tap (12), so that some of the inflating gas flows through the tube (5) instead of the tube (4), reduces the negative pressure produced. When the tap (12) is fully open, the pressure at the mouth may even remain slightly positive throughout the expiratory phase. The maximum negative pressure produced at the mouth during the expiratory phase depends not only on the setting of the tap (12) but also on the flow of inflating gas.

The control (8) sets the inspiratory-expiratory ratio. It is calibrated in terms of 'inspiration % of cycle', i.e. the duration of the inspiratory phase as a percentage of the total respiratory cycle. The control (10) sets the respiratory frequency. A series of concentric calibration scales around the control (10) (see fig. 18.1) allows the absolute duration of the inspiratory phase to be read off for any combination of the control settings.

The tidal volume delivered to the patient is equal to the product of the inspiratory time as read from the 'respiratory frequency' control (10) and the inflating-gas flow rate as read from the flowmeters. A chart (fig. 18.3) fixed to the ventilator shows the relationship between these three parameters. In practice the total minute-volume ventilation must first be decided; a frequency is then selected, and hence the tidal volume is easily calculated. The desired inspiratory-expiratory ratio is then set and the inspiratory time read off the appropriate scale around the control (10). From this inspiratory time and this tidal volume, the necessary inflating-gas flow is read off the chart.

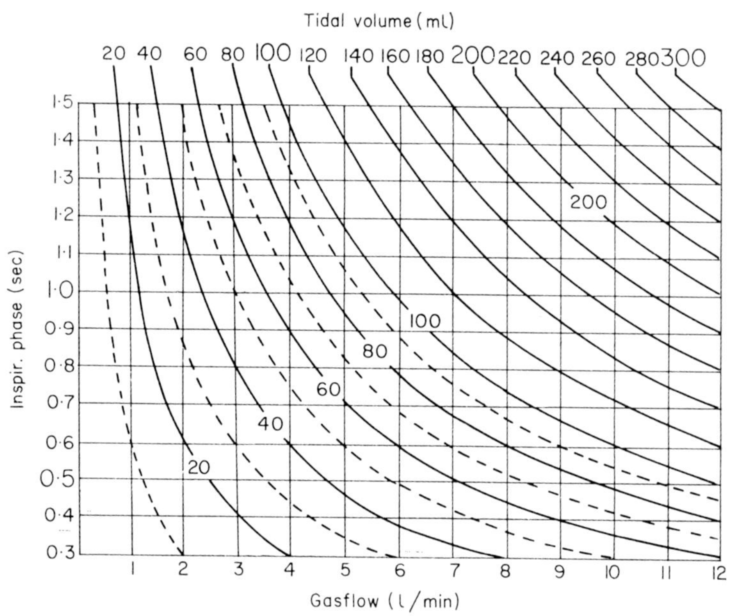

Fig. 18.3. Chart relating tidal volume, inspiratory time, and flow of inflating gas.
Courtesy of G.L.Loos & Co., Amsterdam.

An alternative method of setting the controls is as follows. Having decided the total minute-volume ventilation, the required inspiratory-expiratory ratio is set, the inflating-gas flow rate can then be calculated as:

$$\text{inflating-gas flow} = \frac{\text{total ventilation} \times 100}{\text{`inspiration \% of cycle'}}.$$

The control (10) is now set to the desired frequency and the appropriate tidal volume is delivered automatically.

The frequency can be adjusted between 20 and 55 per min. The inspiratory-expiratory ratio can be adjusted between 1 : 1 and 1 : 3. The ventilator is intended for use with inflating-gas flow rates of up to about 15 litres/min.

A humidifier is available for fitting into the supply line to the ventilator.

The timing circuits run off an a.c. mains supply. Two indicator lights are fitted; one indicates the main electrical supply, the other indicates the inspiratory phase. In the event of a mains failure the indicator lights go out. The valve (14) can then be operated intermittently by finger pressure.

FUNCTIONAL ANALYSIS

Inspiratory phase

In this phase the ventilator operates as a constant-flow generator due to the high pressure and high resistance of the inflating-gas supply.

Change-over from inspiratory phase to expiratory phase

This change-over is time-cycled: it occurs when the solenoid-operated valve (14, 15) opens at a time determined by the electronic timer.

Expiratory phase

In this phase the ventilator operates as a constant-pressure generator, due to the characteristics of the injector (1). The generated pressure is either negative, atmospheric, or slightly positive, depending on how much driving gas flows through the jet of the injector and how much through the auxiliary tube (5).

Change-over from expiratory phase to inspiratory phase

This change-over also is time-cycled: it occurs when the solenoid-operated valve (14, 15) closes at a time controlled by the electronic timer.

REFERENCE

1 Keuskamp D.H.G. (1963) Automatic ventilation in paediatric anaesthesia using a modified Ayre's T-piece with negative pressure during the expiratory phase. *Anaesthesia*, **18**, 46.

CHAPTER 19

The 'Autoanestheton'[1,2]

DESCRIPTION

This ventilator was originally described as a 'physiological ventilator controlled by the patient's own expired carbon-dioxide'.

This apparatus maintains nitrous oxide and oxygen anaesthesia in patients rendered immobile and apnoeic with muscle relaxants. The inflating pressure, and hence the volume exchange, is controlled by the end-expiratory carbon-dioxide concentration. The nitrous-oxide concentration in the mixture is set by the anaesthetist at any desired level, the oxygen concentration being continuously indicated by a paramagnetic oxygen analyser (1) (fig. 19.1).

The anaesthetic gas mixture passes into a 'storage tank' (4) through a solenoid-operated inlet valve (2) actuated by the pressure switch (3). The gas from the storage tank passes through the pressure regulator (5) which reduces the pressure to 10 lb/in^2. A variable pressure regulator (7) reduces this pressure to a suitable level for inflation of the lungs. This is the only factor which is variable and is continuously adjusted automatically by the end-expiratory carbon-dioxide level to suit the patient.

A spring-loaded pneumatically-operated inspiratory-expiratory valve (16) allows the gas to flow into, and so inflate, the lungs. Expiration is passive and the expired gas passes into the atmosphere. The valve (16) is pneumatically opened and closed 15 times per minute by a cam-operated valve (14) in the pneumatic line. The motor (12), operating the cam, is set at 15 r.p.m. The inspiratory phase occupies one-third of the respiratory cycle.

The only variable of the ventilator is the inflating pressure. This pressure is automatically adjusted according to the patient's requirements as follows. During the final 1/5 second of the expiratory phase a small diaphragm pump (11), opened by the cam-operated valve (13), withdraws an 8-ml sample of end-expiratory gas from the endotracheal catheter through the tube (15). This sample is delivered by the diaphragm pump to an infra-red gas analyser (10) for carbon-dioxide estimation. The electrical output of the analyser is compared to a carbon-dioxide value, pre-selected by the control (9), and by means of a servo-system (6) continuously adjusts the inflating pressure at the variable pressure regulator (7).

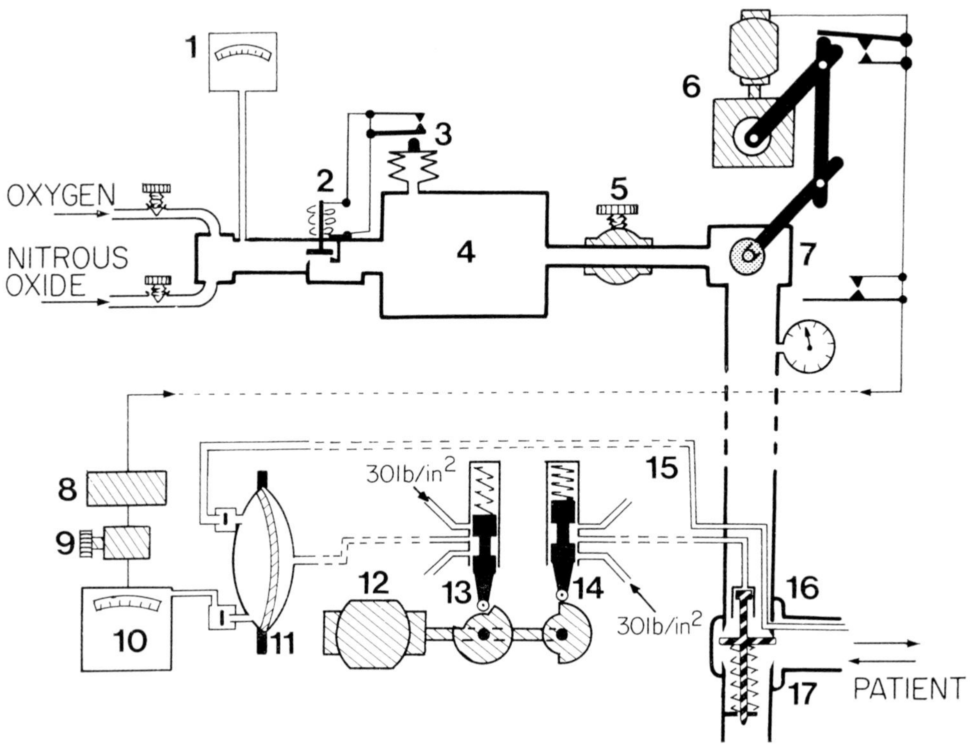

Fig. 19.1. Diagram of the 'Autoanestheton'.

1. Paramagnetic oxygen analyser
2. Solenoid-operated inlet valve
3. Pressure switch
4. Storage tank
5. Pressure regulator
6. Servo-system
7. Variable pressure regulator
8. Amplifier
9. Control for setting carbon-dioxide level
10. Infra-red gas analyser
11. Diaphragm pump
12. Electric motor
13. Cam-operated valve
14. Cam-operated valve
15. Sampling tube
16. Inspiratory–expiratory valve
17. Expiratory outlet

Should, for instance, the carbon-dioxide level in the samples rise above the value to which the apparatus has been set, the inflating pressure is automatically increased within limits. The tidal volume is therefore increased, tending to restore the carbon-dioxide level. Left to itself, the alteration in pressure is limited to a range of 5 cm H_2O. Further increase or decrease needs an adjustment by the anaesthetist. This serves to protect the patient from unchecked changes in delivery pressure which might develop as a result of a fault developing in the apparatus.

The apparatus maintains the arterial carbon-dioxide concentration at a desired level for long periods of time. An indicator warns the anaesthetist when spontaneous respiration starts so that he may give further doses of relaxant.

FUNCTIONAL ANALYSIS

Inspiratory phase

In this phase the ventilator operates as a low-constant-pressure generator. The pressure, which is set by the variable low-pressure regulator (7), is constant for any one inspiratory phase, but is automatically adjusted from one respiration to the next, to maintain a constant end-expiratory carbon-dioxide level.

Change-over from inspiratory phase to expiratory phase

This change-over is time-cycled: the inspiratory time is determined by the rotation of the timing cam (14).

Expiratory phase

In this phase the ventilator operates as a constant, atmospheric, pressure generator: the patient's expired gas passes freely to atmosphere at the outlet (17).

Change-over from expiratory phase to inspiratory phase

This change-over also is time-cycled: the expiratory time is determined by the rotation of the timing cam (14).

REFERENCES

1 Frumin M.J. and Lee A.S.J. (1957) A physiologically oriented artificial respirator which produces N_2O–O_2 anesthesia in man. *J. Lab. clin. Med.* **49**, 617.

2 Frumin M.J. (1957) Clinical use of a physiological respirator producing N_2O amnesia-analgesia. *Anesthesiology*, **18**, 290.

CHAPTER 20

The 'Autovent'

DESCRIPTION

This ventilator (fig. 20.1) is very little bigger than the normal expiratory valve. It is designed for use during anaesthesia with a non-rebreathing circuit. It is fitted in a Magill circuit close to the patient in place of the expiratory valve.

The bobbin (fig. 20.2), in which is fitted a magnet (1) (fig. 20.3), is normally held in

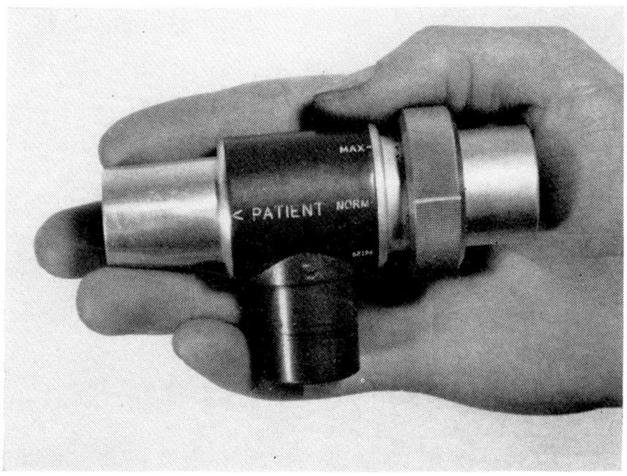

Fig. 20.1. The 'Autovent'.
Courtesy of Department of Medical Illustration, Cardiff Royal Infirmary.

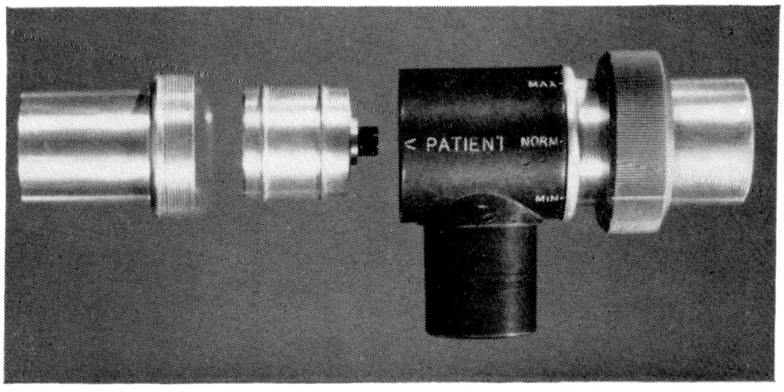

Fig. 20.2. The components of the 'Autovent'.
Courtesy of Department of Medical Illustration, Cardiff Royal Infirmary.

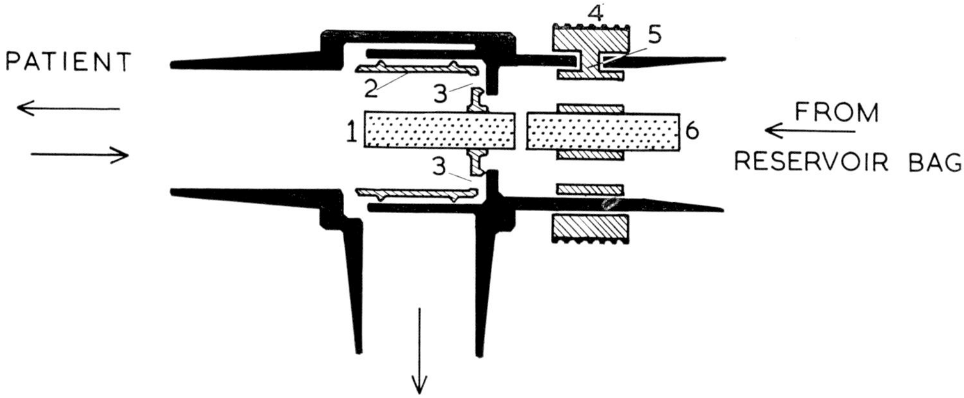

Fig. 20.3. Diagram of the 'Autovent'.

1. Magnet
2. Bobbin
3. Holes
4. Rotatable ring
5. Pin
6. Magnet

the closed position by the attraction between this magnet and the adjustable magnet (6). Pressure in the reservoir bag of the Magill circuit therefore builds up as gas from the anaesthetic apparatus flows into it. When this pressure has increased sufficiently the force exerted on the bobbin overcomes the attraction of the magnets for each other and the bobbin snaps over to the inspiratory position. In this position the bobbin seats against the port to the patient, so closing the pathway to atmosphere. Gas from the reservoir bag then flows, past the adjustable magnet (6), and through the holes (3) in the face of the bobbin, to the patient.

As gas flows to the patient the pressure difference across the bobbin falls. When it has fallen sufficiently the bobbin moves back to the closed, expiratory, position under the attraction of the magnets. Expired gas then flows through the valve to atmosphere.

All the gas flowing into the reservoir bag is delivered to the patient. The flow set on the flowmeters of the anaesthetic apparatus is, therefore, the total minute-volume ventilation of the patient.

The only control on the ventilator is the knurled ring (4); this is connected to the magnet carrier by a pin (5) which slides in a helical slot. The ring (4) can be turned one quarter of a revolution, and alters the position of the adjustable magnet (6) relative to the magnet (1) in the bobbin (2). It therefore sets the pressure in the reservoir bag at which the ventilator cycles to the inspiratory phase and the flow into the patient at which it cycles to the expiratory phase.

Therefore, for any particular total ventilation and any particular lung characteristics, the tidal volume and the frequency depend on the setting of this control. There is no direct control of the inspiratory-expiratory ratio. It may change, however, with changes in the inflating-gas flow, with the setting of the ring (4), and with changes in lung characteristics.

FUNCTIONAL ANALYSIS

Superficially this ventilator closely resembles the 'Minivent'. Its mode of action is also very similar except for an important difference in the change-over from the inspiratory phase to the expiratory phase. Apart from this change-over, therefore, the various elements of the functional analysis are dealt with only briefly here. Provided this difference in the change-over is borne in mind, the reader may find the fuller account of the 'Minivent' helpful in understanding the details of functioning of this ventilator.

Inspiratory phase

In this phase the ventilator operates as a discharging compliance (see p. 98) due to the characteristics of the reservoir bag to which the patient's lungs are then connected.

Change-over from inspiratory phase to expiratory phase

As in the 'Minivent', this change-over occurs when the pneumatic force on the bobbin, tending to hold it in the inspiratory position, falls to less than the magnetic force, tending to restore it to the expiratory position. In both ventilators, the pneumatic force has two components. One fraction of the cross-sectional area of the bobbin is exposed to the pressure difference between the bag and patient ports* and therefore depends only on the inspiratory flow rate and the resistance to flow past the bobbin (the resistance of the holes (3) in the 'Autovent'). The other fraction of the cross-sectional area is exposed to the pressure difference between the bag port and the expiratory port. The pressure at the expiratory port is atmospheric and therefore the pressure difference depends solely on the pressure at the bag port. In the 'Minivent', the two fractions of the cross-sectional area are comparable, so that the change-over depends partly on inspiratory flow and partly on bag pressure—it is a mixture of flow-cycled and pressure-cycled. In the 'Autovent', however, only a very small fraction of the cross-sectional area is exposed (during the inspiratory phase) to the atmospheric pressure at the expiratory port—just a very narrow outer annulus. Therefore the pneumatic force is almost exclusively dependent on the inspiratory flow through the resistance of the holes (3) and the change-over is almost purely flow-cycled.

Expiratory phase

In this phase the ventilator operates as a constant, atmospheric, pressure generator: the patient's expired gas passes to atmosphere at the expiratory port.

Change-over from expiratory phase to inspiratory phase

As in the 'Minivent' this change-over occurs when the pressure in the reservoir bag has risen to a level at which it overcomes the magnetic force tending to hold the bobbin

* This is a simplification of the true situation in the 'Minivent'.

closed. This pressure corresponds to a particular volume in the reservoir bag and therefore is attained in the time, from the start of the previous inspiratory phase, that it takes the inflating-gas flow to supply the tidal volume of gas delivered to the patient during the previous inspiratory phase. But this tidal volume varies with changes of lung characteristics. Therefore this change-over does not fit any of the conventional categories; the simplest way of specifying it is to say that it is time-cycled, but the cycling time is proportional to the previous tidal volume whatever that may happen to have been.

CHAPTER 21

The Bang Ventilator[1]

DESCRIPTION

This apparatus (fig. 21.1) was designed during the Danish 1952 poliomyelitis epidemic.

Compressed air or other oxygen/nitrogen mixture from the cylinder (1) flows at the rate of 7–10 litres/min into the ventilator and distends the reservoir bag (5) which provides a low-pressure supply of gas for inflation of the lungs.

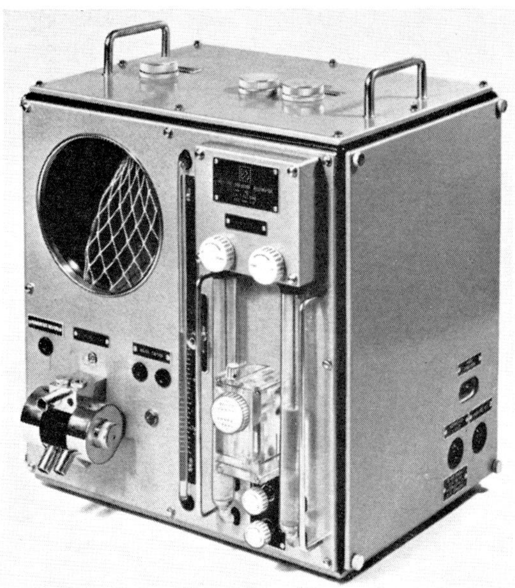

Fig. 21.1. The Bang ventilator.

Courtesy of Dr C. Bang.

Inflation and expiration both take place through the valve (6). This consists of a piston fitting closely into a tube round the ends of which are wound two solenoid coils (7). These, when energized, attract the metal piston to one or other end of the tube. The centre of the piston is cut away so that gas is able to flow through the inspiratory tube

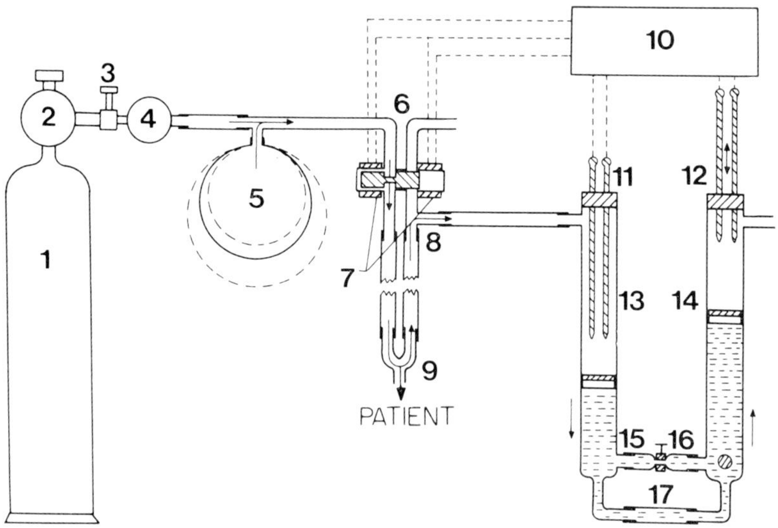

Fig. 21.2. Diagram of the Bang ventilator.

1. Cylinder of compressed gas
2. Cylinder pressure gauge
3. Tap controlling flow rate of gas to reservoir bag
4. Flowmeter
5. Reservoir bag
6. Inspiratory–expiratory valve
7. Solenoid coils
8. Side tube from expiratory tube to manometer
9. Connexion to patient
10. Electrical control circuit
11. Electrodes
12. Electrodes
13. Manometer tube
14. Manometer tube
15. Rubber tubing
15. Clamp on tube (15) controlling duration of expiratory phase
17. Rubber tubing

Courtesy of *The Lancet*.[1]

when the piston is in the left-hand position, and through the expiratory tube when it is in the right-hand position.

Two tubes, one for inflation and one for expiration, pass from the valve and are joined together by a 'Y' connexion (9) near the patient. A side tube (8) from the expiratory tube passes to the manometer, the liquid in which therefore moves with the changes of pressure in the lungs.

The manometer consists of two tubes (13, 14) filled with fluid connected by two pieces of rubber tubing (15, 17). A small metal-faced float lies on the surface of the fluid in each tube. The connecting tube (15) can be partly occluded by the clamp (16). The tube (13) is air-tight and connected to the patient's airway, whilst the tube (14) is open to the atmosphere and contains a one-way ball valve at its base. Thus during the inspiratory phase the liquid flows rapidly into the right-hand tube (14) as the pressure at the mouth rises. During the expiratory phase, however, the fall of the liquid in the right-hand tube is hindered by the pinch-cock (16). Hence, the duration of the expiratory phase can be varied by manipulation of the pinch-cock (16).

The electrodes (11) are adjusted so that contact with the float occurs when the two liquid levels are almost equal again. These electrodes (11) control the left-hand solenoid which, when energized, initiates an inspiratory phase. The height of the electrodes (12) is varied to control the cycling pressure.

The Bang ventilator is one of the earliest examples of a 'minute-volume divider' (see p. 140). The total minute-volume ventilation is nominally equal to the flow of inflating gas from the cylinder (1).

FUNCTIONAL ANALYSIS

Inspiratory phase

In this phase the ventilator operates as a discharging compliance (see p. 98).

Change-over from inspiratory phase to expiratory phase

This change-over is pressure-cycled: the pressure in the manometer which produces cycling is that applied to the patient.

Expiratory phase

In this phase the ventilator operates as a constant, atmospheric, pressure generator: the patient's expired gas passes freely to atmosphere at the expiratory outlet.

Change-over from expiratory phase to inspiratory phase

This change-over is time-cycled: the expiratory time is equal to the time in which enough liquid returns to the left-hand limb of the manometer to close the contacts and produce cycling. This time is uninfluenced by the patient; but if the cycling pressure at the end of the inspiratory phase is raised, by raising the contacts in the right-hand limb, there is more liquid to return to the left-hand limb, and the expiratory phase is therefore lengthened.

REFERENCE

1 BANG C. (1953) A new respirator. *Lancet*, **1**, 723.

CHAPTER 22

The 'Barnet' Mark II Ventilator[1]

DESCRIPTION

This ventilator (fig. 22.1) was designed for ward or anaesthetic use. An electronic timing circuit (26, 28) (fig. 22.2) intermittently energizes a solenoid (15) which controls the action of the inspiratory valve (16) and the expiratory valve (12). A 12-volt nickel-iron battery, housed in the ventilator, supplies the current for this circuit. In normal use it is continuously charged from the a.c. mains. In the absence of such a supply the ventilator will run for 14 hours on a fully-charged battery, a voltmeter being incorporated to show the state of charge.

Fresh gas is delivered through flowmeters at a pressure of between 2 and 60 lb/in^2 and at a flow equal to the desired minute-volume ventilation. It enters the ventilator at the inlet (20). During the expiratory phase this gas is stored in the concertina reservoir bag (6) at a pressure determined by the force exerted by a coil spring (2) acting on the top-plate (3) of the concertina bags (5, 6). A pointer attached to the top-plate (3) protrudes through the outer casing of the ventilator and reflects the movements of the bags (5, 6).

When the inspiratory valve (16) opens, the fresh gas stored in the reservoir bag (6), together with fresh gas entering it, is forced, past the one-way valve (17) and along the inspiratory tube (22), to the patient. When the inspiratory time set by the electronic circuit has elapsed, the solenoid (15) is energized, and the arm (13) is pulled over against the force of the spring (14). The inspiratory valve (16) is closed and the expiratory valve (12) is opened. Expired gas flows, along the expiratory tube (21), past the one-way valve (11) and the expiratory valve (12), into the concertina storage bag (5), and, in certain circumstances, past the one-way valve (7) to atmosphere. The gas accumulated in the bag (5) is discharged to atmosphere past the one-way valve (7) during the next inspiratory phase. When the expiratory time set by the electronic circuit has elapsed, the supply of current to the solenoid (15) is cut off and the spring (14) pulls back the arm (13), opening the inspiratory valve (16) and closing the expiratory valve (12). A ventilation meter may be inserted into the 'expiratory port' (21) to register the ventilation of the patient.

During the expiratory phase the flow of fresh gas into the reservoir bag (6) lifts the top-plate (3) and thereby expands the bag (5), producing a negative pressure within it. The one-way valve (7) prevents air being drawn in through the main expiratory port.

However, air can be drawn in through a second port controlled by the throttle (8). When the throttle (8) is fully closed, the negative pressure is limited to about -10 cm H_2O by the safety-valve (4). When the throttle (8) is fully open no negative pressure is produced within the bag (5). The throttle (8) therefore acts as a 'negative pressure' control.

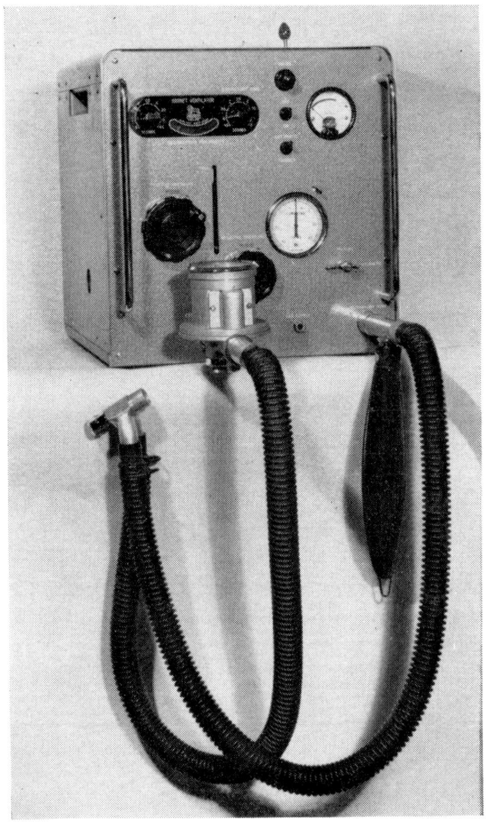

Fig. 22.1. The 'Barnet' Mark II ventilator.

Courtesy of W.Watson & Sons Ltd.

During the inspiratory phase the bag (5) is forced down by the spring (2) and its contents are discharged to atmosphere through the non-return valve (7). This valve also allows the escape of expired gas should the expiratory flow from the patient be at a rate faster than that at which the bag (5) is expanding.

A patient-triggering mechanism can be switched on if desired. An inspiratory effort by the patient produces a negative pressure in the expiratory pathway which moves the diaphragm (9) and so opens the microswitch (10). This interrupts the supply of current to the solenoid (15), terminating the expiratory phase immediately and initiating the next inspiratory phase. The employment of negative pressure during the expiratory phase precludes the use of patient-triggering. If, due to an oversight, both mechanisms are in action at the same time, the negative pressure produced within the bag (5) will operate the patient-triggering device, the expiratory phase will be terminated prematurely, and the lungs will remain partially inflated.

When manual ventilation is desired, the electrical supply must be switched 'off', and the 'automatic/manual' control (19) must be turned to the 'manual' position, so diverting the fresh gas to the reservoir bag (23) which must be brought into the circuit by turning the tap (24). The expiratory valve (12) is held closed when the ventilator is 'off', and expired gas passes back along the inspiratory pathway (22), excess gas being blown off through an expiratory valve which must be included close to the patient. Thus the arrangement of the components in this manual circuit is the same as in the Magill attachment, and therefore rebreathing occurs unless the fresh-gas flow is high enough.

The durations of the inspiratory and expiratory phases may each be varied independently between $\frac{1}{2}$ and $4\frac{1}{2}$ sec by adjustment of the 'inspiratory time' and 'expiratory time' controls (26, 28) of the electronic timing circuit. The respiratory frequency may therefore be varied between 7 and 60 per minute and the inspiratory-expiratory ratio between 1 : 9 and 9 : 1. An 'integrator' (27) on the front panel of the ventilator displays the respiratory frequency which is automatically computed from the settings of these two controls.

In clinical use the fresh-gas supply is connected to the ventilator, the inspiratory time is set to the minimum appropriate for the patient, and the expiratory time is adjusted so as to give a suitable respiratory frequency.

The tidal volume delivered to the patient is the volume of fresh gas entering the ventilator during one complete respiratory cycle. Part of this tidal volume accumulates in the concertina reservoir bag (6) during the expiratory phase, and the rest flows directly to the patient during the inspiratory phase. The amount of gas which can be stored in the bag (6) is limited to 1400 ml by the safety 'cut-off' valve (18), which arrests the flow of fresh gas when the bag is full. As soon as this happens the pressure at the inlet (20) quickly reaches the pressure at which the fresh gas is being supplied, and the bobbins of the flowmeters in the supply line are depressed. In this way the ventilator automatically reduces the flow of fresh gas entering it if the flowmeters are set to deliver more than can be delivered to the patient. A failure to deliver the amount of fresh gas to which the flowmeters are set is shown by the fluctuations of the bobbins and by the bag remaining at or near the top of its stroke. Unless some change in the patient's compliance or the airway resistance can be detected and corrected (e.g. during anaesthesia by the administration of further muscle relaxants or the removal of secretions) attention must be directed to other factors, and either the pressure acting on the bag (6) must be increased or the inspiratory time lengthened. If the latter course is adopted it may be desirable to adjust the duration of the expiratory phase also so that the respiratory frequency, and hence the volume of fresh gas delivered in one complete respiratory cycle,

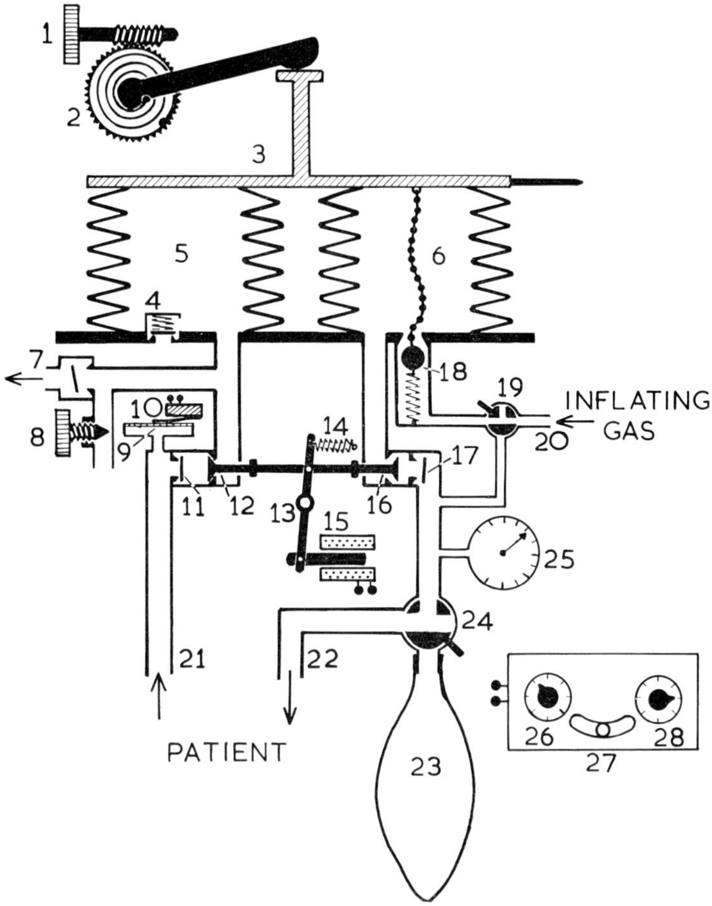

Fig. 22.2. Diagram of the 'Barnet' Mark II ventilator.

1. 'Positive pressure' control
2. Coil spring
3. Top-plate
4. Negative-pressure safety-valve
5. Concertina storage bag (expiratory)
6. Concertina reservoir bag (inspiratory)
7. One-way valve
8. 'Negative pressure' control
9. Patient-triggering diaphragm
10. Microswitch
11. One-way valve
12. Expiratory valve
13. Pivoted lever
14. Spring
15. Solenoid
16. Inspiratory valve
17. One-way valve
18. 'Cut-off' valve
19. 'Automatic/manual' control
20. Inflating-gas inlet
21. Expiratory tube
22. Inspiratory tube
23. Manual reservoir bag
24. Two-way tap
25. Manometer
26. 'Inspiratory time' control
27. 'Integrator' showing frequency
28. 'Expiratory time' control

is unaltered. If the inspiratory time is lengthened but the expiratory time unaltered, then the duration of one respiratory cycle is lengthened and the volume of fresh gas delivered to the ventilator during one cycle is correspondingly increased, with the result that the bag (6) may continue to be overfilled. If these last two adjustments are taken far enough, the tidal volume will enter the patient before the end of the inspiratory phase and the lungs will be held inflated until expiration begins. This will be shown by the bag reaching the bottom of its stroke before the end of the inspiratory phase. In practice this is quite likely to happen. It may be avoided either by shortening the duration of the inspiratory phase (and lengthening the expiratory phase so that the respiratory frequency is unchanged), by reducing the pressure exerted by the spring (2), or by increasing the fresh-gas flow, and hence the tidal volume. Normally, once the fresh-gas flow has been set to equal the desired minute-volume ventilation, the other controls are adjusted so that the bag (6) does not quite reach either limit of its excursion, but 'floats' between these extremes.

FUNCTIONAL ANALYSIS

Inspiratory phase

During this phase the ventilator operates as a pressure generator due to the action of the coil spring (2) on the concertina reservoir bag (6). The pressure probably decreases somewhat as the bag empties and the spring uncoils.

A volume limit occurs when the bag is completely empty and this is quite likely to occur in each inspiratory phase. After this volume limit has been reached the inflating-gas flow constitutes a small-constant-flow generator which continues to inflate the patient slowly for the remainder of the phase.

Change-over from inspiratory phase to expiratory phase

This is time-cycled: the duration of the inspiratory phase is determined by the electronic timing circuit.

Expiratory phase

If the negative-pressure control (8) is set to minimum (fully unscrewed) the ventilator operates as a constant, atmospheric, pressure generator throughout the phase: expiration occurs to atmosphere past the open throttle (8).

If the negative-pressure control (8) is set to maximum (throttle closed) the ventilator operates, at least approximately, as a constant-flow generator with atmospheric and negative-pressure limits (see p. 120). The steady flow of inflating gas into the concertina reservoir bag (6) must produce a nearly-steady expansion of the negative-pressure bag (5) and hence the ventilator approximates to a constant-flow generator. The one-way valve (7) prevents the pressure in the bag rising above atmospheric and the spring-loaded one-way valve (4) prevents it falling below a fixed negative value. Potentially, therefore, there are three successive parts of the expiratory phase: constant, atmospheric, pressure generation; constant-flow generation; and constant, negative, pressure generation.

If the negative-pressure control (8) is partly open, it introduces a leak in parallel with the flow generator which therefore behaves as a high (negative) constant-pressure generator with high series resistance but still with atmospheric-pressure and negative-pressure limits.

Change-over from expiratory phase to inspiratory phase

Basically this is time-cycled: the duration of the expiratory phase is determined by the electronic timing circuit.

If the patient-triggering circuit is switched on the change-over is patient-cycled or time-cycled whichever comes first.

REFERENCE

1 Rochford J., Welch R.F. and Winks D.P. (1958) An electronic time-cycled respirator. *Br. J. Anaesth.* **30**, 23.

CHAPTER 23

The 'Barnet' Mark III Ventilator

This account of the 'Barnet' Mark III is based on a prototype model; the production model differs in a few respects as described on p. 298.

DESCRIPTION

This ventilator (figs. 23.1 and 23.2) is intended for use in the theatre or the ward, and with

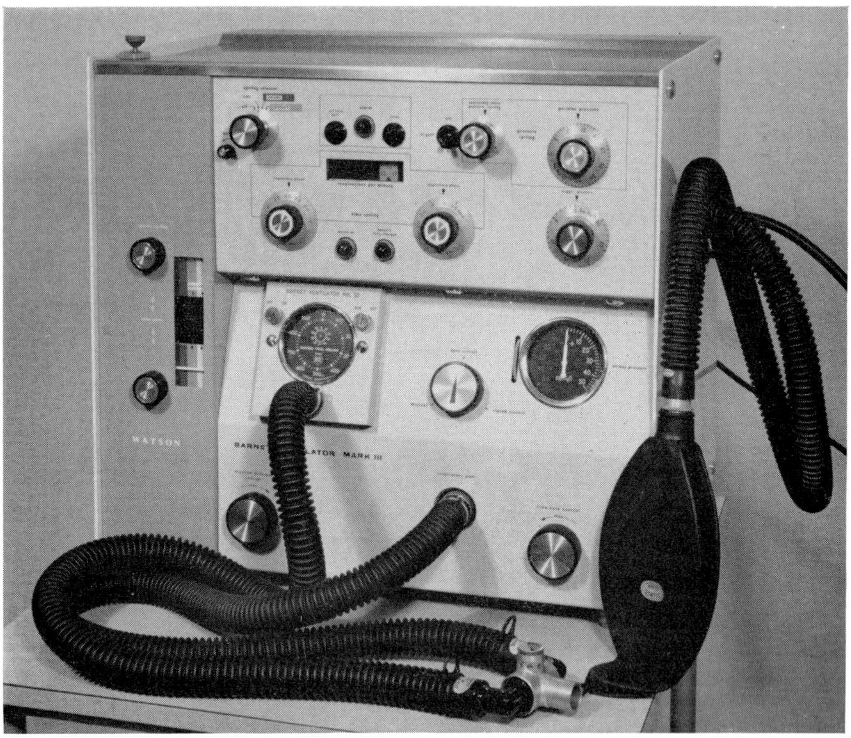

Fig. 23.1. The 'Barnet' Mark III ventilator.
Courtesy of Department of Medical Illustration, Cardiff Royal Infirmary.

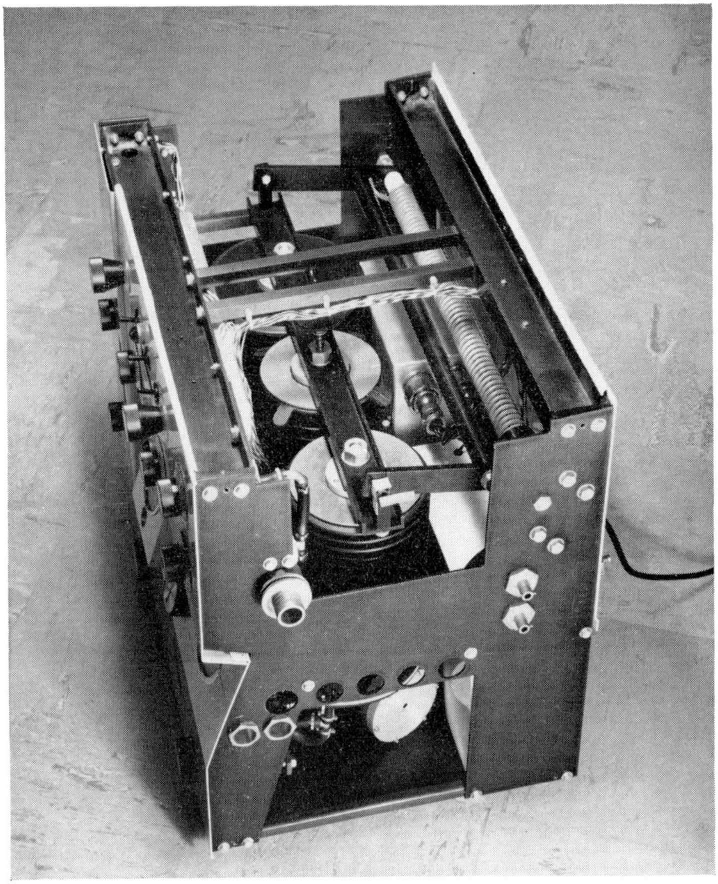

Fig. 23.2. The mechanism of the prototype 'Barnet' Mark III ventilator.
Courtesy of Department of Medical Illustration, Cardiff Royal Infirmary.

either a closed or non-rebreathing circuit. It can be time-, volume-, or pressure-cycled, and it can be patient-triggered. A supply of compressed gas at a pressure of at least 5 lb/in^2 is needed to drive the ventilator. A supply of electricity is also necessary for the electronic control circuits. When the ventilator is connected to an a.c. mains supply a continuous charge is applied to a built-in battery, and, at the same time, current is fed to the control circuits. If such a supply is not available the fully-charged battery allows the ventilator to be run for up to 24 hours.

When the ventilator is used with a non-rebreathing circuit, the inflating gas, which is to be delivered to the patient, is supplied at the port (32) (fig. 23.3). The 'manual/open circuit/closed circuit' control (38) is in the 'open circuit' position in which the poppet valves (39–46) and thc 'gas distribution' valve (47) are in the positions shown in fig. 23.3. The inflating gas therefore passes through the valve (47) to the poppet valve (45) which is in the open position. From the valve (45) the gas flows to the concertina reservoir bag (7). During the expiratory phase the solenoid-operated inspiratory valve (29) is in the closed position and gas flowing into the concertina reservoir bag (7) forces up the top-plate (10) which is common to the three concertina bags (5, 7, and 9), together with the indicator rod (1). The upward movement of the top-plate (10) forces up the levers (3, 3) which are attached to the rod (6), around which is a helical spring. This spring is always under tension, which is increased as the concertina bag (7) is expanded. At the end of the expiratory phase the solenoid valve (29) opens and the solenoid valve (48) closes. The gas contained within the concertina bag (7) is driven, by the force of the spring (6) on the top-plate (10), through the inspiratory valve (29), past the poppet valve (44), and through the poppet valve (43), to the diaphragm valve (51). The pressure of the gas forces over the diaphragm (51) and the gas flows past the 'flow rate control' (52), through the breathing tube (55), to the patient. At the end of the inspiratory phase the inspiratory valve (29) closes and the expiratory valve (48) opens. Expired gas now passes, through the breathing tube (50), the Wright respirometer (49), the expiratory valve (48), the poppet valve (42),

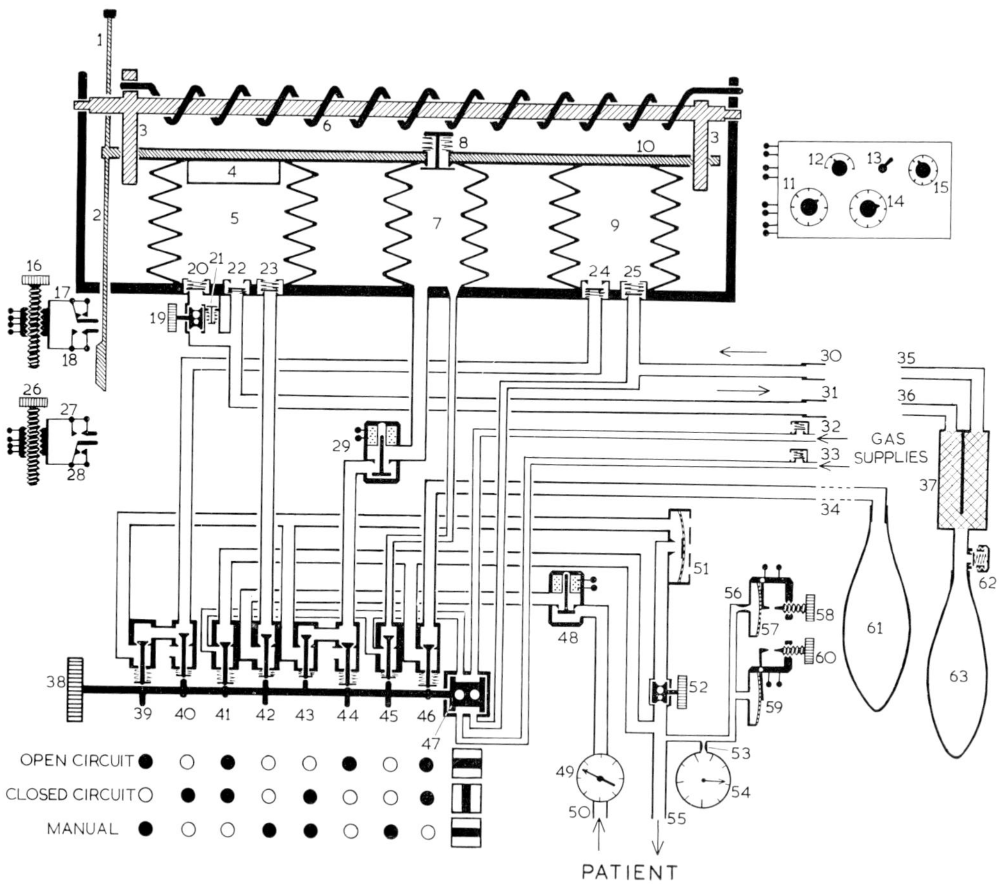

and the one-way valve (23), to the concertina storage bag (5). This concertina bag (5) is being distended by the upward movement of the top-plate (10) brought about by the flow of fresh inflating gas into the concertina bag (7). There is therefore a tendency for a negative pressure to be developed in the concertina bag (5). The amount of negative pressure depends on the setting of the 'negative pressure control' (19). A negative-pressure safety-valve (21) is connected in parallel with the 'negative pressure control' (19) in order to limit the amount of negative pressure that can be developed by the upward movement of the concertina bag (5). When the concertina bag (5) is fully collapsed it is almost filled by the 'inverted top hat' (4). This helps to ensure that negative pressure is quickly developed in the bag (5) at the beginning of the expiratory phase. Without the 'inverted top hat' the first part of the upward movement of the plate (10) would be dissipated in decompressing the relatively-large volume of gas that would then be in the bag.

At the end of the expiratory phase, when the positions of the solenoid valves (29 and 48) are reversed, the top-plate (10) is forced down again by the spring (6), and the expired gas stored in the concertina bag (5) is forced, through the one-way valve (22), and the port (31), to atmosphere.

When the ventilator is to be used for closed-circuit anaesthesia the control (38) is

Fig. 23.3. Diagram of the prototype 'Barnet' Mark III ventilator.

1. Indicator rod
2. Rod
3, 3. Levers bearing on top of plate (10)
4. 'Inverted top hat'
5. Negative-pressure concertina bag
6. Rod with helical spring
7. Open-circuit or driving concertina bag
8. Mechanically-operated excursion-limiting valve
9. Closed-circuit concertina bag
10. Top-plate
11. Time-cycling 'expiratory phase' control
12. 'Cycling selector'
13. 'Trigger on/off' switch
14. Time-cycling 'inspiratory phase' control
15. Pressure-cycling 'expiratory phase' control
16. Volume-cycling 'tidal volume' control
17. Alarm contacts
18. Volume-cycling contacts
19. 'Negative pressure control'
20. One-way valve
21. Negative-pressure safety-valve
22–25. One-way valves
26. Volume-cycling 'tidal volume' control
27. Volume-cycling contacts
28. Alarm contacts
29. Solenoid-operated inspiratory valve
30, 31. Ports
32. Inlet for fresh gas or inflating gas
33. Inlet for driving gas
34–36. Ports
37. Partitioned soda-lime canister
38. 'Manual/open circuit/closed circuit' control
39–46. Poppet valves
47. 'Gas distribution' valve
48. Solenoid-operated expiratory valve
49. Wright respirometer
50. Expiratory tube
51. Diaphragm valve
52. 'Flow rate control'
53. Constriction
54. Manometer
55. Breathing tube
56. Constriction
57. Pressure-cycling diaphragm
58. 'Positive pressure' control
59. Patient-triggering diaphragm
60. 'Trigger pressure' control
61. Manual reservoir bag
62. Spill valve
63. Closed-circuit storage bag

The symbols in the bottom left-hand corner indicate which of the poppet valves (39–46) are open (○) and which are closed (●), and the gas pathway in the 'gas distribution' valve (47) for each of the three positions of the 'manual/open circuit/closed circuit' control (38).

turned to the 'closed circuit' position in which the poppet valves (39–46) and the 'gas distribution' valve (47) are in the positions indicated by the 'closed circuit' key at the bottom of fig. 23.3. The partitioned soda-lime canister (37) and the storage bag (63) are connected by the tubes (35 and 36) to the ports (30 and 31). Driving gas is supplied at the inlet (33) and flows, through the valve (47), to the valve (45), and from this to the concertina bag (7), which, in this mode, operates solely as a 'driving' bag. During the expiratory phase the inspiratory valve (29) is closed, and so the top-plate (10) is forced up by the gas entering the bag (7). Gas from the reservoir bag (63) is drawn, through the one-way valve (25), into the concertina reservoir bag (9).

At the end of the expiratory phase the inspiratory valve (29) opens and the expiratory valve (48) closes. Driving gas contained in the concertina bag (7) now flows, through the inspiratory valve (29), and the open valve (44), to atmosphere. At the same time gas contained in the concertina reservoir bag (9) is forced, through the one-way valve (24), past the closed valve (40), through the open valve (39), the diaphragm valve (51), the 'flow rate control' (52), and the breathing tube (55), to the patient.

At the end of the inspiratory phase the valve (29) closes and the valve (48) opens. Expired gas flows, through the breathing tube (50), the Wright respirometer (49), the expiratory valve (48), the open valve (42), and the one-way valve (23), to the concertina bag (5). During the expiratory phase the top-plate (10) is being forced up by the gas entering the driving bag (7). When the inspiratory phase begins, the concertina bags (5, 7, and 9) are forced down by the spring (6), and the expired gas, which was stored in the concertina bag (5), flows, through the one-way valve (22), the port (31), the connexion (36), and the soda-lime canister (37), to the storage bag (63), where it is stored for the next filling of the concertina bag (9). During this closed-circuit operation of the ventilator the driving gas entering the port (33) does not flow to the patient but is used only to drive the ventilator. Fresh gas to be delivered to the patient is supplied at the port (32) and flows, through the valve (47), to the tube connecting the concertina reservoir bag (9) with the port (30). The spring-loaded valve (62) allows excess gas to be spilled from the breathing circuit.

In summary therefore, in this closed-circuit mode of operation, the concertina bag (7) acts only as a 'driving' bag. During its expansion upwards expired gas is drawn into the negative-pressure bag (5) and inspiratory gas is drawn from the storage bag (63), through the soda-lime (37), into the closed-circuit bag (9). During the collapse of the driving bag (7) the gas in the closed-circuit bag (9) is forced to the patient and the expired gas in the bag (5) is delivered, through the soda-lime (37), to the storage bag (63).

For manual inflation the control (38) is turned to the 'manual' position (see key in fig. 23.3). Fresh gas supplied at the port (32) flows through the valve (47) and the valve (41). It can then pass direct to the breathing tube (55), or, through the poppet valve (46), to the manual reservoir bag (61). Manual compression of the bag (61) forces the gas contained within it, through the port (34), the poppet valve (46), and the breathing tube (55), to the patient. When the reservoir bag (61) is relaxed, gas from the patient flows back, through the tube (55) and the valve (46), to the reservoir bag (61). Since the inspiratory valve (29) and the poppet valves (40 and 44) are open, any gas remaining in, or being delivered to, the concertina bags (7 and 9) flows freely to atmosphere. An expiratory valve near the patient allows excess fresh gas to be blown off. Thus the arrangement of the components in this manual circuit is the same as in the Magill attachment and therefore rebreathing occurs unless the fresh-gas flow is high enough.

Whether the ventilator is used with the non-rebreathing or the closed circuit, it may be cycled in any one of three ways.

If the 'cycling selector' (12) is set to 'time' cycling, the 'inspiratory phase' control (14) and the 'expiratory phase' control (11) in the electronic circuit are used to set the required inspiratory and expiratory times each between $\frac{1}{2}$ and 5 sec. These settings determine the times for which the inspiratory valve (29) and the expiratory valve (48) are open and closed, and hence the durations of the phases. The controls are linked mechanically to an indicator which displays the resultant frequency. A second mechanical linkage between the controls prevents the inspiratory time being set longer than the expiratory time.

If the ventilator is set for 'volume' cycling, then the controls (16 and 26) are used to obtain the desired tidal volume. The reversal of the solenoid valves (29 and 48) from the expiratory to the inspiratory position occurs when the contacts (18) are closed by the upward movement of the rod (2) attached to the plate (10). Similarly, reversal of the valves from the inspiratory to the expiratory position occurs when the contacts (27) are closed by the downward movement of the rod (2). Thus the settings of the 'tidal volume' controls (16 and 26) determine the upper and lower limits of movement of the concertina bags (5, 7, and 9).

When the control (12) is switched to 'pressure' cycling the setting of the 'positive pressure' control (58) determines the pressure which must be reached within the chamber behind the diaphragm (57) in order to close the contacts, and so reverse the solenoid valves (29 and 48). The constriction (56) damps the response of the pressure-cycling mechanism. The expiratory time is controlled electronically. It may be varied by the 'pressure cycling expiratory phase' control (15), which is completely independent of the control (11) used to set the expiratory time in the time-cycled mode.

In addition to the basic cycling mechanisms described above, the electronic timing circuit fixes a limit of $5\frac{1}{2}$ sec to the duration of the inspiratory phase, in both the pressure-cycled and volume-cycled modes, and the same limit to the duration of the expiratory phase in the volume-cycled mode. The 'trigger on/off' switch (13) may be turned to allow the patient to trigger the ventilator, no matter what mode of operation is in use. The negative pressure in the breathing tube (55) acts on the diaphragm (59) to close the contacts. The 'trigger pressure' control (60) determines the sensitivity of this mechanism.

The controls (16 and 26) each carry a second pair of contacts (17 and 28) in addition to the volume-cycling contacts (18 and 27). In the volume-cycled mode, as soon as either of the inner pair of contacts (18 and 27) is operated, the motion of the bags is reversed; therefore the outer contacts are never operated, and the controls (16 and 26) set limits to the excursion of the bags (5, 7, and 9) which cannot be exceeded. In the time-cycled or pressure-cycled modes, on the other hand, the volume-cycling contacts are inoperative and the bags may move far enough to operate one or other of the outer pairs of contacts (17 and 28). If this happens an 'alarm' circuit is triggered which lights a lamp and sounds a buzzer. Therefore, if a large leak develops in the patient circuit, the bags collapse fully during the inspiratory phase, thereby operating the contacts (28) and triggering the alarm circuit. Similarly, a major obstruction will prevent the bags discharging during the inspiratory phase so that during successive expiratory phases they fill further and operate the upper alarm contacts (17). If the controls (16 and 26) are adjusted so that the normal regular excursion of the bags just fails to operate the alarm contacts, then even quite small changes of lung characteristics will cause the excursion of the bags to drift far enough to operate one or other of the alarm contacts.

The pressure in the patient circuit is indicated on the manometer (54), the response of which is damped by the constriction (53).

If the driving-gas flow during closed-circuit operation, or the inflating-gas flow during open-circuit operation, is too great, then, when the top-plate (10) reaches its upper position, the valve (8) is pushed open and excess gas entering the concertina bag (7) spills through it.

If a negative-pressure expiratory phase is used during closed-circuit operation, the diaphragm valve (51) is drawn onto its seating by the negative pressure, and this prevents gas being drawn from the inspiratory pathway during the expiratory phase.

Inspiratory flow may be varied by adjustment of the 'flow rate control' (52).

The production model

In the production model the driving bag (7) is as large as the closed-circuit bag (9). The compression of all three bags is supplemented by a weight. When the ventilator is set to open circuit the closed-circuit bag (9) is coupled in parallel with the negative-pressure bag (5) in order to develop more negative pressure. The effect of these changes is quantitative rather than qualitative. Therefore the account given here should be generally applicable to the production model but not the numerical data of the bag characteristics (fig. 23.4) or of the recordings (figs. 23.5, 6, 7). Where major differences between the functioning of prototype and production model seem likely these have been mentioned in the 'Controls' section.

FUNCTIONAL ANALYSIS

Inspiratory phase

During this phase the 'Barnet' ventilator operates fundamentally as a pressure generator, due to the force exerted by the spring (6) on the cross-sectional area of either the driving (7) or closed-circuit (9) concertina reservoir bags. The force of the spring decreases as the plate (10) falls; therefore the generated pressure decreases as the bags empty (fig. 23.4).

The range of movement of either concertina bag, required to deliver the desired tidal volume, is commonly less than the total available range of movement. Therefore the limits of a given 'tidal stroke' may vary, or be varied, up and down within the overall limits of the full stroke of the bags.

If the tidal stroke is near the top of the available range the generated pressure is generally high, and the ventilator approximates to a flow generator. The approximation is closer on open circuit than on closed circuit because the pressure in the driving bag (7), which then functions as the open-circuit reservoir bag, is generally higher than that in the closed-circuit bag (9) (fig. 23.4). In both cases, however, the generated flow falls off a little during the phase owing to the pressure in the bag falling as the spring (6) relaxes. This is illustrated, in the case of the open circuit, in fig. 23.5: although the flow declines a little

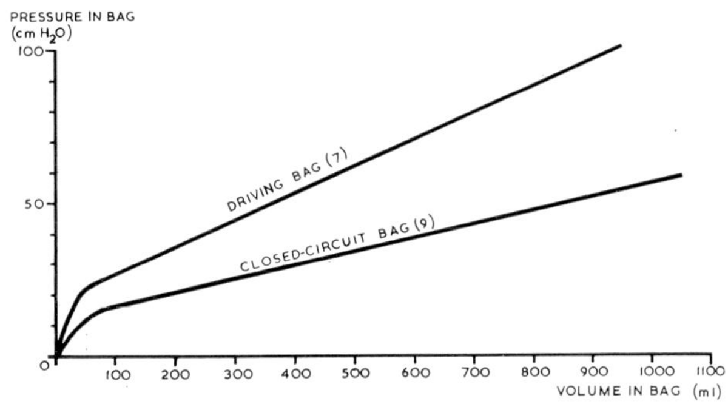

Fig. 23.4. Prototype 'Barnet' Mark III. Pressure-volume characteristics of the driving and the closed-circuit concertina reservoir bags.

during the phase the pattern is barely affected by halving the compliance (b) or doubling the resistance (c) whereas the pattern of pressure is considerably modified.

If the tidal stroke is near the bottom of the available range the generated pressure becomes low towards the end of the phase (fig. 23.4) and it might be expected that the ventilator would exhibit conventional pressure-generating characteristics. In fig. 23.6, however, which was recorded with the ventilator set to closed circuit and with the bags working at the bottom of the available stroke, this is not the case: when the compliance is halved or the resistance doubled the changes which occur in the flow waveform are not typical of a pressure generator. This is a characteristic of the time-cycled mode of operation and the explanation for it is as follows. During the first inflation after the compliance has been suddenly halved, or the resistance suddenly doubled, the pressure pattern within the concertina bag is indeed the same as before and the flow is reduced. Therefore a smaller volume escapes from the bag. During the following expiratory phase the fixed input volume to the bag carries it to a higher level than before so that, in the next inspiratory phase, the generated pressure, though still decreasing during the phase, is at a generally-higher level. Further small increases in the level of working occur over the next

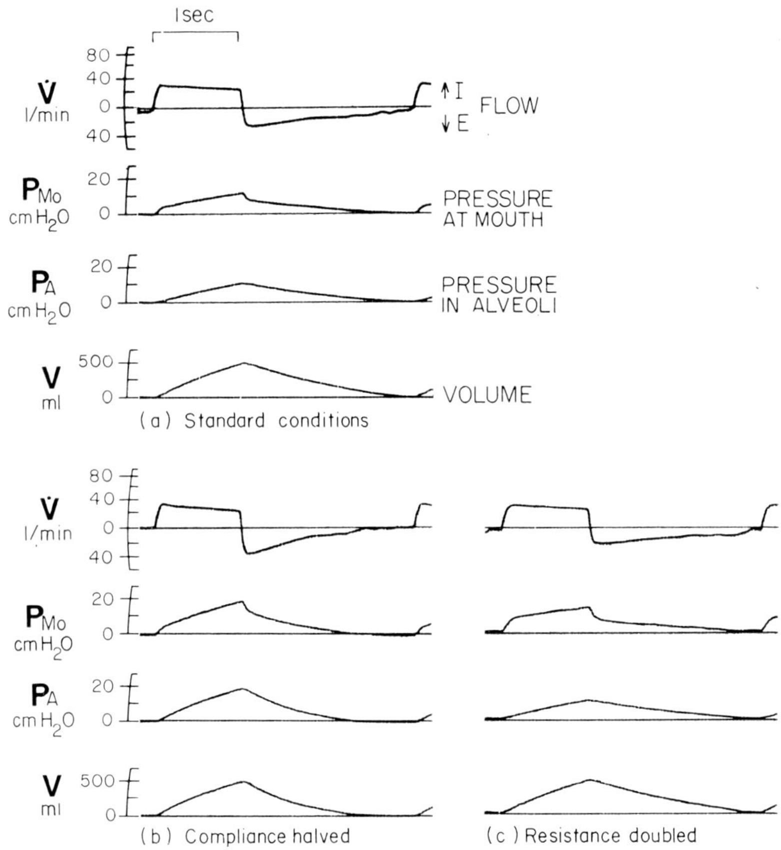

Fig. 23.5. Prototype 'Barnet' Mark III, in the time-cycled, 'open circuit' mode and with the concertina bags working near the top of their range. Recordings showing the effects of changes of lung characteristics.

Standard conditions: 'inspiratory phase', set for an inspiratory time of 1 sec; 'expiratory phase', set for an expiratory time of 2 sec; inflating-gas flow, set (at 11 litres/min) for a tidal volume of 500 ml; 'negative pressure control', minimum; 'flow rate control', set, towards minimum, so that the concertina bags rose almost to the top of their stroke in each expiratory phase.

few cycles until a new equilibrium is established in which the general level of generated pressure is high enough for the volume discharged from the concertina bag during the inspiratory phase to be equal once more to the volume drawn into it during the expiratory phase. Thus the flow waveform is largely restored to what it was before the change of lung characteristics while the mouth-pressure waveform rises higher than before. (The mouth-pressure waveform always differs from the waveform of pressure in the concertina bag because, on closed circuit, the resistance between the bag and the mouth is comparable with the 'standard' airway resistance between the mouth and the alveoli.)

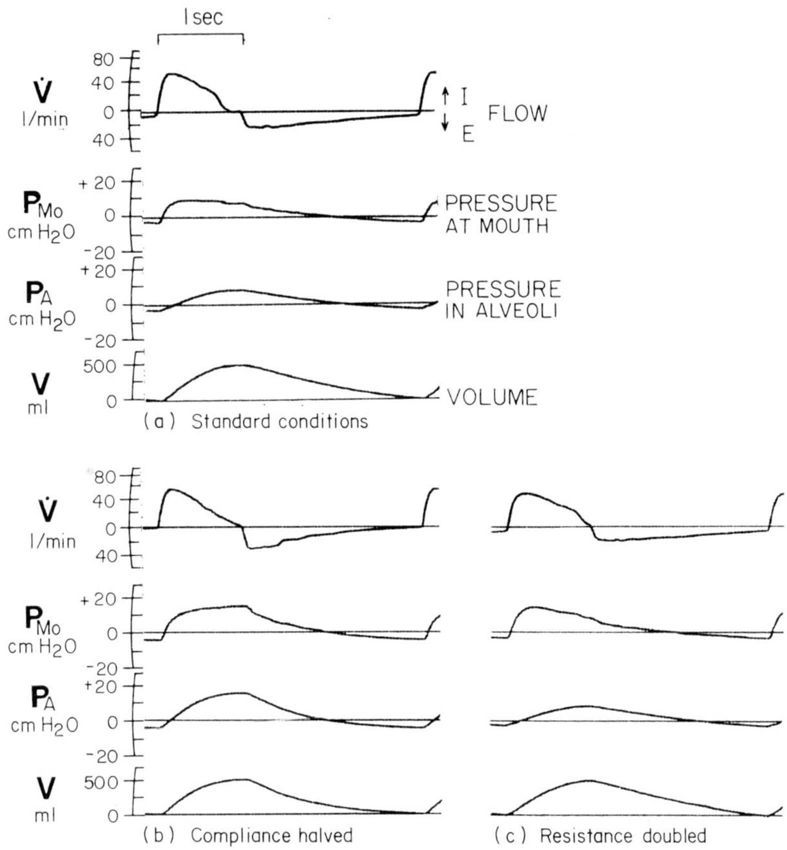

Fig. 23.6. Prototype 'Barnet' Mark III, in the time-cycled, 'closed circuit' mode and with the concertina bags working near the bottom of their range. Recordings showing the effects of changes of lung characteristics.

Standard conditions: 'inspiratory phase', set for an inspiratory time of 1 sec; 'expiratory phase', set for an expiratory time of 2 sec; 'flow rate control', maximum; driving-gas flow set (at 17 litres/min) for a tidal volume of 500 ml; 'negative pressure control', set for an end-expiratory alveolar pressure of -3 cmH_2O.

Thus, in the time-cycled mode of operation, with the bags working towards the lower end of their stroke, the ventilator operates as a (decreasing) pressure generator in the sense that the pattern of pressure is not immediately changed by a decrease in compliance or increase in resistance; but the response of the ventilator to the consequent reduction in flow and tidal volume is such as to produce a gradual increase in generated pressure over a few cycles of operation until the tidal volume and flow pattern are more or less restored.

In the volume-cycled mode of operation, not illustrated here, the position of the working range within the limits of the total available stroke is fixed and no such gradual compensation can occur; the pressure falls off in a predetermined manner with respect to bag volume. The only effect of decreasing compliance or increasing resistance, apart from decreasing the flow, is to increase the time over which the fall in pressure is spread and therefore to prolong the inspiratory phase.

Alternatively, whatever mode of cycling is in use, the ventilator may be regarded as a discharging compliance during this phase (see p. 98).

Change-over from inspiratory phase to expiratory phase

This change-over can be either time-cycled by the electronic timer, volume-cycled by the electrical contacts (27), or pressure-cycled by the pressure-sensitive contacts (57), the choice being controlled by the setting of the 'cycling selector' switch (12).

In the volume-cycled mode the change-over occurs when the concertina bags have been compressed through a preset stroke volume. In the closed circuit the tidal volume is equal to the stroke volume except for losses in the compliance of the breathing tubes and through any leaks. In the open circuit the same losses may occur but the tidal volume is increased by the volume of fresh gas which enters during the inspiratory phase. If the concertina bags fail to complete their preset stroke, perhaps because of a very large increase in airway resistance, then an overriding electronic time-cycling mechanism comes into play, reversing the solenoid valves (29, 48) to the expiratory position after about $5\frac{1}{2}$ sec, so that the ventilator cannot remain indefinitely in the inspiratory position.

In the pressure-cycled mode the action is significantly different from that in most other pressure-cycled ventilators. Because of the restriction (56) in the inlet to the pressure-sensitive switch (57), the pressure behind the diaphragm does not rapidly follow pressure changes at the inspiratory port (55) or at the mouth; it does so only with an appreciable time lag. In fact the compliance of the diaphragm, combined with the resistance of the restrictor, constitutes a miniature 'lung' which is 'inflated' in parallel with the patient. The time constant of this 'miniature lung' appears to be comparable with, or rather longer than, that of the 'standard lung' used in the recordings. The consequence of this is that the inspiratory phase does not end at the moment when the pressure at the mouth reaches some critical level but, instead, at the moment when the pressure in the pressure switch reaches a critical level which is related to the pressure at the mouth only in a very complex manner, depending upon lung characteristics and the characteristics of the mode of action of the ventilator during the inspiratory phase. Therefore, for a particular setting of the 'positive pressure' control (58), the pressure at the mouth at the moment when cycling occurs may vary from time to time with changes in the compliance and airway resistance of the patient. For instance, in one test, not illustrated here, when the compliance was halved the mouth and alveolar pressures rose much higher than before so that, although the tidal volume was reduced, the reduction was much less than would have occurred with the more usual type of pressure cycling.

If the pressure behind the diaphragm fails to reach the cycling pressure, perhaps because of a leak, the overriding time-cycling mechanism comes into play after about $5\frac{1}{2}$ sec just as in the volume-cycled mode.

The time-cycled mode was used for recording figs. 23.5 and 23.6 and it is clear that changes of lung characteristics had no effect on the inspiratory time. In fig. 23.5 the high generated pressure makes the ventilator operate effectively as a flow generator during the inspiratory phase so that the change-over is effectively also volume-cycled. The same cannot be said when the generated pressure is low, as in fig. 23.6, because, when this recording was made, the immediate effect of a change of lung characteristics was a change of flow and of tidal volume. However, by the time the sample recordings of fig. 23.6(b) and (c) were taken, the generated pressure had increased to a sufficient extent to restore the tidal volume.

In the volume-cycled mode, if the bags are working near the top of their stroke, the ventilator approximates to a flow generator in the inspiratory phase, and therefore the change-over is also effectively time-cycled.

Expiratory phase

During this phase the lungs are connected to the negative-pressure bag (5) which is being expanded for at least the majority of the expiratory phase by the refilling of the driving bag (7). This expansion acts as a near-constant-flow generator but several other factors influence the flow from the patient and the pressure at the mouth.

In the first part of the expiratory phase it commonly arises that the flow from the patient exceeds that generated by the expansion of the bag (5) and the excess spills to atmosphere past the one-way valve (22). In this period the ventilator operates as a constant-pressure generator, the generated pressure being slightly positive due to the opening pressure of the one-way valves (22, 23). However, the resistance of the expiratory pathway within the ventilator, in series with this pressure generator, is greater than the 'standard' airway resistance so that the initial flow is rather small and is slow to decay.

Once the flow from the patient has fallen to equal the flow generated by the expansion of the bag, there follows the second part of the expiratory phase in which the flow-generating action is unmodified. This part of the phase normally continues for only a short period while the pressure in the bag falls from the small positive value (about 1·5 cmH_2O) required to open the one-way valves (22, 23) to the small negative value (about $-0{\cdot}5$ cmH_2O) required to open the one-way valve (20).

Once the one-way valve (20) has opened, the third part of the expiratory phase commences in which the flow generator may have a leak in parallel with it. However, if the 'negative pressure control' is set to maximum, the leak is negligible, so that the ventilator continues to operate as a constant-flow generator until the end of the phase or until the negative-pressure limit set by the spring-loaded valve (21) comes into play. On the other hand, if the 'negative pressure control' is at any other setting there will be some appreciable leak through the one-way valve (20). A flow generator with a leak in parallel is equivalent to a pressure generator (negative in this case) with a resistance in series (see

p. 85), so that the flow gradually falls off as the pressure in the bag falls towards the equivalent generated pressure. The magnitude of the generated pressure depends on the size of the leak and the size of the generated flow. If the leak is large ('negative pressure control' set to minimum) and the generated flow is not large (driving- or inflating-gas flow small, so that the rate of expansion of the negative-pressure bag is small) the generated pressure is no more negative than the opening pressure of the one-way valve (20), about $-0{\cdot}5$ cmH_2O. If the leak is small however, and the generated flow is large, the system behaves like a generator of quite a large negative pressure but with a large series resistance.

The three parts of the phase are apparent in most of the accompanying recordings. In fig. 23.5 the first part, in which the ventilator generates a constant pressure of about $+1{\cdot}5$ cmH_2O, is demonstrated by the way in which the expiratory flow rises rapidly to a peak and then decays, both the magnitude of the peak and the rate of decay being altered when the lung characteristics are altered, particularly when the compliance is halved. The second part of the phase, in which the flow-generating action operates unmodified, is represented by a levelling out of the flow curve at about 12 litres/min before falling off again during the third part of the phase when the ventilator generates a pressure of about $-0{\cdot}5$ cmH_2O.

In fig. 23.6 the ventilator was set to 'closed circuit' with the bags working near the bottom of their stroke. Both these factors tend to increase the generated expiratory flow which in fact was about 22 litres/min. In addition, because some negative pressure was developed during the expiratory phase, the end-inspiratory alveolar pressure was less than in fig. 23.5. One consequence of this combination of conditions is that only when the compliance is halved (fig. 23.6b) does passive expiration produce an initial flow in excess of the generated flow: therefore only in fig. 23.6b does the first, positive-pressure-generating, part of the phase occur. Under the standard conditions (fig. 23.6a), and when the airway resistance has been doubled (fig. 23.6c), the phase starts with the constant-flow-generating part of the phase and this also occurs very briefly in fig. 23.6b after the initial period of high flow. In all three conditions the remainder of the phase is occupied by the third, constant (negative) pressure generating, part of the phase. The settings of the controls for fig. 23.6 are such that the magnitude of the generated pressure is about -5 cmH_2O with, of course, considerable series resistance. Therefore in (a) (b) and (c) in fig. 23.6, while this pressure is being generated, the flow declines as the alveolar pressure approaches the generated pressure. Only in fig. 23.6b, however, with the compliance halved, is the decline fast enough for the flow to have reached zero, and therefore for the alveolar pressure to have reached the generated pressure, by the end of the phase.

In fig. 23.7f the 'negative pressure control' has been set high and the ventilator approximates to a constant-flow generator for all the later part of the phase. It can be seen that the flow declines only slightly while the mouth and alveolar pressures run down to about -6 cmH_2O. This recording also makes clear that the generated flow is slow to build up to its full value on closed circuit. This is because, at the start of the expiratory phase, the contents of the driving bag (7) are at atmospheric pressure and have to be compressed before the plate (10) starts its upward movement so expanding the negative-pressure bag (5).

If the controls are set in such a way that the bags reach the top of their stroke before the end of the expiratory phase, so that excess driving gas or inflating gas escapes through the valve (8), then clearly the expiratory-flow-generating action is cut short. For the remainder of the phase, in these circumstances, the alveolar pressure cannot become any more negative but, if it is still positive, passive expiration can continue past the one-way valves (23, 22). This situation is not illustrated here.

Change-over from expiratory phase to inspiratory phase

In both the 'time-cycled' and the 'pressure-cycled' modes the change-over from expiration to inspiration is electronically time-cycled, although separate controls are provided for each mode for presetting the cycling time. In the 'volume-cycled' mode the change-over occurs when the bags have been raised through a preset stroke by the steady driving-gas or inflating-gas flow. This occurs in a preset time, uninfluenced by lung characteristics, and therefore the end of the expiratory phase is also time-cycled in the 'volume-cycled' mode. The only difference is that the cycling time cannot be directly set but is determined by the preset stroke and the driving-gas or inflating-gas flow.

In all three modes it is possible to introduce patient-triggering by setting the 'trigger' switch (13) to 'on' and the 'trigger pressure' control to a pressure slightly more negative than that being developed by the action of the negative-pressure bag (5). In these circumstances the change-over is either time-cycled or patient-cycled whichever event occurs first. However, if an appreciable negative pressure is being developed normally, a reduction in compliance, at least in the time-cycled mode, can result (as in fig. 23.6b) in the development of a bigger negative pressure which could operate the trigger mechanism a little before the time-cycling mechanism comes into play. The trigger mechanism could of course, if desired, be used deliberately to provide (negative) pressure cycling from expiration to inspiration.

CONTROLS

This ventilator can be operated with open or closed circuit and with either time, volume, or pressure cycling from the inspiratory phase to the expiratory phase. This provides six main modes of operation together with variations depending upon whether or not negative pressure is used, whether or not patient-triggering is used, and whether the bags work near the top or bottom of their stroke. Clearly, therefore, the following account must be highly selective. The time-cycled mode, combined with closed-circuit operation, has been chosen for the customary detailed treatment, while other modes are discussed much more briefly afterwards.

Time-cycled, closed-circuit mode

Total ventilation

This cannot be directly controlled but is equal to the product of tidal volume and respiratory frequency.

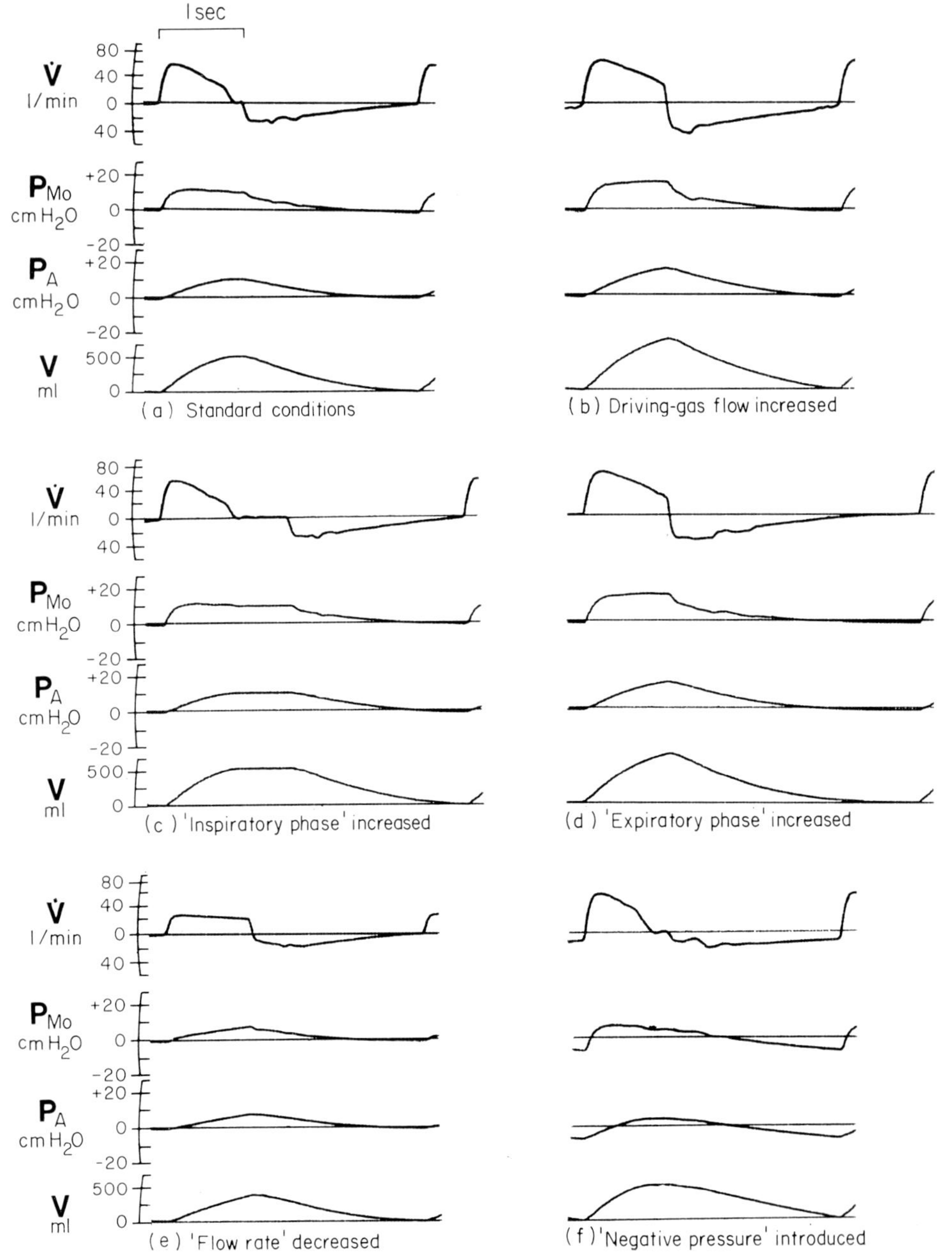

Tidal volume

This is equal, apart from losses in the compliance of the circuit and through any leaks, to the volume discharged from the closed-circuit concertina bag (9) during its downstroke, which, in the long run, must be equal to the volume drawn into it on the upstroke. This, in turn, is approximately proportional to the volume of driving gas supplied to the driving concertina bag (7) during the expiratory phase. Therefore the tidal volume is approximately proportional to the driving-gas flow and variation of this flow provides the primary means of controlling the tidal volume (fig. 23.7b). However, when the driving-gas flow is increased this may lead to the driving bag becoming full before the end of the expiratory phase so that some driving gas escapes through the valve (8). If this happens before the desired increase of tidal volume has been achieved it may be possible to increase the tidal volume further by increasing the setting of the 'flow rate control' (52). This decreases the resistance to inspiration so that the bags fall to a lower level by the end of the inspiratory phase leaving room for an increased upstroke in the expiratory phase. In fig. 23.7, however, the 'flow rate control' was already at maximum and the tidal volume indicated in fig. 23.7b (750 ml) was the maximum that could be obtained from the prototype ventilator tested by means of adjustment of the driving-gas flow and the 'flow rate control' but with otherwise 'standard' conditions. In the production model the use of a weight to supplement the compression of the concertina bags should give a larger maximum tidal volume in these circumstances.

As well as being approximately proportional to the driving-gas flow, the stroke of the bags is also approximately proportional to the expiratory time and hence variations in this time produce nearly-proportional changes in tidal volume (fig. 23.7d).

Although (in the prototype) driving bag (7) is of smaller cross-sectional area than the closed-circuit bag (9) the volume of driving gas added to the driving bag during expiration is comparable to or, when the bags are working near the top of their stroke, considerably greater than the (tidal) volume drawn into the closed-circuit bag. This is because the pressure in the driving bag rises from atmospheric throughout the expiratory phase whereas the pressure in the closed-circuit bag first falls from some positive pressure to atmospheric. Therefore the driving gas, which flows continuously, has to supply about a tidal volume of gas (or considerably more if the bags are near the top of their stroke) in only the expiratory part of the respiratory cycle. Consequently the driving-gas flow is

---

Fig. 23.7. Prototype 'Barnet' Mark III, in the time-cycled, 'closed circuit' mode. Recordings showing the effects of changes in the settings of the controls.

(a) Standard conditions as in fig. 23.6. except for 'negative pressure control' set to minimum.

(b) Driving-gas flow increased, from 17 to 27 litres/min, so that the concertina bags rose almost to the top of their range during the expiratory phase.

(c) 'Inspiratory phase' increased for an inspiratory time of 1·5 sec.

(d) 'Expiratory phase' increased for an expiratory time of 3 sec.

(e) 'Flow rate control' setting decreased $\frac{5}{8}$ turn.

(f) 'Negative pressure control' setting increased $\frac{1}{2}$ turn.

greater than the total ventilation to a substantial and variable degree and, in the closed-circuit mode, the ventilator cannot be thought of as a minute-volume divider.

Tidal volume is not much affected by changes of lung characteristics. If the bags are working near the bottom of their stroke then the generated pressure is low and a drop in compliance or rise in resistance does lead to an immediate fall in tidal volume—but only a temporary fall because, as explained in the functional analysis, concertina bag (9) gradually fills a little higher each respiratory cycle until the generated pressure has been increased far enough for the downstroke of the bag once more to equal the upstroke. If, on the other hand, the bags are working at the top of their stroke (not illustrated here for the closed circuit) they cannot rise any further to increase the generated pressure. However, the generated pressure and inspiratory resistance are then already high: in the prototype tested it can be seen from fig. 23.4 that a tidal volume of 500 ml could be delivered with a closed-circuit-bag pressure falling from 57 to 36 cmH_2O during the phase. Therefore the ventilator approximates to a time-cycled flow generator and moderate changes of lung characteristics have little effect on the tidal volume.

Respiratory frequency and inspiratory-expiratory ratio

These are both determined by the inspiratory and expiratory times both of which are entirely determined by the electronic timer and can be separately varied. They are not in any way influenced by lung characteristics.

If the bags are normally working with their tidal stroke about the middle of the available range, increasing the inspiratory time allows more gas to flow out of the closed-circuit bag in each respiratory cycle, so that the tidal stroke gradually drifts down until the generated pressure is reduced sufficiently to compensate for the increased time, and a new stable state is reached. Then the lower pressures in the driving bag will result in a somewhat bigger linear stroke of all the bags and hence a bigger tidal volume from the closed-circuit bag, delivered at a lower average inspiratory flow. Under the 'standard' conditions (fig. 23.7a) the bags were already 'bottoming': inspiratory flow was zero for the last 0·1 sec of the inspiratory phase. Therefore when the inspiratory time was increased (fig. 23.7c) this merely increased the period of held inflation of the lungs.

When the expiratory time is increased the upstroke of the bags is increased and this results in a nearly-proportional increase in tidal volume (fig. 23.7d) unless, as a result of the change, the bags reach the top of their stroke before the end of the phase and gas escapes at the valve (8).

Inspiratory waveforms

This ventilator offers a true choice of inspiratory waveforms by means of the 'flow rate control' (52). With this set to maximum, as in fig. 23.7a, the resistance to inspiration is a minimum and the ventilator operates as a decreasing-pressure generator. The inspiratory flow is initially large and declines rapidly as the alveolar pressure rises and the bag pressure declines. On the other hand, if the setting of the 'flow rate control' is decreased (fig. 23.7e) the resistance to inspiration is increased and the tidal stroke of the bags gradually drifts upwards; therefore, after a few cycles, the generated pressure is increased to the point at which the ventilator approximates to a flow generator. Admittedly the generated flow decreases during the phase but the decrease in flow is very much less (fig. 23.7e) than with the 'flow rate control' at maximum, and with the bags working at the bottom of their stroke (fig. 23.7a). In moving the tidal stroke of the bags upwards the refilling of the closed-circuit bag (which is brought about by the flow of driving gas to the driving bag) is made less efficient and the tidal volume falls, as in fig. 23.7e, unless this is corrected by increasing the driving-gas flow.

Expiratory waveforms

The expiratory waveforms vary somewhat with lung characteristics and with the settings of most of the controls but these settings are generally determined by other requirements. Therefore, for given values of all the other ventilatory parameters, including particularly the end-expiratory alveolar pressure, there is generally no choice of expiratory waveforms. Usually the expiratory flow declines throughout the phase (unless large negative pressures are being developed) but the initial, peak, flow is never large and the flow has often not fallen to zero by the end of the phase.

Pressure limits

Neither pressure limit can be rigidly controlled but, having set all the other controls, the end-expiratory pressure can be varied, by means of the 'negative pressure control', and this has only a small effect on other parameters: in fig. 23.7f increasing the 'negative pressure control' setting by 180° decreased the end-expiratory alveolar pressure from 0 to -6 cmH_2O. When the 'negative pressure control' is at minimum, changes of lung characteristics have little effect on the end-expiratory pressure (fig. 23.5) but, when an appreciable negative pressure is being developed (fig. 23.6), a decrease in the compliance makes the end-expiratory pressure more negative (fig. 23.6b).

The peak, end-inspiratory, alveolar pressure is not directly determined but exceeds the end-expiratory pressure by an amount equal to the tidal volume divided by the compliance.

Sequence of adjustment

On the basis of the foregoing the logical sequence of adjustment of the controls in the time-cycled closed-circuit mode would appear to be as follows.

1 Set 'inspiratory time' and 'expiratory time' to give the desired frequency and inspiratory-expiratory ratio.

2 Set the driving-gas flow, and the 'flow rate control', to give the desired tidal volume with the bags working over the desired portion of the available range of movement, depending on the inspiratory waveform required.

3 Set the 'negative pressure control' to give the desired end-expiratory pressure. This may need to be followed by some slight readjustment of driving-gas flow and of the 'flow rate control'.

Changes of lung characteristics may require some readjustment of the 'negative pressure control' but only a very large fall in compliance or rise in resistance will need to be compensated by adjustment of the 'flow rate control'.

Time-cycled, open-circuit mode

The main difference on changing from the closed-circuit to the open-circuit mode, while on time-cycling, is that the ventilator becomes a minute-volume divider: providing there is no escape of gas through the valve (8), the total ventilation is equal to the inflating-gas flow apart from losses due to circuit compliance and to any leaks. Therefore, having set the respiratory frequency, by means of the inspiratory and expiratory time controls, the tidal volume is also determined. Then it is necessary to adjust the 'flow rate control' so that the tidal stroke of the bags occupies the desired portion of the total available stroke. No blowing off can be allowed if the minute-volume-dividing action is to be maintained. Finally the pressure levels are set by the 'negative pressure control', although the amount of negative pressure which can be developed on open circuit is much less than on closed circuit, especially when the bags are working near the top of their stroke. This is because the flow of gas to the driving bag is much less than on closed circuit—nominally equal to the total ventilation instead of much larger—and so the flow generated by the negative bag is much less. In fig. 23.5, with the bags working near the top of their stroke on open circuit, the generated flow is only about 12 litres/min; whereas, in fig. 23.6, with the bags near the bottom of their stroke on closed circuit, but delivering the same tidal volume at the same frequency, the generated flow is about 22 litres/min. In the production model, when the ventilator is set to 'open circuit', the closed-circuit concertina bag (9) is switched in parallel with the negative-pressure bag (5) so that the expiratory generated flow should be much higher than in the prototype. The maximum amount of negative pressure available should also be greater.

Changes in lung characteristics may require some readjustments of the 'negative pressure control' but the much higher generated pressures in the open circuit (fig. 23.4) will maintain the tidal volume in the face of any likely change in compliance or resistance.

Volume-cycled mode

In this mode the tidal stroke of the bags and its position within the total available range is preset by means of the volume-cycling contacts (18, 27), while timing is determined indirectly by the settings of the other controls and by lung characteristics.

In the closed circuit the preset stroke fully determines the tidal volume (apart from circuit compliance and leakage losses). Expiratory time is controlled by means of the driving-gas flow which determines the speed of the upstroke. Inspiratory time is varied by means of the 'flow rate control' which is the main determinant of the speed of the down-stroke. The two controls together set the respiratory frequency and inspiratory-expiratory ratio.

In the open circuit the ventilator operates as a minute-volume divider with the total ventilation nominally equal to the inflating-gas flow. Then the setting of the volume-cycling contacts determines the expiratory time (the time it takes the preset inflating-gas flow to drive the plate (10) through its upstroke) while the 'flow rate control' sets the inspiratory time. In practice it may prove more convenient to think, first, of the volume-cycling contacts as the main determinant of the tidal volume, and hence, in combination with the preset total ventilation, of the respiratory frequency, and, second, of the 'flow rate control' as the main determinant of the inspiratory-expiratory ratio. However, since the tidal volume exceeds the stroke volume of the driving bag by the volume of inflating gas which enters during the inspiratory phase, the tidal volume (and hence the respiratory frequency) and the inspiratory-expiratory ratio are both influenced by both controls and more than one adjustment of each will generally be necessary if this approach is used.

In both the open circuit and the closed circuit, negative pressure is controlled by the 'negative pressure control', but its adjustment may require some change of the 'flow rate control' setting to restore the inspiratory time, if the bags are working near the bottom of their stroke. Changes of lung characteristics will influence the end-expiratory negative pressure a little and also, especially if the bags are working near the bottom of their stroke, the inspiratory time.

Pressure-cycled, closed-circuit mode

In this mode the expiratory time is fully controlled by an electronic circuit and can be adjusted by means of the 'expiratory phase pressure cycling' control (15). This then provides a rough determination of respiratory frequency.

In the closed circuit the tidal volume is primarily controlled by the 'positive pressure' control, which varies the pressure which has to be built up behind the diaphragm (57) in order to close the contacts. However, the driving-gas flow must be set high enough (considerably more than the desired total ventilation) to ensure that the closed-circuit bag is expanded to the extent of the desired tidal volume during the expiratory phase. If the driving-gas flow is set higher than necessary the working range of the bags will gradually rise to the top of the available stroke and excess driving gas will escape through the valve (8) at the end of each expiratory phase. If the driving-gas flow is set too low the bags will reach the bottom of their stroke before the cycling pressure has been reached behind the diaphragm. Since the pressure can then rise no further the inspiratory phase will continue until the overriding time-cycling mechanism comes into play at about $5\frac{1}{2}$ seconds. Providing this 'bottoming' of the bags does not occur, the inspiratory time, and hence the inspiratory-expiratory ratio, and the exact value of the respiratory frequency, can be controlled by means of the 'flow rate control'.

Since the time-constant of the pressure-cycling mechanism is of the same order as that of the lungs of a normal intubated patient, variations in inspiratory flow rate (due either to adjustment of the 'flow rate control', or to variation in the position of the working range of the bags and hence in the generated pressure) have remarkably little effect on the tidal volume—much less than with the more conventional type of pressure cycling which responds immediately to the pressure at the mouth. Changes of lung characteristics do affect the tidal volume but to a lesser extent than with the conventional type of pressure-cycling.

Pressure-cycled, open-circuit mode

In the open circuit the cycling pressure, as adjusted by the 'positive pressure' control, is still the main determinant of the tidal volume. However, since the ventilator operates as a minute-volume divider on open circuit, provided no loss occurs through the valve (8), it may be preferable first to set the inflating-gas flow to slightly above the desired total ventilation (to allow for losses in circuit compliance). Then, having set the expiratory time, the cycling pressure can be adjusted to produce a compatible tidal volume while the 'flow rate control' is set so that this is done in the desired inspiratory time.

CHAPTER 24

The Beaver Mark III Ventilator

DESCRIPTION

This ventilator (fig. 24.1) is designed for ward use. The basic mechanism consists of an electric motor which alternately compresses and expands a concertina reservoir bag. In the Mark III this mechanism (fig. 24.2) is essentially the same as that of earlier models,[1] but reliability has been improved by substituting an induction motor for the commutator type used previously, and by fitting an improved speed control.

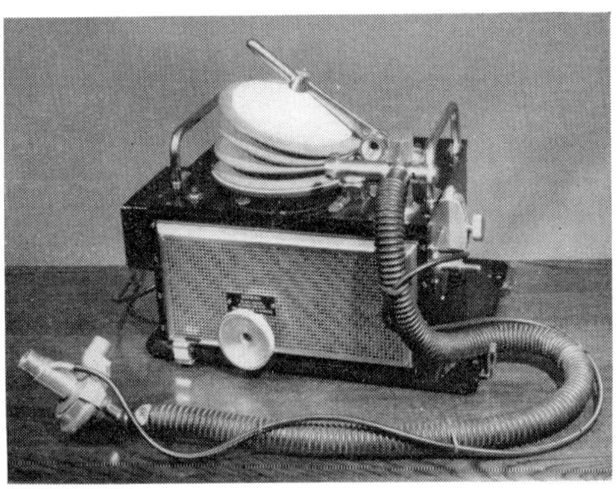

Fig. 24.1.

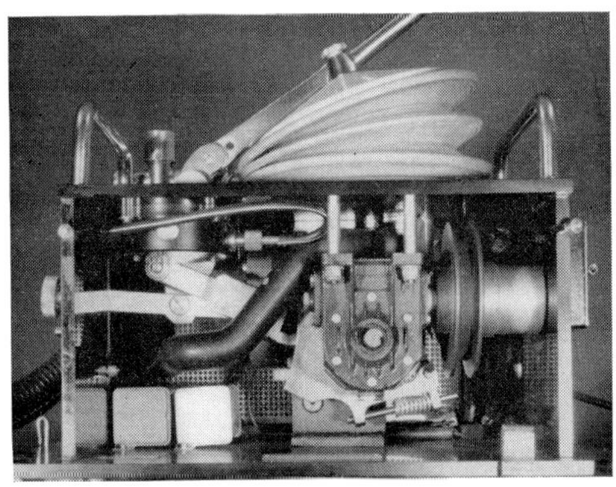

Fig. 24.2.

Fig. 24.1. The Beaver Mark III ventilator.
Courtesy of Department of Medical Illustration, Cardiff Royal Infirmary.

Fig. 24.2. The mechanism of the Beaver Mark III ventilator.
Courtesy of Department of Medical Illustration, Cardiff Royal Infirmary.

The a.c. mains electric motor (16) (fig. 24.3) is connected by a belt drive to an expanding pulley (18) mounted on the shaft of a gear-box (17). On the output shaft of this gear-box there is an eccentric (15), the rotation of which imparts a to-and-fro movement to the pitman (14). This motion is transmitted, through the connecting rod (13) and the lever (9), to the top-plate (11) of the concertina reservoir bag (10).

During the upward movement of the top-plate (11) the concertina reservoir bag is expanded and air is drawn in freely through the one-way valve (6) and the wire-gauze filter (5) until the pitman (14) reaches the limit of its movement and the expiratory phase ends. The inspiratory phase now begins and the bag (10) is compressed. Its contents are forced through the delivery tube (1) to a Beaver inflating valve (see p. 778) which is fitted

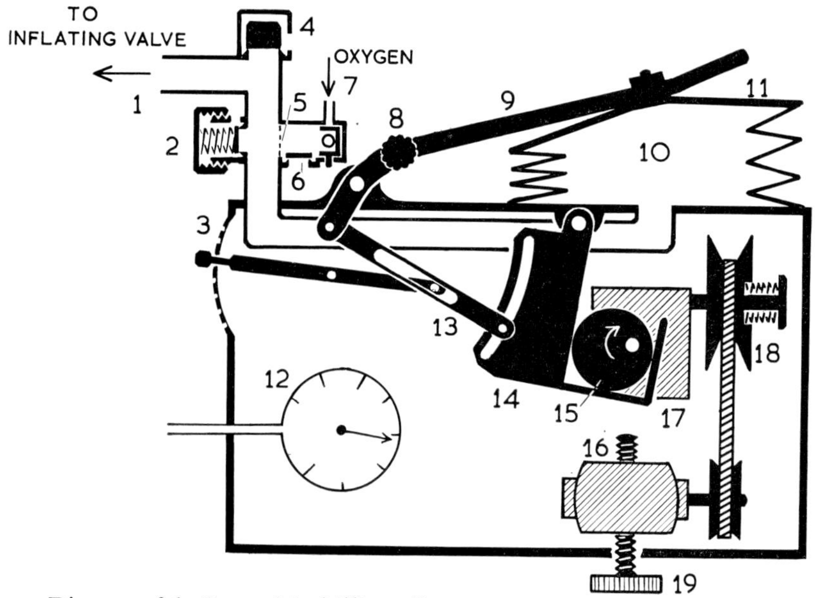

Fig. 24.3. Diagram of the Beaver Mark III ventilator.

1. Delivery tube
2. Adjustable blow-off valve
3. 'Tidal volume' control
4. Safety-valve
5. Wire-gauze filter
6. Air-inlet valve
7. Oxygen inlet
8. Removable link-pin
9. Pivoted lever
10. Concertina reservoir bag
11. Top-plate
12. Manometer
13. Connecting rod
14. Pitman
15. Eccentric
16. Induction motor
17. Gear-box
18. Expanding pulley
19. 'Respiration rate' control

near the patient. The inspiratory phase ends when the motion of the pitman is again reversed. Expired gas now flows freely to atmosphere through the inflating valve and the bag (10) is refilled.

The distance between the constant-speed electric motor (16) and the gear-box (17) can be varied by the 'respiration rate' control (19). The closer the motor is to the gear-box, the greater is the effective diameter of the expanding pulley (18) and the slower the movement of the pitman (14), and vice versa.

The excursion of the pitman is fixed, but the 'tidal volume' control (3) alters the point of contact between the quadrant of the pitman (14) and the connecting rod (13). The amplitude of the motion imparted to the lever (9) is therefore variable. The greater the distance of the point of contact from the pivot of the pitman, the greater is the movement of the connecting rod (13). The lever (9) is pivoted in such a way that it magnifies the motion of the connecting rod (13) which it is transferring to the top-plate (11). When the 'tidal volume' control is set so that the connecting rod (13) is in contact with the lowest part of the pitman, the excursion of the concertina reservoir bag (10) is at its maximum. The range of tidal volume is 200–1200 ml.

The maximum pressure is limited to 35 cmH_2O by the dead-weight safety-valve (4), but may be set at a lower level by adjustment of the blow-off valve (2). The pressure is shown on the manometer (12), which is directly connected to the patient outlet of the Beaver inflating valve.

Oxygen may be added at the inlet (7).

If the screw link-pin (8) is removed, the mechanical drive is disconnected and the top-plate (11) may be moved up and down by hand.

FUNCTIONAL ANALYSIS

Inspiratory phase

During this phase the Beaver operates fundamentally as a non-constant flow generator because the constant-speed induction motor drives the concertina reservoir bag through a preset pattern of movement at a preset speed. The waveform of flow (fig. 24.5a) bears a

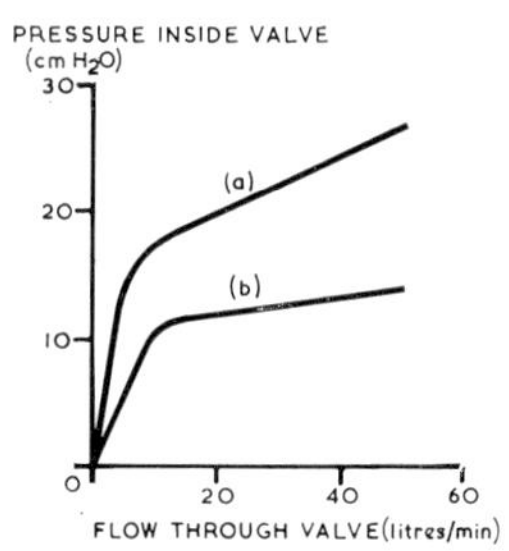

Fig. 24.4. Beaver Mark III. Pressure-flow characteristics of the valve assembly.
(a) With the blow-off valve closed and therefore only the safety-valve operative.
(b) With the blow-off valve opened $6\frac{1}{2}$ turns as for the recordings in fig. 24.6e.

resemblance to a half cycle of a sine wave but is rather more peaky. However, this fundamental action is modified a little by the action of the safety-valve (4) which, according to the static characteristics shown by curve (a) in fig. 24.4, must open to some extent in every inspiratory phase. Nevertheless, in the conditions used to obtain the recordings of fig. 24.5, changes in lung characteristics have less effect on the flow waveform than on the mouth-pressure waveform.

If the adjustable blow-off valve (2) is opened, a more-precise pressure limit is set on the fundamental flow-generating action. This is illustrated by curve (b) in fig. 24.4 for which the blow-off valve was unscrewed $6\frac{1}{2}$ turns. This same setting was used to record fig. 24.6e; there it can be seen that the flow is at first the same as it was with the blow-off valve closed (fig. 24.6a) but that, once the mouth pressure reaches the limit of about 10 cmH_2O set by the blow-off valve, no further rise of mouth pressure occurs and the flow is generally less than with the blow-off valve closed.

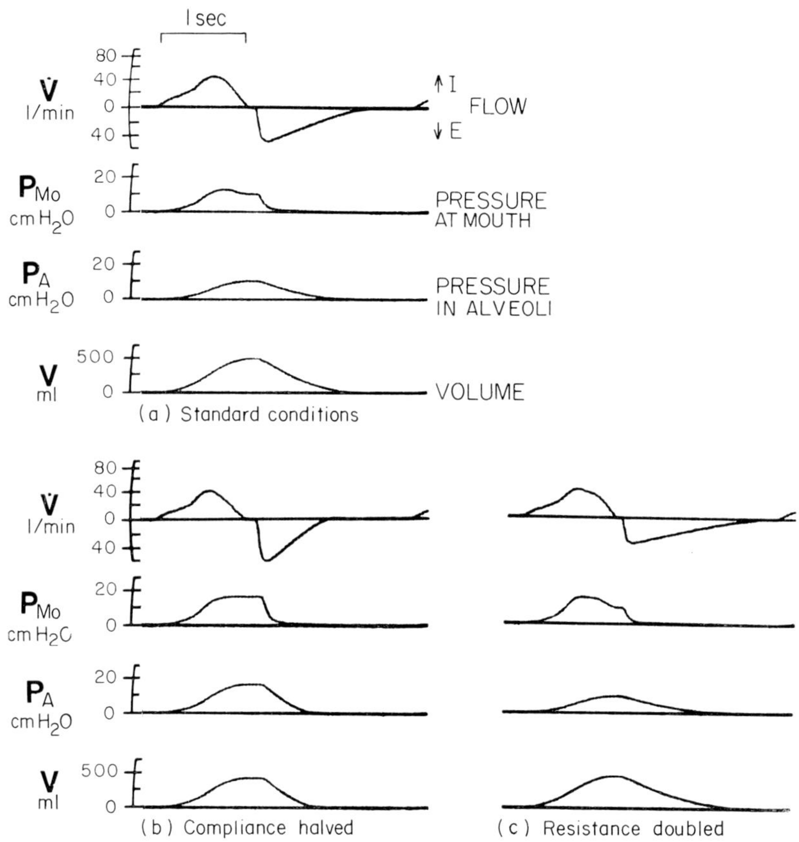

Fig. 24.5. Beaver Mark III. Recordings showing the effects of changes of lung characteristics. Standard conditions: blow-off valve, fully closed; fresh-gas flow, nil; 'respiration rate', set between 'C' and 'D' to produce a respiratory frequency of 20/min; 'tidal volume' control, set to '3' to produce a tidal volume of 500 ml. For these recordings, and those of fig. 24.6, air instead of oxygen was used to calibrate the pneumotachograph since the Beaver normally inflates the lungs with air. In order to be fully consistent air was also used as the 'fresh gas' in fig. 24.6 so that the pneumotachograph calibration should still be valid.

Any steady fresh-gas flow from a Rotameter supplied at the inlet (7) operates as a constant-flow generator in parallel with the main near-sine-wave-flow generator. The increased flow into the patient is just detectable in fig. 24.6d where a fresh-gas flow of 5 litres/min was introduced.

Change-over from inspiratory phase to expiratory phase

This change-over is both volume-cycled and time-cycled in the sense that the constant-speed motor drives a preset volume of gas out of the concertina bag in a preset time.

However, the tidal volume exceeds the stroke volume of the bag to the extent of any fresh gas which enters the system during the phase; at the same time it falls short of this combined volume to the extent of any loss through the safety-valve or blow-off valve. This loss increases with increasing mouth pressure and therefore the tidal volume is decreased by a decrease in compliance (fig. 24.5b) or an increase in resistance (fig. 24.5c) although the inspiratory time is unaltered.

Expiratory phase

In this phase the Beaver operates as a constant, atmospheric, pressure generator, atmospheric pressure being applied at the expiratory port of the Beaver valve. The resistance between this point and the mouth is small so that the pressure at the mouth rapidly falls almost completely to atmospheric at the beginning of the expiratory phase, whatever the lung characteristics (fig. 24.5). On the other hand, the flow waveform is considerably influenced by changes of lung characteristics.

Change-over from expiratory phase to inspiratory phase

This change-over is time-cycled. It occurs when the concertina bag has been re-expanded to a preset extent at a preset speed by the constant-speed motor. In fig. 24.5 it can be seen that, despite changes of lung characteristics, the expiratory phase always ends at a fixed time after it began, not immediately some critical pressure has been reached at the mouth, nor immediately some critical volume has come out of the lungs.

CONTROLS

Total ventilation

This is not directly controlled but is equal to the product of the separately-controllable tidal volume and respiratory frequency.

Tidal volume

This is directly controlled by the 'tidal volume' control (3) which alters the stroke volume of the concertina bag (fig. 24.6b). However, the tidal volume exceeds the stroke volume of the bag to the extent of the volume of fresh gas entering the system during the inspiratory phase and therefore the tidal volume is increased a little when the fresh-gas flow is increased (fig. 24.6d). Furthermore, the tidal volume falls short of the combination of stroke volume and fresh-gas volume to the extent of any loss through the safety-valve or blow-off valve. Therefore opening the blow-off valve decreases the tidal volume (fig. 24.6e). In addition, any change which raises the mouth pressure during the inspiratory phase increases the loss through the safety-valve and so decreases the tidal volume to some extent. This can arise from increasing the respiratory frequency, and so increasing the generated flow (fig. 24.6c), or as a result of a decrease of compliance (fig. 24.5b) or increase of resistance (fig. 24.5c), but in none of these instances is the effect large.

When the tidal volume is increased by means of the 'tidal volume' control (3) there is no change of respiratory frequency so the increase of total ventilation is proportional.

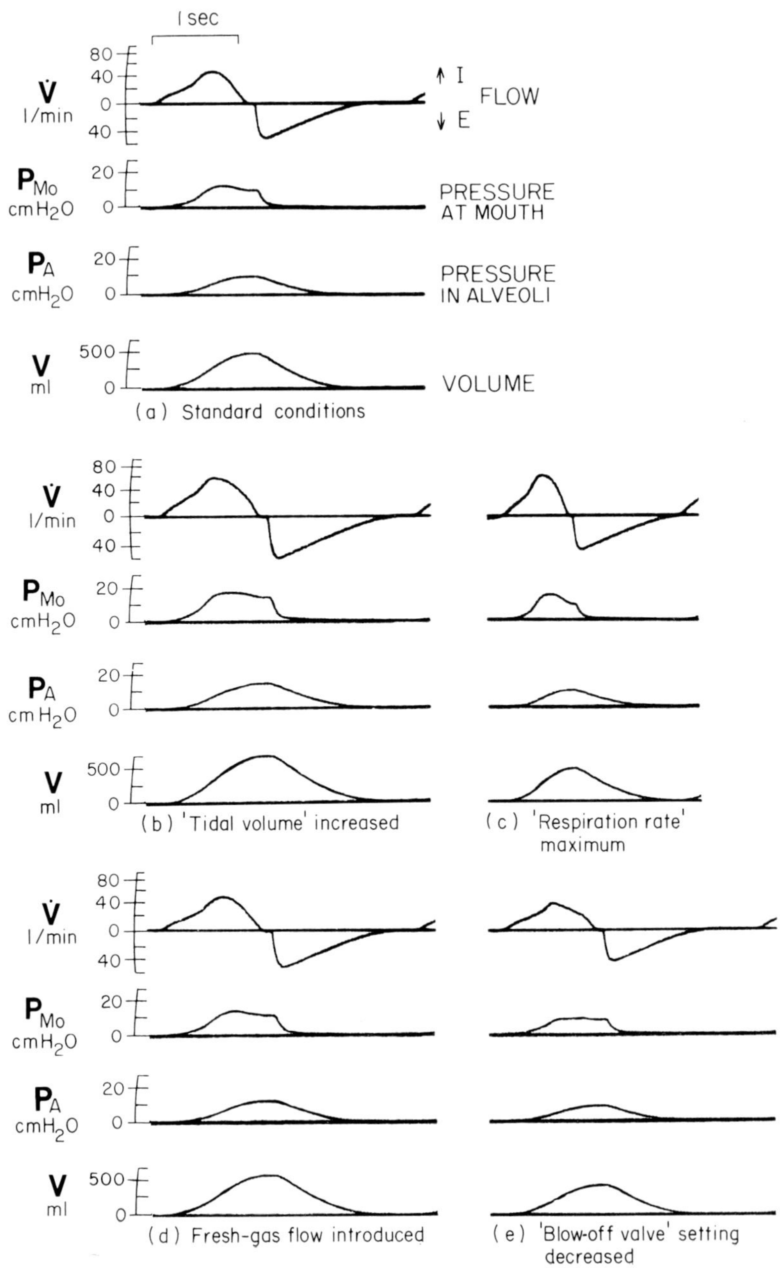

Respiratory frequency

This is directly controlled by the variable-gear 'respiration rate' control (19) and is quite unaffected by any other control or by changes of lung characteristics. When the respiratory frequency is increased by means of adjusting this control the inspiratory flow and hence the mouth pressure during inspiration is increased and so also is the loss through the safety-valve. Therefore the tidal volume is decreased and the increase in total ventilation is less than in proportion to the tidal volume.

Inspiratory-expiratory ratio

This is virtually fixed at about 1 : 1·5 and cannot be directly controlled. In fact a slight variation occurs because the Beaver valve does not change to the inspiratory position immediately the concertina bag starts its compression stroke, nor does the valve reverse immediately the compression stroke ends. These delays vary a little with different conditions and, as a result, some small but insignificant variations in the inspiratory-expiratory ratio can be found in fig. 24.6.

Inspiratory waveforms

This ventilator offers some slight but real choice of inspiratory waveforms. With the blow-off valve fully closed the ventilator makes a close approximation to a flow generator, the waveform being roughly sinusoidal with the peak flow about the middle of the phase (fig. 24.5a).

On the other hand, if the blow-off valve is opened by several turns, the pressure limit thereby set converts the action to that of a constant-pressure generator for the later part of the phase. If the 'tidal volume' control setting is increased to compensate for the increased loss, the tidal volume can be restored to its original level but the peak of the flow waveform will occur earlier in the phase, rather as in fig. 24.6e in which no compensation has been made for loss through the valve. In this second mode of operation however, the tidal volume, and therefore the total ventilation, will be much more dependent on lung characteristics.

Expiratory waveforms

Since the ventilator operates as a constant, atmospheric, pressure generator during the expiratory phase there is no choice of waveform. The pressure waveform is determined by

---

Fig. 24.6. Beaver Mark III. Recordings showing the effects of changes in the settings of the controls.

(a) Standard conditions as in fig. 24.5.
(b) 'Tidal volume' setting, increased from '3' to '6' to produce a tidal volume of 750 ml.
(c) 'Respiration rate', increased to maximum to produce a respiratory frequency of 29/min.
(d) Fresh-gas flow of 5 litres/min of air introduced at (7) (fig. 24.3).
(e) Blow-off valve, unscrewed 6½ turns from the fully-closed position.

the ventilator and the flow waveform results from the effect of this pressure waveform on the lungs.

Pressure limits

Since the Beaver operates as a constant, atmospheric, pressure generator during the expiratory phase, the alveolar pressure normally falls to this level by the end of the phase. It does so in all the recordings in figs. 24.5 and 24.6; it will fail to do so only when the airway resistance is very high or the expiratory time very short. The peak alveolar pressure, at the end of the inspiratory phase, is not directly controlled; it is determined by the fact that it must exceed the minimum, at the end of the expiratory phase, by an amount equal to the tidal volume divided by the compliance.

REFERENCE

1 BEAVER R.A. (1953) Pneumoflator for treatment of respiratory paralysis. *Lancet*, **1**, 977.

CHAPTER 25

The Beaver Electronic Ventilator[1]

DESCRIPTION

This ventilator (figs. 25.1 and 25.2) is designed for ward use. It consists essentially of a solenoid-valve (fig. 25.3) operated by an electronic timing circuit. When the solenoid (3) is energized by the timing circuit, the inspiratory valve (1) is opened and the expiratory valve (2) is closed. Compressed air is now delivered to the patient. After a time set by the timing circuit, the electrical supply to the solenoid (3) is cut off. The inspiratory valve (1) closes and the expiratory valve (2) opens. Expired gas escapes freely to atmosphere. The expiratory phase lasts until the timing circuit again energizes the solenoid.

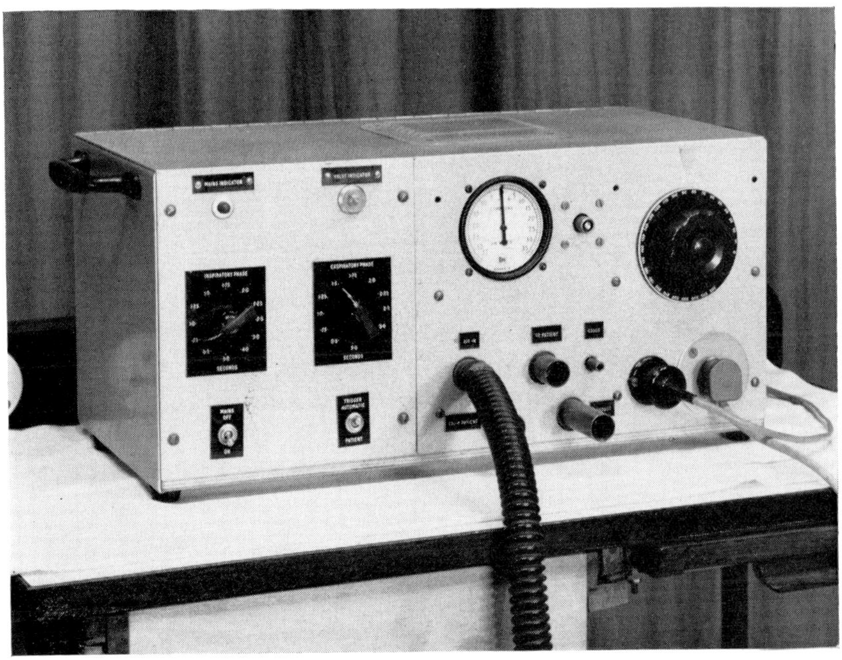

Fig. 25.1. The original Beaver electronic ventilator.

Courtesy of Dr A.Beaver.

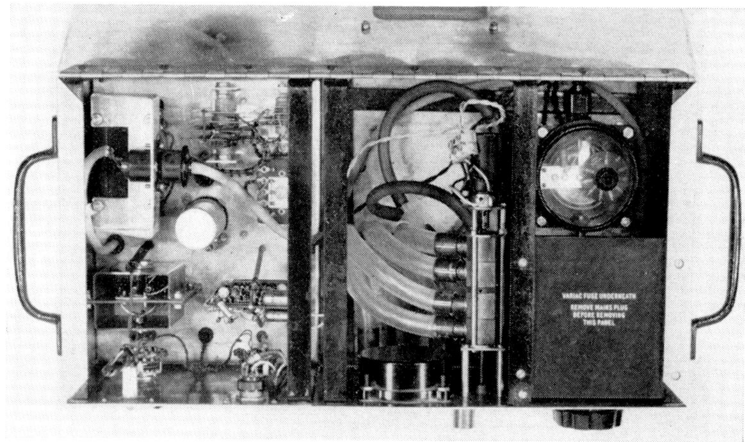

Fig. 25.2. The mechanism of the original Beaver electronic ventilator.

Courtesy of Dr A. Beaver.

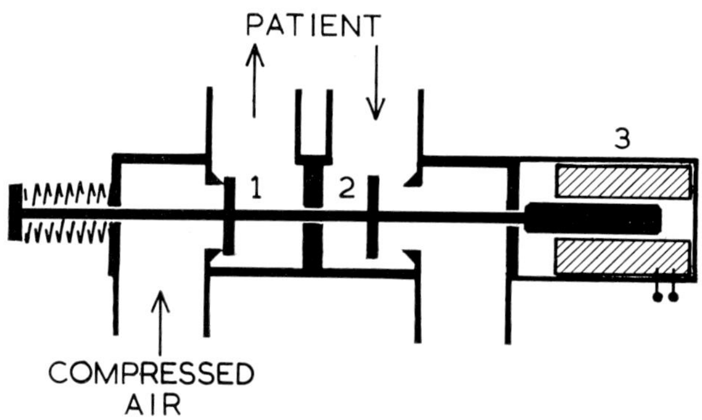

Fig. 25.3. Diagram of the solenoid-operated valve of the Beaver electronic ventilator.
1. Inspiratory valve 2. Expiratory valve 3. Solenoid

In this ventilator the source of compressed air is a vacuum cleaner, connected to the a.c. mains through a variable transformer. Adjustment of this transformer varies the voltage supplied to the cleaner and thereby controls the flow of compressed air delivered from the cleaner.

The electronic circuit is designed to give inspiratory and expiratory times which can each be adjusted between 0·5 and 5·0 seconds. A pressure-operated switch can be brought into circuit to provide for patient-triggering. Then the expiratory phase is cut short if the patient makes an inspiratory effort which closes a one-way valve in the expiratory pathway and produces a negative pressure of at least 0·5 cmH_2O before the preset expiratory time has elapsed. In the original model (fig. 25.1) the solenoid valve (3) was incorporated in the main body of the ventilator, but a modified version[2] has the valve connected in the breathing circuit near the patient.

FUNCTIONAL ANALYSIS

Inspiratory phase

In this phase the patient is connected to a vacuum cleaner the characteristics of which are likely to be such that the ventilator operates as a constant-pressure generator. The generated pressure can be made low by reducing the voltage supplied to the vacuum-cleaner motor.

Change-over from inspiratory phase to expiratory phase

This change-over is time-cycled: it occurs when the solenoid (3) is de-energized in a preset time determined by the electronic timer.

Expiratory phase

In this phase the ventilator operates as a constant, atmospheric, pressure generator: the patient's expired gas passes freely to atmosphere through the valve (2).

Change-over from expiratory phase to inspiratory phase

This change-over is time-cycled or patient-cycled whichever occurs first: it occurs when the solenoid (3) is energized, either in a preset time due to the operation of the electronic timer, or when the patient makes an inspiratory effort thereby operating the pressure-sensitive switch.

REFERENCES

1 ATHERLEY D.W. and BEAVER R.A. (1963) An improved ventilator. *Lancet*, **2**, 1257.
2 CUNDY J.M. (1965) An easily sterilised distal solenoid respiratory valve. *Lancet*, **1**, 1256.

CHAPTER 26

The Bennett Model AP–4 'Pressure Breathing Therapy Unit'

DESCRIPTION

This portable ventilator (fig. 26.1) is designed for ward or domestic use. There are several versions available which differ in their external design and in their working voltage.

A small a.c. mains electric motor (11) (fig. 26.2) drives a high-pressure blower (9) which draws in room air through a filter (10) and delivers it, through another filter (8), to

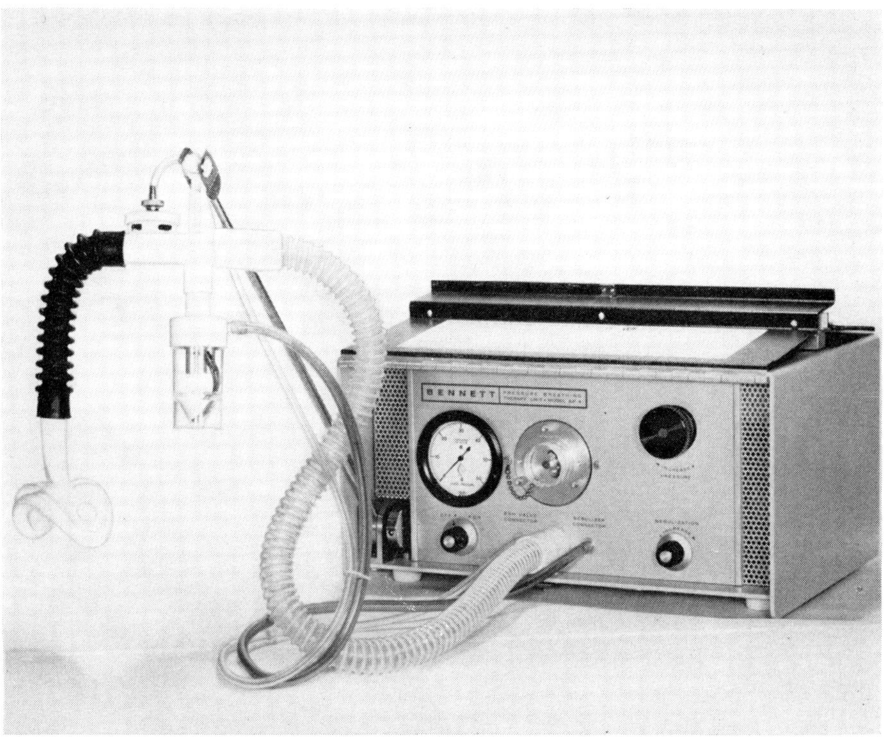

Fig. 26.1. The Bennett Model AP–4 'Pressure Breathing Therapy Unit'.
Courtesy of Bennett Respiration Products Inc. and Puritan Compressed Gas Corporation.

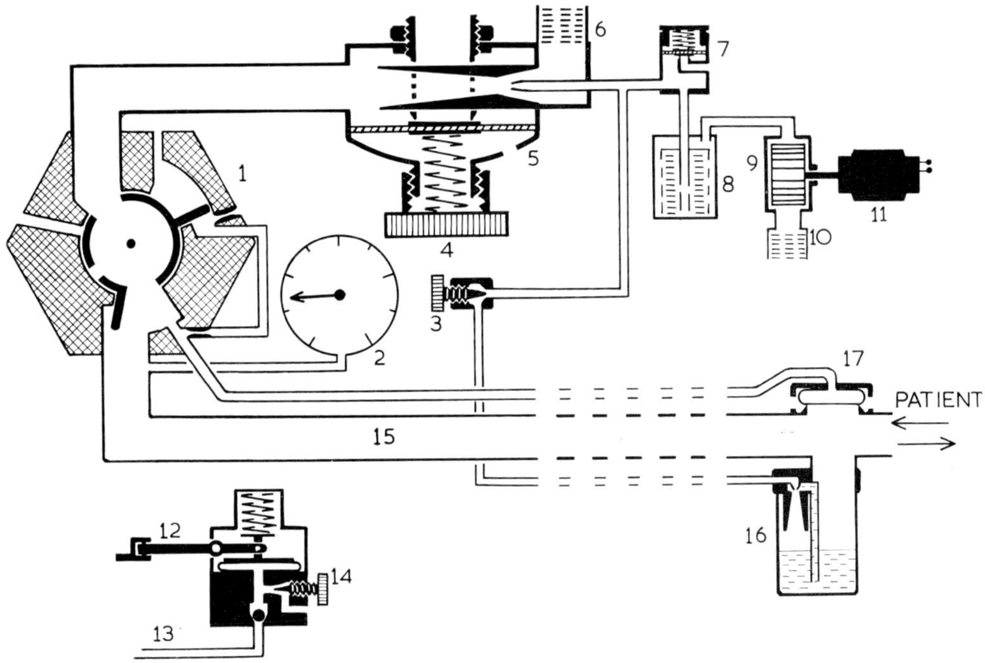

Fig. 26.2. Diagram of the Bennett Model AP-4 'Pressure Breathing Therapy Unit'.

1. Bennett valve
2. Manometer
3. 'Nebulization' control
4. 'Pressure' control
5. Pressure-limiting valve
6. Filter
7. Safety-valve
8. Filter
9. High-pressure blower
10. Filter
11. Electric motor
12. Lever
13. Connecting tube
14. Expiratory-time control
15. Breathing tube
16. Nebulizer
17. Expiratory valve

the adjustable pressure-limiting valve (5) and the nebulizer control (3). The air delivered by the blower drives an injector incorporated in the pressure-limiting valve (5) which entrains, through the filter (6), four times the driving flow of air. At normal inflating pressures the maximum unrestricted flow delivered to the patient is about 90 litres/min.

When the patient makes an inspiratory effort the negative pressure produced in the breathing tube (15) opens the 'Bennett' valve (1). The pressure in the lower chamber of the Bennett valve inflates the capsule (17) of the expiratory valve, and air from the pressure-limiting valve (5) flows, through the Bennett valve (1) and the breathing tube (15), to the patient. As the pressure in the breathing tube (15) increases towards the pressure set by the pressure-limiting valve (5) the flow through the Bennett valve (1) decreases until, when the flow has fallen to 4 litres/min, the Bennett valve closes and the inspiratory phase ends.

When the Bennett valve closes, the capsule (17) of the expiratory valve immediately collapses since it is connected to atmosphere through the centre of the Bennett valve.

Expired gas now flows freely through the expiratory valve to atmosphere. The expiratory phase continues until the patient makes another inspiratory effort.

The pressure in the breathing circuit at which the ventilator cycles from the inspiratory phase to the expiratory phase is set by adjusting the 'pressure' control (4). The pressure in the breathing tube is shown on the manometer (2). The 'nebulization' control (3) can be set to deliver a continuous flow of air from the blower to the nebulizer (16).

This ventilator is designed principally for patient-triggered use. In an emergency it is possible to cycle the ventilator by removing the dust-cover of the Bennett valve and operating the valve manually.

Fully-automatic cycling may be obtained by removing the dust-cover of the Bennett valve and fitting a special 'Automatic Cycling Attachment' (12, 13, 14). The connecting tube (13) ends in a needle which is inserted into the breathing tube (15). The arm (12) opens the Bennett valve after a time set by the control (14).

FUNCTIONAL ANALYSIS

Inspiratory phase

At the start of this phase the mode of operation depends upon the characteristics of the injector; probably these make the ventilator a fairly-high-constant-pressure generator with high series resistance so that it approximates to a constant-flow generator. Well before the end of the phase, however, the pressure limit, set by the control (4) on the pressure-limiting valve (5), comes into play and thereafter the ventilator becomes a low-constant-pressure generator.

Change-over from inspiratory phase to expiratory phase

This change-over is flow-cycled: it occurs when the flow through the Bennett valve (1) has fallen to 4 litres/min. At this predetermined flow there is a given pressure drop, from the generated pressure in the pressure-limiting valve (5) to the mouth. Therefore the mouth pressure at the change-over is unaffected by changes of lung characteristics and the ventilator is also effectively pressure-cycled (see p. 108).

Expiratory phase

In this phase the ventilator operates as a constant, atmospheric, pressure generator: atmospheric pressure is 'generated' at the expiratory valve (17).

Change-over from expiratory phase to inspiratory phase

This change-over is normally only patient-cycled. If the 'Automatic Cycling Attachment' (12, 13, 14) is in use, the change-over may be time-cycled, by the decay of pressure in the capsule through the needle valve (14), or patient-cycled, whichever comes first.

CHAPTER 27

The Bennett Model BA–4 'Anesthesia Ventilator'

DESCRIPTION

This ventilator (fig. 27.1) is designed primarily for closed-circuit anaesthetic use. It is driven by compressed gas, supplied at a pressure of 40–60 lb/in^2, which entrains air through the injector (39) (fig. 27.2) for economy. It operates as a fully-automatic or as a patient-triggered ventilator with automatic override with or without a negative-pressure phase. A Bennett valve (36) allows the driving gas to flow intermittently into the rigid plastic pressure chamber (47) compressing the concertina reservoir bag (48).

Before the driving gas is turned on, the capsules (1, 4, 21, 23, 25, 27, 41, 44, and 49) of the valves are collapsed, and the valves are in their resting positions. The Bennett valve is in the closed (clockwise) position (see Inset fig. 27.2). Driving gas supplied to the inlet (42) flows, through a sintered-bronze filter, to the inflating-pressure-control mechanism (40) and the pressure regulator (9) of the control circuit. From the pressure regulator (9) it flows, through the channel (5, 5) of the pneumatic valve (4) and the 'sensitivity' control (12), to the chamber (35) of the Bennett valve. However, the flow from the 'sensitivity' control (12) is so restricted, that, as there is a leak to atmosphere from the chamber (35), the pressure in this chamber can never rise sufficiently to move the Bennett valve. Meanwhile, when the ventilator is set for automatic cycling, driving gas also flows from the pressure regulator (9), through the 'rate' control (11), to the bottom of the pneumatic valve (1), where, as the channel (7, 7) of the pneumatic valve (4) is closed, pressure begins to rise. This rise in pressure continues, at a rate determined by the setting of the control (11), until it is sufficient to force the valve (1) into its 'down' position, thereby opening the channel (2, 2) in parallel with the 'sensitivity' control (12). This allows an additional flow of driving gas, through the channel (2, 2), past the capsule (10), to the chamber (35) of the Bennett valve. The flow is determined by a constriction in the line leading to the channel (2, 2). As this flow continues, pressure rises within the capsule (10) and the chamber (35) of the Bennett valve, until, after a delay dependent on the capacity of the capsule (10), it is sufficient to rotate the drum to its open (anti-clockwise) position (shown in the main diagram, fig. 27.2).

The flow of driving gas and entrained air from the 'pressure' control (40) through the Bennett valve now distends the capsule (44), closing the relief port of the rigid plastic

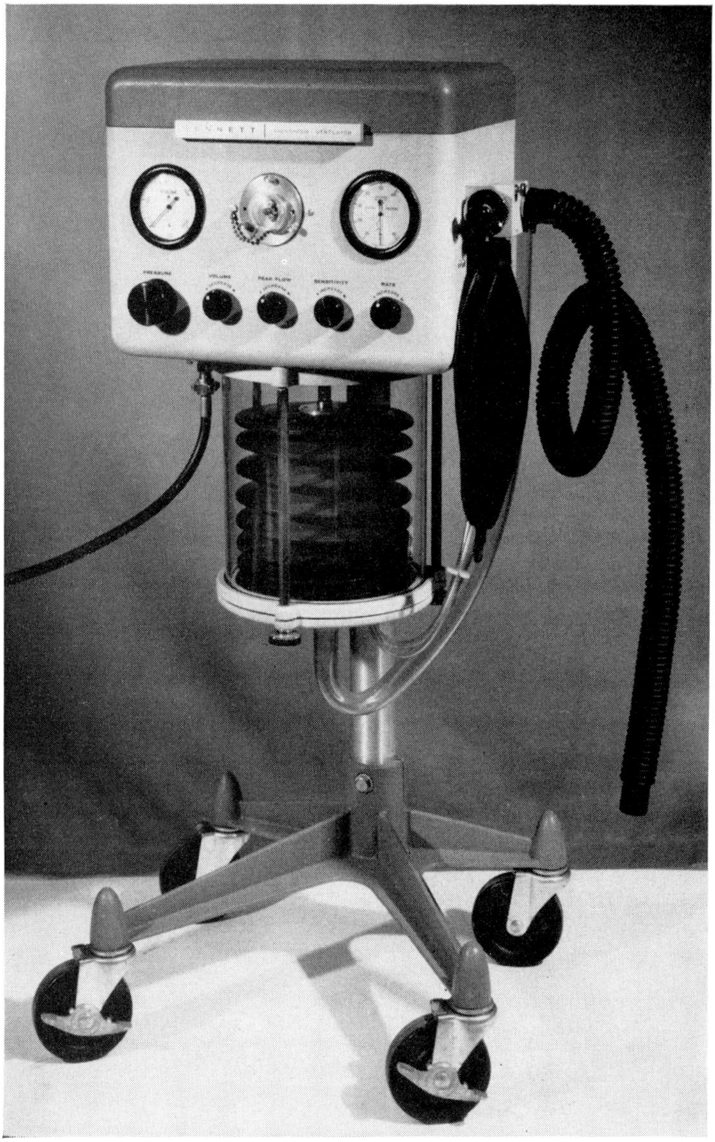

Fig. 27.1. The Bennett Model BA–4 'Anesthesia Ventilator'.
Courtesy of Department of Medical Illustration, Cardiff Royal Infirmary.

pressure chamber (47), and the capsule (49) of the spill valve. The concertina reservoir bag (48) is compressed and the gas within it is forced to the patient. The flow of driving gas through the Bennett valve produces a pressure difference across its lower vane which holds the valve open. As the contents of the concertina reservoir bag (48) are discharged the left-hand end of the beam (14), to which it is connected by the string (28), is pulled down and the piston in the cylinder (29) is forced down by the rack-and-pinion mechanism (15). Since the Bennett valve is open, the capsule (21), which is connected to its outlet, is distended, and the orifice (20) is thereby closed. This prevents any leak of air from the cylinder (29) and the pressure within it rises. This rise is proportional to the movement of the concertina bag and the pressure gauge (43) interprets this movement as a volume reading.

In addition, as soon as the Bennett valve opens, the supply of gas from the central chamber (36) to the bottom of the pneumatic valve (4), and through this to the capsule (23), rapidly forces the valve (4) into its 'down' position and closes the orifice (22). As soon as the valve (4) is in the 'down' position a number of conditions change. Firstly, free connexion is established between the bottom of the valve (1) and atmosphere, through the channel (7, 7), and then through both the channel (3, 3) and the orifice (26). Therefore the pressure in the capsule (1) falls rapidly to atmospheric, and the valve (1) is returned to its 'up' position by its spring. Secondly, the flow of driving gas through the channel (5, 5) to the 'sensitivity' control (12) is cut off. Thirdly, there is a flow from the pressure regulator (9), through the channel (6, 6), partly past the constriction (19) and the ball valve (33) to atmosphere, and partly to the capsule (25) which is inflated, occluding the orifice (24). This allows the capsule (27) to be inflated gradually by gas flowing through the constriction (8) until it occludes the orifice (26). Once this has occurred the escape of gas from the bottom of the valve (1), through the channel (7, 7), is prevented and, since the channel (3, 3) has already been closed by the rise of the valve stem (1), the pressure in (1) begins to rise again via the 'rate' control (11) and a new timing cycle is begun. The situation is now that illustrated in fig. 27.2. The timing cycle determines the duration of a complete respiratory cycle. The end of the timing cycle therefore corresponds to the end of the expiratory phase. During the cycle the change-over from the inspiratory phase to the expiratory phase occurs in one of two ways.

(*A*) *When the ventilator is 'volume-cycled'*. The pinion (15) is connected by the lever (16) to the eccentric (17) which is moved anti-clockwise as inflation proceeds. This movement draws up the stop (31) against the pull of its spring. The 'volume' control (30) is regulated so that when the required volume, as indicated on the gauge (43), has been delivered the stop (31) pivots the weighted arm (32) and thus allows the ball valve (33) to close. Driving gas flowing from the channel (6, 6) of the valve (4), past the constriction (19), can no longer escape to atmosphere through the valve (33), and, since the orifice (22) is closed, the capsule (41) is now distended. The flow of driving gas from the 'pressure' control (40) to the Bennett valve is therefore arrested.

Because the return of the valve (1) to its 'up' position blocked the channel (2, 2), and the channel (5, 5) is blocked as the valve (4) is 'down', there is no flow of gas to the chamber (35) of the Bennett valve, and the pressure within the chamber (35) is atmospheric. However, leakage of driving gas from the central chamber (36) of the Bennett valve into the chamber (34) causes a rise in pressure there, limited by the size of the orifice connecting this chamber (34) to atmosphere. So long as flow continues through the

Bennett valve the pressure difference across the lower vane caused by the flow is sufficient to hold the valve open in spite of this pressure rise in the chamber (34). But as soon as flow ceases and there is no pressure difference across the lower vane, the pressure in the chamber (34) moves the valve clockwise to the closed position.

(*B*) *When the ventilator is 'pressure-cycled'*. The cessation of flow through the Bennett valve, which initiates cycling, occurs when the pressure in the chamber (47) reaches that set by the 'pressure' control (40).

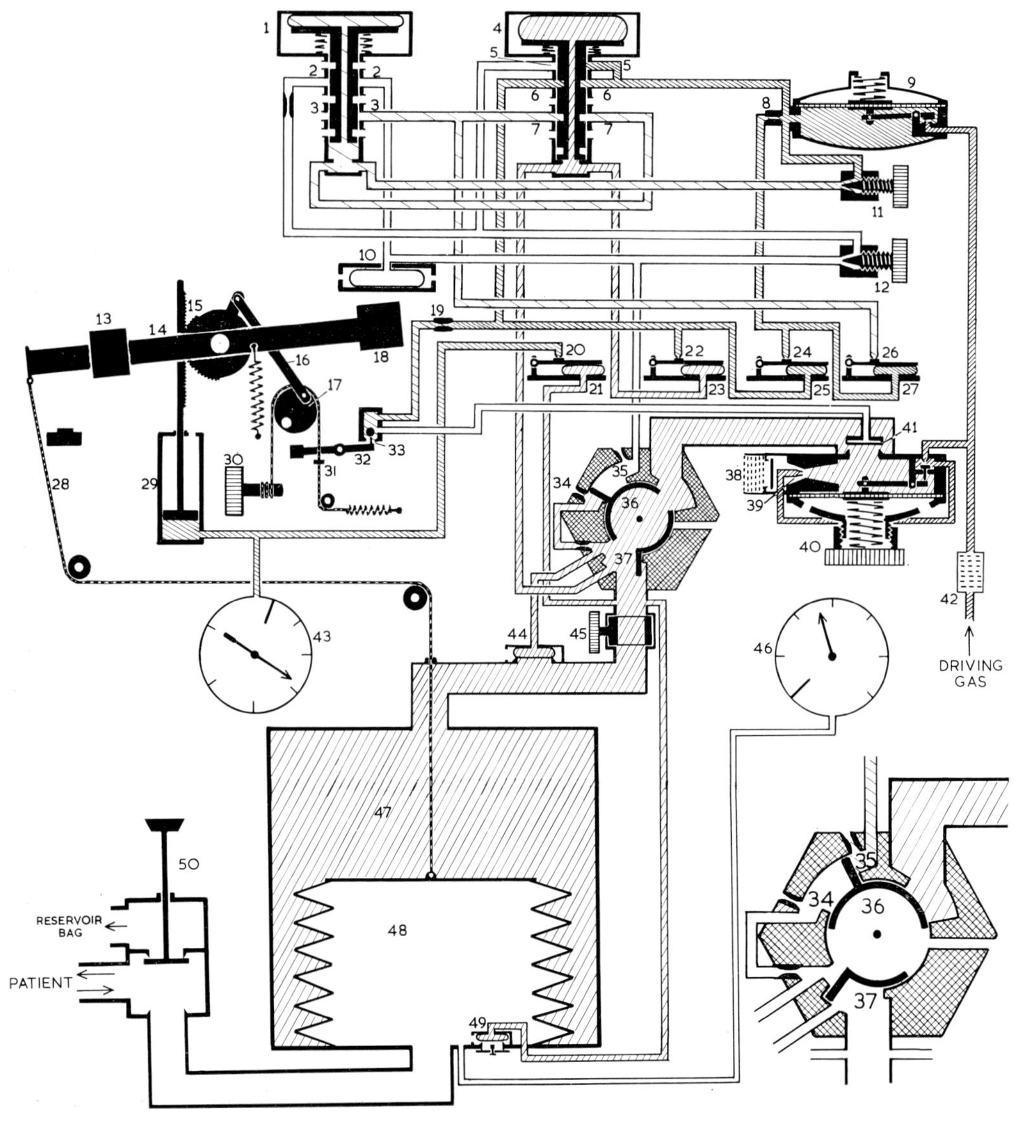

Whichever method of cycling is used the closure of the Bennett valve establishes a free pathway through it between the capsule (44) and atmosphere, and the capsule collapses. The pressure in the chamber (47) immediately falls to atmospheric and expiratory flow from the patient into the concertina reservoir bag (48) commences. The fall in pressure in the chamber (47) allows the capsules (21) and (49) to collapse. The collapse of the capsule (21) opens the orifice (20), and thereby releases the pressure in the volumetric system (29, 43). The collapse of the capsule (49) frees the spill valve of the concertina bag so that, once the bag has re-expanded, excess respiratory gas can escape to atmosphere. As the concertina bag expands, the end of the beam (14) which carries the fixed weight (18) moves down, and the movement of the eccentric (17) is reversed. The stop (31), which, if the ventilator was volume-cycled, was holding up the lever (32), moves downward; the weighted lever (32) pivots, and the valve (33) opens. This allows the capsule (41) to collapse ready for the next inflation.

As the pressure in the chamber (47) falls the pressure in the base of the valve (4) and the capsule (23) also falls, the Bennett valve being in its closed position. The valve (4) returns to its 'up' position, and the supply through the channel (6, 6) to the capsule (25) is shut off. As the orifice (22) is now open, the capsule (25) collapses quickly, thereby opening the orifice (24) which in turn allows the capsule (27) to collapse—but nothing comes out of the orifice (26) as the valve (4) is now 'up' and the valve (1) is only part-way 'down'. The ventilator is now back in its resting position, except that the valve (1) is part-way through its timing cycle.

If negative pressure is desired the weight (13) is slid towards the pivot of the beam (14) thereby increasing the effect of the weight (18). This only exerts its effect until such time as the concertina bag (48) is fully expanded. If it is desired to maintain negative pressure

---

Fig. 27.2. Diagram of the Bennett Model BA-4 'Anesthesia Ventilator'.

1. Pneumatic valve
2, 2. Channel
3, 3. Channel
4. Pneumatic valve
5, 5. Channel
6, 6. Channel
7, 7. Channel
8. Constriction
9. Pressure regulator
10. Capsule
11. 'Rate' control
12. 'Sensitivity' control
13. Sliding weight
14. Beam
15. Rack and pinion
16. Lever
17. Eccentric
18. Fixed weight
19. Constriction
20. Orifice
21. Capsule
22. Orifice
23. Capsule
24. Orifice
25. Capsule
26. Orifice
27. Capsule
28. String
29. Cylinder
30. 'Volume' control
31. Stop
32. Weighted arm
33. Ball valve
34. Chamber
35. Chamber
36. Bennett valve
37. Chamber
38. Sintered-bronze filter
39. Injector
40. 'Pressure' control
41. Capsule
42. Driving-gas inlet
43. 'Volume' gauge
44. Capsule
45. 'Peak flow' control
46. 'System pressure' manometer
47. Rigid plastic pressure chamber
48. Concertina reservoir bag
49. Capsule
50. 'Ventilator/bag' tap

throughout the expiratory phase, excess anaesthetic gas must be spilled during the inspiratory phase through a blow-off valve in the anaesthetic circuit and only the pressure-cycling mode of operation may be used. The reservoir bag (48) then empties completely during each inspiratory phase and cycling to expiration follows almost immediately afterwards. However, the bag does not reach its upper limit during the expiratory phase.

Patient-triggering

During the expiratory phase the Bennett valve is in the closed (clockwise) position (see Inset fig. 27.2). When the valve (4) is 'up' there is a supply of gas from the pressure regulator (9), through the channel (5, 5), to the 'sensitivity' control (12), the setting of which, in conjunction with the fixed orifice of the chamber (35), determines the pressure maintained in the chamber (35) which is tending to open the Bennett valve. If the patient makes an inspiratory effort the negative pressure produced is transmitted to chamber (37) of the Bennett valve. The pressure above the lower vane is atmospheric, and when the sum of the pressure differences across the two vanes is sufficient, the valve is rotated to the open position and inflation commences. The negative inspiratory pressure required to do this therefore depends on the pressure reached in the chamber (35), which is determined by the setting of the 'sensitivity' control (12). If the patient fails to make an inspiratory effort or if patient-triggering is not being used, then the ventilator will cycle from the expiratory phase to the inspiratory phase at a preset time after the start of the previous inspiratory phase.

A new respiratory cycle starts when the downward movement of the valve (1) is complete, and almost instantaneously the valve (1) moves up again. After a short fixed delay, due mainly to the time taken to inflate the capsule (27) through the constriction (8), the valve (1) is forced down again in a time directly dependent on the setting of the 'rate' control (11). In effect, therefore, this control determines the duration of a complete respiratory cycle.

The duration of the inspiratory phase is the time taken for the ventilator either (a) to deliver the volume set by the control (30) which alters the position of the stop (31), or (b) to reach the inflating pressure set on the 'pressure' control (40). In either case, the expiratory phase occupies the remainder of the complete respiratory cycle.

If, for any reason, the inspiratory phase takes a longer time than that allowed by the setting of the 'rate' control (11) for a complete respiratory cycle, then the Bennett valve remains open, and the valve (4) remains in its 'down' position. In this circumstance the valve (1) will have moved down before the inspiratory phase is completed. However, before this downward movement is completed the exhaust channel (3, 3) starts to open. The valve (1) is now pressure-balanced and remains in this position without cycling taking place until the Bennett valve eventually closes and the valve (4) moves up. Only then can gas from the pressure regulator (9) flow through the channels (5, 5) and (2, 2) in order gradually to build up pressure in the capsule (10) and the chamber (35), thereby turning on the Bennett valve again. A certain minimum expiratory time is thus assured.

The 'peak flow' limiting control (45) allows the resistance of the inspiratory pathway to be increased if it is desired to limit the inspiratory flow. The 'system pressure' manometer (46) indicates the pressure in the concertina bag. The tap (50) allows manual ventilation. A removable filter (38) is fitted to the air-entrainment port of the injector (39).

The manufacturers recommend that in clinical practice the controls should be set in the following sequence:— set the rate, then adjust the tidal volume, and finally set the pressure and the flow so that the inspiratory phase occupies a suitable part of the total cycle.

FUNCTIONAL ANALYSIS

Inspiratory phase

The second-stage reducing valve of the pressure-control mechanism (40) delivers a preset pressure throughout the inspiratory phase irrespective of the flow drawn from it. This pressure is not applied directly to the patient but to the outside of the concertina reservoir bag (48). The pressure drop across the wall of this bag depends on the setting of the sliding weight (13) on the beam (14) but, for any given setting, the pressure drop is constant throughout the compression of the bag. Fundamentally, therefore, the ventilator operates as a constant-pressure generator during the inspiratory phase, the generated pressure being equal to the pressure supplied by the pressure-control mechanism (40) less the pressure drop across the wall of the bag (48). However, the actual mode of operation depends on the setting of the 'peak flow' control (45).

When this control is set for maximum peak flow (fig. 27.3) the resistance within the apparatus is at a minimum. Therefore the required tidal volume can usually be delivered in the required inspiratory time with a generated pressure which is little in excess of the peak pressure needed in the alveoli. Therefore the ventilator does indeed operate as a constant-pressure generator. However, with the 'peak flow' control (45) at maximum there is still some resistance between the pressure-control mechanism (40), where the pressure is effectively generated, and the mouth. Therefore the pressure at the mouth (fig. 27.3) does not rise immediately to the full generated pressure; instead, after an initial rise, it gradually approaches the generated pressure as the flow falls. Nevertheless, it is clear from fig. 27.3 that, when the compliance is halved (b), the flow falls off much more rapidly.

When the 'peak flow' control (45) is set for near-minimum flow on the other hand, the resistance within the ventilator becomes high and the generated pressure must be set high in order to deliver the required tidal volume in the required time. In this situation, of relatively-high generated pressure with high series resistance, the mode of operation is much more nearly that of a flow generator. This can be seen in fig. 27.4 where changes of lung characteristics have more effect on the mouth-pressure waveform than on the flow waveform.

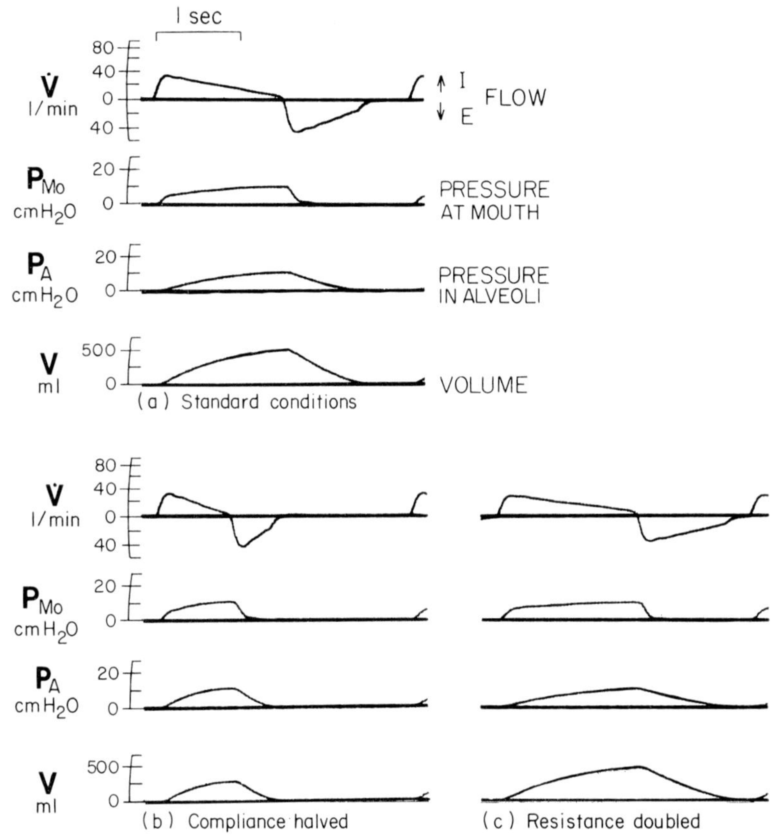

Fig. 27.3. Bennett Model BA–4 'Anesthesia Ventilator'. Recordings showing the effects of changes of lung characteristics: flow-cycled, pressure-generating mode, with no blow-off valve in the patient circuit, and therefore with excess gas escaping through the spill valve (49).

Standard conditions: driving gas, oxygen at 60 lb/in^2; 'sensitivity', minimum; 'volume', maximum; 'peak flow', maximum; negative pressure, minimum; fresh-gas flow, 0·5 litre/min; 'rate', set for a frequency of 20/min; 'pressure', set for a tidal volume of 500 ml. Note that for this standard frequency and tidal volume the 'standard' inspiratory-expiratory ratio of 1 : 2 could not be achieved.

In both modes of operation, at the start of the inspiratory phase, there is a slight oscillation in the flow and mouth-pressure waveforms which can be attributed to the inertia of the weights (13) and (18) which have to be accelerated when inspiratory flow starts.

Change-over from inspiratory phase to expiratory phase

This change-over is fundamentally flow-cycled; it occurs when the flow through the Bennett valve has fallen to a critical low level. But this can arise in two quite different ways.

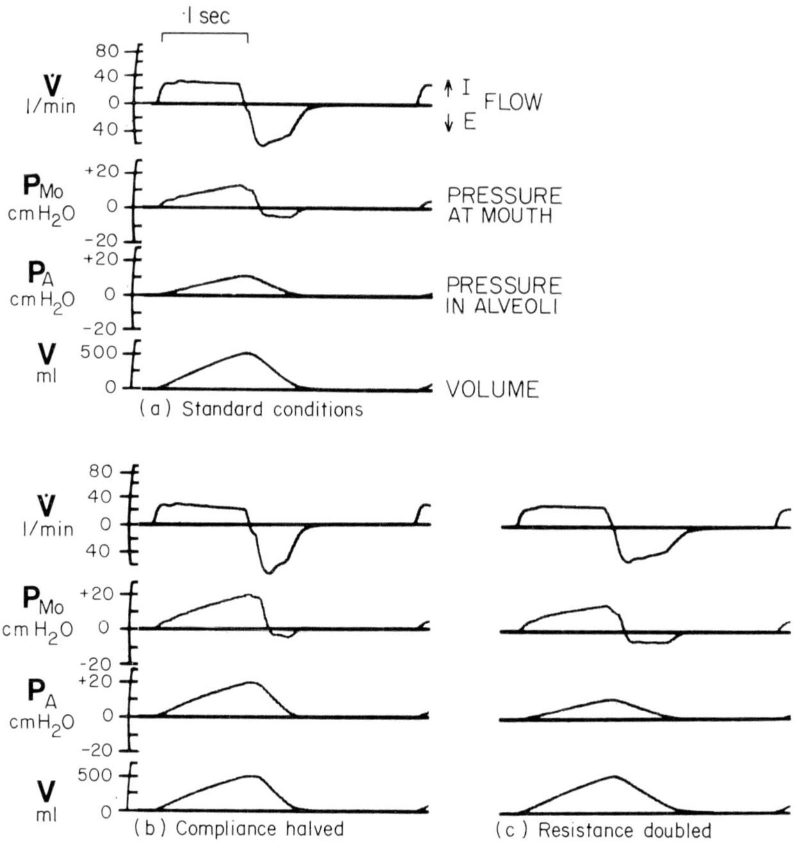

Fig. 27.4. Bennett Model BA–4 'Anesthesia Ventilator'. Recordings showing the effects of changes of lung characteristics: volume-cycled, flow-generating mode, with no blow-off valve in the patient circuit and therefore with excess gas escaping through the spill valve (49).

Standard conditions: driving gas, oxygen at 60 lb/in^2; 'sensitivity', minimum; 'pressure', maximum; negative pressure, maximum; fresh-gas flow, 0·5 litre/min; 'rate', set for a frequency of 20/min; 'volume', set for a tidal volume of 500 ml; 'peak flow', set, near minimum, for an inspiratory-expiratory ratio of 1 : 2.

Firstly, the flow may fall to the critical level because the pressure in the alveoli is approaching the generated pressure. In this case the change-over is truly flow-cycled. But, for a given flow through the ventilator, the pressure difference, between the mouth and the generated pressure, is determined entirely by the ventilator and is uninfluenced by the lung characteristics. Therefore the change-over is also effectively pressure-cycled by the pressure at the mouth. This can be seen in fig. 27.3: when the lung characteristics are changed, neither the flow, nor the pressure at the mouth (at the end of the inspiratory phase), is changed.

Although the pressure at the mouth at the end of the inspiratory phase, i.e. the cycling pressure, is independent of lung characteristics it does depend on the generated pressure. In fact it is only slightly less than the generated pressure because the critical flow at which the Bennett valve closes is so small. Therefore the cycling pressure changes when the generated pressure is changed either by adjusting the 'pressure' control (40) or by adjusting the sliding weight (13) which alters the pressure drop across the walls of the concertina reservoir bag (48). Therefore to understand the functioning of this ventilator it is preferable to consider the change-over as flow-cycled. The flow at the mouth exceeds the flow through the Bennett valve to the extent of the fresh-gas flow to the breathing circuit. Therefore the cycling flow (at the mouth) can be varied by adjusting the fresh-gas flow, but the setting for this will normally be decided on quite different grounds.

The second way in which the flow through the Bennett valve may fall to the critical level is as a result of the pressure source being cut off by the inflation of capsule (41) consequent upon the closure of ball valve (33) when a preset volume has been expelled from the concertina reservoir bag (48). In this case the change-over is effectively volume-cycled and fig. 27.4 shows that changes of lung characteristics do not alter the tidal volume. When volume cycling is combined with flow generation in the inspiratory phase the change-over is also effectively time-cycled. In fact, in fig. 27.4, the inspiratory time is slightly prolonged when the compliance is halved or the resistance doubled because the BA-4 does not operate as a perfect flow generator.

When volume cycling was combined with pressure generation in the inspiratory phase (recordings made but not reproduced here) the generated pressure required to deliver the standard volume (500 ml) in the standard inspiratory time (1 sec) to the standard model lung was not greatly in excess of the peak alveolar pressure under standard conditions. Therefore, when the compliance was halved, the alveolar pressure approached the generated pressure, and the flow fell to the critical level for cycling, well before the full 500 ml had been delivered. A similar effect may occur in ventilators which are fundamentally pressure-cycled but which become effectively volume-cycled by means of a volume limit in a bag-in-bottle arrangement; but in these ventilators an unwanted change from volume cycling to pressure cycling, consequent upon a decrease in compliance, can be avoided by setting the cycling pressure high. To avoid this trouble in the Bennett BA-4, the generated pressure must be set high, by means of the 'pressure' control (40), and the inspiratory time regulated by adjusting the inspiratory resistance by means of the 'peak flow' control (45). In other words to ensure volume cycling the BA-4 must be run in the flow-generating mode in the inspiratory phase.

When flow cycling was combined with flow generation in the inspiratory phase ('peak flow' at minimum) the setting of the 'pressure' control (40) which made the change-over occur when a tidal volume of 500 ml had been delivered to the lungs, was such that the inspiratory time was about 4 sec. To reduce this time to a more normal value would have required an increase in the setting of the 'peak flow' control to lower the inspiratory resistance so that the ventilator operated more nearly as a pressure generator.

Thus, when flow cycling is used it will usually be necessary to set the 'peak flow' at or near maximum, so that the ventilator operates as a pressure generator in the inspiratory phase; whereas when volume cycling is used it will usually be desirable to set the 'peak flow' at or near minimum, so that the ventilator approximates to a flow generator.

Expiratory phase

During the first part of this phase, while the concertina reservoir bag (48) is expanding, this ventilator operates as a constant, negative, pressure generator as a result of the constant net force, produced by the weights (13) and (18), expanding the bag (48). When the net force is at a minimum (sliding weight (13) at the extreme left) negative pressure is not detectable at the mouth (fig. 27.3). This is because there is some apparatus resistance (from the mouth to the bag (48) and from the pressure chamber (47) to atmosphere by way of valve (44)) through which there is some flow so long as the bag is expanding. On the other hand, when the net force acting on the reservoir bag is at a maximum (sliding weight (13) at the extreme right) negative pressure is clearly shown at the mouth (fig. 27.4). In both cases (figs. 27.3 and 27.4) the pronounced effects of changes of lung characteristics on the flow waveforms in this first part of the phase can clearly be seen.

During the later part of the phase, when the bag (48) is fully expanded, constant, atmospheric, pressure is generated at the spill valve (49); in figs. 27.3 and 27.4 the mouth pressure is always zero for the later part of the phase.

Change-over from expiratory phase to inspiratory phase

This change-over is either patient-cycled or time-cycled whichever mechanism operates first. An inspiratory effort by the patient opens the Bennett valve by means of the negative pressure applied to the right-hand side of the lower vane (37). The timing mechanism opens the Bennett valve by the application of pressure to the upper vane (35), normally at a preset time after the start of the previous *inspiratory* phase not, as in many ventilators, after the start of the expiratory phase. Therefore, in the purely time-cycled mode of change-over it is normally the whole respiratory period which is determined by the ventilator and any increase or decrease in inspiratory time resulting from changes in lung characteristics (or from changes of control settings) is accompanied by a precisely-compensating decrease or increase in expiratory time. This can be seen very clearly by comparing (b) with (a) in fig. 27.3.

However, if the inspiratory phase is very prolonged, as a result of a change in lung characteristics or in the settings of the controls, then the respiratory period is prolonged to a time somewhat greater than the inspiratory time. The mechanism is explained in the 'Description' above.

CONTROLS

The following analysis and the recordings in fig. 27.5 refer to the volume-cycled, flow-generating mode of operation with no patient-cycling and with no blow-off valve in the breathing circuit; excess fresh gas escapes through the spill valve (49) during expiration. Some notes on other modes of operation follow on p. 341.

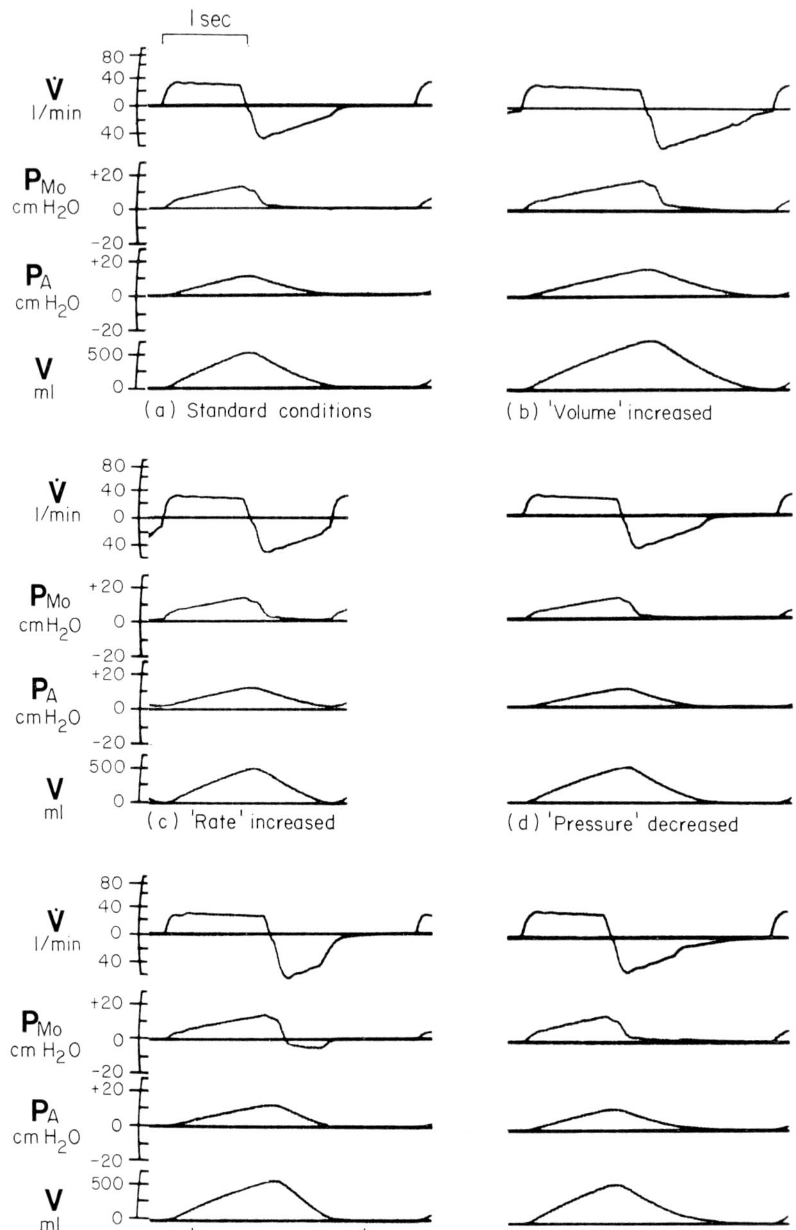

(a) Standard conditions (b) 'Volume' increased (c) 'Rate' increased (d) 'Pressure' decreased (e) 'Negative pressure' increased (f) Fresh-gas flow increased

Total ventilation

This cannot be directly controlled but is equal to the product of tidal volume and respiratory frequency both of which can be directly controlled.

Tidal volume

This can be directly controlled by adjusting the stroke volume of the concertina reservoir bag (48) by means of the 'volume' control (30). However the tidal volume exceeds this stroke volume by the volume of fresh gas which enters the patient circuit during the inspiratory phase. Therefore increasing the fresh-gas flow produces some increase in tidal volume (fig. 27.5f). Similarly, if the inspiratory time is increased, either by decreasing the generated pressure by means of the 'pressure' control (40) or by increasing the resistance to inspiration by decreasing the setting of the 'peak flow' control (45), then the tidal volume is increased—but the effect is negligible, as in fig. 27.5d, unless the fresh-gas flow is high.

The tidal volume is also increased when 'negative pressure' is increased by moving weight (13) to the right (fig. 27.5e). This is because, although the linear excursion of the top-plate of the reservoir bag (48) is unaltered, the greater tension in the wire (28) results in a bigger pressure drop across the bag wall and hence a greater compression of the convolutions of the bag wall and therefore an increased volume displacement from the bag. Increasing the 'negative pressure' from minimum to maximum (fig. 27.5e) increased the tidal volume by about 10%.

When the tidal volume is deliberately increased by means of the 'volume' control (30) the inspiratory time is necessarily increased (fig. 27.5b). This changes the inspiratory-expiratory ratio but not the respiratory frequency.

Changes of lung characteristics of course have no effect on the tidal volume (fig. 27.4).

Respiratory frequency

The respiratory period, and hence the respiratory frequency, is fully determined by the timing mechanism (1, 4). It can therefore be directly controlled by the 'rate' control (11)

Fig. 27.5. Bennett Model BA–4 'Anesthesia Ventilator'. Recordings showing the effects of changes in the settings of most of the controls: volume-cycled, flow-generating mode, with no blow-off valve in the patient circuit and therefore with excess gas escaping through the spill valve (49).

(a) Standard conditions as for fig. 27.4 except that the negative pressure here was at minimum.

(b) 'Volume' increased for tidal volume of 800 ml.

(c) 'Rate' increased for frequency of 30/min.

(d) 'Pressure' decreased 2 turns out of a total of $4\frac{1}{4}$.

(e) 'Negative pressure' increased to maximum.

(f) Fresh-gas flow increased to 4 litres/min.

and is unaffected by changes of lung characteristics (fig. 27.4) or by the settings of other controls (fig. 27.5). The only exception to this is that if the inspiratory period becomes very prolonged then the action of the timing mechanism is temporarily arrested for a short while in each cycle so that the respiratory period is prolonged to a time somewhat greater than the inspiratory period. The mechanism is explained in the 'Description' above but does not come into play in any of the recordings shown in figs. 27.3, 27.4 or 27.5.

Since it is the respiratory period which is determined by the timing mechanism, changing the frequency by adjusting the 'rate' control (11) does not affect the inspiratory time and so the inspiratory-expiratory ratio is altered (fig. 27.5c).

Inspiratory-expiratory ratio

This cannot be directly controlled but, for a given respiratory frequency, and hence a given respiratory period, the inspiratory time, and hence the inspiratory-expiratory ratio, can be independently adjusted. Thus the inspiratory time can be increased by reducing the generated flow. This can be achieved either by decreasing the pressure delivered from the pressure-control mechanism by means of the 'pressure' control (40) (fig. 27.5d) or by increasing the resistance to inspiration by decreasing the setting of the 'peak flow' control (not illustrated in fig. 27.5). However, if the respiratory frequency is altered this will alter the inspiratory-expiratory ratio (fig. 27.5c) and a further adjustment of the generated flow will be necessary if the inspiratory-expiratory ratio is to be restored.

In addition, increasing the tidal volume by means of the 'volume' control (30) increases the inspiratory time and so alters the inspiratory-expiratory ratio (fig. 27.5b). Increasing the 'negative pressure' has the same effect in a smaller degree (fig. 27.5e), partly because of the resultant small increase in tidal volume (explained above) and partly because of the increased pressure drop across the wall of the reservoir bag (48) which leads to some reduction in flow.

Since, for the recordings shown in fig. 27.4, the ventilator was operating as a fairly close approximation to a flow generator (with volume cycling) changing the lung characteristics did not have much effect on the inspiratory time or inspiratory-expiratory ratio.

Inspiratory waveforms

With the ventilator operating as a constant-flow generator the flow waveform is determined by the ventilator and the pressure waveforms result from the interaction of this flow waveform with the lung characteristics. The magnitude of the flow can be adjusted by means of the 'pressure' control (40) (fig. 27.5d) or the 'peak flow' control (45) but these choices may already have been made in order to deliver a given tidal volume in a given inspiratory time. By decreasing the 'pressure' and increasing the 'peak flow' it is possible to change the mode of operation from that of a flow generator towards that of a pressure generator. However, to make any appreciable difference the pressure delivered by the pressure-control mechanism (40) (less the pressure drop across the walls of the reservoir bag) must be set to not much more than the minimum required to deliver the preset tidal volume. Then any large fall in compliance may lead to flow cycling before the preset tidal volume has been delivered.

Expiratory waveforms

During this phase it is primarily the pressure waveform at the mouth which is determined by the ventilator while the flow and alveolar-pressure waveforms depend on the effect of the mouth-pressure waveform on the lungs. The negative pressure generated during the first part of the phase, while the reservoir bag is still expanding, can be adjusted by the sliding weight (13). This does not affect the end-expiratory alveolar pressure, which must be no lower than atmospheric for excess fresh gas to escape through the spill valve. However, increasing the 'negative pressure' does result in most of the tidal volume coming out of the lungs rapidly at the start of the expiratory phase (fig. 27.5e) rather than more gradually over a longer portion of the phase (fig. 27.5a).

Pressure limits

During the expiratory phase the alveolar pressure normally falls to equal the atmospheric pressure which is generated at the spill valve (49) in the later part of the phase. It will fail to do so only if the airway resistance is very high or if, as in fig. 27.5c, the expiratory time is too short. The peak alveolar pressure in the inspiratory phase is not directly controlled; it exceeds the minimum pressure at the end of the expiratory phase by an amount equal to the tidal volume divided by the compliance.

Other modes of operation

The above analysis refers to the volume-cycled, flow-generating mode of operation with no patient cycling and with no blow-off valve in the patient circuit.

A full set of recordings has not been made of the flow-cycled, pressure-generating mode (with no blow-off valve) but it is clear that the principal effects of changing to this mode are that the tidal volume is primarily controlled by the 'pressure' control (40) and that (as can be seen in fig. 27.3) the tidal volume and inspiratory time (and hence the inspiratory-expiratory ratio) become dependent on compliance.

If the patient is making inspiratory efforts, and if the sensitivity control (12) is suitably set, the respiratory frequency becomes controlled by the patient, except that the timing mechanism sets a minimum frequency.

If negative pressure is to be produced in the alveoli it must be maintained at the mouth throughout the expiratory phase and therefore the reservoir bag (48) cannot be allowed to expand to its upper limit. As the manufacturers acknowledge, it follows from this that the volume-cycling mechanism cannot be used, and that excess fresh gas cannot escape past the spill valve (49); therefore fresh gas must be vented in the inspiratory phase through a blow-off valve in the patient circuit. Some recordings were made, but are not reproduced here, of the ventilator operating in this mode. They showed that most of the respiratory parameters depended in a complex way on several of the controls and on lung characteristics; the main features may be summarized as follows.

The 'pressure' control must be set at least high enough to vent the required volume of excess fresh gas in each cycle through the blow-off valve; therefore the reservoir bag (48) must reach the bottom of its stroke in each inspiratory phase leading to immediate cycling of the Bennett valve.

Respiratory frequency is still directly controlled by the ventilator (subject to the provisos mentioned above) and may be adjusted by the 'rate' control (11).

Tidal volume is not directly controlled but is determined by the pressure limits in combination with the lung characteristics. Since negative-pressure generation continues throughout the expiratory phase, the minimum alveolar pressure in each expiration is usually close to the generated, negative pressure. The peak mouth pressure in the inspiratory phase depends on the setting of the blow-off valve and, unless it is an ideal pressure-limiting valve which most anaesthetic expiratory valves are not, on the flow of escaping fresh gas through the valve. The peak alveolar pressure is less than the peak mouth pressure by an amount equal to the product of airway resistance and end-inspiratory flow. Therefore the tidal volume is dependent on many factors but the main means of control are by increasing the peak alveolar pressure by screwing down the blow-off valve (provided that the 'pressure' setting (40) is high enough) or by making the minimum pressure more negative by adjusting the sliding weight (13). Varying the relative magnitudes of these adjustments will vary the mean pressure.

Inspiratory time, and hence inspiratory-expiratory ratio, is influenced by many factors but can be adjusted by means of the 'peak flow' control (45) or the 'pressure' control (40). In the latter case some change of peak alveolar pressure, and hence of tidal volume, results.

CHAPTER 28

The Bennett Model PR–2 'Respiration Unit'

DESCRIPTION

This compact ventilator (fig. 28.1) is designed for ward use. Oxygen at a pressure of 40–70 lb/in^2 operates the ventilator and is delivered to the patient with or without entrained air. It operates as a fully-automatic or as a patient-triggered ventilator with automatic override, with or without a negative-pressure phase.

The diagram (fig. 28.2) is drawn as at the beginning of the inspiratory phase. The gas which powers the ventilator enters at the inlet (5), passes through a sintered-bronze filter, and flows to three units:— the pressure regulator (6), the inflating-pressure-control mechanism (13), and the phase-selector mechanism (19).

In the resting position the small capsules at the tops of the pneumatic valves (2, 3, 4) are collapsed and the valve springs hold the valves in the 'up' position. When the ventilator is set for automatic cycling, driving gas at the reduced pressure leaves the regulator (6) and flows, past a constriction, through the 'rate' control needle valve (8), and, through the valve (3) which is in the 'up' position, to the 'expiration time' control needle valve (10), and hence to the valve (4). The escape of gas from the valve (4) through the valve (3) is prevented as the valve (3) is 'up', and therefore the distension of the capsule (4) pushes down the valve stem of (4) in a time determined by the setting of the 'rate' control (8) and the 'expiration time' control (10). As soon as the valve (4) is forced down, a free pathway is opened through its stem between the regulator (6) and the chamber (15) of the Bennett valve, and the pressure within this chamber rises rapidly. This moves the drum of the Bennett valve, in an anti-clockwise direction, to the position shown in which there is a free pathway through the Bennett valve from the inflating-pressure-control mechanism (13) to the long delivery tube (27), past the expiratory-valve assembly (32), and then through a very short tube to the patient. The capsule (31) of the expiratory valve (32) is connected to the outlet port (26) of the Bennett valve, and is therefore held inflated.

At the same time, the pressure within the Bennett valve is transmitted to the bottom of the pneumatic valve (3). The pressure builds up rapidly in the capsule (3) and distends it, thus forcing the valve stem down against its spring. This cuts off the supply of driving gas from the needle valve (8), through the needle valve (10), to the pneumatic valve (4),

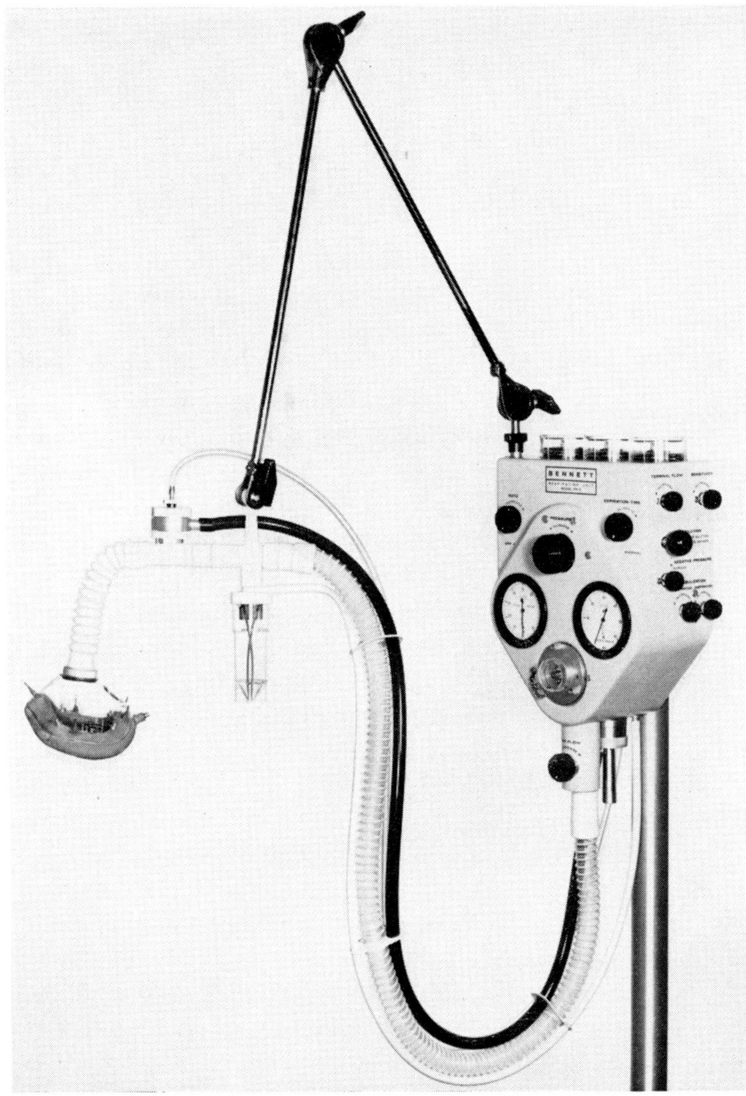

Fig. 28.1. The Bennett Model PR–2 'Respiration Unit'.
Courtesy of Bennett Respiration Products Inc. and Puritan Compressed Gas Corporation.

and opens a pathway from the valve (4) to atmosphere. The valve (4) therefore returns to its resting position and cuts off the supply of driving gas to the chamber (15). The pressure on the upper side of the vane in the chamber (15) falls to atmospheric through the constriction (16). Meanwhile the pressure on the under side has risen since it is in connexion with the breathing circuit. Even though the pressure difference across the upper vane is tending to move the Bennett valve in a clockwise direction, it is still held 'open' by the pressure difference across the lower vane caused by the flow of gas through the valve. When the flow through the Bennett valve to the patient has ceased, in one of the ways to be described later, there is no longer a pressure difference across the lower vane, and therefore the pressure below the vane in the chamber (15) can now rotate the valve in a clockwise direction. There is now a free connexion between the capsule (31) of the expiratory valve (32) and atmosphere through the centre of the Bennett valve and the injector (29). The capsule (31) collapses, the inspiratory phase ends, and expired gas flows to atmosphere past the flap (30) of the expiratory valve (32).

There are two ways in which flow through the Bennett valve may be brought to an end.

(a) The pressure in the lungs rises until it has approached the pressure set by the 'pressure control' (13) closely enough for the flow through the Bennett valve to have fallen to 1 litre/min. Since the pressure drop across the lower vane is now insufficient to hold the Bennett valve open, the valve closes and flow through it stops completely. This occurs in a time which depends on the lung characteristics.

(b) The flow of gas to the Bennett valve is cut off when the capsule (12) is inflated and thereby closes the outlet port of the pressure-control mechanism (13). This occurs in a preset time determined by the slow inflation of capsule (2) via the 'rate' control (8). The sequence of events is as follows. With the valve (3), in the 'down' position, gas flows, through the needle valve (8) and the valve (3), to the valve (2) until the pressure there is sufficient to move it to the 'down' position. This allows gas to flow directly from the regulator (6) through the valve (2) to the capsule (12).

When the Bennett valve closes, the free pathway between the capsule of the pneumatic valve (3) and the delivery tube (27) allows the pressure in the capsule (3) to fall rapidly. Its spring returns the valve (3) to the 'up' position, thus connecting the base of valve (2) to atmosphere and allowing the valve (2), if it is 'down', to return to the 'up' position. If inflation was ended by distension of the capsule (12), the gas in the capsule (12) now escapes, past the constriction (9) and through the valve (3), to atmosphere; the capsule (12) collapses and the outlet port of the pressure-control mechanism (13) is reopened.

There are two modes in which the next inspiratory phase may be initiated.

(a) The capsule (4) is inflated via the needle valves (8) and (10) until, after a time determined by the settings of these valves, the valve (4) reaches the bottom of its stroke. Pressure from the regulator (6) is now applied, through the valve (4), to the chamber (15), and the Bennett valve is opened.

(b) If the 'sensitivity' control (7) is open, then there is a supply of gas during the expiratory phase from the regulator (6), through the valve (2), the 'sensitivity' control (7), and the valve (3), to the chamber (15) of the Bennett valve. Therefore there is always a pressure tending to turn the Bennett valve anti-clockwise. However, the pressure in the chamber (15) is limited by the escape of gas through the orifice (16). Therefore the

Bennett valve will not open until the force tending to turn it is supplemented by a pressure difference across its lower vane.

The ventilator is patient-triggered if, before it has been cycled in mode (a), an inspiratory effort by the patient supplies this pressure difference. The degree of inspiratory effort required of the patient may be varied by adjustment of the 'sensitivity' control (7).

The phase-selector mechanism (19) performs a number of functions.

Firstly, it allows negative pressure to be applied during the expiratory phase. During the inspiratory phase the capsule (24) is distended by gas flowing from the outlet port (26) of the Bennett valve. The distended capsule (24) opens the hinged valve (23), through which the driving gas can escape to atmosphere; this prevents any build-up of pressure behind the diaphragm (22), and the ball valve (20) is therefore held, by its spring, on its right-hand seating. When the expiratory phase starts the capsule (24) collapses, the hinged valve (23) closes, and pressure builds up behind the diaphragm (22). The diaphragm (22) is moved over, and pushes the ball valve (20) onto its left-hand seating. Therefore during the expiratory phase driving gas flows, past the ball valve (20) and through the 'negative pressure' control valve (17), to the injector (29). By this means negative pressure is applied at the expiratory valve (32). The needle valve (17) controls the flow of gas to the injector and hence the negative pressure produced.

Secondly, it allows a nebulizer (33), if attached to the expiratory-valve assembly (32), to be brought into action. The flow to the nebulizer during the inspiratory and expiratory phases is controlled by the 'nebulization, inspiration' needle valve (18) and the 'nebulization, expiration' needle valve (21) respectively.

Finally, if for any reason, such as a leak in the breathing circuit or an unduly slow equalization of pressure across the Bennett valve, the valve fails to rotate clockwise soon enough and thus end the inspiratory phase, the 'terminal flow' needle valve (25) may be

---

Fig. 28.2. Diagram of the Bennett Model PR–2 'Respiration Unit'.

1. 'Control pressure' gauge
2. Inspiratory-timing pneumatic valve
3. Change-over pneumatic valve
4. Expiratory-timing pneumatic valve
5. Driving-gas inlet
6. Pressure regulator supplying timing mechanism
7. Patient-triggering 'sensitivity' control
8. 'Rate' control
9. Constriction
10. 'Expiration time' control
11. Push-pull air 'dilution' control
12. Capsule
13. Inflating-pressure-control mechanism
14. 'System pressure' gauge
15. Chamber
16. Escape orifice with constriction
17. 'Negative pressure' control
18. 'Nebulization, inspiration' control
19. Phase-selector mechanism
20. Ball valve
21. 'Nebulization, expiration' control
22. Diaphragm
23. Hinged valve
24. Capsule
25. 'Terminal flow' control
26. Outlet port of Bennett valve
27. Delivery tube
28. 'Peak flow' limiting control
29. Injector for expiratory negative pressure
30. Flap valve over expiratory port
31. Capsule
32. Expiratory-valve assembly
33. Nebulizer

opened. This allows driving gas to flow through an injector, where it entrains air, into the breathing circuit. The flow through the Bennett valve can now fall to a low-enough level to permit clockwise rotation of the valve, while the flow to the patient is still relatively high.

A 'peak flow' control (28) in the delivery tube (27) allows the resistance to inspiration to be increased if it is desired to limit the inspiratory flow.

The position of the push-pull 'dilution' control (11) on the inflating-pressure-control mechanism (13) determines whether or not air is entrained by the driving gas. The

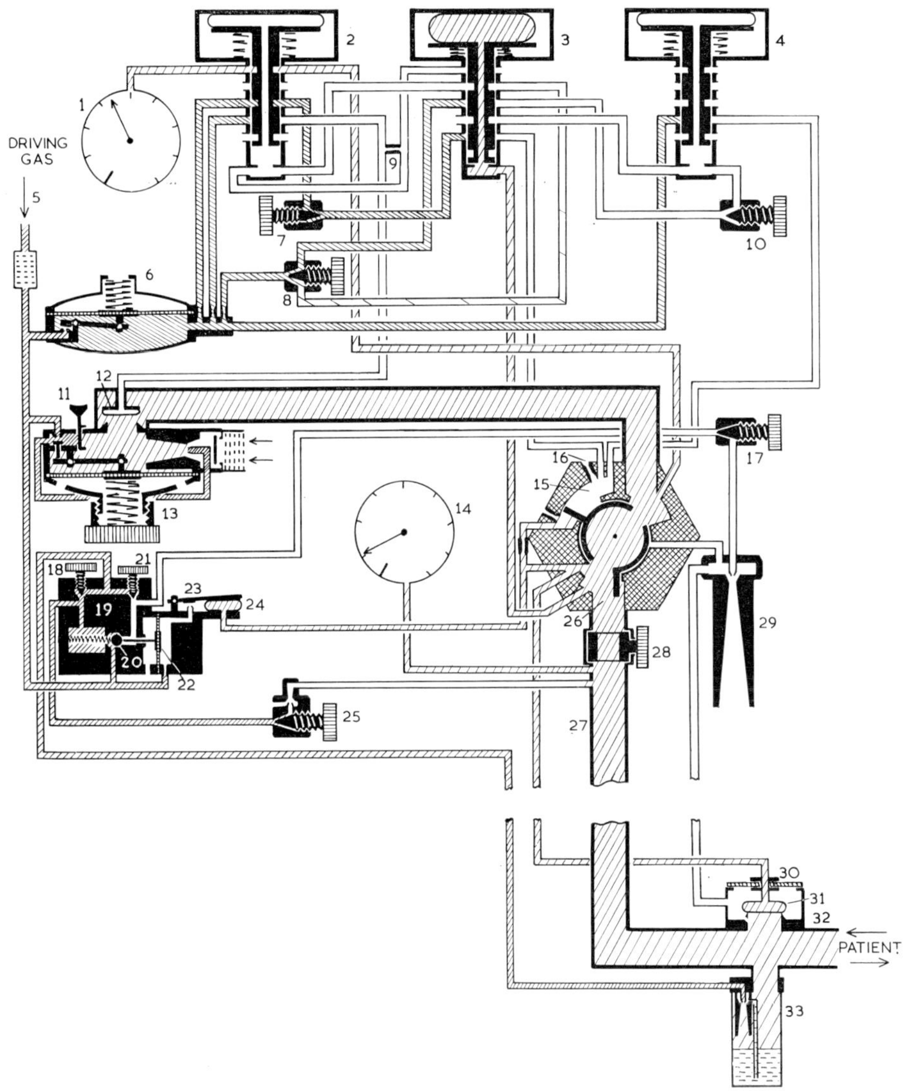

manufacturers state that, if the driving gas is oxygen and the control is pushed in, the oxygen concentration in the mixture delivered to the patient is approximately 40%, but variations from this may occur.[1,2]

The manometer (1) ('control pressure' gauge) is connected to the input side of the Bennett valve and indicates the pressure delivered by the pressure-control mechanism (13). The manometer (14) ('system pressure' gauge) is connected to the delivery tube (27) below the 'peak flow' control (28) and indicates 'mouth' pressure irrespective of the mode of cycling.

A small adjustable positive pressure may be achieved during the expiratory phase by fitting a 'retard' mechanism to the expiratory-valve assembly (32).

The filters, which are fitted in the driving-gas inlet (5) and in the air-entrainment port of the pressure-control mechanism (13), can be removed for cleaning.

FUNCTIONAL ANALYSIS

Inspiratory phase

Fundamentally this ventilator is a constant-pressure generator during the inspiratory phase because the second-stage reducing valve in the inflating-pressure-control mechanism (13) supplies a preset pressure irrespective of the flow from it. However, the actual mode of operation of the ventilator depends on the setting of the 'peak flow' limiting control (28).

When this control (28) is set for maximum peak flow (fig. 28.3 curve (a) and fig. 28.4) the resistance within the apparatus is at a minimum and the ventilator does indeed operate as a constant-pressure generator. However, there is some resistance between the pressure-control mechanism (13) and the mouth, so that the pressure at the latter is somewhat dependent on flow (fig. 28.3 curve (a)) and does not rise immediately to the full

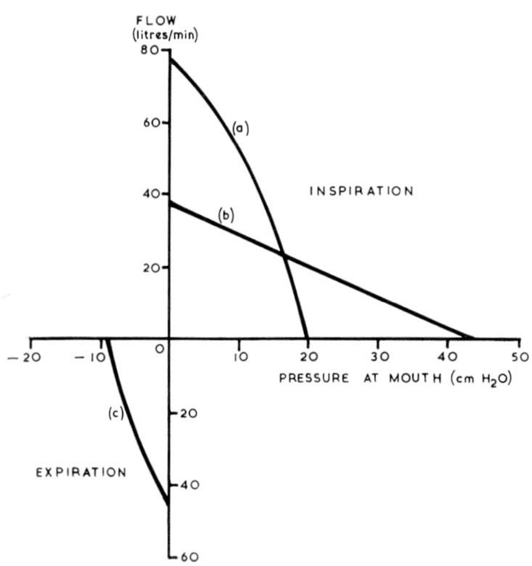

Fig. 28.3 Bennett Model PR–2 'Respiration Unit'. Pressure-flow characteristics of the positive pressure ('inspiration') and negative pressure ('expiration') systems.

Curve (a): 'peak flow' control, maximum, and 'pressure' control, intermediate, as used for fig. 28.4.

Curve (b): 'pressure' control, maximum, and 'peak flow' control, near minimum, as used for figs. 28.5. and 28.6.

Curve (c): 'negative pressure', maximum.

For all three curves the conditions were as follows: driving gas, oxygen at 50 lb/in^2; 'dilution', 100% oxygen; 'terminal flow' and 'nebulization' controls, off.

generated pressure (fig. 28.4). Instead, after an initial rise, it gradually approaches the generated pressure as the flow falls. Nevertheless, it is clear from fig. 28.4 that the flow waveform is considerably affected by changes of lung characteristics; for instance when the compliance is halved the flow falls off more rapidly.

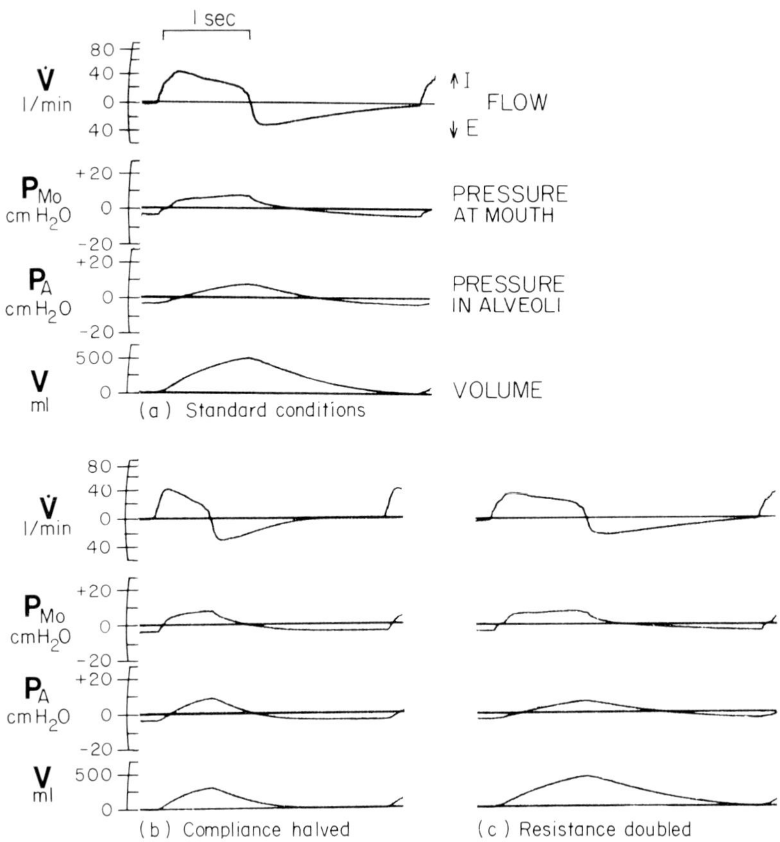

Fig. 28.4. Bennett Model PR–2 'Respiration Unit' in the pressure-generating, flow-cycled mode. Recordings showing the effects of changes of lung characteristics.

Standard conditions: driving gas, oxygen at 50 lb/in^2; 'dilution', 100% oxygen; 'sensitivity', minimum; 'nebulization, expiration', off; 'peak flow', maximum; 'expiration time', 'normal'; 'terminal flow', maximum; 'negative pressure', set for about -3 cmH_2O in the alveoli at the end of the expiratory phase; 'pressure' and 'nebulization, inspiration', set for a tidal volume of 500 ml in an inspiratory time of 1 sec; 'rate', set for an expiratory time of 2 sec, producing a frequency of 20/min and an inspiratory-expiratory ratio of 1 : 2.

On the other hand, when the 'peak flow' control (28) is set for near-minimum flow, the resistance within the ventilator becomes high and the generated pressure must be set high in order to deliver the tidal volume in the required time. In this situation, of relatively-high generated pressure with high series resistance, the mode of operation is much more nearly that of a flow generator (fig. 28.3 curve (b)). This can also be seen in fig. 28.5 where changes of lung characteristics have more effect on the mouth-pressure waveform than on the flow waveform.

The functioning is complicated by the leak at the 'terminal flow' needle valve (25) and by the additional inputs of gas when the 'nebulization, inspiration' (18) and 'terminal flow' controls are turned on. However, these do not affect the conclusions that, at least within the ranges of lung characteristics tried here, the ventilator approximates to a constant-pressure generator when the 'peak flow' control is set for maximum flow and to a constant-flow generator when it is set for minimum flow.

Change-over from inspiratory phase to expiratory phase

Fundamentally this change-over is flow-cycled; it occurs when the flow through the Bennett valve has fallen to a critical low level. However, this can arise in two quite different ways.

Firstly, the flow may fall to the critical level simply because the pressure generator has been cut off by the inflation of capsule (12), by means of the timing mechanism (2, 3, 8), at a preset time after the start of the inspiratory phase. In this case the change-over is effectively time-cycled and fig. 28.5 shows that changes of lung characteristics do not alter the inspiratory time although they do alter the mouth pressure at the end of the inspiratory phase. When time cycling is combined with pressure generation in the inspiratory phase (not illustrated here) changes of lung characteristics do alter the tidal volume; but, when time cycling is combined with flow generation, as in fig. 28.5, the almost-constant flow for a fixed time results in the delivered volume reaching a given value at the end of the phase, irrespective of lung characteristics. That is, the phase is also effectively volume-cycled.

Secondly, the flow may fall to the critical level because the pressure in the lungs is approaching the generated pressure. The flow at the mouth, at the moment of change-over, will usually differ from the critical flow through the Bennett valve, because some flow may be entering from the nebulizer (33) and from the 'terminal flow' needle valve (25) and some may be escaping through the entrainment orifice of this valve. However, the difference between the two flows, and therefore the actual flow at the mouth at the moment of change-over, depends entirely on the ventilator and the settings of its controls; it is uninfluenced by the lung characteristics. Therefore the change-over may be said to be flow-cycled by the flow at the mouth. The actual flow at the mouth which ends the inspiratory phase depends on the settings of the 'nebulization, inspiration' and 'terminal flow' controls.

However, if all the flows within the ventilator are fixed, then so also is the pressure drop from the pressure generated at the pressure-control mechanism (13) to the pressure at the mouth. Therefore the pressure at the mouth at the moment of change-over is determined entirely by the ventilator and is uninfluenced by the lung characteristics. Therefore the change-over may equally well be said to be pressure-cycled by the pressure

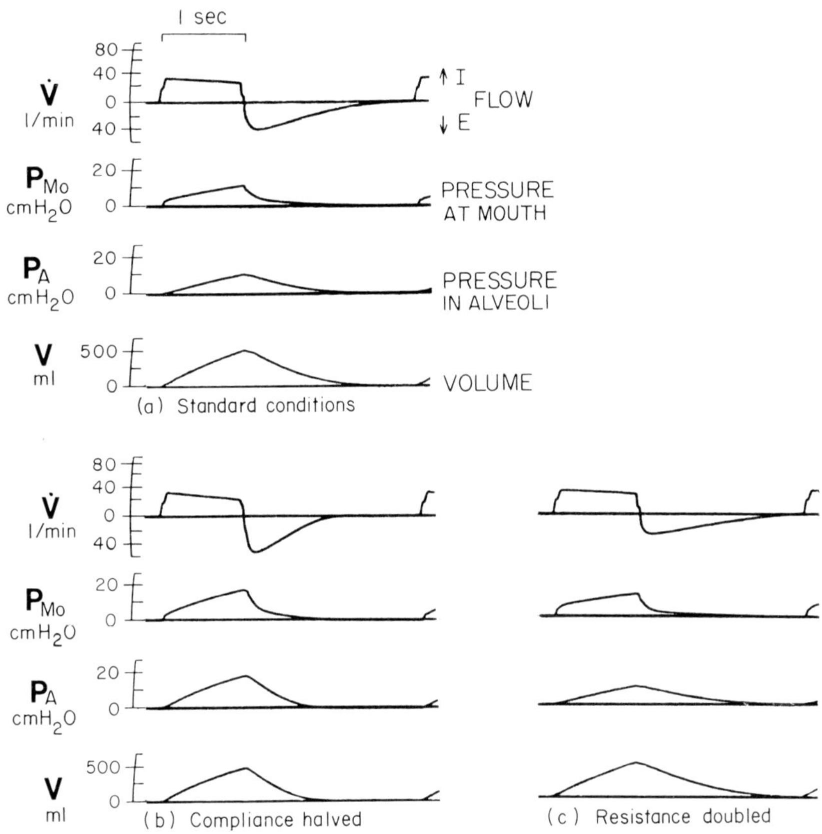

Fig. 28.5. Bennett Model PR–2 'Respiration Unit' in the flow-generating time-cycled mode, without negative pressure. Recordings showing the effect of changes of lung characteristics.

Standard conditions: driving gas, oxygen at 50 lb/in^2; 'dilution', 100% oxygen; 'sensitivity', 'terminal flow', 'negative pressure', and 'nebulization' controls, off; 'pressure', maximum; 'rate' and 'expiration time', set for a frequency of 20/min and an inspiratory-expiratory ratio of 1 : 2; 'peak flow', set (near minimum) for a tidal volume of 500 ml.

at the mouth. This can be seen in fig. 28.4: when the lung characteristics are changed, neither the pressure at the mouth nor the flow (at the end of the inspiratory phase) is changed.

Most ventilators are pressure-cycled, volume-cycled, or time-cycled. Therefore, in comparing this ventilator with others, it is probably preferable to consider the change-over as pressure-cycled. The 'terminal flow' control can then be regarded as the cycling-pressure control because it alters the amount by which the cycling pressure at the mouth falls short of the generated pressure. However the cycling pressure will also be altered when the generated pressure is altered by the 'pressure' control (13). Therefore, to understand the functioning of this ventilator without regard to others, it is preferable to consider the change-over as flow-cycled. Then the 'terminal flow' control can be regarded as the cycling-flow control because it alters the flow at the mouth at which cycling occurs. The 'nebulization, inspiration' control also has some effect on both the flow and the pressure at the mouth at the moment of the change-over but it will normally be set in accordance with nebulization requirements.

The time-cycling mode of change-over can be eliminated by turning the 'rate' control (8) to 'off'. Then the change-over will be purely flow-cycled; but it should be borne in mind that, as explained below, the change-over from the expiratory phase to the inspiratory phase will then be only patient-cycled. On the other hand when the time-cycling mode of change-over is brought into operation, by turning up the 'rate' control (8), the flow-cycling mode is not eliminated but remains potentially in operation. Then the change-over occurs either after the lapse of a preset time or when the flow at the mouth has fallen to a preset level, whichever event occurs first.

Expiratory phase

With the 'negative pressure' control turned off (fig. 28.5) the ventilator operates as a constant, atmospheric, pressure generator in this phase with expired gas escaping to atmosphere past the flap (30) of the expiratory valve (32).

The pressure at the mouth does not immediately fall to atmospheric in the tracings in fig. 28.5 because the resistance of the valve is in series with the generated pressure. However, changes in lung characteristics, particularly halving the compliance (fig. 28.5b), can be seen to alter the flow waveform.

With the 'negative pressure' control turned on (fig. 28.4) the injector (29) is brought into operation. The characteristics of this are such that the ventilator operates as a constant, negative, pressure generator with some series resistance (fig. 28.3 curve (c)). Since the series resistance is greater than with atmospheric-pressure generation the pressure at the mouth is a little slower to fall to the generated pressure; but again the changes of flow waveform with changes of lung characteristics are clear (fig. 28.4).

Change-over from expiratory phase to inspiratory phase

If the 'rate' control (8) is turned to 'off' this change-over is solely patient-cycled: the Bennett valve opens only in response to an inspiratory effort from the patient. This is not illustrated in figs. 28.4, 28.5, or 28.6.

When the 'rate' control is turned on, the Bennett valve can also be opened by the application of gas pressure to the upper surface of the vane in chamber (15) at the time determined by the timing mechanism (4, 8, 10). Therefore the change-over is either patient-cycled or time-cycled whichever event occurs first. With the model lung, only the time-cycling mechanism could operate and in figs. 28.4 and 28.5 it can be seen that the expiratory time is uninfluenced by changes of lung characteristics.

Additional note on the time-cycling mechanism
When the timing mechanism is examined closely certain complications are discovered. It is only the descents of the valve stems (2) and (4) which are accurately timed. In general, there is some delay between the opening or closing of the Bennett valve and the start of the descent of valve stems (2) or (4) respectively. In addition there is some delay between the completion of the descent of valve stem (2) and the closing of the Bennett valve. These delays vary somewhat with the settings of some of the controls and with lung characteristics. However, the delays are always short and therefore the variations in total inspiratory and expiratory times are small. They can be detected in some of the tracings in figs. 28.5 and 28.6 but they are too small to be of clinical importance and have therefore been ignored in the functional analysis above and in the 'Controls' section below.

CONTROLS

In the following discussion it is assumed that both change-overs are time-cycled as in fig. 28.6. Furthermore, in all the tracings in fig. 28.6 the ventilator was operating as a flow generator during the inspiratory phase ('peak flow' near minimum) although in the text some mention is made of the effects of using the pressure-generating mode.

If the change-over from the inspiratory phase to the expiratory phase is flow-cycled then, in addition to the variations described below, the respiratory frequency and the inspiratory-expiratory ratio will depend on lung characteristics and on the settings of some of those controls which, in the time-cycled mode of operation, do not affect these parameters.

Total ventilation
This cannot be directly controlled but is equal to the product of tidal volume and respiratory frequency.

Tidal volume
In the flow-generating time-cycled mode of operation the tidal volume can be deliberately controlled by adjusting the generated flow, either by the 'pressure' control (fig. 28.6b) or by the 'peak flow' control (fig. 28.6d).

However, the tidal volume is also affected by some of the other controls. Increasing the 'rate' decreases the inspiratory time and hence the tidal volume (fig. 28.6c). If this were not accompanied by a change in the inspiratory-expiratory ratio there would be no change in total ventilation but, in thc conditions of fig. 28.6, the change of ratio is in such a direction that there is some drop in total ventilation along with the drop in tidal volume. If the 'terminal flow' (fig. 28.6e) or 'nebulization, inspiration' control settings are increased the main generated flow is supplemented and so the tidal volume is increased.

Since during the inspiratory phase there is a preset flow for a preset time the change-over is effectively volume-cycled and the tidal volume is unaffected by changes of lung characteristics (fig. 28.5).

In the pressure-generating time-cycled mode (not illustrated here) the tidal volume can still be controlled by the 'pressure' and 'peak flow' controls. However any decrease in

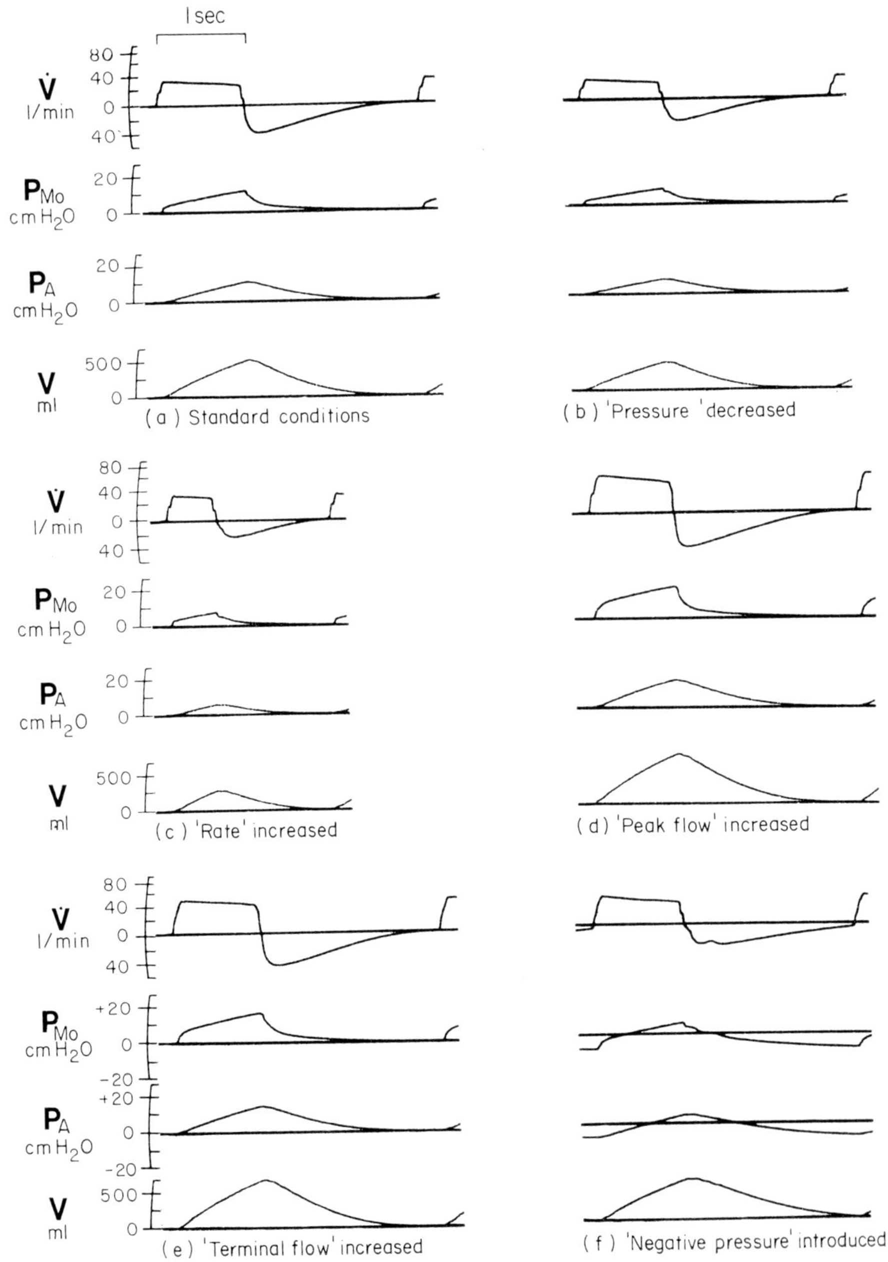

compliance or increase in resistance will now result in a decrease in tidal volume. The tidal volume is influenced by other controls in the same way as in the flow-generating mode except that it is not very sensitive to changes in the settings of the 'terminal flow' and 'nebulization, inspiration' controls. This is because their flow-generating action is largely swamped by the main pressure-generating action. However, the tidal volume is dependent on the setting of the 'negative pressure' control because this affects the pressure swing in the alveoli.

Respiratory frequency

In the time-cycled mode of operation this is directly controlled by the 'rate' control (8) and is uninfluenced by changes of lung characteristics (fig. 28.5). It is decreased by increasing the setting of the 'expiration time' control (10) because this lengthens the expiratory time without altering the inspiratory time (not shown in fig. 28.6).

When the 'rate' control was adjusted to increase the frequency from 20/min to about 30/min (fig. 28.6c) the inspiratory-expiratory ratio was changed from 1 : 2 to 1 : 2·3. The reason for this is as follows. In order to achieve the inspiratory-expiratory ratio of 1 : 2 for the 'standard conditions', the 'expiration time' control had been set above 'normal' thereby introducing a resistance at the needle valve (10) in series with the expiratory-timing valve (4). When the setting of the 'rate' control was decreased, this decreased the resistance of needle valve (8) which is in series with both timing valves. But the effect on the total resistance in series with the expiratory-timing valve, and hence on the expiratory time, was smaller than that on the resistance in series with the inspiratory-timing valve (2), and hence on the inspiratory time.

Increasing the 'rate' setting also reduces the tidal volume because the inspiratory time, the time for which the lungs are exposed to the generated flow (fig. 28.6c) or generated pressure, is reduced.

Inspiratory-expiratory ratio

This can be adjusted by means of the 'expiration time' control (10) but, since this merely alters the expiratory time (not shown in fig. 28.6), the frequency is also altered. If the frequency is then restored by means of the 'rate' control (8) some further change in the inspiratory-expiratory ratio will result (see above) and further adjustments of the two controls may be necessary to achieve a given pattern of timing exactly. Even then the

---

Fig. 28.6. Bennett Model PR–2 'Respiration Unit' in the flow-generating time-cycled mode. Recordings showing the effects of changes in the settings of some of the controls.

(a) Standard conditions as in fig. 28.5.
(b) 'Pressure' decreased for 'control pressure' of 30 cmH_2O.
(c) 'Rate' increased to maximum.
(d) 'Peak flow' increased.
(e) 'Terminal flow' increased to maximum.
(f) 'Negative pressure' set to maximum.

changed inspiratory time will result in a changed tidal volume which will require adjustment by means of the 'pressure' (13) or 'peak flow' (28) controls if the total ventilation is to be unaltered.

Since both change-overs are time-cycled the inspiratory-expiratory ratio is not affected by changes of lung characteristics (fig. 28.5).

Inspiratory waveforms

These can be varied by means of the 'peak flow' control. At the maximum peak-flow setting the ventilator approximates to a constant-pressure generator (fig. 28.4); near the minimum setting it approximates to a constant-flow generator (figs. 28.5 and 28.6), but then the 'pressure' control must be set high to obtain an adequate flow and hence an adequate tidal volume.

Expiratory waveforms

These depend on whether atmospheric pressure is generated at the expiratory valve (32) or a negative pressure at the injector (29). The choice between these two and the choice of the degree of negative pressure may well be made on other grounds but, when the negative-pressure generator is brought into use, by means of the 'negative pressure' control (17), the apparatus resistance to expiration is increased and so the decay of expiratory flow is more gradual (fig. 28.6f).

Pressure limits

Since the ventilator operates as a pressure generator, either atmospheric or negative, during the expiratory phase, the alveolar pressure usually falls to this pressure by the end of the phase. It does so in all the tracings reproduced here. It will fail to do so only if the expiratory time is too short or the resistance to expiration is too great.

When the ventilator is operating as a pressure generator in the inspiratory phase the alveolar pressure again approaches the generated pressure. But in this phase the approach is not at all close because the resistance of the ventilator, and hence the time constant of the system, is greater in inspiration than in expiration while the available time is less. Therefore the positive-pressure limit in the alveoli falls short of the generated pressure to an extent dependent on lung characteristics (see fig. 28.4).

When the ventilator is operating as a flow generator the tidal volume is virtually fixed because of the fixed inspiratory time. Then the peak alveolar pressure in the inspiratory phase is determined by the fact that it must exceed the minimum pressure in the expiratory phase by an amount equal to the tidal voulme divided by the compliance. In this situation the main effect of adjusting the 'negative pressure' control is to move the whole alveolar-pressure waveform up or down without greatly changing its shape (fig. 28.6f). This control may therefore be regarded as providing a direct control of mean pressure.

REFERENCES

1 Fairley H.B. and Britt B.A. (1964) The adequacy of the air-mix control in ventilators operated from an oxygen source. *Can. med. Ass. J.* **90**, 1394.
2 Mayrhofer O. and Steinbereithner K. (1967) Some observations on the function of the Bird Mk 8 ventilator. *Br. J. Anaesth.* **39**, 519.

CHAPTER 29

The Bird Ventilators

The progressive development of the original Bird Mark 7 ventilator has given rise to a large series of ventilators, all of which operate on the same basic principle. They differ considerably in the limits of various respiratory parameters and the refinement of certain controls. A series of attachments is available for use in conjunction with these ventilators. The Bird Mark 2 and Mark 6 ventilators operate on different principles from the Mark 7. The Bird Mark 3 Chemomechanical Console is a manually-operated chemotherapy unit and is not, therefore, described here. For convenience the entire range of ventilators is listed here in three groups; this is the order in which they are described.

Group A. Variations of the Bird Mark 7 ventilator.

Mark 7.

Mark 8 = Mark 7 with negative-pressure expiratory phase.

Mark 9 = Mark 8 with higher inspiratory flows and cycling pressures.

Mark 10 = preset Mark 7, with flow accelerator and without 'air-mix'.

Mark 14 = Mark 7 with higher inspiratory flows and cycling pressures, flow accelerator, oxygen enrichment, and vernier sensitivity, and without 'air-mix'.

Mark 17 = Mark 14 with 'chest-volume' cycling and without vernier sensitivity.

Group B. Attachments for use with ventilators of Group A.

Mark 4 'Anesthesia Assistor/Controller' attachment.

'Infant J circuit'.

'Q circle Breathing Arrangement'.

Bird Spirometer.

Group C. Other Bird ventilators.

Mark 2.

Mark 6.

THE BIRD MARK 7 VENTILATOR

DESCRIPTION

This compact ventilator (fig. 29.1) is designed for non-rebreathing use in the ward. The driving gas, with or without entrained air, is delivered to the patient. The ventilator can be cycled automatically or be patient-triggered.

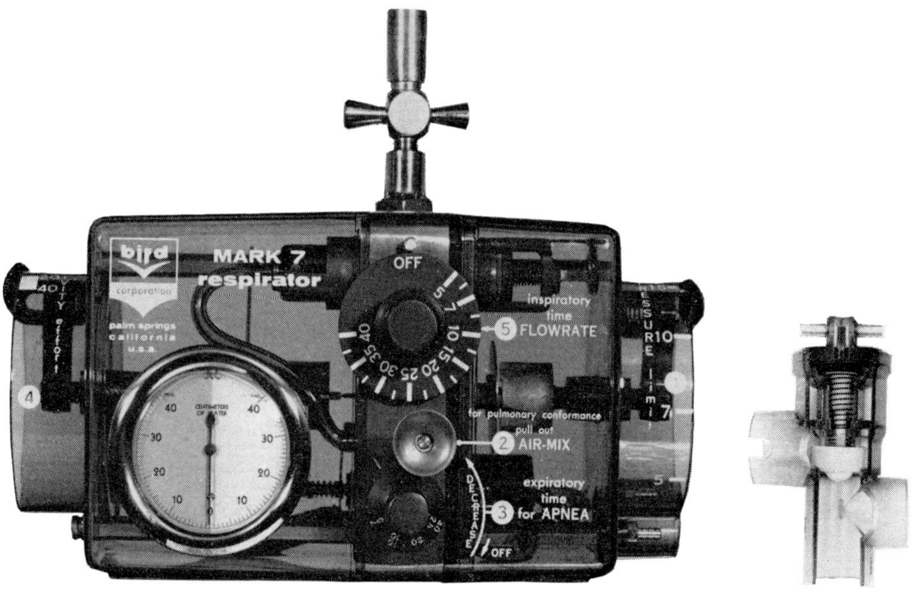

Fig. 29.1. The Bird Mark 7 ventilator and expiratory-valve assembly.
Courtesy of the Bird Corporation.

Oxygen or compressed air at a pressure between 25 and 100 lb/in^2 is supplied at the inlet (3) (fig. 29.2a) and flows through the 'inspiratory time flowrate' control (2) to the ceramic sliding valve (13). The valve (13) has two outlet ports (12) and (21). The port (21) is connected by a small-bore tube (23), running inside the breathing tube, to the chamber above the diaphragm (27) (fig. 29.2b) in the expiratory-valve assembly. The pressure on the diaphragm (27) forces down the small push rod (28) against the force of the spring (29) and so holds the expiratory valve (30) closed. The port (12) of the sliding valve is connected by the tube (4) to the 'air-mix' control (1) which can be set so that the driving gas either passes directly to the main chamber (7) of the ventilator, as shown in fig. 29.2a, and hence to the patient, or through an injector (5), thereby entraining air. If the injector is not in use, the one-way valve (6) prevents gas from the main chamber (7) escaping through the injector to atmosphere.

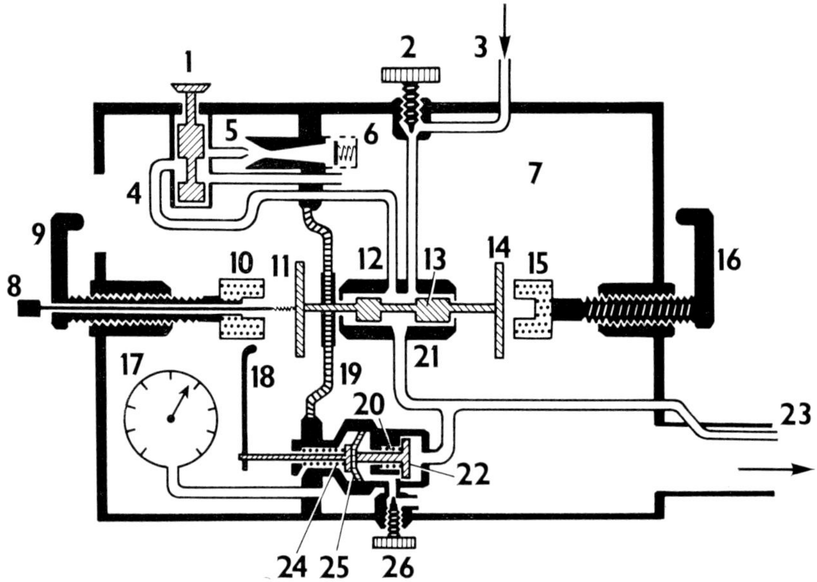

Fig. 29.2a

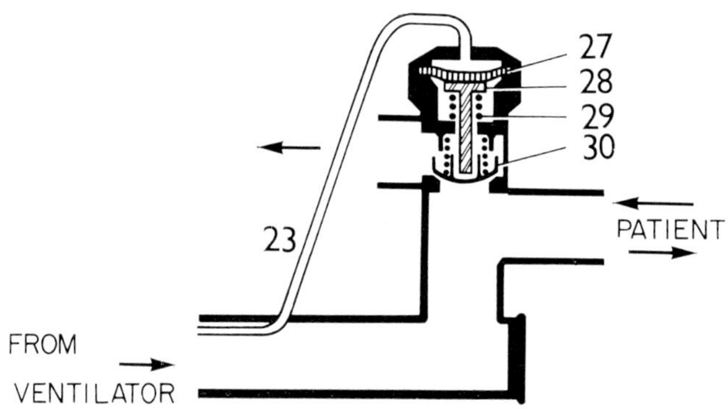

Fig. 29.2b.

Figs. 29.2a and 29.2b. Diagrams of the Bird Mark 7 ventilator and expiratory-valve assembly.

1. 'Air-mix' control
2. 'Inspiratory time flowrate' control
3. Driving-gas inlet
4. Connecting tube
5. Injector
6. One-way valve
7. Main chamber
8. Manual-cycling control
9. 'Sensitivity effort' control
10. Magnet
11. Soft-iron plate
12. Outlet
13. Ceramic sliding valve
14. Soft-iron plate
15. Magnet
16. 'Inspiratory pressure limit' control
17. Manometer
18. Striking arm
19. Diaphragm
20. Spring
21. Outlet
22. Piston
23. Small-bore tube
24. Spring
25. Diaphragm
26. 'Expiratory time' control
27. Diaphragm
28. Push rod
29. Spring
30. Expiratory valve

In any injector the total flow falls as the downstream pressure rises. The characteristics of the particular injector (5) in this ventilator and its one-way valve (6) are such that the flow falls steeply within the range of inflation pressures in the chamber (7). The characteristics of the equivalent injector in the Mark 8 ventilator are shown in fig. 29.5. The manufacturer refers to this steep fall as a 'pneumatic clutch'. During the inspiratory phase therefore, the total inspiratory flow falls, but the oxygen content of the mixture increases, as inflation proceeds.[1,2]

During the inspiratory phase the sliding valve (13) is held in the position shown in fig. 29.2 by the attraction of the magnet (15) for the soft-iron plate (14). Since the expiratory valve (30) is closed, gas flows to the patient and pressure builds up in the main chamber (7) to the right of the diaphragm (19). As soon as the pressure in the main chamber (7) has risen sufficiently for the force applied to the sliding valve by the diaphragm to exceed the pull of the magnet (15) on the plate (14), the sliding valve snaps over. The pull of the magnet (10) for the plate (11) now holds the sliding valve in this expiratory position, and the supply of compressed gas is cut off. The expiratory phase now begins.

The chamber above the diaphragm (27) is now connected through the narrow-bore tube (23), the sliding valve (13), and the 'air-mix' control (1), either with the main chamber (7) or with atmosphere, depending on the setting of the 'air-mix' control (1). The positive pressure behind the diaphragm (27) falls and the diaphragm (27) is forced upwards by the spring (29). The expiratory valve (30) is no longer held closed, and expired gas and gas from the main chamber (7) therefore escape freely through it to atmosphere.

The rods on which the magnets (10, 15) are mounted have screw threads, so that the position of either magnet may be altered by adjusting the graduated controls (9) and (16). The maximum positive pressure during the inspiratory phase is determined by the position of the magnet (15) set by the 'inspiratory pressure limit' control (16). The nearer the magnet (15) is to the plate (14), the higher the pressure which must be reached in order to overcome the force of attraction between them. The 'inspiratory pressure limit' control (16) therefore sets the pressure at which the ventilator cycles from the inspiratory phase to the expiratory phase. For any particular compliance and airway resistance the setting of this control determines the tidal volume, whilst the combined settings of the 'inspiratory time flowrate' control (2) and the 'inspiratory pressure limit' control (16) determine the duration of the inspiratory phase.

The duration of the expiratory phase is controlled by the 'expiratory timer' (20, 22, 24, 25, 26) which is connected to the port (21) of the sliding valve (13). During the inspiratory phase thc pressure of the driving gas overcomes the force of the compression spring (20), and so forces over the piston (22), which in turn pushes out the diaphragm (25) against the pressure of a second spring (24). The diaphragm carries with it the rod and striking arm (18). At the start of the expiratory phase the pressure behind the piston (22) is released through the sliding valve (13) and the 'air-mix' control (1). The piston (22) is returned to its resting position by the spring (20). The diaphragm (25) however can only return, under the influence of the spring (24), at a speed which depends on the escape of the gas behind it through the 'expiratory time' control (26). As the diaphragm (25) returns, the striking arm (18) impinges on the plate (11) and forces it away from the magnet (10). This action continues until the plate (14) reaches a point at which the attraction of the magnet (15) is strong enough to flick over the sliding valve (13) and so start the next inspiratory phase. The duration of the expiratory phase therefore, provided the ventilator is not triggered by the patient, depends on the setting of the 'expiratory time' control (26).

The position of the magnet (10) can be varied by the 'sensitivity effort' control (9). The further away the magnet (10) is from the plate (11) the less is its pull on the plate and the less the force required to overcome it and so cycle the ventilator from the expiratory phase to the inspiratory phase. This force can be reduced to a level at which, should the patient make an inspiratory effort during the expiratory phase, cycling is immediately effected by the slight negative pressure produced in the main chamber (7). The sensitivity of the ventilator to patient-triggering is dependent on the precise setting of the control (9). If the patient does not make any spontaneous inspiratory effort, the ventilator cycles automatically in the usual way.

A small rod (8) runs through the centre of the control (9) and the magnet (10). By pushing or pulling this rod, and thereby changing the position of the sliding valve (13), the ventilator can be cycled manually at any time.

A manometer (17) indicates the pressure in the main chamber (7). The inspiratory pressure may be varied between 5 and 60 cmH_2O. The 'sensitivity effort' control (9) may be adjusted so that the negative pressure required to trigger the ventilator is very slight indeed, or it may be set as high as -5 cmH_2O to prevent patient-triggering. The expiratory time can be varied between 0·5 and 15 seconds. The way in which inspiratory flows vary with pressure depends on the injector characteristics and is similar to that shown in fig. 29.5, for the Mark 8. By adjustment of the various controls, frequencies of up to 80 per minute can be obtained. If the supply of driving gas should fail at any time, and the patient makes an inspiratory effort which produces a negative pressure of -2 cmH_2O, air is drawn in through the one-way valve (6). The expiratory flow may be retarded by fitting a 'multiorificed' cap to the exhaust port of the expiratory-valve assembly. The restriction imposed on the expiratory flow depends on the size of the orifice left open for use. A nebulizer for inhalation therapy is available for use with this ventilator.

FUNCTIONAL ANALYSIS

Detailed laboratory tests have been made on a Bird Mark 8 ventilator but not on a Mark 7. The main difference is that the Mark 8 provides negative pressure in the expiratory phase. If this is borne in mind the detailed functional analysis and discussion of the controls of the Mark 8 can be read to gain information on many of the details of action of the Mark 7. For the sake of completeness, however, a simplified functional analysis of the Mark 7 is given here.

Inspiratory phase

If the 'air-mix' control (1) is pushed in, the patient is connected to the inlet pressure of 25 lb/in^2 or more, via the resistance of the 'inspiratory time flowrate' control (2). The ventilator therefore operates as a flow generator. Ideally the generated flow would be constant but a number of factors (see the account of the Mark 8) cause it to vary systematically during the phase.

If the 'air-mix' control is pulled out, the patient is inflated by the injector (5). Assuming that the characteristics are similar to those of the injector in the Mark 8 (fig. 29.5) the ventilator operates as a pressure generator. Ideally the generated pressure would be constant but a number of factors (see the Mark 8) cause it to vary. It is quite low at the lower settings of the 'inspiratory time flowrate' control (2).

Change-over from inspiratory phase to expiratory phase

This change-over is pressure-cycled: it occurs when the force due to the pressure on the right of the diaphragm (19), which is nearly the same as the mouth pressure, is sufficient to overcome the force of attraction of the magnet (15) for the soft-iron plate (14).

Expiratory phase

During this phase the ventilator operates as a constant, atmospheric, pressure generator: expiration to atmosphere occurs through the expiratory valve (30).

Change-over from expiratory phase to inspiratory phase

This change-over is time-cycled or patient-cycled whichever occurs first: the change-over occurs when the slide valve (13) is moved to the right, either by the striking arm (18) in a preset time due to the controlled decay of pressure to the right of the diaphragm (25), or by the force due to the negative pressure on the right of the diaphragm (19) when the patient makes an inspiratory effort.

THE BIRD MARK 8 VENTILATOR

DESCRIPTION

The Bird Mark 8 (fig. 29.3) is essentially the same as the Bird Mark 7, except that provision is made for the use of negative pressure during the expiratory phase.

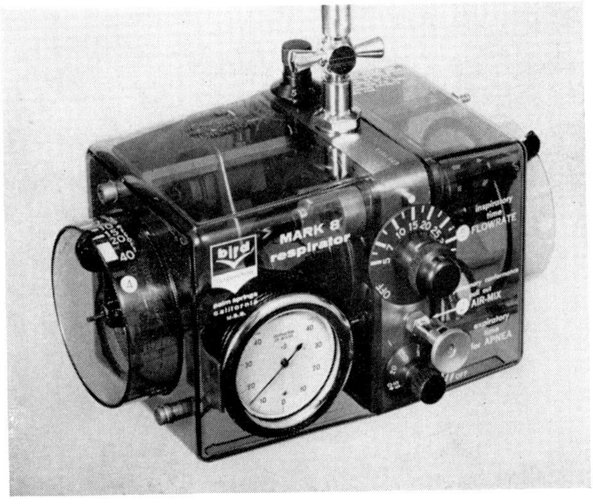

Fig. 29. 3. The Bird Mark 8 ventilator.

Courtesy of the Bird Corporation.

A small-bore tube (32) (figs. 29.4a and 29.4b) supplies driving gas to an injector (31) in the expiratory-valve assembly during the expiratory phase. The flow of gas through the injector produces a negative pressure, the magnitude of which depends on the flow of driving gas, which is set by the 'negative pressure generator' control (4). During the inspiratory phase the high pressure of the gas behind the diaphragm (7) pushes over the piston (8) against the force of its spring, and so cuts off the supply of driving gas to the injector (31). During the expiratory phase the spring returns the piston (8) and driving gas flows to the injector (31). If negative pressure is used the position of the magnet (10) must be suitably adjusted to prevent the ventilator being cycled prematurely by this negative pressure. However, if the 'inspiratory effort' control (9) is set correctly, the ventilator may still be patient-triggered satisfactorily.

When more than 1–2 cmH_2O negative pressure is used the negative-pressure injector (31) entrains gas from the delivery tube as well as from the patient. Air is drawn in past the one-way valve (6) and, if the inflating gas is oxygen, the oxygen concentration of the next inspiration is reduced, even if the 'air-mix' control is pushed in.

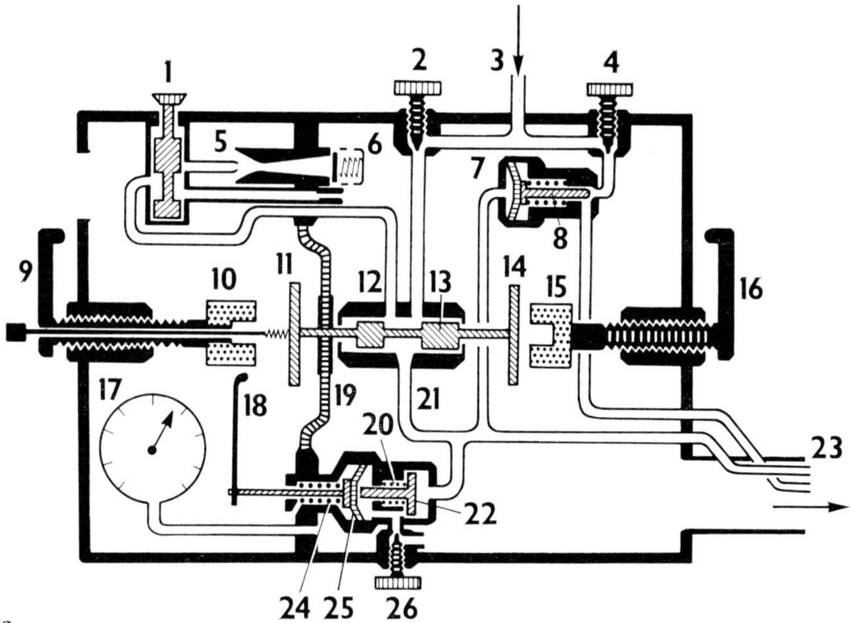

Fig. 29.4a.

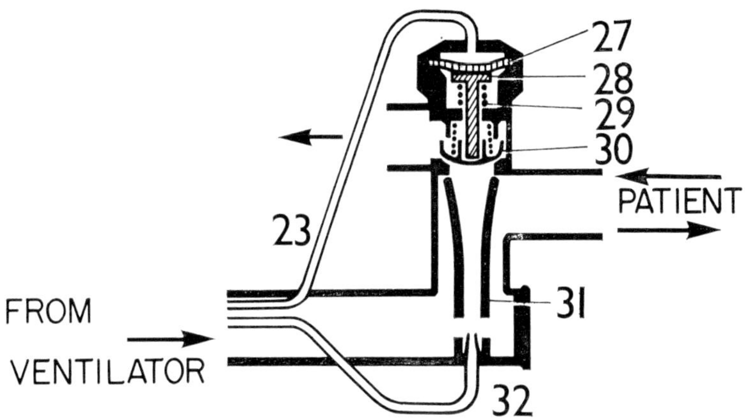

Fig. 29.4b.

Figs. 29.4a and 29.4b. Diagrams of the Bird Mark 8 ventilator and expiratory-valve assembly.

1. 'Air-mix' control
2. 'Inspiratory time flowrate' control
3. Driving-gas inlet
4. 'Negative pressure generator' control
5. Injector
6. One-way valve
7. Diaphragm
8. Piston
9. 'Inspiratory effort' control
10. Magnet
11. Soft-iron plate
12. Outlet
13. Ceramic sliding valve
14. Soft-iron plate
15. Magnet
16. 'Inspiratory pressure limit' control
17. Manometer
18. Striking arm
19. Diaphragm
20. Spring
21. Outlet
22. Piston
23. Small-bore tube
24. Spring
25. Diaphragm
26. 'Expiratory time' control
27. Diaphragm
28. Push rod
29. Spring
30. Expiratory valve
31. Injector
32. Small-bore tube

FUNCTIONAL ANALYSIS

Inspiratory phase

With the 'air-mix' control pushed in, the lungs are connected to the high-pressure driving gas (3) via the high resistance of the 'flowrate' control needle valve (2). In these conditions the ventilator operates fundamentally as a constant-flow generator during the inspiratory phase. This is largely confirmed by curves (a) and (f) in fig. 29.5 which shows the characteristics of the inspiratory and expiratory mechanisms of the ventilator. The slight fall-off in flow with increasing pressure must be attributed to a small leak in the ventilator tested; the effect was less in another model.

With the ventilator cycling regularly the fundamental action is modified a little. When the slide valve (13) first opens to initiate the inspiratory phase, pressure has to

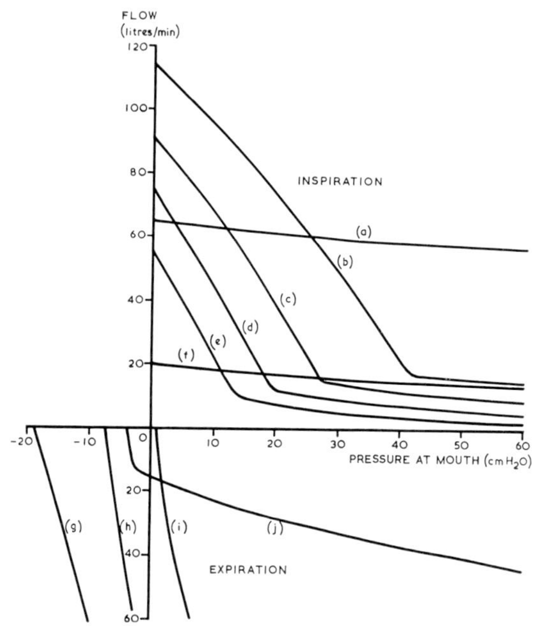

Fig. 29.5. Bird 'Mark 8'. Static flow-pressure characteristics of the inspiratory and expiratory mechanisms when connected to a supply of gas at 50 lb/in^2.

Curve (a) 'Air-mix', pushed in; 'flowrate', maximum.
Curve (b) 'Air-mix', pulled out; 'flowrate', maximum.
Curve (c) 'Air-mix', pulled out; 'flowrate', '29'.
Curve (d) 'Air-mix', pulled out; 'flowrate', '14'.
Curve (e) 'Air-mix', pulled out; 'flowrate', '8½'.
Curve (f) 'Air-mix', pushed in; 'flowrate', '22'.
Curve (g) 'Negative pressure', '−10'.
Curve (h) 'Negative pressure', '−5'.
Curve (i) 'Negative pressure', '0'.
Curve (j) 'Negative pressure', maximum; 'retard' cap fitted, with smallest side hole open.

build up in the high-pressure tubing distal to the slide valve (mostly tube (23)) before the flow reaches its full value. Similarly, when the slide valve (13) closes due to the build-up of pressure on the right of the diaphragm (19), the pressure in the high-pressure tubing takes an appreciable time to fall to the level at which the expiratory valve is allowed to open; during this time therefore the flow into the patient gradually declines. Therefore, as can be seen in the recordings of fig. 29.6, the flow is not constant throughout the inspiratory phase but takes about 0·2 sec to reach its maximum level and decreases

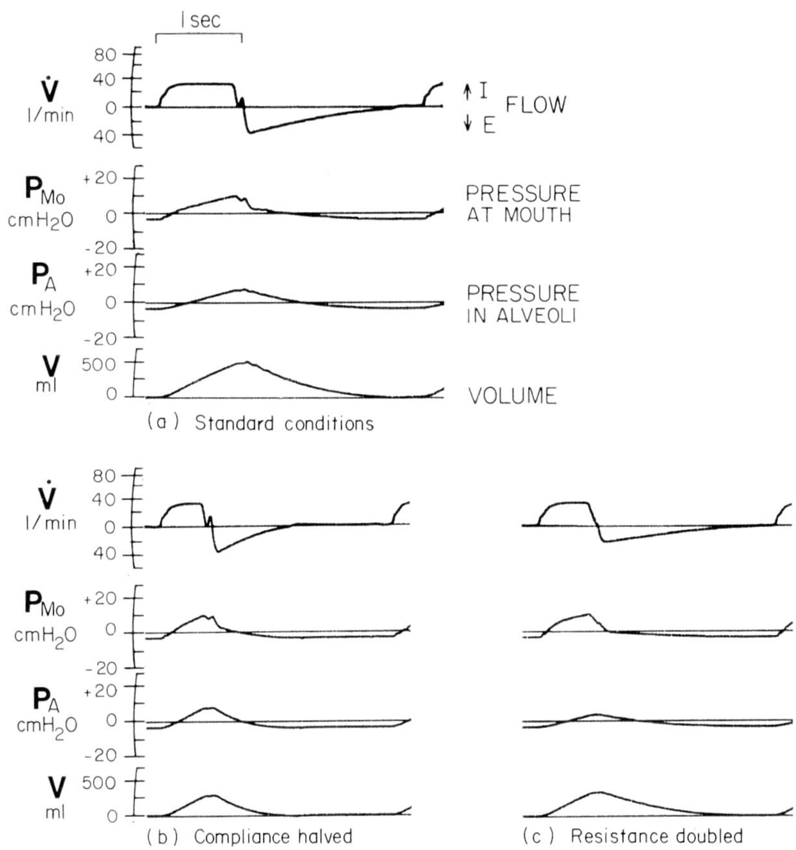

Fig. 29.6. Bird 'Mark 8', with no air entrainment ('air-mix' control pushed in). Recordings showing the effects of changes of lung characteristics.

Standard conditions: driving gas, nitrogen at 50 lb/in^2; 'retard', not used; other controls set to produce a tidal volume of 500 ml at a frequency of 20/min with an inspiratory-expiratory ratio of 1 : 2 and an end-expiratory alveolar pressure of -3 cmH_2O; namely 'inspiratory pressure limit', '7½'; 'expiratory time', '7'; 'flowrate', '38'; 'negative pressure', less than '3'; 'sensitivity', '-3'.

towards zero for the last 0·1 sec. In another model the build-up and decline were slower, taking about 0·3 sec each. However, the build-up and decline are determined by characteristics of the ventilator and are not influenced by the patient, so the ventilator can still be regarded as a flow generator although the pattern of flow is a little more complex than the static characteristics suggest. In fig. 29.6 changes of lung characteristics alter the duration of the phase (for reasons explained below) but the pattern of flow is the same in all cases in the following sense. The flow always builds up in the same way at the start of the phase to the same maximum level, and always decays in the same way at the end of the phase; reductions of duration are at the expense of the central, steady flow, section of the phase. The origin of the oscillations in the flow waveform during the decline is not known but may possibly be associated with the inertia of the three spring-loaded pistons (8, 22, 28).

When the 'air-mix' control is pulled out the lungs are inflated via the injector (5). The characteristics for inflation under these conditions are shown in curves (b) to (e) in fig. 29.5. They show quite a steep fall in flow as pressure rises. In addition to the usual fall of flow as pressure rises, for each setting there is a certain minimum flow which is fairly-well maintained even at very high pressures. This is mainly due to the flow-generating characteristics of the supply to the nebulizer which was fitted to the model tested. (These parts of the characteristics do not come into play in any of the recordings of figs. 29.7 or 29.8.)

At the maximum setting of the 'flowrate' control (2), curve (b), fig. 29.5, the ventilator is equivalent to a fairly-high-constant-pressure generator (about 50 cmH_2O) with considerable series resistance. Therefore, for moderate airway pressures it would approximate to a constant-flow generator as with the 'air-mix' control pushed in. At the lower settings, however, curves (d) and (e), which correspond approximately to the settings used for recordings fig. 29.7 and most of fig. 29.8 respectively, the ventilator must be regarded as a low-pressure generator with some series resistance. Therefore the recordings might be expected to show an inspiratory flow waveform which declined during the phase as the mouth pressure built up, the decline varying with lung characteristics. However, with the 'air-mix' control pulled out, the build-up of driving pressure in tube (23) is even slower than with it pushed in, taking 0·5 sec to reach 90% of its maximum. Therefore, for most of the phase, the supply to the injector is gradually increasing, so that the equivalent generated pressure is also increasing, towards its maximum, at the same time as the mouth pressure is increasing. The net result (fig. 29.7) is a flow waveform with a relatively-flat top. However, the height of the flat top (the magnitude of the flow for the greater part of the phase) is reduced by about 15% when the compliance is halved (b) or the resistance doubled (c).

Change-over from inspiratory phase to expiratory phase

Fundamentally this change-over is pressure-cycled. It is initiated when the pressure on the right of the diaphragm (19) becomes sufficient to overcome the pull of the magnet (15)

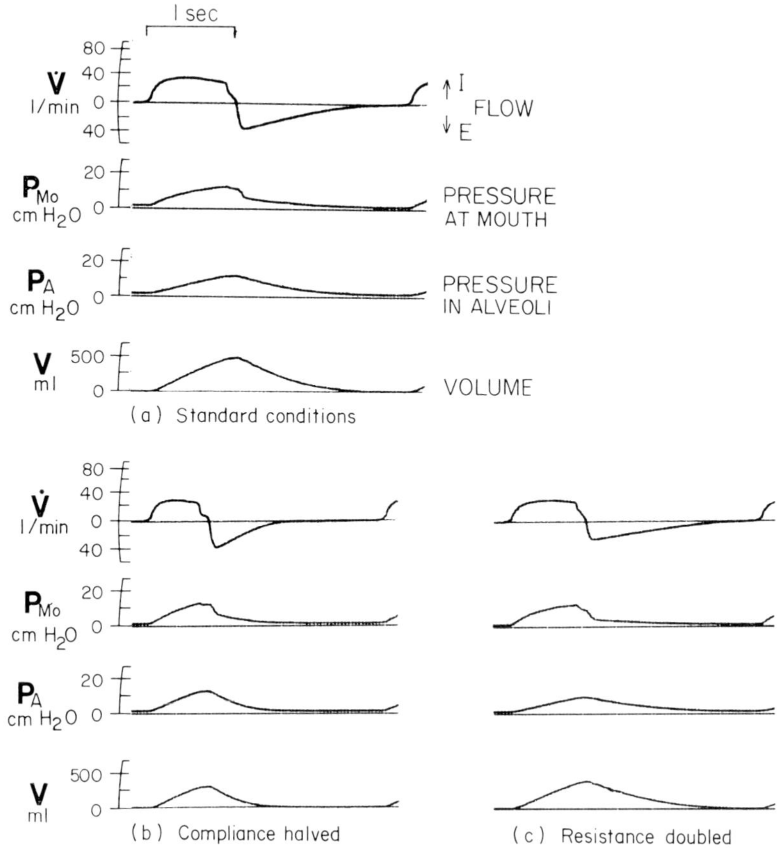

Fig. 29.7. Bird 'Mark 8', with air entrainment ('air-mix' control pulled out). Recordings showing the effects of changes of lung characteristics.

Standard conditions: driving gas, nitrogen at 50 lb/in^2; 'retard', not used; 'negative pressure', off; other controls set to produce a tidal volume of 500 ml at a frequency of 20/min with an inspiratory-expiratory ratio of 1 : 2; namely 'inspiratory pressure limit', '10'; 'expiratory time', less than '7'; 'flowrate', '15'; 'sensitivity', minimum.

on the soft-iron plate (14). However, as explained above, there is then a short, fixed delay, during which the pressure in the tube (23) decays, before the expiratory valve is allowed to open and the change-over actually to occur. In figs. 29.6 and 29.7 it can be seen that, despite changes of lung characteristics, the inspiratory flow always starts to decline when the mouth pressure has reached the same critical value, and that in all cases the phase finally ends 0·1 sec later.

Expiratory phase

With the 'negative pressure' control (4) turned off (fig. 29.7) the ventilator operates as a constant, atmospheric, pressure generator throughout this phase. The resistance of the expiratory-valve assembly is about half the 'standard' airway resistance so that the pressure at the mouth does not fall immediately to zero at the beginning of the expiratory phase, but the flow waveform shows typical changes when the lung characteristics are altered.

From the characteristics in fig. 29.5 it is evident that when the 'negative pressure' control is turned on (curves (g) and (h)) the ventilator must still be regarded as a constant-pressure generator (now negative) with only a little more series resistance than with the 'negative pressure' control turned off (curve (i)). This is confirmed by the recordings of fig. 29.6 in which the expiratory flow curves with negative pressure are very similar to the corresponding ones, without negative pressure, in fig. 29.7. The sudden slight drop in flow, towards the end of the expiratory phase in fig. 29.6a and about half-way through the phase in fig. 29.6b, corresponds to the moment at which the pressure at the entrainment port of the negative-pressure injector becomes sufficiently negative to start entraining air through the one-way valve (6) in the ventilator, causing a drop in the flow entrained from the lungs. A corollary of this is that the inflating gas in the next inspiratory phase contains a higher proportion of air than otherwise and, even with the 'air-mix' control pushed in, 100% oxygen cannot be delivered. This phenomenon has been studied in detail by Stoddart.[2]

If the negative-pressure control is set to maximum and, at the same time, the 'retard' cap is fitted over the expiratory port, (curve (j) in fig. 29.5) the system makes a fair approximation to a constant-flow generator for all positive mouth pressures. However this involves the usage of 25 litres/min of driving gas during the expiratory phase.

Change-over from expiratory phase to inspiratory phase

This change-over occurs when the force tending to move the slide valve (13) to the right is sufficient to overcome the attraction of the magnet (10) for the soft-iron plate (11), so that the slide valve suddenly moves to the right and thereby initiates a fresh inspiratory phase. Two factors affect the force tending to move the slide valve to the right during the expiratory phase. Firstly, the escape of gas from behind the diaphragm (25) past the 'expiratory time' needle valve (26) allows the striking arm (18) to press increasingly on the soft-iron plate (11). Secondly, any pressure difference across the diaphragm (19) helps or hinders the force exerted by the striking arm (18) depending on the direction of the pressure difference. The relative importance of these two factors in bringing about the change-over depends on the circumstances.

A common situation is with the ventilator operating as a constant-pressure generator during expiration and with the time constant of the system (lungs plus ventilator) fairly short, so that the mouth pressure, and hence the pressure on the right of the diaphragm, falls to the generated pressure early in the expiratory phase and then remains constant. In this situation moderate changes of lung characteristics do not alter the pressure difference existing across the diaphragm (19) in the last part of the phase, the termination of which is therefore brought about solely by the preset decay of pressure in the timing mechanism (20, 22, 24, 25, 26), i.e. the change-over is purely time-cycled. This is the situation illustrated in figs. 29.6 and 29.7: the mouth pressure always falls to the generated pressure before the end of the phase and, when the lung characteristics are changed, the expiratory time is unaltered.

One way in which pressure difference across the diaphragm can influence the change-over is if, in the common situation just described, the 'sensitivity' control (9) is set so that a small negative pressure (or a pressure slightly more negative than that being generated) when applied to the right of the diaphragm is sufficient to trigger the movement of the slide valve to the right. In this situation an inspiratory effort by the patient can bring about the change-over which is therefore time-cycled or patient-cycled whichever occurs first.

A second way in which pressure difference can influence the change-over arises if the expiratory resistance is very high, either because of a very high respiratory resistance in the patient or because the 'retard' cap is in use. In these circumstances the mouth pressure continues to decline slowly throughout any normal length of expiratory phase. The hindrance, which the pressure difference across the diaphragm (19) offers to the initiation of the change-over, progressively decreases throughout the phase. Therefore, if the compliance becomes reduced the hindrance decreases more rapidly during the phase, and the striking arm (18) will overcome the hindrance earlier. In other words the change-over is no longer purely time-cycled but is influenced by the fall of pressure on the right of the diaphragm. This situation is not fully illustrated here but, by comparing (f) with (a) in fig. 29.8, it can be seen that, when the 'retard' cap is brought into use, the fall in mouth pressure becomes slower and the expiratory phase is prolonged.

CONTROLS

Total ventilation

This cannot be directly controlled but is equal to the product of tidal volume and respiratory frequency.

Tidal volume

This is indirectly controlled by adjustment of the cycling pressure by means of the 'inspiratory pressure limit' control (16) (fig. 29.8b). However, when the setting of this is increased, not only is the tidal volume increased but so also is the inspiratory time (fig. 29.8b) unless a compensating increase is made in the setting of the 'flowrate' control.

The tidal volume is also affected by several of the other controls. When the setting of the negative-pressure control (4) is increased (fig. 29.8e) the alveolar pressure is made more negative by the end of expiration without much alteration of the end-inspiratory alveolar pressure; the tidal volume is therefore increased. Increasing the 'flowrate' setting increases the pressure drop across the airway resistance and hence leads to cycling at a lower alveolar pressure and so to a reduced tidal volume (fig. 29.8d). Bringing the 'retard' cap into use (fig. 29.8f) or decreasing the 'expiratory time' setting in the presence of high expiratory resistance (not illustrated) may prevent the alveolar pressure from falling fully to the generated pressure in the expiratory phase and so reduce the tidal volume a little.

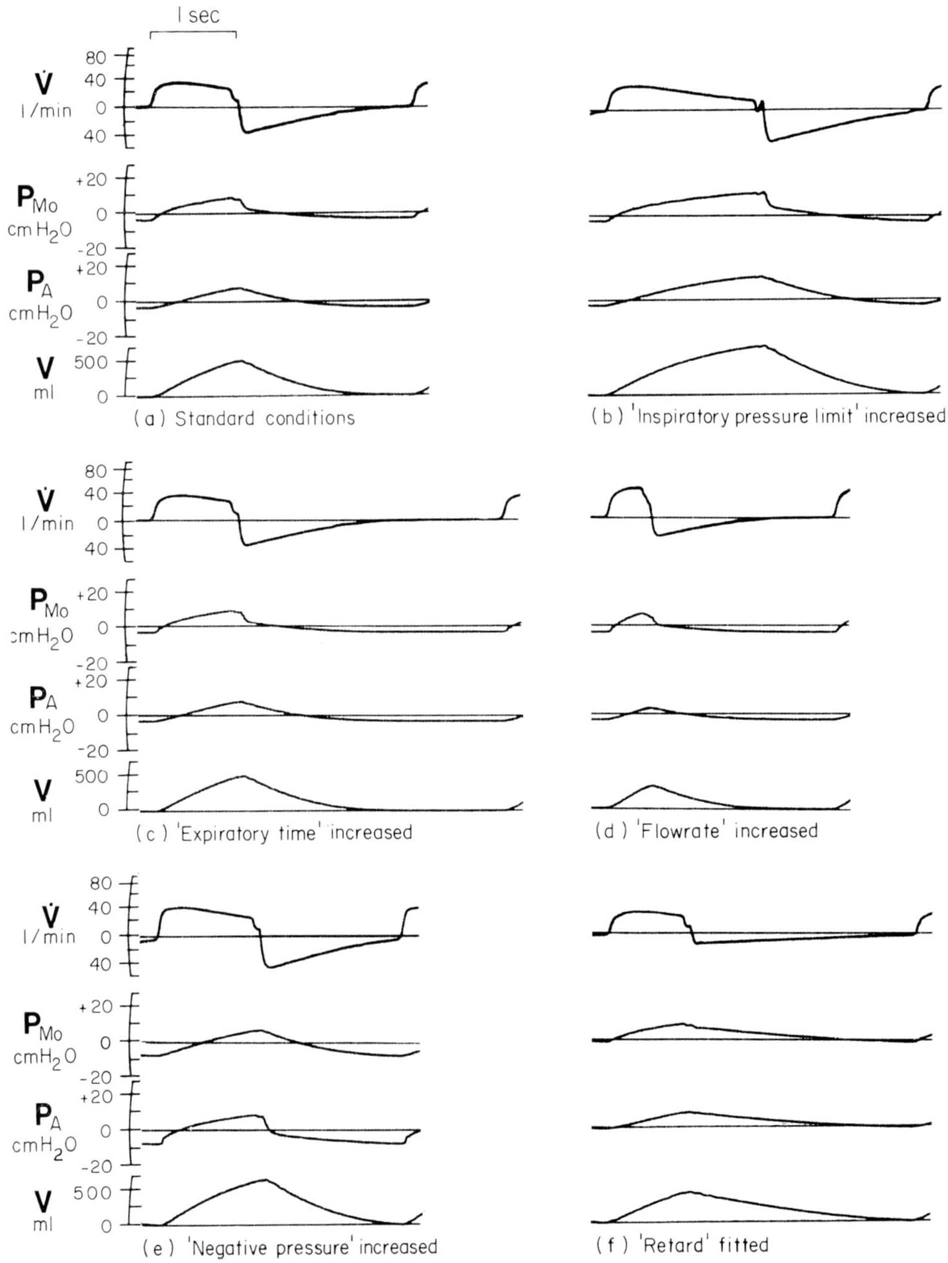

Since the tidal volume is indirectly determined by means of the cycling pressure it is considerably reduced by a decreased compliance or increased resistance (figs. 29.6 and 29.7).

Respiratory frequency and inspiratory-expiratory ratio

Neither of these parameters can be directly controlled but both are determined by the separately-variable inspiratory and expiratory times.

The inspiratory time cannot be directly controlled but the principal means of influencing it indirectly is by means of the 'flowrate' control whose full title on the ventilator is 'inspiratory time FLOWRATE'. Increasing the inspiratory flow by means of this control decreases the inspiratory time but it also increases the pressure drop across the airway resistance and hence decreases the tidal volume (fig. 29.8d). Therefore a compensatory increase of the 'inspiratory pressure' control is required to change the inspiratory time without changing the tidal volume.

The inspiratory time is influenced by any change of tidal volume, either deliberate (fig. 29.8b), or incidental to a change of control setting (fig. 29.8e and f), or resulting from a change in lung characteristics (figs. 29.6 and 29.7).

The expiratory time can usually be directly controlled by the 'expiratory time' control (fig. 29.8c) but it is influenced by other controls. Thus, increasing the 'negative pressure' setting increases the pressure difference across the diaphragm (19) aiding the return of the slide valve to the right and causing this to occur earlier, shortening the expiratory time (fig. 29.8e) unless the 'sensitivity' control (9) is adjusted to compensate. Similarly, adding the 'retard' cap to the expiratory valve delays the fall in pressure at the mouth (on the right of the diaphragm) and prolongs the expiratory phase (fig. 29.8f).

Normally, when the ventilator is purely time-cycled, the expiratory time is, of course, uninfluenced by changes of lung characteristics (fig. 29.6 and 29.7). However, when the 'retard' cap is in use, or if the airway resistance is very high, the fall of mouth pressure, even in the later part of the phase, becomes dependent on lung characteristics and hence so does the expiratory time (see the functional analysis above).

Since all the controls have some influence on either the inspiratory or expiratory

---

Fig. 29.8. Bird 'Mark 8', with air entrainment ('air-mix' control pulled out). Recordings showing the effects of changes in the settings of the controls.

(a) Standard conditions as in fig. 29.6 except that the 'air-mix' control was pulled out and the settings of the controls required to produce the standard pattern of ventilation were as follows: 'inspiratory pressure limit', '7'; 'expiratory time', between '7' and '15'; 'flowrate', '8½'; 'negative pressure', less than '3'; 'sensitivity', '−3'.

(b) 'Inspiratory pressure limit' increased to '10' to produce a tidal volume of 750 ml.

(c) 'Expiratory time' increased to greater than '15' to produce an expiratory time of 3 sec.

(d) 'Flowrate' increased to '15'.

(e) 'Negative pressure' increased to '−5'.

(f) 'Retard' cap fitted with next-to-smallest side hole open.

time, the respiratory frequency and inspiratory-expiratory ratio are both dependent on all the controls—and also on lung characteristics.

Inspiratory waveforms

If the 'air-mix' control is pushed in, the ventilator operates as a flow generator with the flow constant for most of the phase at a level which is uninfluenced by lung characteristics (fig. 29.6). If the 'air-mix' control is pulled out, so that the injector (5) is brought into use, the ventilator operates fundamentally as a pressure generator. However, for reasons explained in the functional analysis above, the result is usually still a relatively-flat-topped waveform of flow, although the height of the flat top varies with lung characteristics (fig. 29.7). However, if the inspiratory time is made long (1·5 sec or more) by using a low setting of the 'flowrate' control or, as in fig. 29.8b, by using a high setting of the 'inspiratory pressure limit' control, then the inspiratory flow does fall off gradually during a large part of the phase. Thus the two positions of the 'air-mix' control do provide some limited choice of inspiratory flow waveform but the choice of position will often be dictated by considerations of economy of driving gas or of the oxygen content desired in the gas delivered to the patient.

Expiratory waveforms

Normally the ventilator operates as a constant-pressure generator during the expiratory phase so that the expiratory flow starts high and then declines exponentially in a manner dependent upon the lung characteristics. However, a radically-different expiratory flow waveform can be achieved by setting the 'negative pressure' control high and the 'retard' device to give a high resistance to expiration. Then the ventilator approximates to a constant-flow generator as explained in the functional analysis above.

Pressure limits

The peak inspiratory pressure at the mouth is equal to the cycling pressure; the peak alveolar pressure is less than this by an amount equal to the airway resistance multiplied by the inspiratory flow. During the expiratory phase the ventilator normally operates as a constant-pressure generator, so that the alveolar pressure usually falls to the generated pressure by the end of the phase, and therefore the end-expiratory and end-inspiratory alveolar pressures are largely independent.

THE BIRD MARK 9 VENTILATOR

DESCRIPTION

This ventilator (fig. 29.9) is a development of the Bird Mark 8. It differs from the Mark 8 in that much higher inspiratory flows and pressures are available. The 'air-mix' control is replaced by one which allows 'low range' or 'high range' flows to be selected. The upper limit of flow on the 'low range' is 200 litres/min at a back-pressure of about 34 cmH_2O; on the 'high range' the limit is 272 litres/min at about 55 cmH_2O. Inspiratory positive pressures approaching 260 cmH_2O can be achieved with this ventilator.

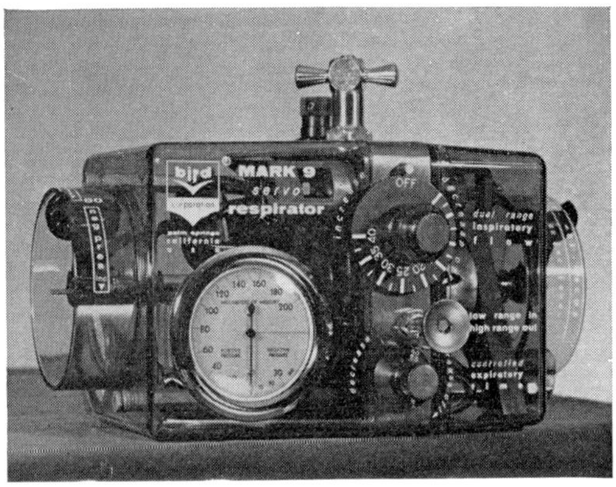

Fig. 29.9. The Bird Mark 9 ventilator.

Courtesy of the Bird Corporation.

FUNCTIONAL ANALYSIS

This should be very similar to that of the Mark 8 ventilator with the following exceptions. In the inspiratory phase, in the absence of the 'air-mix' control, pure constant-flow generation will not be available; the ventilator will always operate as a pressure generator although the generated pressure may be high. The maximum cycling pressure is much higher than in the Mark 8.

THE BIRD MARK 10 VENTILATOR

DESCRIPTION

This ventilator (fig. 29.10) is a development of the Mark 7, which is designed for use with a minimum of supervision. Only two controls are readily adjustable, one for the inspiratory flow, marked 'Air' (2) (fig. 29.11), and the other for expiratory time, marked

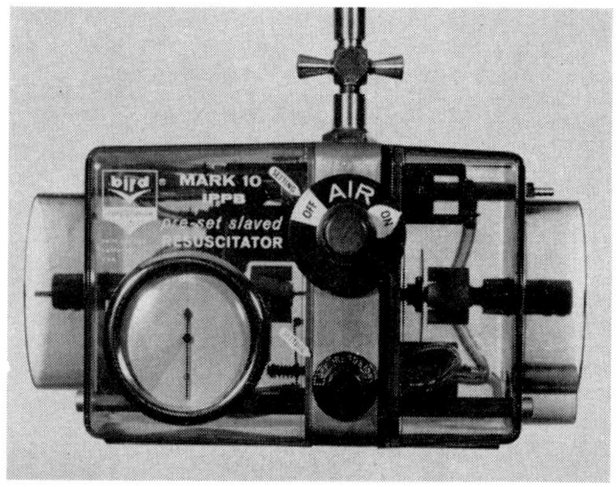

Fig. 29.10. The Bird Mark 10 ventilator.

Courtesy of the Bird Corporation.

'Resus' (26). The remaining controls are preset. The cycling pressure is preset at 15 cmH_2O. There is no 'air-mix' control; the driving gas flows directly to the injector (5), the characteristics of which are such as to give 40–60% entrained air in the inflating-gas mixture. The sensitivity for triggering is preset to -2 cmH_2O.

Normally the ventilator cycles from the inspiratory phase to the expiratory phase when sufficient pressure has built up behind the diaphragm (19) to force over the ceramic sliding valve (13). In the event of the development of an accidental leak this cycling will be delayed, the extent of the delay being dependent on the magnitude of the leak. If the leak is big enough, the machine might be arrested in inflation. However this is prevented by the 'flow accelerator' mechanism (1, 4, 7) which, after a delay, increases the flow of driving gas to the injector (5).

At the start of the inspiratory phase the driving gas flows through the inner main jet of the injector (5). The piston (7) is pushed over against the force of its spring by the pressure of the driving gas behind its diaphragm. This allows the inflating gas to flow from the preset 'lapse period' control (1), through a channel in the piston (7), to the chamber beneath the piston (4). Pressure builds up here until, after a time determined by the flow through the 'lapse period' control (1), the piston (4) moves upwards against the force of its spring. Additional inflating gas can now flow through the outer secondary jet of the injector (5). The increased flow from the injector is still-further enhanced by the increased entrainment of air, and consequently the build-up of pressure in the main chamber of the ventilator to the preset cycling pressure of 15 cmH_2O is accelerated.

The 'lapse period' control (1) is normally preset so that if the pressure of the driving gas is 50 lb/in² the 'flow accelerator' operates after a delay of 4 seconds. This delay time is 3 seconds if the supply pressure is 55 lb/in², and 5 seconds if it is 45 lb/in². Although usually not necessary, some adjustment of this 'lapse period' control (1) is possible using a special key.

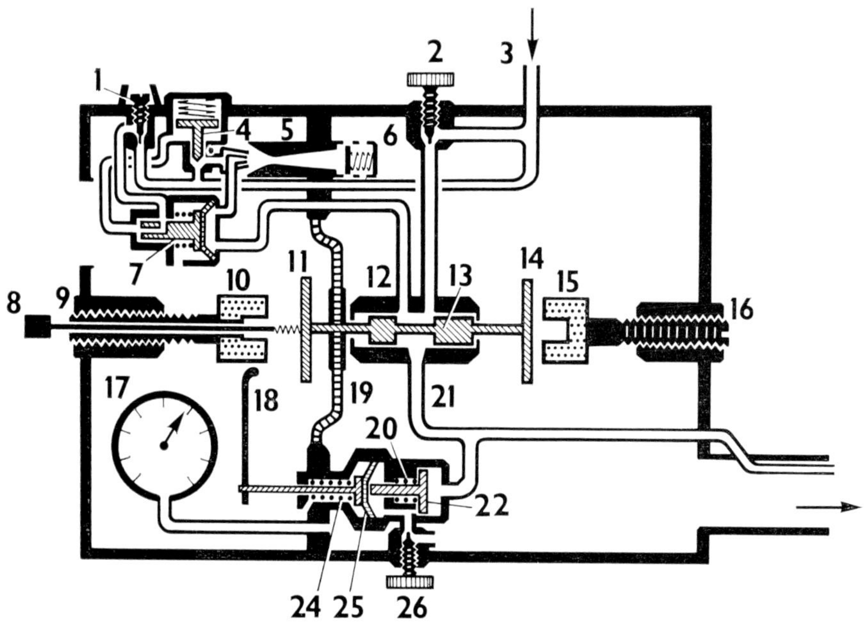

Fig. 29.11. Diagram of the Bird Mark 10 ventilator.

1. Preset 'lapse period' control
2. 'Air' control
3. Driving-gas inlet
4. Piston
5. Injector
6. One-way valve
7. Piston
8. Manual-cycling control
9. Preset 'sensitivity effort' control
10. Magnet
11. Soft-iron plate
12. Outlet
13. Ceramic sliding valve
14. Soft-iron plate
15. Magnet
16. Preset cycling-pressure control
17. Manometer
18. Striking arm
19. Diaphragm
20. Spring
21. Outlet
22. Piston
24. Spring
25. Diaphragm
26. 'Resus' control

At the end of the inspiratory phase the supply of driving gas through the sliding valve (13) is cut off, and the piston (7) returns to its resting position. The supply of driving gas to the chamber below the piston (4) is now cut off, and the chamber is connected to atmosphere through the channel in the piston (7). The piston (4) returns to its resting position and the inflating gas is no longer supplied to the secondary jet of the injector (5). Apart from this, the functioning of this ventilator during the expiratory phase is identical with that described for the Mark 7 ventilator.

Should it be necessary, the preset cycling pressure and the patient-triggering sensitivity can be altered by resetting the controls (16) and (9) respectively using special tools.

FUNCTIONAL ANALYSIS

The functioning of this ventilator is similar to that of the Mark 7 (or the Mark 8 with negative pressure switched off) with the following exceptions. Since the patient is always inflated via the injector, the ventilator will always operate as a pressure generator. However, when the 'flow accelerator' comes into action, the generated pressure increases to a new level. The cycling pressure, patient-triggering sensitivity, and time of onset of the increase of generated pressure are all preset.

THE BIRD MARK 14 VENTILATOR

DESCRIPTION

This ventilator (fig. 29.12) is a development of the Bird Mark 7 which incorporates the 'flow accelerator' (leak-compensating) mechanism of the Mark 10. It can deliver high inspiratory flows (approaching 200 litres/min) and can be set for high cycling pressures

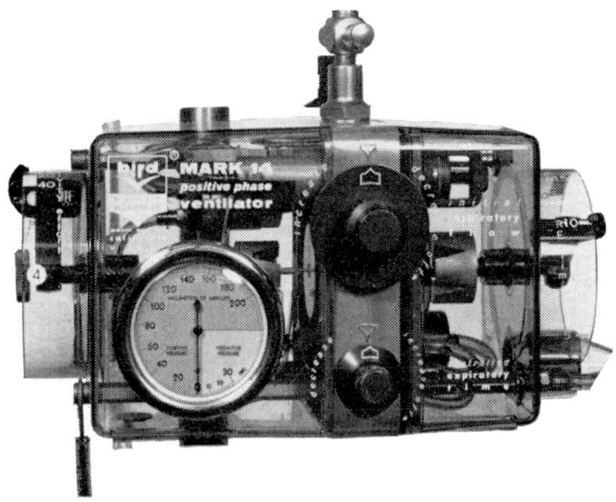

Fig. 29.12. The Bird Mark 14 ventilator.

Courtesy of the Bird Corporation.

(up to 95 cmH_2O). There is no 'air-mix' control: inflation always occurs via the injector. All controls are adjustable, including the speed of onset of the 'flow-accelerator' mechanism, and the patient-triggering sensitivity control is fitted with a vernier for ease of setting. The inflating gas may be enriched with oxygen by supplying a continuous flow of oxygen to the chamber containing the entrainment port of the injector.

FUNCTIONAL ANALYSIS

Qualitatively this is the same as for the Mark 10 ventilator but higher cycling pressures are available. In addition the cycling pressure, the patient-triggering sensitivity, and the time at which the 'flow accelerator' comes into operation are all adjustable instead of preset.

THE BIRD MARK 17 VENTILATOR

DESCRIPTION

The Mark 17 (fig. 29.13) incorporates all the features of the Mark 7, together with the automatic-leak-compensation and oxygen-enrichment facilities of the Mark 14 and a volume-cycling device operated by a 'sentinel' band round the patient's chest (fig. 29.14).

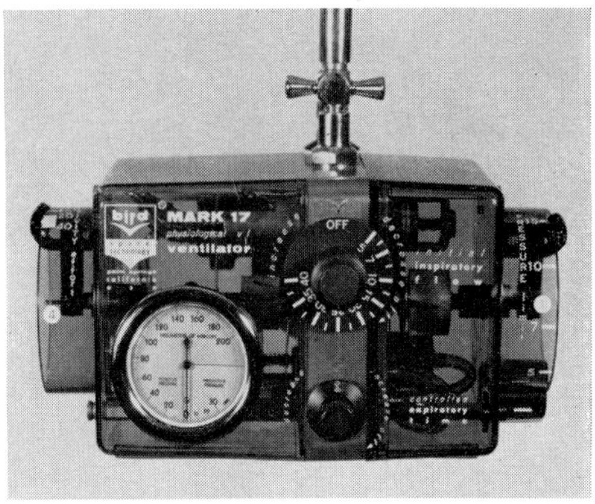

Fig. 29.13. The Bird Mark 17 ventilator.
Courtesy of the Bird Corporation.

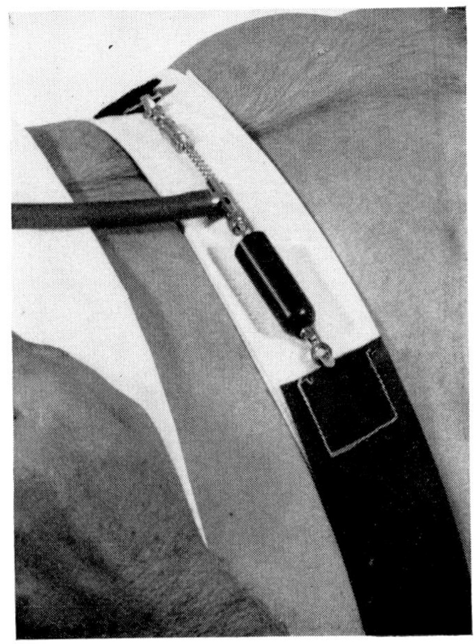

Fig. 29.14. 'Sentinel band' of the Bird Mark 17 ventilator.
Courtesy of the Bird Corporation.

The maximum inspiratory flow, with the 'flow accelerator' (1, 4, 7, fig. 29.15) in use, is 163 litres/min at a back pressure of 42 cmH_2O. The maximum cycling pressure is 120 cmH_2O.

The volume-cycling device consists essentially of a servo-mechanism which, when a preset circumferential expansion of the chest has occurred, automatically terminates the inspiratory phase.

During the inspiratory phase gas from the main chamber of the ventilator flows past a constriction to the chamber above the diaphragm (2). This chamber is connected to the 'sentinel valve' assembly (28–32) on the chest band.

When the chest band has been fitted to the patient, the 'sentinel valve' (29–31) is adjusted by rotating the stretch screw (28) so that during the inspiratory phase there is a free connexion, through the valve, between the chamber above the diaphragm (2) and atmosphere. As the chest continues to expand during the inspiratory phase the pull

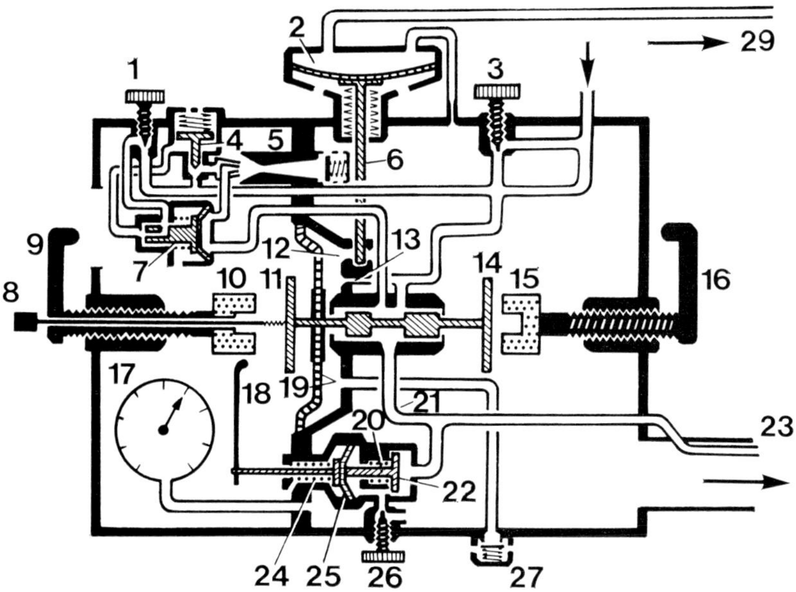

Fig. 29.15a

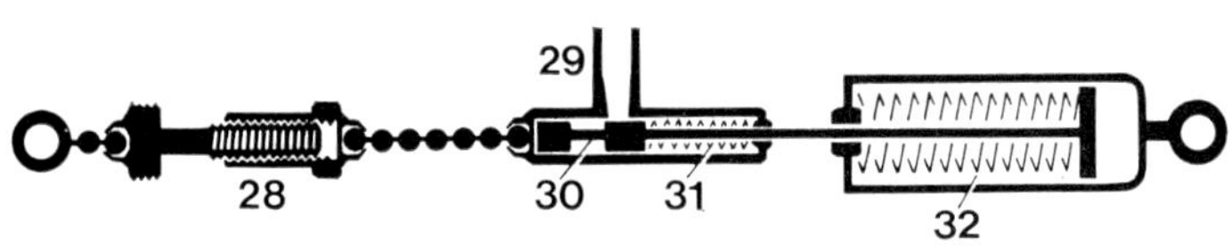

Fig. 29.15b.

Figs. 29.15a and 29.15b. Diagram of the Bird Mark 17 ventilator and 'sentinel band'.

1. 'Terminal inspiratory flow' control
2. Diaphragm
3. 'Initial inspiratory flow' control
4. Piston
5. Injector
6. Push rod
7. Piston
8. Manual-cycling control
9. 'Sensitivity effort' control
10. Magnet
11. Soft-iron plate
12. Small chamber
13. Restricted connexion
14. Soft-iron plate
15. Magnet
16. 'Inspiratory pressure limit' control
17. Manometer
18. Striking arm
19. Diaphragm
20. Spring
21. Outlet
22. Piston
23. Small-bore tube
24. Spring
25. Diaphragm
26. 'Expiratory time' control
27. Safety-valve limiting pressure in small chamber (12)
28. Stretch screw
29. Connexion to chamber (2) of ventilator
30. Sliding bobbin
31. Spring
32. Spring

exerted by compression of the spring (32) increases steadily, overcoming the force of the spring (31), and drawing the sliding bobbin of the valve over to its extreme closed position. The pressure of gas now pushes down the diaphragm (2) and the rod (6) against the force of its spring. The lower end of the rod (6) now blocks the channel between the main chamber of the ventilator and the small chamber (12) beside the cycling diaphragm (19). There is a constant 'bleed' of driving gas (2·5 litres/min) through the constriction (13) to the chamber (12). Therefore, as soon as the outlet from the chamber (12) is blocked, the pressure within it rises rapidly, moving over the diaphragm (19) and cycling the ventilator to expiration.

As soon as the patient's chest begins to collapse, the sentinel valve reopens and pressure above the diaphragm (2) falls. The rod (6) is returned to its resting position by its spring, the chamber (12) is reconnected with the main chamber of the ventilator, and pressure in the chamber (12) falls to atmospheric. A safety-valve (27) eliminates any possibility of the pressure within the chamber (12) ever rising high enough to rupture the diaphragm (19).

Should the tension of the chest band be reduced as a result of breakage or displacement, the spring (32) ceases to exert a pull on the sliding bobbin. In this event, the spring (31) holds the bobbin in its resting position in which the valve is closed. Cycling from the inspiratory phase to the expiratory phase is no longer dependent on the expansion of the chest, but occurs when the pressure above the diaphragm (2), which, in these circumstances, follows the pressure in the main chamber of the ventilator, is sufficient to move the rod (6) down. This pressure depends on the characteristics of the spring below the diaphragm. The spring normally fitted allows cycling to occur when the pressure reaches 19 cmH_2O, but two alternative springs are available which allow cycling at 23 and 27 cmH_2O respectively.

FUNCTIONAL ANALYSIS

The functioning of this ventilator is similar to that of the Mark 14 except for the provision of volume-cycling. Because of the many unusual factors of the volume-cycling mechanism a complete, theoretical, functional analysis is given here.

Inspiratory phase

In this phase the ventilator operates as a pressure generator due to the injector characteristics. For the first part of the phase the generated pressure is, ideally, constant (see Mark 8) but, after a delay which can be adjusted by means of the 'terminal inspiratory flow' control (1), the generated pressure increases progressively towards a new level.

Change-over from inspiratory phase to expiratory phase

The Bird Mark 17 is designed so that this change-over can be made to occur when the volume of gas in the lungs rises to a critical level. When this critical volume is reached the tube (29) is occluded by the thickened end of bobbin (30). This usually results in rod (6) being pushed down, shutting off chamber (12), and allowing the pressure within it to rise rapidly to a level at which the diaphragm (19) and the slide valve are moved to the left and the inspiratory phase is ended. Thus the change-over is volume-cycled.

However, there are two conditions which must be satisfied if the change-over is to occur in the manner just described. The first is that, when the critical lung volume is reached, the pressure in the main chamber shall be greater than 19 cmH_2O (for the standard spring around push rod (6)). If the pressure is less than this, the rod (6) will not be pushed down until the lungs have been inflated beyond the critical volume and the pressure in the main chamber has reached 19 cmH_2O. In other words the change-over becomes pressure-cycled after the critical volume has been exceeded.

The second condition is that the pressure in the main chamber shall not have reached the cycling pressure set by the 'inspiratory pressure limit' control (16) before the critical volume is reached. If the cycling pressure is reached first, the change-over becomes pressure-cycled before the critical volume has been reached.

In conventional volume-cycling mechanisms the cycling volume is sensed somewhere in the ventilator and there is always the possibility that some different, usually lesser, volume reaches the patient's lungs. This possibility is eliminated in the Mark 17 volume-cycling mechanism which is unique in sensing the volume in the patient's chest. However it should be noted that cycling occurs at a particular *absolute* lung volume and not after a particular *change* of lung volume. Therefore, if the end-expiratory lung volume were to increase—perhaps because an increase in resistance prevented complete expiration—the end-inspiratory lung volume would be unaltered and the tidal volume would be decreased. In addition, the sensing of lung volume is indirect and any change which might occur in the relationship between lung volume and chest circumference would alter the end-inspiratory lung volume at which cycling occurred.

Expiratory phase

In this phase the Mark 17, like the Marks 7, 10, and 14, operates as a constant, atmospheric, pressure generator: expired gas flows to atmosphere through the expiratory valve.

Change-over from expiratory phase to inspiratory phase

As in the Marks 7, 9, 10, and 14, this change-over is time-cycled or patient-cycled whichever occurs first.

THE BIRD MARK 4

'ANESTHESIA ASSISTOR/CONTROLLER' ATTACHMENT

DESCRIPTION

This unit (fig. 29.16) is basically a 'bag-in-bottle' assembly designed to allow a Bird Mark 7, Mark 8, or Mark 10 ventilator to be used for anaesthesia. The Mark 7, 8, or 10 ventilator is the source of driving gas and acts as the main control unit of the combination.

The driving-gas inlet of a Mark 7, 8 or 10 ventilator is connected to the Mark 4

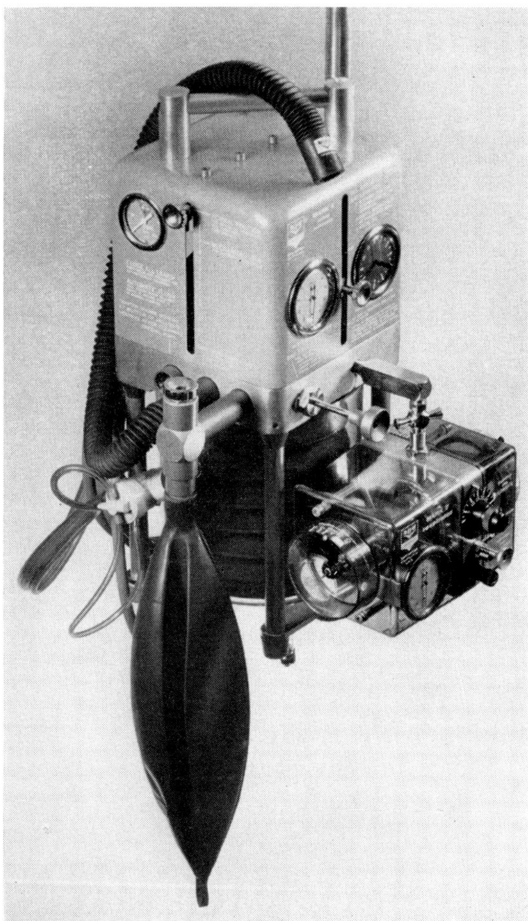

Fig. 29.16. The Bird Mark 4 attachment connected to the Bird Mark 7 ventilator.
Courtesy of the Bird Corporation.

assembly by a rigid gas-tight union, through which driving gas, supplied at the inlet (1) (fig. 29.17) of the Mark 4 assembly, flows to the ventilator.

The inflating valve of the Mark 7, 8, or 10 ventilator is fitted to the port (21) of the rigid plastic pressure chamber (20) which contains the concertina reservoir bag (17). During the inspiratory phase the bag (17) is compressed and its contents are forced past the 'bag switch-over' slide valve (10), and, together with fresh gas entering at the inlet (9), through the delivery tube (8), to the patient. The manometer (11) indicates the pressure in the breathing circuit. The safety-valve (14) limits this pressure to 70 cmH_2O. It is not operative when manual ventilation is performed. When the ventilator cycles to the expiratory phase, the pressure chamber (20) is connected to atmosphere through the inflating valve. The pressure in the chamber (20) falls and expired gas flows through the tube (8) to the concertina reservoir bag (17).

The tube (18), the perforated lower end of which rests on the weighted base (19) of the concertina bag (17), can slide up and down freely through the fixed top-plate and therefore follows the movements of the bag. When the concertina bag (17) is at the bottom of its stroke, excess gas flows up through the tube (18) and spills through the one-way valve (12). When the base-plate (19) starts its upward movement, it takes with it the tube (18). Gas from the reservoir bag (17) continues to spill through the valve (12) until this valve is closed by meeting the sliding weight (13), the resting position of which is set by the 'excess gas leak' control (15). When the sliding stop (15) is set in its lowest position, the valve (12) is closed as soon as the base-plate (19) begins to rise. The inspiratory phase now commences. Further upward movement of the tube (18) now raises the weight (13), and the valve (12) is held closed throughout the inspiratory phase. This phase continues until the pressure in the rigid plastic chamber (20) reaches the cycling pressure set on the driving ventilator.

The full effect of the 'spill' mechanism described above can only be understood in conjunction with a consideration of the fresh-gas flow and the anaesthetic circuit in which the assembly is used. If the 'excess gas leak' control (15) is set so that the weight (13) rests in its lowest position, then excess gas can only spill during the expiratory phase after the concertina reservoir bag (17) has re-expanded and any negative pressure produced within it, by the fall of the base-plate (19), has been abolished.

If the control (15) is raised, then excess gas can continue to spill while the base-plate (19) is beginning its upward movement and the time available for spillage is accordingly increased.

During the expiratory phase a negative pressure is produced in the reservoir bag (17) so long as the weighted base-plate (19) is falling. If the amount of gas spilled during one respiratory cycle exceeds the amount of fresh gas admitted during that cycle, then the base-plate (19) never reaches the lower limit of its stroke and, until it has moved upwards sufficiently to open the valve (12), a negative pressure is maintained in the bag (17). In an extreme case, in which the fresh-gas flow is very small, or the stop (15) is set very high, the lower limit of the excursion of the base-plate (19) rises progressively with each respiration. When this lower limit becomes sufficiently raised for the bag (17) to empty completely during the inspiratory phase any further rise in the lower limit is accompanied by a progressive decrease in tidal volume. To prevent this, and the ultimate cessation of ventilation which would ensue, an 'automatic bellows refill' mechanism (2, 3, 4, 5) is provided. If the concertina bag (17) is completely emptied the weight (13) is raised high enough to strike one end of the pivoted rod (5) and so open the valve (2). Driving gas can now flow from the inlet (1) to the chamber above the upper piston of the 'flush timer' (4). The piston is forced down, pushing down the diaphragm and the lower piston, thereby opening the valve (3). Driving gas now flows freely into the reservoir bag (17). The resultant downward movement of the weight (13) immediately releases the pivoted rod (5) and the valve (2) is closed by its spring. The upper piston is returned to its resting position by its spring. The time taken for the diaphragm, and hence the lower piston, to return to their resting positions, depends on the rate at which the pressure above the diaphragm can fall. This rate is preset by a locked needle valve.

The combined ventilator may be pressure- or volume-cycled from the inspiratory to the expiratory phase. It is pressure-cycled if the cycling pressure set on the driving ventilator is reached before the concertina reservoir bag (17) has reached the limit of its upward movement set by the volume limit (7). On the other hand, once the bag has reached the limit of its upward excursion, then inflation ceases and the pressure within the chamber (20) rises rapidly to the cycling pressure, and the inspiratory phase ends. At the start of the expiratory phase, the pressure in the chamber (20) falls rapidly to atmospheric, or, if the Mark 8 ventilator is being used as the driving unit, to the negative pressure set. The rate at which the bag (17) re-expands depends on (a) the rate at which the pressure in the rigid chamber (20) falls, (b) the weight (19) in the bottom of the bag, and (c) the resistance of the respiratory pathway.

Until the bag (17) is fully expanded the pressure within it is less than that in the chamber (20) due to the weight (19) (see fig. 29.18). When the bag has fully expanded the pressure within it will rise until at a pressure of 1 cmH_2O the valve (12) opens and any further gas entering the bag during the remainder of the expiratory phase spills to atmosphere.

The amount of rebreathing and the quantity of gas spilled when the bag is compressed depend on the setting of the 'excess gas leak' control (15) together with the flow of fresh gas and the place in the breathing circuit at which it enters.

When used with a totally-closed circuit the control (15) is set in its lowest position and the fresh-gas flow adjusted to the minimum required to ensure that the bag is fully expanded at the start of the inspiratory phase. If the fresh-gas flow is increased, the excess gas is spilled only before the bag moves up.

For non-rebreathing anaesthetic use the inlet (9) is plugged, and the fresh gas is supplied to the circuit near the patient. The fresh-gas flow is set to equal the desired minute volume, and the resting position of the weight (13) is raised sufficiently to allow an equivalent amount of gas to spill through the valve (12).

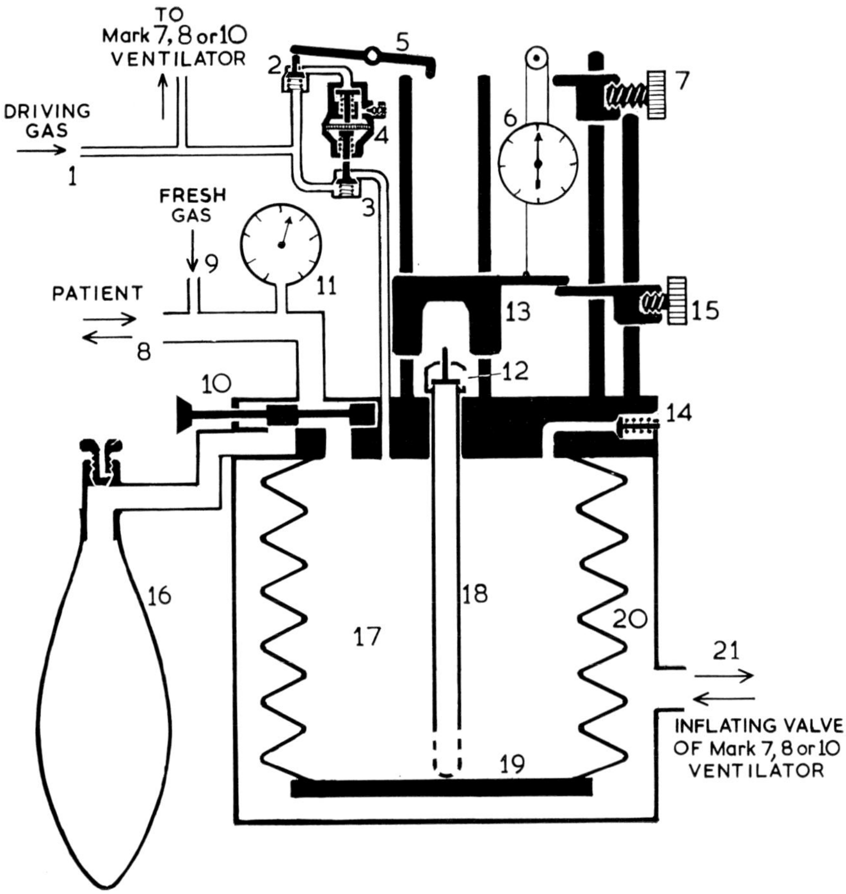

Fig. 29.17. Diagram of the Bird Mark 4 attachment.

1. Driving-gas inlet
2. Valve
3. Valve
4. 'Flush timer'
5. Pivoted rod
6. 'Spirometer'
7. 'Volume limiting' control
8. Breathing tube
9. Fresh-gas inlet
10. 'Bag switch-over' control
11. Manometer
12. 'Excess gas bleed' valve
13. Sliding weight
14. Safety-valve
15. 'Automatic excess gas leak' control
16. Reservoir bag
17. Concertina reservoir bag
18. 'Escapement' tube
19. Weight
20. Rigid plastic pressure chamber
21. Port for fitting expiratory-valve assembly of driving ventilator

The 'spirometer' (6) consists of a rotating disc, graduated from 0–12, which is connected to the weight (13) by a string. Any movement of the weight (13) is therefore indicated by rotation of the disc. The amount and rate of rotation therefore give an indication of the movement of gas into and out of the concertina reservoir bag (17) during such time as the valve (12) is closed. One division of the disc represents a volume of about 100 ml, but the main purpose is not so much to give absolute measurements as to indicate changes in the patient's compliance, the airway resistance, or the fresh-gas flow, or the development of a leak.

The 'bag switch-over' control (10) consists of a sliding tap which is pulled outwards to connect the reservoir bag (16) with the breathing circuit for manual inflation. This reservoir bag incorporates an adjustable leak.

FUNCTIONAL ANALYSIS

This analysis, the 'Controls' section which follows, and the recordings of figs. 29.20 to 29.22 refer to a Bird Mark 4 driven by a Bird Mark 8 with the 'air-mix' control pulled out for economy of driving gas.

Inspiratory phase

The Mark 8 on its own operates usually as a fairly-low-pressure generator with some series resistance, but with a gradual build-up of the generated pressure at the start of the phase. This results in a flow which rises rapidly at the beginning of the phase and then stays relatively steady at a level dependent upon lung characteristics. The interposition of the concertina bag (17) of the Mark 4, between the Mark 8 and the patient, has little effect because of its shallow and nearly-flat pressure-volume characteristic (fig. 29.18).

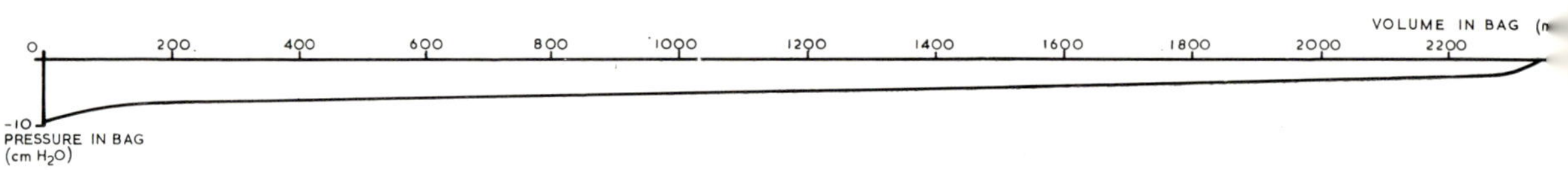

Fig. 29.18. Bird Mark 4. Pressure-volume characteristic of the concertina reservoir bag. The 'excess gas leak' control was set at its lowest position so that the weight, (13) in fig. 29.17, acted on the bag for all volumes except above 2250 ml.

However, the pattern of flow delivered to the patient is considerably modified by the process of spilling excess gas from the patient circuit during the inspiratory phase.

At the start of the phase the pressure within the concertina bag (17) is rapidly raised above the opening pressure (1 cmH_2O) of the one-way valve (12) (unless a large negative pressure has been developed in the previous expiratory phase). For the first part of the phase, therefore, part of the flow from the Mark 8 is used in spilling excess gas through the one-way valve (12) and only part in inflating the patient. If the valve were capable of passing large flows for little more pressure drop than the opening pressure, the ventilator would operate as a constant (1 cmH_2O) pressure generator for this part of the phase. In fact however, the resistance of the pathway for the escape of gas is quite high (fig. 29.19), and any increase in the flow through the valve must be associated with an increase in the pressure in the concertina bag. The consequence of this is that, as the pressure generated by the Mark 8 increases towards its maximum, the pressure in the concertina bag increases, thereby increasing the spill of excess gas. But the increase in pressure in the concertina bag, which is essentially the same as that at the mouth, results in a flow into the lungs which rises rapidly to a relatively-steady level—the rise in alveolar pressure with

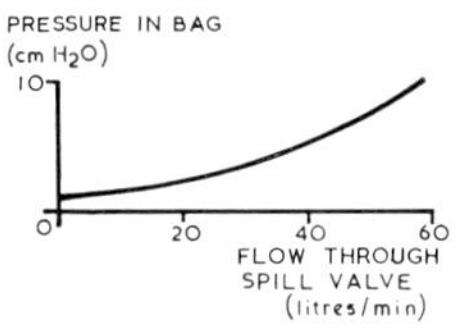

Fig. 29.19. Bird Mark 4. Pressure-flow characteristic of the one-way 'excess gas bleed' valve, (12) in fig. 29.17.

time is more or less matched by the rise in mouth (and bag) pressure. This can be seen clearly in fig. 29.21 where, because of the high fresh-gas flow (5 litres/min), spillage of excess gas goes on for about 0·4 sec. In fig. 29.20, where the fresh-gas flow was only 0·5 litre/min, spillage of fresh gas goes on for only about 0·1 sec and a steady level of flow is barely established before the one-way valve (12) is closed.

During this first part of the phase the volume of gas driven out through the one-way valve (12) must, in the long run, equal the volume of fresh gas entering the patient circuit in one respiratory cycle (after making allowance for any leaks and for uptake by the patient). Therefore the duration of this first part of the phase is determined by the time it takes the Mark 8 to supply this volume of gas, together with the small volume of gas which enters the patient during this part of the phase.

Although the characteristics of the one-way valve (12), and of the Mark 8 as a whole, are such that the flow into the lungs happens to be fairly steady in both the first and second parts of the inspiratory phase, the ventilator does not operate as a flow generator in either part, and the magnitudes of the flows do alter somewhat when the lung characteristics are changed, as can be seen from figs. 29.20 and 29.21.

As explained in the functional analysis of the Mark 8, the flow declines in the last 0·1 sec of the inspiratory phase after the sliding valve has shut off the supply of driving gas. This is reflected faithfully in the flow into the lungs from the Mark 4 in the recordings of fig. 29.20, in which the pressure-cycling mechanism of the Mark 8 operated normally. In fig. 29.21, however, the volume limit (7) of the Mark 4 was brought into play. When this was reached, it prevented any further upward movement of the base of the concertina bag, but some further, rapidly-diminishing, flow occurred because the build-up of pressure outside the bag, towards the cycling pressure, compressed the convolutions of the bag. This decline of flow at the end of the phase lasted about 0·3 sec.

Change-over from inspiratory phase to expiratory phase

Provided the volume limit (7) is not reached, this change-over is nominally pressure-cycled as in the Mark 8. As explained in the functional analysis of that ventilator, the

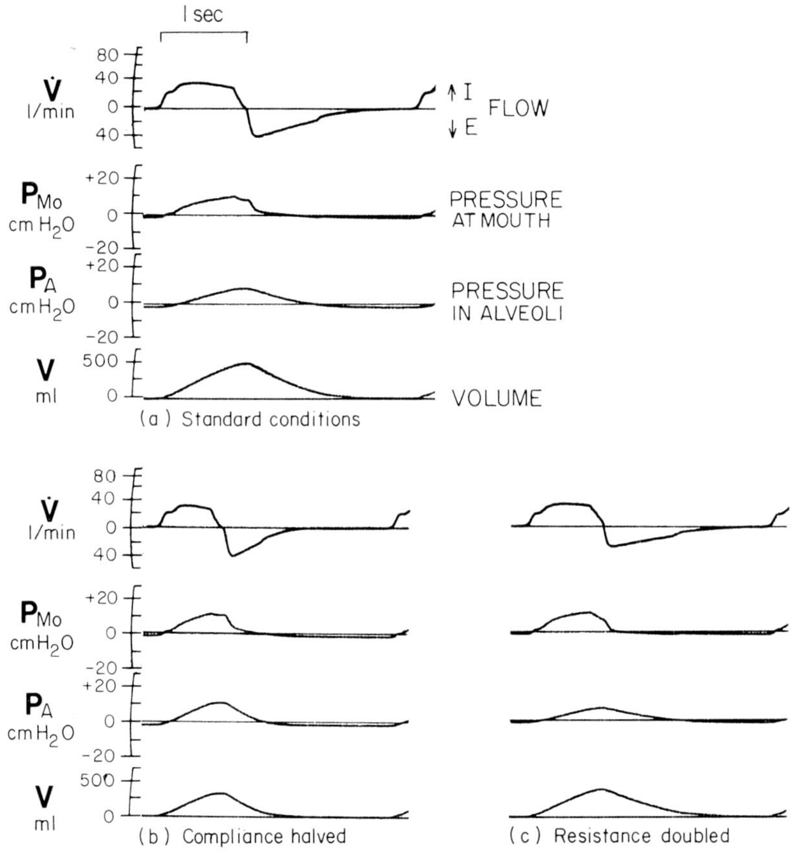

Fig. 29.20. Bird Mark 4, driven by Bird Mark 8 and operating in the pressure-cycled mode with a small fresh-gas flow. Recordings showing the effects of changes of lung characteristics.

Standard conditions: driving gas, oxygen at 50 lb/in^2; 'air-mix' control, pulled out to produce air entrainment in the Mark 8; 'retard', not used; 'excess gas leak', at position 'II'; 'mechanical stop' ('volume limit'), at 'normal' (in its highest position); fresh-gas flow, 0·5 litre/min; 'negative pressure' (on the Mark 8), off; other controls on the Mark 8 set to produce a tidal volume of 500 ml at a frequency of 20/min with an inspiratory-expiratory ratio of 1 : 2; namely 'inspiratory pressure limit', '16'; 'expiratory time', less than '7'; 'flow-rate', '25'; 'sensitivity', minimum.

inspiratory flow starts to decline as soon as the pressure in the Mark 8 casing reaches a critical level, and the change-over occurs at a preset time interval later. This is the case in fig. 29.20, although the mouth pressure at the moment at which the flow starts to decline is slightly different for the different lung characteristics. This is because of the resistance between the mouth and the casing of the Mark 8 and the slightly-different flows.

When the volume limit (7) is brought into use, as in fig. 29.21, the change-over becomes approximately volume-cycled. Once the volume limit is reached further movement

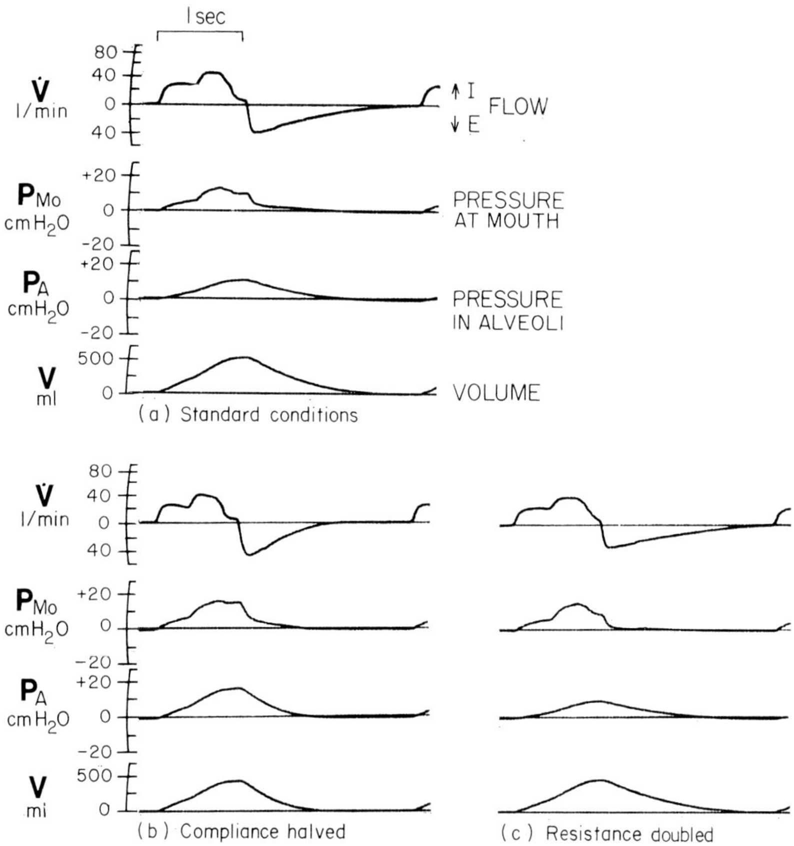

Fig. 29.21. Bird Mark 4, driven by Bird Mark 8 and operating in the volume-limited mode with a large fresh-gas flow. Recordings showing the effects of changes of lung characteristics.

Standard conditions: driving gas, oxygen at 50 lb/in^2; 'air-mix' control, pulled out to produce air entrainment in the Mark 8; 'retard', not used; 'excess gas leak', at position 'II'; fresh-gas flow, 5 litres/min; 'negative pressure' on Mark 8, off; 'mechanical stop' ('volume limit'), set for a tidal volume of 500 ml; 'inspiratory pressure limit', '25', to ensure reaching volume limit with halved compliance; 'sensitivity', '25'; 'expiratory time', set, at less than '7', for an expiratory time of 2 sec; 'flowrate', set, at '35', for an inspiratory time of 1 sec.

of the base of the concertina bag is prevented, and the pressure outside the bag builds up fairly rapidly to the cycling pressure set on the Mark 8. In fig. 29.21 the delay is about 0·3 sec. Therefore the change-over is volume-cycled in only a restricted sense of the term: it occurs at a nearly-constant time interval after the concertina bag has been compressed to a preset volume. Two factors alter the tidal volume delivered to the patient when the lung characteristics are altered. Firstly, when the compliance is halved (fig. 29.21b), the pressure inside the bag at the end of the phase is higher and the convolutions of the bag are compressed less by the pressure outside the bag, so the tidal volume is reduced a little.

This concerns that part of the tidal volume delivered to the lungs between the moment at which the one-way valve (12) is closed, by making contact with the weight (13), and the end of the phase. Secondly, the other part of the tidal volume, that which is delivered between the start of the phase and the moment at which the one-way valve (12) is closed, is affected. During this part of the phase, halving the compliance or doubling the resistance leads to higher mouth and bag pressures, so that a larger fraction of the flow from the Mark 8 is used in driving excess gas through the one-way valve, and a smaller fraction in driving gas into the patient. Therefore this part of the tidal volume is reduced. This effect would, however, be negligible with a small fresh-gas flow.

Expiratory phase

As with the Mark 8 alone, the Mark 4 normally acts as a constant-pressure generator throughout the expiratory phase. The weight (19) serves to generate a small negative pressure (fig. 29.18) even when the 'negative pressure' control on the Mark 8 is turned off, as in figs. 29.20 and 29.21. The only complication is that the weight (13) contributes about 1 cmH_2O to the negative pressure generated so that when, during the descent of the concertina bag, the weight is 'caught' by the stop of the 'excess gas leak' control (15), the generated pressure is suddenly made 1 cmH_2O less negative, leading to a sudden drop in the expiratory flow. When the fresh-gas flow is small, as in fig. 29.20, this occurs only when almost the whole of the tidal volume has come out of the lungs, since the small volume of excess gas entering during the respiratory cycle carries the concertina bag only a little distance below the point at which the weight (13) is caught by the stop (15). When the fresh-gas flow is high, on the other hand, as in fig. 29.21, the bag is carried well down by the end of the phase and the weight (13) is caught early in the phase, when only a much smaller fraction of the tidal volume has come out and therefore when the alveolar pressure and expiratory flow are still quite high. Because of this, the percentage change of pressure difference across the airway, and hence the percentage change of expiratory flow, is much smaller: the change is barely detectable in fig. 29.21.

Change-over from expiratory phase to inspiratory phase

As with the Mark 8 alone, this change-over is commonly time-cycled, as in figs. 29.20 and 29.21, although, by suitable setting of the sensitivity control, it could be made to respond to an inspiratory effort by the patient if this were made before the time-cycling mechanism effected the change-over.

CONTROLS

Only the volume-limited mode of operation, with a small fresh-gas flow, is illustrated (fig. 29.22) and considered in detail here, although some mention is made of the pressure-cycled mode and the effect of high fresh-gas flows.

Total ventilation

This cannot be directly controlled but is equal to the product of tidal volume and respiratory frequency.

Tidal volume

That part of the tidal volume which is delivered after the one-way valve (12) has been closed, by making contact with the weight (13), is directly controlled by the 'mechanical stop' or 'volume limit' control (7). This therefore provides the primary means of adjusting the tidal volume although, when the 'mechanical stop' is raised to increase the tidal volume, the inspiratory time is also increased (fig. 29.22b) unless a compensating adjustment is made to the 'flowrate' control. This part of the tidal volume may conveniently be called the 'regulated' part. The other part of the tidal volume, which is delivered before the one-way valve (12) closes, is not directly controlled and is subject to variation. It will therefore be referred to as the 'unregulated' part.

When the fresh-gas flow is small and the 'negative pressure' control on the Mark 8 is turned off (fig. 29.22a), this unregulated part of the tidal volume is only a small fraction of the total, so that variations in the unregulated part have little influence on the whole. Then the total tidal volume is controlled almost completely by the 'mechanical stop' (7) and is uninfluenced by lung characteristics, apart from a small effect arising from compression of the convolutions of the concertina bag as explained in the functional analysis above. On the other hand, if the 'negative pressure' control on the Mark 8 is turned on, or if the fresh-gas flow is made large, the unregulated part of the tidal volume may become a substantial fraction of the total tidal volume, which is therefore not precisely controlled by the 'mechanical stop'. These two situations are now considered in detail.

When the 'negative pressure' control on the Mark 8 is turned on, the concertina bag is pulled down further during the expiratory phase and a substantial negative pressure is developed in the bag which helps to keep the one-way valve (12) closed. Therefore, at the beginning of the inspiratory phase, there is a period in which the whole of the flow from the Mark 8 is used in driving gas into the lungs. This period lasts until the pressure inside the concertina bag has risen to the opening pressure of the one-way valve (12), after which excess gas escapes in the same way as when the 'negative pressure' control is off. The gas which enters the lungs during the initial period represents an increase in the unregulated part of the tidal volume which therefore becomes a substantial fraction of the total tidal volume. Thus, when negative pressure is introduced, the total tidal volume is increased (fig. 29.22e) and it can be expected that the fraction, and therefore the total, will be influenced by changes in lung characteristics and in the setting of the 'flowrate' control. This is because these factors influence the time it takes, at the beginning of the inspiratory phase, to raise the pressure inside the concertina bag to the opening pressure of the valve (12).

When the fresh-gas flow is increased (to 5 litres/min in fig. 29.22f) the concertina bag is again carried down further during the expiratory phase, just as when the 'negative pressure' control on the Mark 8 is turned on. In this case, however, it is due to the increased volume of fresh gas which enters the system during both the expiratory phase and the later part of the inspiratory phase (after the one-way valve (12) has been closed

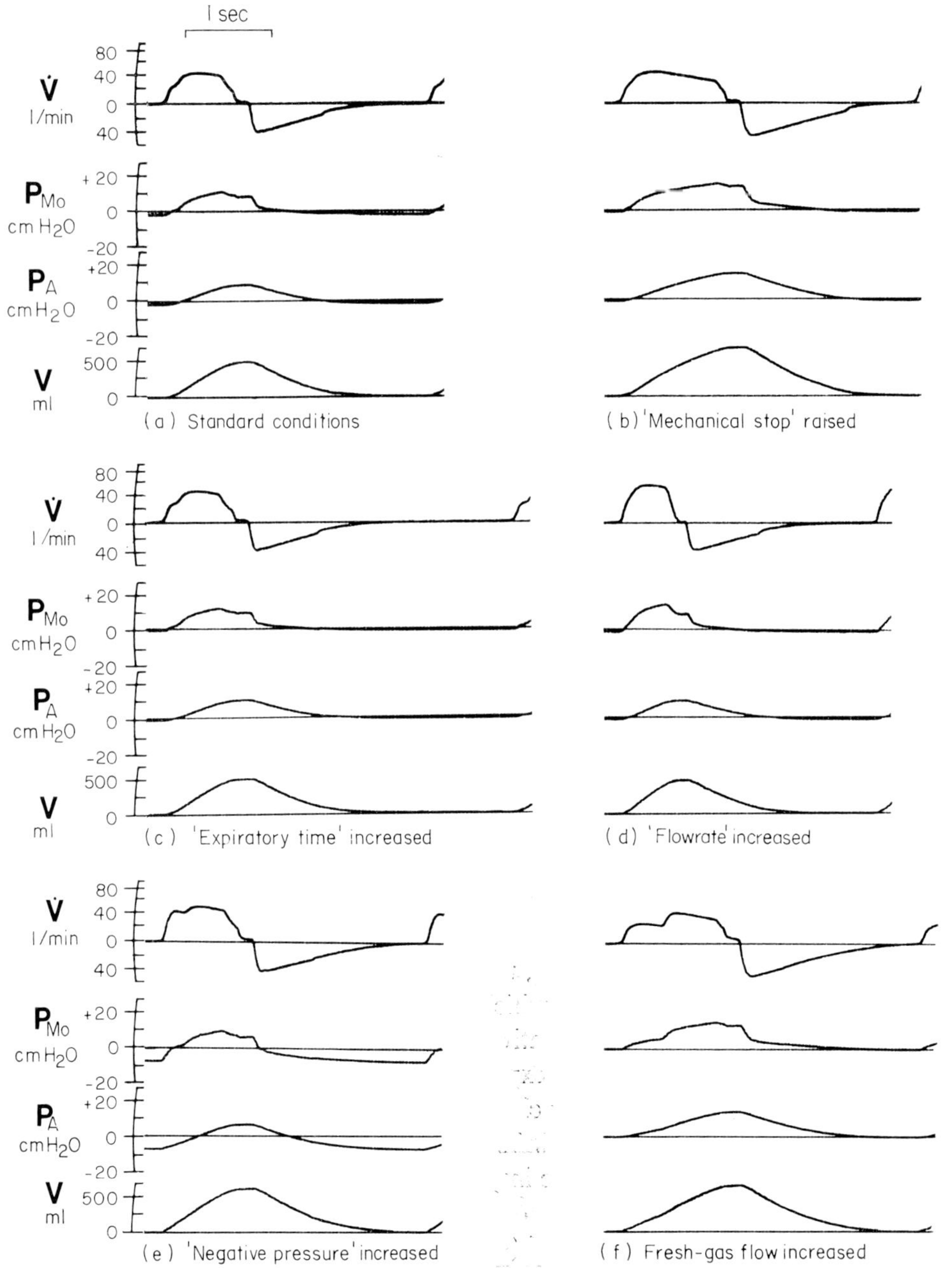

by making contact with the weight (13)). Therefore, at the start of the inspiratory phase, the pressure in the concertina bag is immediately raised above the opening pressure of the one-way valve (12) and the period, in which the flow from the Mark 8 is shared between inflating the lungs and discharging excess gas, commences immediately. However, because a much larger volume of gas has to be spilt in each inspiratory phase, the period of spilling lasts longer and, during this time, a greater volume of gas is delivered to the lungs. That is, the unregulated part of the tidal volume is increased and, with it, the total tidal volume (fig. 29.22f). Since this unregulated part of the tidal volume is influenced by lung characteristics (see the functional analysis above and fig. 29.21) the total tidal volume is less-closely controlled by the 'mechanical stop' than when the fresh-gas flow is small.

In the pressure-cycled mode the tidal volume is determined indirectly by the compliance and the difference between the inspiratory and expiratory pressures to which the lungs are subjected. Therefore the tidal volume varies considerably with lung characteristics (fig. 29.20) and the primary means of controlling it is the 'inspiratory pressure limit' control on the Mark 8. The tidal volume is also increased when negative pressure is introduced, and it is sensitive to the 'flowrate' setting which affects the difference between the cycling pressure and the end-inspiratory alveolar pressure. However, the tidal volume is not influenced by changes of fresh-gas flow.

Respiratory frequency and inspiratory-expiratory ratio

Neither of these parameters can be directly controlled but both are determined by the separately-variable inspiratory and expiratory times.

As with the Mark 8, the inspiratory time can be indirectly regulated by means of the 'flowrate' control (fig. 29.22d) but is also influenced by any change in tidal volume, either deliberate (fig. 29.22b) or incidental to a change of control setting (fig. 29.22f and, to a small extent, 29.22e).

The expiratory time is usually directly controlled by the 'expiratory time' control (fig. 29.22c) but it is also sensitive to pressures in certain circumstances as discussed in detail in relation to the Mark 8. None of the changes of control settings in fig. 29.22, or

---

Fig. 29.22. Bird Mark 4, driven by Bird Mark 8 and operating in the volume-limited mode with a small fresh-gas flow. Recordings showing the effects of changes in the settings of the controls.

(a) Standard conditions as in fig. 29.21 except that the fresh-gas flow was only 0·5 litre/min and the 'sensitivity' control was set to 'minimum' to prevent premature cycling from the expiratory phase to the inspiratory phase.

(b) 'Mechanical stop' ('volume limit'), raised to produce a tidal volume of 750 ml.

(c) 'Expiratory time', increased to produce an expiratory time of 3 sec.

(d) 'Flowrate', increased to '40'.

(e) 'Negative pressure', increased to '−3'.

(f) Fresh-gas flow, increased to 5 litres/min.

of lung characteristics in fig. 29.21, had more than a very small effect on the expiratory time.

Thus all the controls, except perhaps the 'negative pressure' control, affect either the inspiratory or expiratory time and hence both the respiratory frequency and the inspiratory-expiratory ratio.

Inspiratory waveforms

With the fresh-gas flow low, the inspiratory flow normally rises in about 0·1 sec to a level which is maintained fairly steady for most of the phase and, if the volume limit is not in action, is followed by a decline in the last 0·1 sec or so. A substantially-different waveform occurs when the fresh-gas flow is made high and the volume limit is brought into play (compare fig. 29.21a with fig. 29.20a) but the choice of fresh-gas flow and use of the volume limit may be dictated by other considerations. Since the ventilator is not a flow generator, the flow waveform varies somewhat with lung characteristics.

Expiratory waveforms

As with the Mark 8, the Mark 4 normally operates approximately as a constant-pressure generator throughout the expiratory phase so that the expiratory flow rises rapidly to a peak and then declines in a manner dependent on lung characteristics. The flow can be made more-nearly constant throughout the phase by using negative pressure and the 'retard' cap, but this is not illustrated here.

Pressure limits

Since the ventilator operates as a constant-pressure generator during the expiratory phase, the alveolar pressure normally falls to the generated pressure by the end of the phase. It does so in all the recordings in figs. 29.20 to 29.22; it will fail to do so only if the airway resistance is very high, or the 'retard' cap is in use, or the expiratory time is very short. The minimum, end-expiratory, alveolar pressure can therefore be directly controlled by means of the 'negative pressure' control on the Mark 8, although this results in a change in tidal volume (fig. 29.22e). The peak, end-inspiratory, alveolar pressure is not directly controlled and even its indirect determination is complex. The simplest statement that can be made about it is that it exceeds the end-expiratory alveolar pressure by an amount equal to the tidal volume divided by the compliance. However, it must be remembered that the tidal volume is not, in general, rigidly controlled and is influenced by many factors.

In the pressure-cycled mode the peak, end-inspiratory, alveolar pressure is largely independent of the end-expiratory pressure. It is primarily controlled by the cycling pressure, but falls short of this by an amount dependent on the inspiratory flow and on the total resistance between the alveoli and the main chamber of the Mark 8.

THE BIRD 'INFANT J CIRCUIT'

DESCRIPTION

This attachment (fig. 29.23) is designed to permit cycling of the driving ventilator at frequencies up to 120/min and control of the degree of nebulization in the inflating gas mixture.

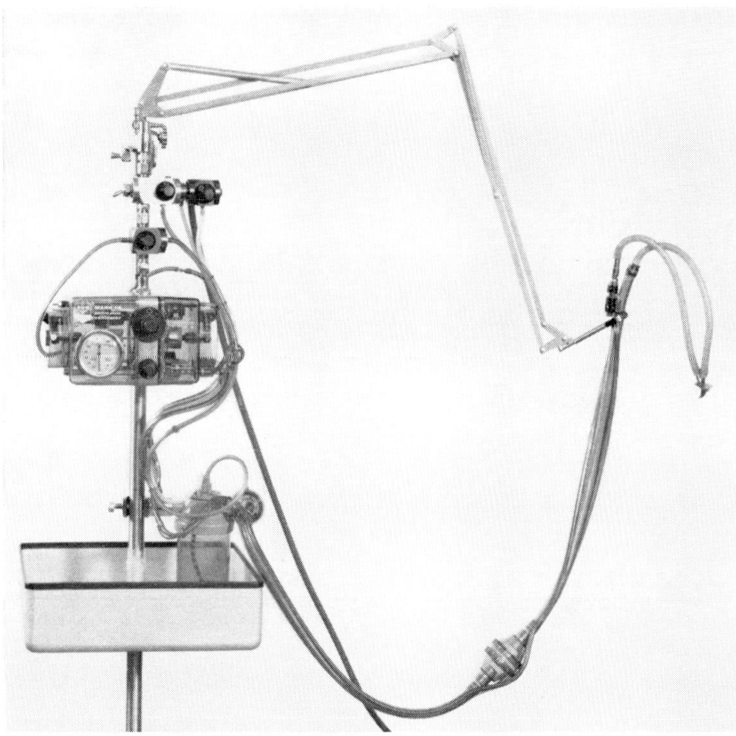

Fig. 29.23. The Bird 'Infant J Circuit'.

Courtesy of the Bird Corporation.

It is intended for use with a Bird Mark 8 ventilator which has been modified by adding a vernier to the sensitivity control and a Bird 500 ml in-line nebulizer, and substituting a much finer negative-pressure control.

The main component is a reversible injector (14, 15, 16) (fig. 29.24). It is normally supplied with a 'parallel flow booster cartridge' (3, 4), to control the operation of the nebulizer. Alternatively, it can be supplied with a twin 'parallel booster', as shown in fig. 29.24 (3, 4, 5, 6), in which the second 'booster' (5, 6) permits adjustable oxygen enrichment of the inflating gas mixture.

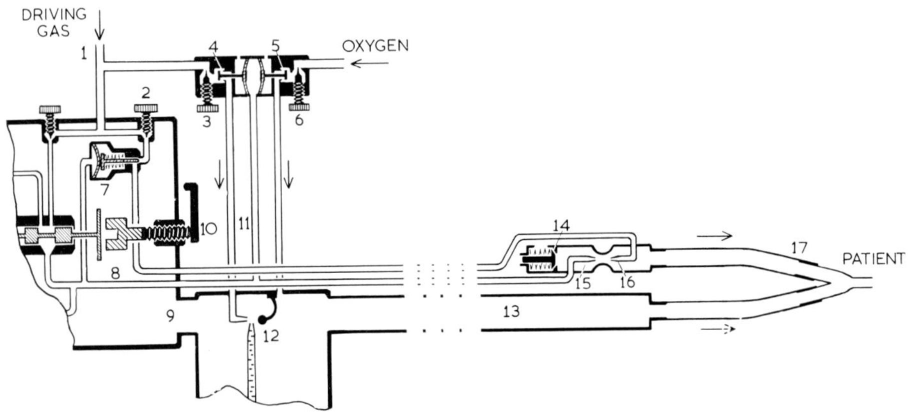

Fig. 29.24. Diagram of the Bird 'Infant J Circuit'.

1. Driving-gas inlet
2. Vernier negative-pressure control
3. Needle valve
4. Valve
5. Valve
6. Needle valve
7. Valve
8. Connecting tube
9. Delivery port
10. Positive-pressure control
11. Connecting tube
12. Nebulizer
13. Delivery tube
14. Spring-loaded expiratory valve
15. Inspiratory jet
16. Expiratory jet
17. Breathing tube

When the patient makes an inspiratory effort the ventilator cycles to the inspiratory position (fig. 29.24) in the usual way. The vernier adjustment on the sensitivity control makes it easier to set the ventilator to trigger at a pressure only slightly more negative than that being generated during the expiratory phase (see below).

There are four sources of gas flow during the inspiratory phase all contributing to the inflation of the lungs. Firstly, gas at high pressure flows, at a rate of up to 15 litres/min, through the connecting tube (8) and the inspiratory jet (15) of the double injector, and then through the breathing tube (17) to the patient. The entrainment effect of the injector ensures that, despite the rise in pressure in the breathing tube (17) during the phase, the pressure in the chamber behind the inspiratory jet (15) is negative or, if positive, is small enough to ensure that the spring-loaded expiratory valve (14) remains closed. At the same time the rise in pressure in the connecting tube (8) is transmitted through the tube (11) to the chamber between the two diaphragms of the twin parallel booster, forcing the diaphragms outwards. The valves (4) and (5) are opened. There is now a second flow of gas: driving gas flows from the main supply line (1), at a rate controlled by the needle valve (3), through the valve (4), to the nebulizer (12). If desired, a third flow of gas may be obtained: supplemental oxygen may be admitted to the nebulizer through the valve (5) at a rate controlled by the needle valve (6). These three flows come direct from supply-line pressure (the injector (15) does not entrain any gas). The fourth flow is the conventional inflating flow from the delivery port (9) of the Mark 8 ventilator. Since the manufacturer's instructions say that, when connected to the J circuit, the ventilator should be operated with the 'air-mix' control pulled out, this fourth flow comes via the injector in the Mark 8. As is explained in the account of the Mark 8, the build-up of flow from this injector is rather slow but the three additional flows should give a more rapid start to inflation, thereby permitting the high respiratory frequencies mentioned above.

All flows continue until the pressure in the main chamber of the ventilator reaches the cycling pressure set on the positive-pressure control (10), and the ventilator cycles to the expiratory position. The flows to the inspiratory jet (15) and from the delivery port (9) of the Mark 8 ventilator are immediately cut off. The pressure between the diaphragms of the flow booster falls to that in the breathing tube (17) and the valves (4) and (5) close, cutting off the flows through them. The fall in pressure in the connecting tube (8) allows the valve (7) to open and driving gas flows, at a rate controlled by the needle valve (2), to the expiratory jet (16) of the double injector. The expiratory valve (14) is opened and expired gas flows, together with driving gas from the expiratory jet (16), through it to atmosphere. The amount of negative pressure produced in the expiratory pathway depends on the setting of the negative-pressure control (2).

The expiratory phase continues until the patient makes a further inspiratory effort, or, if he fails to do so, until the ventilator cycles in the usual way after a time set by the expiratory-time control.

The nebulizer (12) holds 500 ml of liquid and is intended solely for humidification. If it is desired to add any medication to the inspiratory gas a second small 'therapy nebulizer' is fitted into the circuit on the patient side of the 'in-line' nebulizer using a Bird 'chemotherapy bifurcation'.

It would seem advisable to keep the tube (17) short since inflation occurs partly through this tube and at the start of the inspiratory phase it must contain expired gas—unless sufficient negative pressure is developed during the expiratory phase to entrain a flow of gas through the one-way valve over the throat of the injector in the Mark 8 (6 in fig. 29.4) and along the delivery tube (13) sufficient to wash out this tube (17).

FUNCTIONAL ANALYSIS

Inspiratory phase

The Bird J circuit driven by a Mark 8 incorporates four sources of inflating flow. The compliance of some of the patients to which it is connected may well be little more than the internal compliance of the ventilator. The rather slow build-up and decay processes noted in the Mark 8 on its own will occupy a substantial fraction of the very short inspiratory times that may occur.

In view of these factors and their possible interactions it is not possible to make confident theoretical predictions of the mode of operation in this phase. It is unlikely to be a pure flow generator; it is most likely to be some complex form of non-constant-pressure generator.

Change-over from inspiratory phase to expiratory phase
This change-over is pressure-cycled as in the Mark 8 on its own.

Expiratory phase
In this phase the ventilator operates as a constant-pressure generator, usually negative, due to the characteristics of the injector (16) and of the expiratory valve (14).

Change-over from expiratory phase to inspiratory phase
This change-over is time-cycled or patient-cycled whichever occurs first, as in the Mark 8 on its own.

THE BIRD 'Q CIRCLE BREATHING ARRANGEMENT'

DESCRIPTION

Despite its name this arrangement (fig. 29.26) is not a closed circle system but a non-rebreathing circuit which allows the expiratory-valve assembly of the Mark 8 ventilator (27–32 in fig. 29.4) to be sited up to 4 feet from the patient, without increasing the dead space. This is achieved by using separate inspiratory and expiratory tubes (5, 6) (fig. 29.25). As a result the mechanical dead space of the circuit is actually less than with direct connexion of the patient's airway to the expiratory valve. The dead space is 0·57 ml in the adult version and 0·28 ml in the infant version.

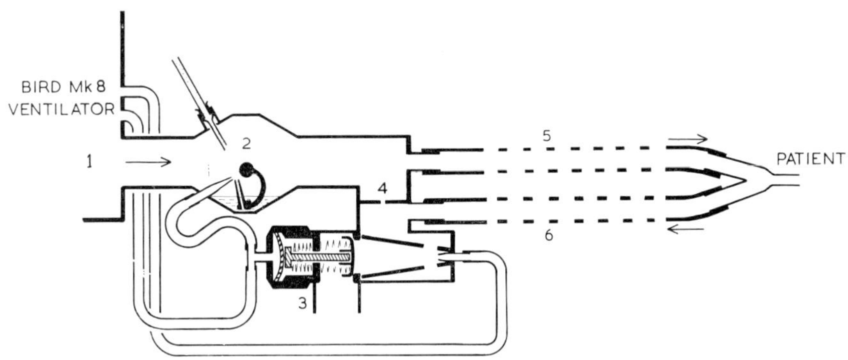

Fig. 29.25. Diagram of the Bird 'Q Circle Breathing Arrangement'.

1. Delivery port of Bird Mark 8 ventilator
2. Nebulizer
3. Expiratory-valve assembly
4. Partition
5. Inspiratory tube
6. Expiratory tube

The nebulizer (2) and the expiratory-valve assembly (3) are fitted directly to the delivery port (1) of the Mark 8 ventilator or connected to it by a length of breathing tube. During the inspiratory phase gas is delivered to the patient through the tube (5). During the expiratory phase expired gas can only pass along the tube (6) and escape to atmosphere through the expiratory-valve assembly (3). A small hole in the partition (4) between the inspiratory and expiratory pathways in the valve assembly (3) allows any condensation from the nebulizer to drain into the expiratory side of the assembly, whence it can be drained off through a special port (not shown in fig. 29.25).

A similar arrangement, permitting a lesser separation between the expiratory-valve assembly and the patient, is available for the Mark 7 ventilator.

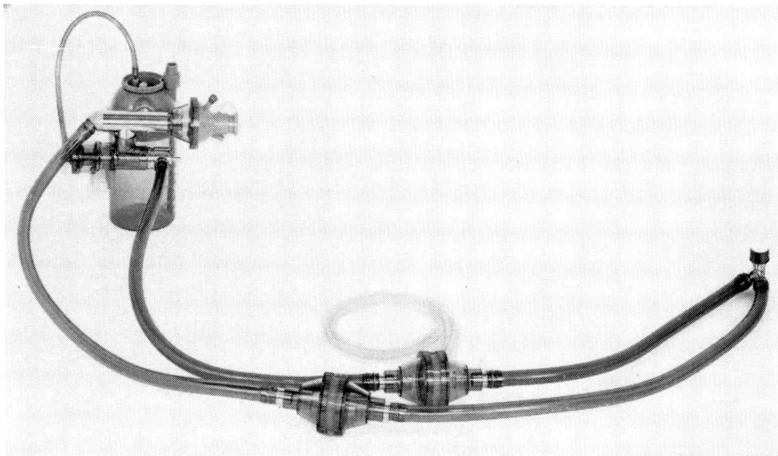

Fig. 29.26. The Bird 'Q Circle Breathing Arrangement'. Water traps are included in the inspiratory and expiratory tubes.

Courtesy of the Bird Corporation.

FUNCTIONAL ANALYSIS

The use of this circuit should have no appreciable effect on the functional analyses of the Mark 7 or Mark 8 ventilators.

THE BIRD SPIROMETER

DESCRIPTION

This apparatus (fig. 29.27), which is adaptable for use with all Bird ventilators of the Mark 7 to Mark 17 family, admits the expired gas from the patient to a calibrated concertina bag and discharges it to atmosphere during the next inspiratory phase.

Inflating gas from the ventilator goes direct, or via nebulizers, to a Y-piece close to the

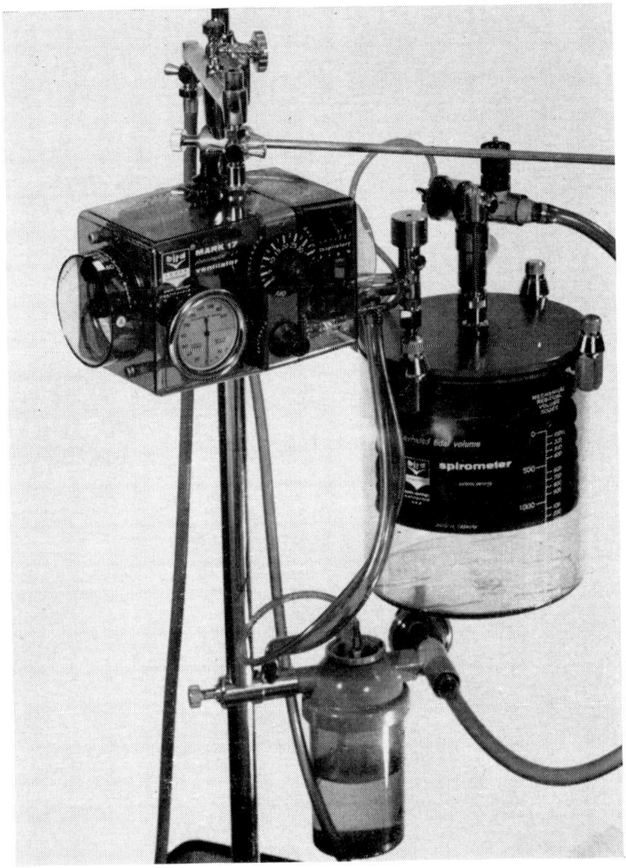

Fig. 29.27. The Bird Spirometer fitted to the Bird Mark 17 ventilator.
Courtesy of the Bird Corporation.

patient; expired gas comes from the Y-piece to the port (1) (fig. 29.28) and the standard expiratory-valve assembly (without negative-pressure injector) (6, 7) on the top of the spirometer.

The high-pressure line (11) to the expiratory-valve assembly has a branch connected to the 'flow booster cartridge' (9, 10). Therefore, during the inspiratory phase, the pressure on the diaphragms (7, 9) holds the expiratory valve (6) closed and the valve (10) open. The needle valve (12) is permanently connected to the 50 lb/in^2 driving-gas supply of the main ventilator, and driving gas flows to the injector (17), where it entrains air and enters the rigid plastic chamber (16). The rate of flow is set by the needle valve (12) so that the concertina bag is compressed fully, and all the expired gas stored in it is discharged to atmosphere through the one-way valve (2), before the end of the inspiratory phase.

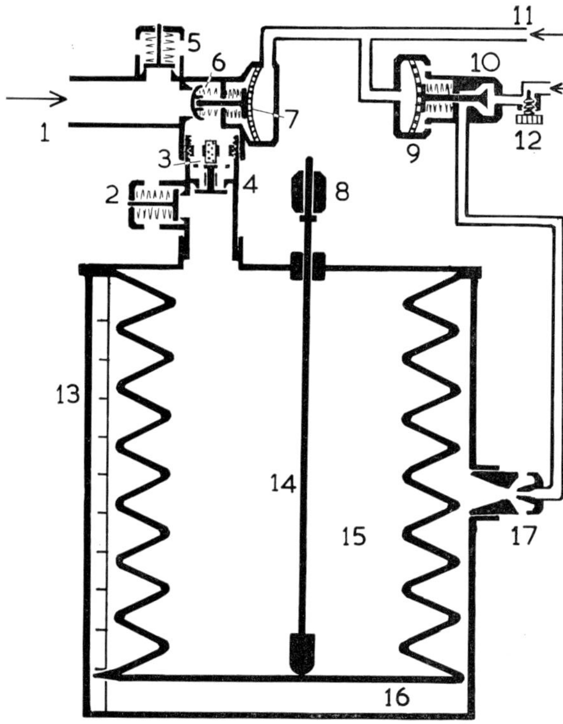

Fig. 29.28. Diagram of the Bird Spirometer.

1. Port
2. One-way valve
3. Magnet
4. Valve
5. Safety-valve
6. Expiratory valve
7. Diaphragm
8. Weight
9. Diaphragm
10. Valve
11. High-pressure line
12. Needle valve
13. Scale
14. Sliding rod
15. Concertina bag
16. Rigid plastic chamber
17. Injector

During the expiratory phase pressure in the line (11) falls (see the account of the Bird Mark 7 in which the corresponding line is numbered (23) (fig. 29.2)). Therefore the valve (10) closes and the valve (6) opens; the flow of driving gas to the injector (17) is cut off and expired gas flows, past the magnetic valve (3, 4), into the concertina bag (15).

The magnet (3) is normally set so that, with the concertina bag (15) fully compressed, as it should be at the start of the expiratory phase, the valve (4) opens when there is a positive pressure above it of 0·5 cmH_2O irrespective of any negative pressure in the bag (15). The valve subsequently closes when the pressure drop across it, due to the flow of expired gas into the bag, falls to 1 cmH_2O. This helps to ensure that there is a short period at the end of the expiratory phase during which expiratory flow into the bag is stopped, so that a steady reading of expired volume is indicated by the pointer on the scale (13). The weight of the bag generates some small negative pressure within it, which decreases as the bag expands. This negative pressure can be supplemented by adding weights (8) to the top of the sliding rod (14). These weights are marked with the volume of gas which, if the inlet (1) is open to atmosphere, they will cause to be drawn into the bag (15) before the magnetic valve (3, 4) snaps shut.

The maximum capacity of the concertina bag is 2400 ml. The safety-valve (5) is normally set to 40 cmH_2O but can be replaced by an airtight cap if higher inflating pressures are to be delivered by those Bird ventilators capable of so doing.

FUNCTIONAL ANALYSIS

The use of this spirometer will have only a small effect on the functional analysis of any Bird ventilator with which it is used, and that only during the expiratory phase. During that phase the action will be primarily that of a pressure generator, the generated pressure being slightly negative to begin with but progressively tending towards atmospheric as the concertina bag expands. Once the resultant expiratory flow falls to the critical level at which the pressure drop across the valve (4) is 1 cmH_2O, the valve shuts and the ventilator becomes a zero-flow generator for the remainder of the phase.

THE BIRD MARK 2 VENTILATOR

DESCRIPTION

This compact apparatus (fig. 29.29) is designed to compress intermittently the reservoir bag of an anaesthetic circuit.

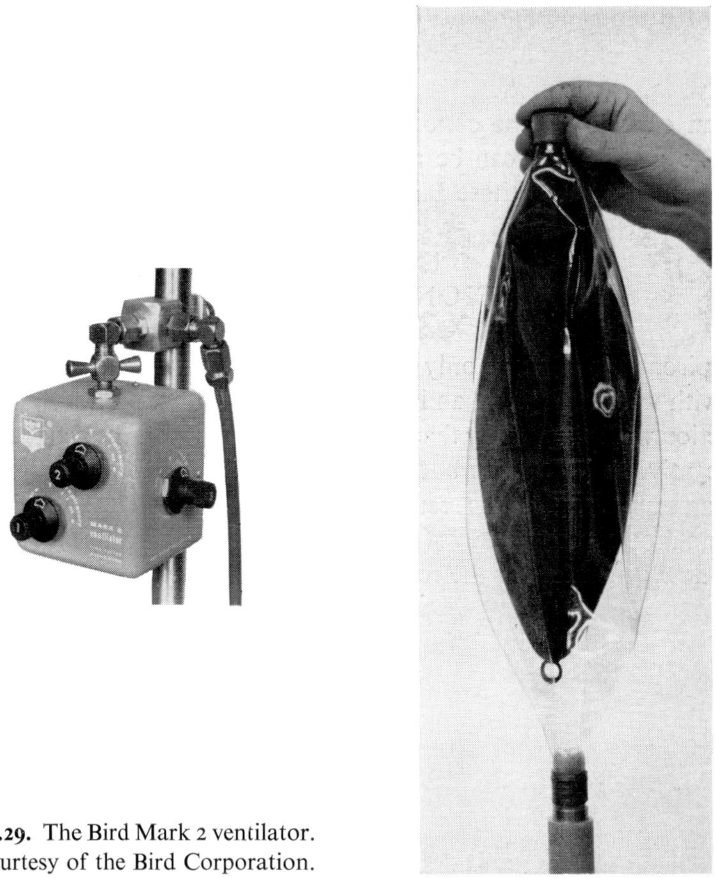

Fig. 29.29. The Bird Mark 2 ventilator. Courtesy of the Bird Corporation.

The neck of the transparent plastic bag (4) (fig. 29.30) is sealed round the neck of the anaesthetic reservoir bag (3). The inlet (7) of the control unit (6–15) is connected to a supply of compressed gas at a pressure of 50 lb/in². There is then a flow of gas, through the filter (8) and the 'expiratory time' control (11), so that pressure builds up behind the diaphragm (10) and opens the valve (9) against the force of its spring. Driving gas can now flow, through the valve (9), the 'inspiratory flow/pressure' control (6), and the injector (16), where it entrains air, to the plastic bag (4). The reservoir bag (3) is compressed and the gas within it is delivered to the patient.

At the same time there is a flow of driving gas from the valve (9), past the 'inspiratory time' control (12), to the chamber behind the diaphragm (14). Pressure in this chamber rises since the escape valve (13) is held closed by the pressure of driving gas above its diaphragm. When the pressure behind the diaphragm (14) has risen sufficiently, the valve (15) is opened against the force of its spring. Driving gas flowing from the 'expiratory time' control (11) now escapes to atmosphere, and pressure in the chamber behind the diaphragm (10) falls. The valve (9) closes, cutting off the flow of driving gas to the

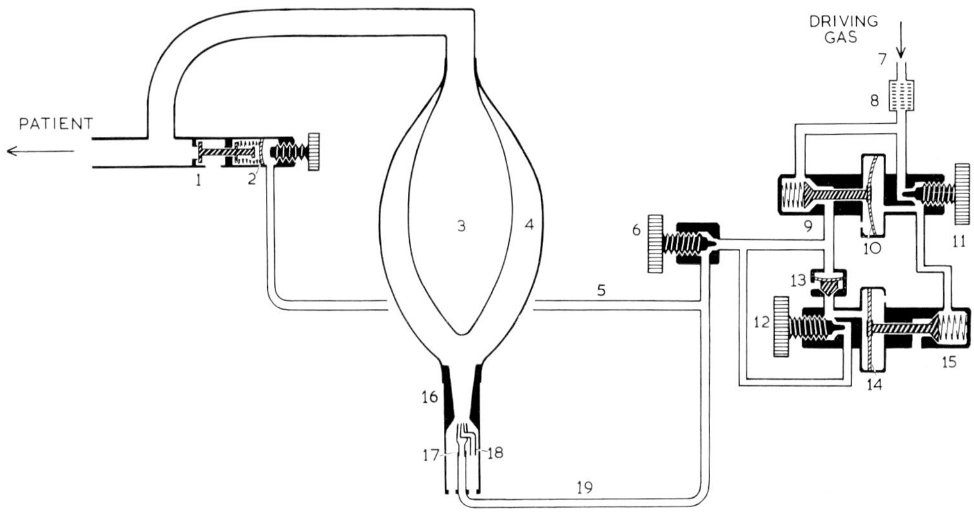

Fig. 29.30. Diagram of the Bird Mark 2 ventilator.

1. Valve
2. Diaphragm
3. Reservoir bag
4. Transparent plastic bag
5. Connecting tube
6. 'Inspiratory flow/pressure' control
7. Driving-gas inlet
8. Filter
9. Valve
10. Diaphragm
11. 'Expiratory time' control
12. 'Inspiratory time' control
13. Escape valve
14. Diaphragm
15. Valve
16. Injector
17. Nipple
18. Nipple
19. Connecting tube

injector (16). Gas within the plastic bag (4) now escapes to atmosphere through the entrainment ports of the injector, and the reservoir bag (3) refills with expired or fresh gas depending on the anaesthetic circuit in use. Pressure in the tube (19) falls, the escape valve (13) opens, pressure behind the diaphragm (14) falls, and the valve (15) closes. Pressure can now build up again behind the diaphragm (10) at a rate determined by the setting of the 'expiratory time' control (11). The expiratory phase ends when this pressure is sufficient to reopen the valve (9).

The duration of the inspiratory phase depends on the setting of the 'inspiratory time' control (12) which determines the time needed for the pressure behind the diaphragm (14) to rise sufficiently to open the valve (15). The duration of the expiratory phase depends on the setting of the 'expiratory time' control (11). The inspiratory-expiratory ratio is set by adjusting the durations of the inspiratory and expiratory phases.

The volume of gas delivered to the patient is the volume delivered from the bag during the inspiratory phase together with fresh gas entering the circuit during the phase. The volume delivered from the bag is limited by one of three factors—(a) the driving unit cycles, after a time set by the control (12), from its inspiratory position to its expiratory position, (b) the bag (3) is completely collapsed, or (c) before either of these events occurs, the pressure within the plastic bag (4) reaches a level which prevents further flow from the injector (16) into the bag, and driving gas flows out through the entrainment ports of the injector.

For normal use the tube (19) is fitted to the centre nipple (17) of the injector assembly which allows the inflating pressure to be varied between 4 and 40 cmH_2O. If higher pressures are required the connecting tube (19) is fitted to the other nipple (18) of the injector assembly, thereby bringing a different jet into action. This allows the inflating pressure to be adjusted up to 65 cmH_2O. A 'muffler' can be fitted over the entrainment ports of the injector assembly to reduce noise.

The 'pressure/flow' control (6) determines the flow of driving gas to the injector (16) during the inspiratory phase. This in turn determines the pressure which must be reached in the bag (4) before further flow of driving gas into the bag is prevented. It therefore determines the maximum inflating pressure which can be achieved. At the same time this control regulates the inspiratory flow rate from the reservoir bag (3) to the patient.

During automatic ventilation excess gas spills during the expiratory phase through the valve (1) of the 'automatic gas balance valve' assembly (1, 2, and the screw control). The valve (1) is held closed during the inspiratory phase by the pressure of driving gas behind the diaphragm (2). During the expiratory phase the valve opens at a pressure of 5 cmH_2O. Therefore spill occurs only at the beginning of the expiratory phase, when rapid flow through the resistance of the expiratory pathway (from the valve (1), through the bag (3) and the injector (16), to atmosphere) produces sufficient pressure drop to open the valve (1).

If manual ventilation is to be performed the 'automatic gas balance valve' (1, 2) must be locked in its closed position by its screw control, and the three controls (6, 11 and 12) must be closed. A standard blow-off valve must be included in the breathing circuit. The plastic bag (4) and the reservoir bag (3) can then be squeezed as a single unit.

If the supply of driving gas is cut off, the patient can breathe spontaneously from the reservoir bag (3) since the outer plastic bag (4) is in free communication with atmosphere through the entrainment ports of the injector.

The Bird Mark 2 can be used on its own as a resuscitator by plugging the injector (16) into a face mask. It may be used as a power source to drive a Bird Mark 4 or Mark 6 ventilator. The Mark 4 is available with a Mark 2 unit built into it; this combination is called simply the Bird Mark ventilator.

Note on the operation of the 'Automatic gas balance valve' (1, 2)

This valve is designed to fulfill the functions of the more-conventional spill valves in other closed-circuit ventilators, namely to spill enough excess gas during each expiratory phase to balance the volume of fresh gas which enters the circuit in each complete respiratory cycle. However, the mode of operation is quite different from that of the conventional spill valves and is therefore discussed at some length.

Throughout the expiratory phase, atmospheric pressure is applied at the entrainment ports of the injector assembly (16) so that the flow from the patient rises suddenly to a peak and then declines. Therefore it can be only at the beginning of the expiratory phase that sufficient pressure drop will occur, across the resistance of the expiratory pathway from the valve (1) to the injector (16), to open the valve (1).

The volume of gas spilt through the valve in each expiratory phase depends on the pattern of flow out of the lungs. This pattern of flow depends on the effects on the patient's lungs of the atmospheric pressure at the entrainment ports of the injector (16) and the +5 cmH_2O pressure limit imposed at the valve (1). Therefore the pattern of flow, and hence the volume of gas spilt, will vary with the volume in the lungs at the end of the inspiratory phase and with lung characteristics. In general, therefore, the escape of excess gas through the valve (1) in each respiratory cycle will not automatically exactly balance the inflow of fresh gas during the cycle.

If the escape of excess gas exceeds the inflow of fresh gas the reservoir bag (3) will progressively empty until it is flattened shortly before the end of each inspiratory phase so that the tidal volume will be reduced. This will reduce the expiratory flow and hence the escape of excess gas. A balance will be achieved when the reservoir bag (3) is flattened early enough in the inspiratory phase for the reduced excess-gas escape to balance the fresh-gas inflow. In this situation the lungs will be held inflated for the last part of the inspiratory phase.

The sequence of events just described can be prevented, or at least limited, by partly closing the screw control of the 'automatic gas balance valve' assembly (1, 2) so that the opening of the valve (1) is restricted and the escape of excess gas is reduced to the point at which it just balances the fresh-gas inflow. However, any subsequent alteration in lung characteristics or deliberate change of tidal volume (by increasing the 'inspiratory flow' (6) or 'inspiratory time' (12) control settings) will upset the balance and necessitate readjustment of the screw control of the 'automatic gas balance valve'.

If the escape of excess gas is less than, instead of more than, the inflow of fresh gas the reservoir bag (3) will progressively fill until it becomes taut at the end of the expiratory phase and the alveolar pressure will not be able to fall to atmospheric. Therefore the end-expiratory lung volume will be increased. Therefore the subsequent end-inspiratory volume will be increased (unless the alveolar pressure was previously coming fully into equilibrium with the generated pressure in the inspiratory phase) and the expiratory flow will be more rapid. This will increase the escape of excess gas and eventually a balance will be achieved with the inflow of fresh gas, but with the alveolar pressure failing to fall to atmospheric by the end of the expiratory phase. If this situation is to be avoided the screw control of the 'automatic gas balance valve' (1, 2) must be unscrewed and, if this is not sufficient, the fresh-gas flow must be reduced.

FUNCTIONAL ANALYSIS

Inspiratory phase

During this phase the ventilator operates as a constant-pressure generator due to the characteristics of the injector. The generated pressure can be set low. If the bag (3) becomes completely collapsed before the end of the phase the ventilator will then operate as a constant-flow generator, the generated flow being the flow of fresh gas into the patient circuit. This condition will continue, either until the end of the phase, or until the mouth pressure rises to the pressure generated by the injector, whichever event occurs first. If the latter occurs first, the ventilator then reverts to constant-pressure generation with some of the fresh gas flowing into the bag (3).

Change-over from inspiratory phase to expiratory phase

This change-over is time-cycled: it occurs when the pressure behind the diaphragm (14) has risen to a critical level in a preset time from the beginning of the inspiratory phase which can be adjusted by the 'inspiratory time' control (12).

Expiratory phase

Throughout this phase constant, atmospheric, pressure is generated at the entrainment ports of the injector assembly (16). In addition, an upper pressure limit of $+5$ cmH_2O is imposed at the valve (1). In the early part of the phase this pressure limit will normally be reached. Therefore the ventilator operates first as a constant, positive, pressure generator at (1) and then as a constant, atmospheric, pressure generator at (16).

Change-over from expiratory phase to inspiratory phase

This change-over also is time-cycled: it occurs when the pressure behind the diaphragm (10) has risen to a critical level in a preset time from the beginning of the expiratory phase which can be adjusted by the 'expiratory time' control (11).

THE BIRD MARK 6 VENTILATOR

DESCRIPTION

This ventilator consists essentially of a concertina reservoir bag which is contained in a rigid plastic pressure chamber and forms part of a non-rebreathing circuit. It may be driven by any Bird ventilator, but the manufacturers recommend that it be used in conjunction with a Mark 2/6, Mark 9, or Mark 14 model. The simplest combination is that of the Mark 6 driven by the Mark 2/6 (fig. 29.31) and it is this combination which is described here.

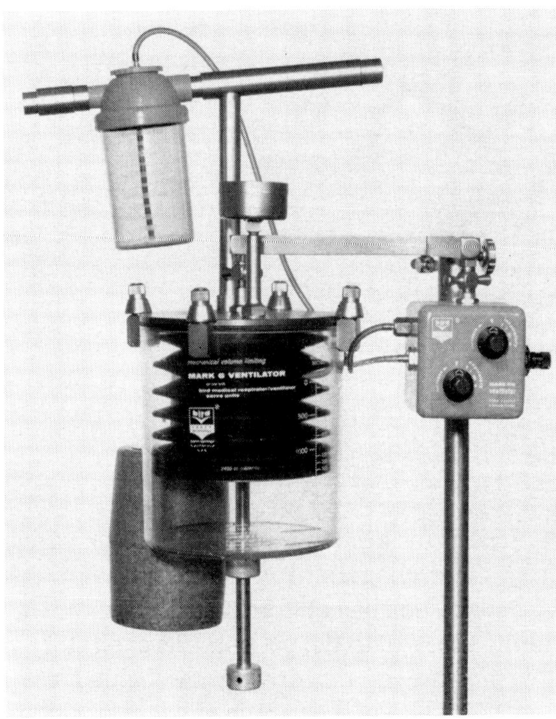

Fig. 29.31. The Bird Mark 6 ventilator driven by the Bird Mark 2/6.
Courtesy of the Bird Corporation.

The Mark 2/6 is basically the same as the Mark 2 (see p. 406) but modified so that the supply of driving gas to the injectors is no longer adjustable. Instead there is an adjustable supply to a nebulizer during the expiratory phase.

During the inspiratory phase driving gas can be supplied to either one of two injectors (9) (fig. 29.32). For a given supply pressure the choice between these two injectors

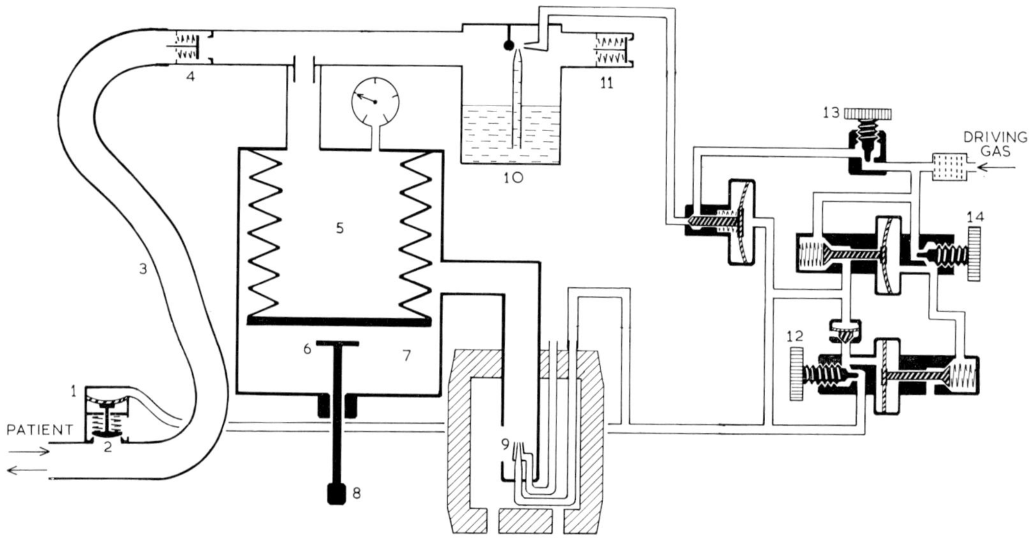

Fig. 29.32. Diagram of the Bird Mark 6 ventilator driven by the Bird Mark 2/6.

1. Diaphragm
2. Expiratory valve
3. Breathing tube
4. One-way valve
5. Concertina bag
6. Plate
7. Rigid plastic pressure chamber
8. Volume control
9. Injector
10. Nebulizer
11. One-way valve
12. Inspiratory-time control
13. Nebulizer-flow control
14. Expiratory-time control

is the only control the user has over the speed of inflation. The driving gas, together with entrained air, flows from the driving unit to the rigid plastic pressure chamber (7) and compresses the reservoir concertina bag (5) forcing the gas within it, through the one-way valve (4) and the breathing tube (3), to the patient. The expiratory valve (2) is held in the closed position by the pressure of the driving gas behind the diaphragm (1). The volume contained in the reservoir bag is determined by the position of the plate (6) set by the control (8). The inspiratory time depends on the setting of the control (12). At the end of the inspiratory phase pressure above the diaphragm (1) falls, the expiratory valve (2) is no longer held closed, and expired gas can flow through it to atmosphere. The concertina bag (5) refills with air drawn in through the one-way valve (11) to which a bag-entrainment system may be fitted to allow the use of special gas mixtures. Driving gas also flows from the driving unit to the nebulizer (10) during the expiratory phase so that the gas stored in the bag (5) is humidified. The expiratory time depends on the setting of the control (14).

FUNCTIONAL ANALYSIS

Inspiratory phase

In this phase the ventilator operates fundamentally as a constant-pressure generator due to the characteristics of the injectors (9). In practice the generated pressure may fall a little during the phase due to the pressure-drop across the wall of the concertina bag increasing as the convolutions are compressed. The volume of gas in the reservoir bag at the start of the phase sets a volume limit which will commonly be reached before the end of the phase. Once this volume limit is reached the ventilator operates as a zero-flow generator for the remainder of the phase: the lungs are held inflated.

Change-over from inspiratory phase to expiratory phase

This change-over is time-cycled: as in the Mark 2 it occurs at a time, after the start of the inspiratory phase, which is controlled by the pneumatic timer (12, 14).

Expiratory phase

In this phase the ventilator operates as a constant, atmospheric, pressure generator: the patient's expired gas passes freely to atmosphere at the expiratory valve (2).

Change-over from expiratory phase to inspiratory phase

This change-over also is time-cycled: it occurs at a time, after the start of the expiratory phase, which is controlled by the pneumatic timer (12, 14).

REFERENCES

1 HARRISON G.A. (1967) The high oxygen mixtures delivered by the air-mix control of the Bird Mark 7 ventilator. *Br. J. Anaesth.* **39**, 659.

2 STODDART J.C. (1966) Some observations on the function of the Bird Mark 8 ventilator. *Br. J. Anaesth.* **38**, 977.

CHAPTER 30

The Blease 'All Purpose Pulmoflator' 'Deansway Three' (D.3)

DESCRIPTION

The original Blease 'Pulmoflator'[1] was a pioneer of ventilators in Britain. Over the years a range of models has been developed for use in a wide variety of circumstances. Basically the ventilator comprises an electrically-driven air compressor and a complex spring-and-ratchet device which controls the flow from the compressor to a rigid plastic pressure chamber containing a reservoir bag.

The model (figs. 30.1 and 30.2) described here is the D.3. As in all the current models, an Edwards Speedivac Model ES 150 rotary pump, having a volume flow rate of 150 litres/min, is used as the air compressor. This pump and the spark-proof electric motor by which it is driven are housed in the lower compartment of the ventilator cabinet.

Air from the compressor enters through the inlet (52) (fig. 30.3) and flows through the tap (26) to the main chamber (40) which contains the control mechanism. The tap (26) has two outlets which lead to the jet (51) and the diffuser tube (46) of an injector. The proportion of compressed air which enters the main chamber by either route is determined by the setting of the tap (26). There is always a free connexion between the main chamber (40) and the rigid plastic pressure chamber (5). As pressure rises in both these chambers, the concertina reservoir bag (4) is compressed and the gas within it is forced past the spring-loaded one-way valve (8) to the 'open/closed circuit' control tap (20). When this tap (20) is set to 'open circuit' (as in fig. 30.3) the gas flows directly to the patient through the inspiratory tube (23). When it is set to 'closed circuit', the gas from the concertina bag (4) is forced into a second rigid plastic pressure chamber (2) containing the reservoir bag (3) which is part of an anaesthetic closed circuit. The gas within the reservoir bag (3) is forced through the breathing tube (1) to the patient. The concertina reservoir bag (4) has a weight in its base, and when the tap (20) is set to 'closed circuit' air is drawn into the bag during the expiratory phase through the air filter (11) and the one-way valves (10, 9). Whichever circuit is chosen fresh gas to be delivered to the patient is supplied at the inlet (21). When the tap (20) is set to 'open circuit' this fresh gas flows through the 'manual/automatic ventilation' control tap (27) to the storage bag (12), from which it is drawn into the bag (4) during the expiratory phase. If the tap (20) is set to 'closed circuit' the fresh gas flows straight from the tap, through the ventilator, to an

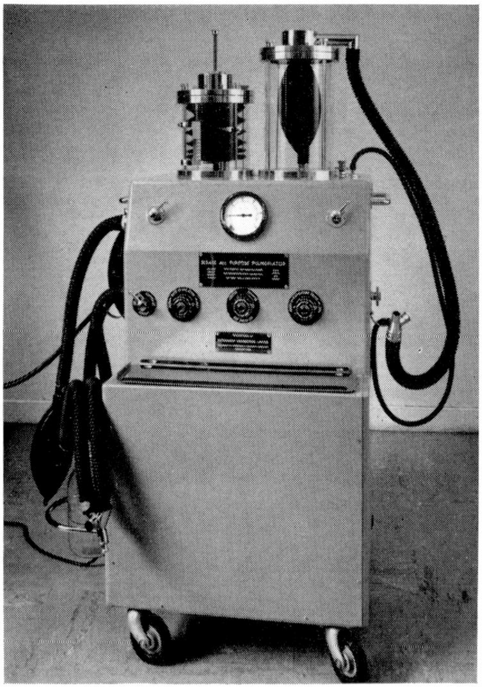

Fig. 30.1.

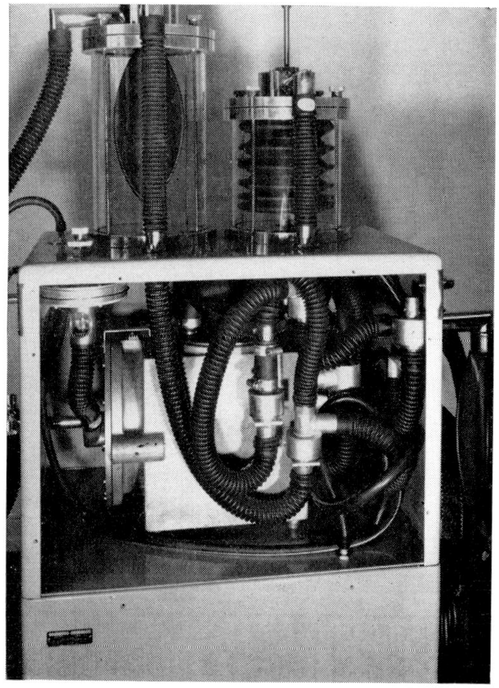

Fig. 30.2.

Fig. 30.1. The Blease 'All Purpose Pulmoflator' 'Deansway Three' (D.3).
Courtesy of Department of Medical Illustration, Cardiff Royal Infirmary.

Fig. 30.2. The mechanism of the Blease 'All Purpose Pulmoflator' 'Deansway Three' (D.3).
Courtesy of Department of Medical Illustration, Cardiff Royal Infirmary.

outlet (16) from which a connexion must be made to the closed-circuit system.

As the pressure within the main chamber (40) rises, the diaphragm (34) is forced outwards, compressing the spring (31). The diaphragm takes with it the rod (35), the movement of which is transferred through the linkage (36) to the spring (39). The tension thereby developed in the spring (39) exerts a pull on the ratchet wheel (41), but the wheel is prevented from rotating by the sprung pawl (44). When the rod (35) has moved over far enough, one end of the rod (42) trips the lever (43) and releases the pawl (44). The tension of the spring (39) now pulls the ratchet wheel (41) sharply anti-clockwise, allowing the other sprung pawl (37) to engage. The rod (45) connects the ratchet wheel to the exhaust valve (49) which is now held open. The movement of the rod (45) is guided by the lever mechanism (47).

The compressed air stored in the main chamber (40) and the compressed air entering it during the expiratory phase now escape freely through the valve (49). The pressure within the main chamber (40) falls rapidly to atmospheric. If the tap (20) is set to 'open circuit' expired gas from the patient flows, through the expiratory tube (22), the taps (20) and (28), the one-way valve (50), the main chamber (40), and out to atmosphere through the port (49). If the tap (20) is set to 'closed circuit' expired gas flows back to the reservoir bag (3), and the gas displaced from the pressure chamber (2) flows back through the taps (20) and (28) to the main chamber (40).

During the outward movement of the diaphragm (34) the air contained in the chamber (32) escapes freely to atmosphere through the one-way valve (24). Once pressure in

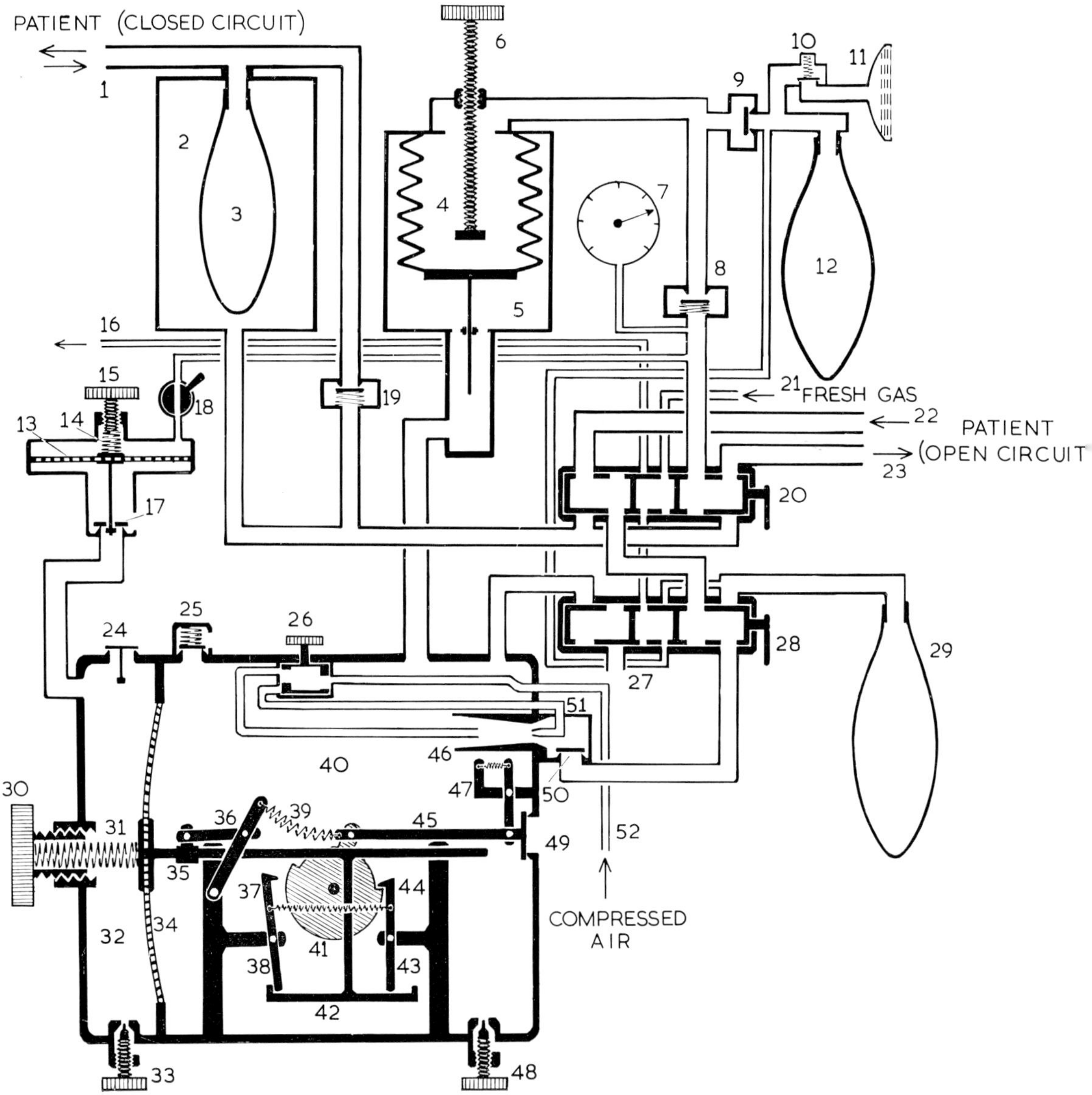

the main chamber (40) has fallen, the diaphragm (34) is gradually returned to its former position by the spring (31). The rate of this return is determined by the setting of the needle valve (33) which controls the flow of air into the chamber (32). The reversed movement of the rod (35) now compresses the spring (39), through the linkage (36). When the rod (42) has moved far enough to strike the lever (38) and release the pawl (37), the force exerted by the spring (39) returns the ratchet wheel (41) clockwise to its former position and the valve (49) is closed. The next inspiratory phase begins. The 'inflation pressure' control (30) alters the force exerted by the spring (31) on the diaphragm (34) and hence determines the cycling pressure. On the model tested the cycling pressure at the mouth was found to be 38 cmH_2O when this control was set to 'maximum'. In addition, the valve (25) provides a safety limit when the ventilator is set to 'automatic'. Adjustment of the 'rate of inflation' control (48) allows a variable amount of the compressed air entering the main chamber (40) to escape. Its setting therefore determines the time required for the cycling pressure to be reached, i.e. the duration of the inspiratory phase. Since the 'expiratory pause' control (33) regulates the flow of air into the chamber (32) during the expiratory phase, its setting determines the duration of the expiratory phase. The pressure in the delivery tube from the concertina reservoir bag (4) is indicated on the manometer (7).

When the tap (20) is set to 'open circuit', fresh gas in excess of the ventilation spills

---

Fig. 30.3. Diagram of the Blease 'All Purpose Pulmoflator' 'Deansway Three' (D.3).

1. Closed-circuit breathing tube
2. Rigid plastic pressure chamber
3. Reservoir bag
4. Concertina reservoir bag
5. Rigid plastic pressure chamber
6. Adjustable stop for limiting tidal volume
7. Manometer
8. One-way valve
9. One-way valve
10. One-way valve
11. Air filter
12. Storage bag for fresh gas
13. Diaphragm
14. Compression spring
15. 'Trigger negative pressure' control
16. Fresh-gas outlet to closed circuit
17. Inlet valve
18. 'Trigger on/off' control
19. One-way valve
20. 'Open/closed circuit' control
21. Fresh-gas inlet
22. Expiratory tube
23. Inspiratory tube
24. One-way outlet valve
25. Safety-valve
26. 'Expiratory pressure' control
27. Outlet for compressed air during manual ventilation
28. 'Manual/automatic ventilation' control
29. Reservoir bag for manual inflation
30. 'Inflation pressure' control
31. Compression spring
32. Chamber
33. 'Expiratory pause' control
34. Diaphragm
35. Rod
36. Link mechanism
37. Sprung pawl
38. Lever
39. Compression/expansion spring
40. Main chamber
41. Ratchet wheel
42. Trip rod
43. Lever
44. Sprung pawl
45. Rod
46. Diffuser tube of injector
47. Valve guide mechanism
48. 'Rate of inflation' control
49. Exhaust valve
50. One-way valve
51. Jet of injector
52. Compressed-air inlet

through the one-way valve (50) into the main chamber (40) during the expiratory phase. When the tap (20) is set to 'closed circuit', excess fresh gas flows past the one-way valve (19) and then spills in the same way.

The stop (6) may be adjusted to set an upper limit to the tidal volume delivered from the concertina reservoir bag (4).

The 'manual/automatic' tap (28) allows manual inflation to be performed by compression of the reservoir bag (29), the fresh gas flowing directly into this bag. If the tap (20) is set to 'open circuit', the gas stored in the bag (29) is directed to the patient through the expiratory tube (22); the excess gas must be blown off through an expiratory valve at the Y-piece near the patient. If the tap (20) is set to 'closed circuit' then this gas is directed into the pressure chamber (2), and the reservoir bag (3) is in turn compressed. During manual inflation the compressed air entering the main chamber (40) escapes continuously to atmosphere through the outlet (27) of the tap (28).

The setting of the 'expiratory pressure' control (26) determines the proportions of compressed air entering the main chamber (40) through the jet (51) of the injector and the diffuser tube (46). If all this compressed air flows through the jet (51) then there is maximum entrainment through the one-way valve (50) and maximum negative pressure is developed in the breathing circuit during the expiratory phase. As the proportion of compressed air directed through the diffuser tube (46) is increased by adjustment of the tap (26), so the negative pressure applied decreases. In the extreme situation all the compressed air enters through the diffuser tube (46) and a positive pressure is maintained in the breathing circuit throughout the expiratory phase. During the inspiratory phase the rise in pressure in the main chamber (40) holds the one-way valve (50) closed, irrespective of the setting of the tap (26).

The 'trigger' control (18) allows the patient-triggering mechanism to be brought into use. If during the expiratory phase the patient makes an inspiratory effort, a negative pressure is produced in the chamber above the diaphragm (13). The diaphragm moves up against the force exerted on it by the spring (14) and the exhaust valve (17) is opened. This allows an immediate entry of air into the chamber (32), and hence an immediate change of the cycling mechanism from the expiratory to the inspiratory position. The negative pressure required to trigger the ventilator in this way depends on the setting of the 'trigger negative pressure' control (15) which alters the force exerted by the spring (14) on the diaphragm (13). The range of triggering pressures is $-1{\cdot}5$ to $-6{\cdot}0$ cmH_2O. This allows negative pressure to be used during the expiratory phase without precluding the use of patient-triggering. The duration of the expiratory phase may be varied between 0·5 sec and more than 1 min. A prolonged expiratory time may be set, when ventilation is being assisted, so as to ensure ventilation if the patient does not make an inspiratory effort within the set time.

For ward use the tap (20) must be set to 'open circuit'. During the expiratory phase air is drawn through the filter (11) and the one-way valves (10, 9) into the concertina reservoir bag (4). If oxygen is added at the fresh-gas inlet (21) it is stored in the bag (12) during the inspiratory phase to be drawn into the concertina reservoir bag (4), along with air, during the expiratory phase.

Other models

There are five other models in the standard range of Blease 'Deansway Pulmoflators'. Each model incorporates the cycling mechanism already described, positive and negative phases, and patient-triggering. They vary in the details of their breathing circuits, the additional facilities they incorporate, and whether or not they are combined with a complete anaesthetic apparatus.

FUNCTIONAL ANALYSIS

Non-rebreathing circuit

Inspiratory phase

Fundamentally this ventilator is a flow generator during the inspiratory phase because the compressor is a positive-displacement pump (see p. 85), driven by a constant-speed motor. There is therefore a constant flow of gas to the ventilator irrespective of the pressures developed. However, this fundamental action is modified by a number of factors.

Firstly, the compressibility of the gas in the large main chamber (40) and in the pressure chamber (5), together with the high distensibility of the large diaphragm (34), comprises a substantial compliance which has to be inflated in parallel with the patient. Secondly, unless the 'rate of inflation' control is at its maximum, its needle valve (48) is partly open, constituting a leak in parallel with the patient. Thirdly, the characteristics of the weighted reservoir bag (4) have some effect on the functioning.

The consequences of these factors are as follows. After the ratchet mechanism (41) operates, and the exhaust valve (49) closes, there is some delay while the pressure in the pressure chamber (5) builds up sufficiently to overcome the weight in the concertina bag. During this delay there is usually no flow into the patient and the delay simply forms an extension of the expiratory period. However, if the fresh-gas flow exceeds the total ventilation, the storage bag (12) becomes taut towards the end of the expiratory phase and the excess spills past the one-way valves (9) and (8); during the last part of the expiratory phase proper the excess goes to waste, but during the delay the one-way valve (50) is closed by the rising pressure in the main chamber and therefore the fresh gas flows into the patient. In fig. 30.4b and c, where the fresh-gas flow did indeed exceed the patient's ventilation, an initial pulse of inflating flow can be seen in what would otherwise have been part of the expiratory phase.

Even when the weight in the concertina bag is overcome, and inflation proper commences, there is still a further period of time, while the pressure in the pressure chamber

(5) and the main chamber (40) is built up, before the flow rises to its full value. Once this point has been reached the flow stays fairly steady, at a level which is not greatly affected by changes of lung characteristics (compare b and c with a in figs. 30.4 and 30.5), so long as the concertina bag (4) can be freely compressed. In the pressure-cycled mode of operation this is so until the end of the phase, when the flow rapidly reverses to expiration (fig. 30.4). In the volume-limited mode of operation, however, further complications ensue when the bottom of the concertina reservoir bag (4) hits the adjustable stop (6) of the stroke-volume control. After this event the pressure in the pressure chamber continues to rise until it attains the cycling pressure. In so doing it compresses the convolu-

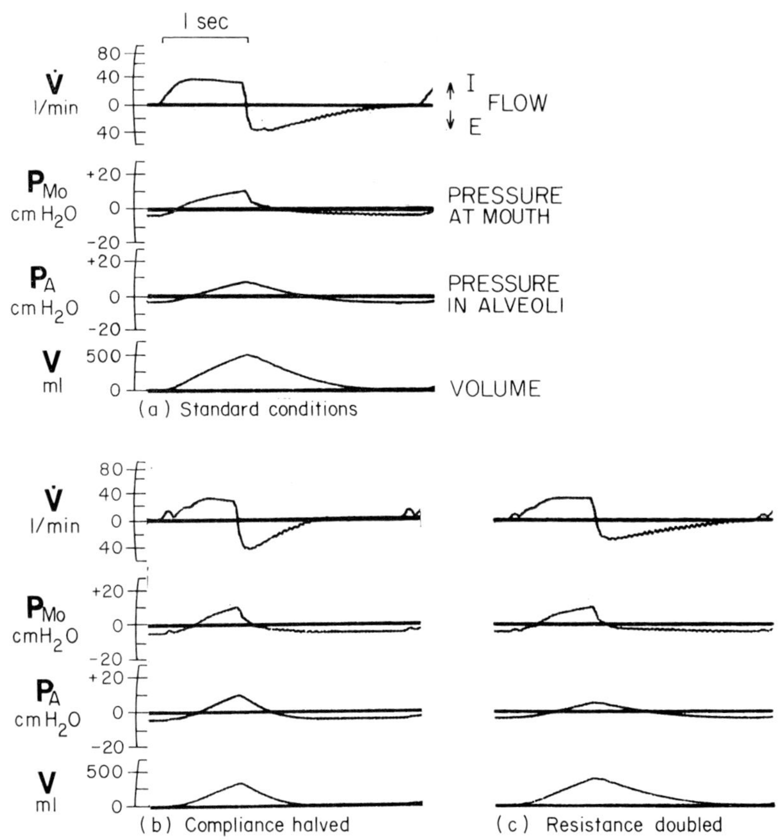

Fig. 30.4. Blease 'Pulmoflator' D.3, with non-rebreathing circuit, in the pressure-cycled mode of operation. Recordings showing the effects of changes of lung characteristics.

Standard conditions: volume control maximum; fresh-gas flow 10·5 litres/min oxygen; 'expiratory pressure' control set for a minimum alveolar pressure of -3 cmH_2O; 'inflation pressure' and 'rate of inflation' controls set to produce a tidal volume of 500 ml in an inspiratory time of 1 sec; 'expiratory pause' control set to produce an expiratory time of 2 sec and hence a respiratory frequency of 20/min and an inspiratory-expiratory ratio of 1 : 2.

tions of the concertina bag producing some further small flow into the patient as shown in fig. 30.5.

An alternative view of the mode of operation during the inspiratory phase is to consider the ventilator as primarily inflating its own compliance. The resultant increasing pressure is applied to the concertina bag (4) and the patient is inflated incidentally. On this view the ventilator becomes an increasing-pressure generator like the Engström; if the inspiratory waveforms of fig. 30.5 are compared with those of fig. 52.6 for the Engström they will be seen to have many similarities. However, changes of lung charac-

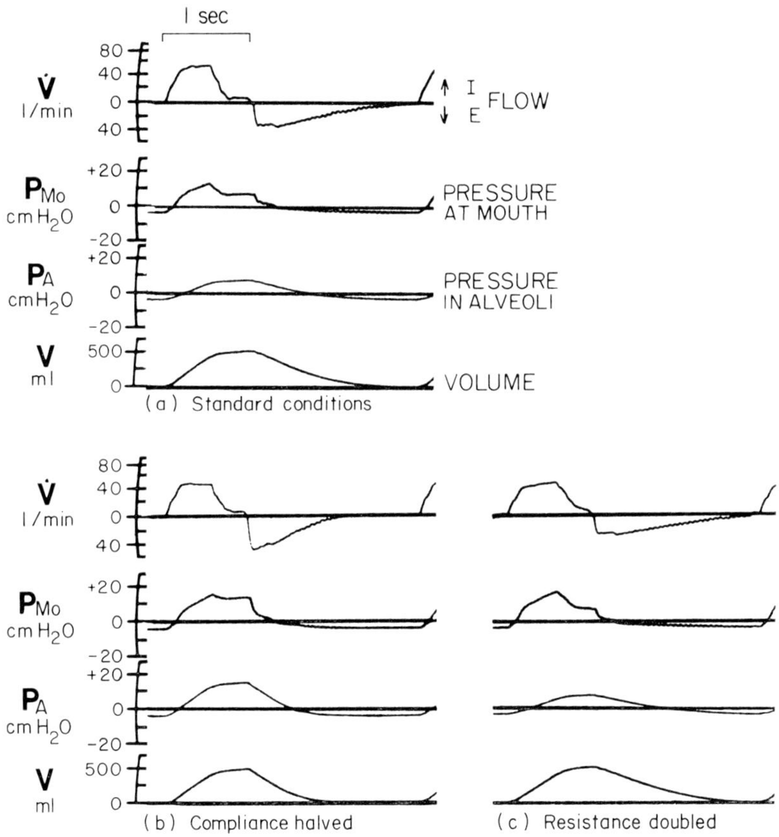

Fig. 30.5. Blease 'Pulmoflator' D.3, with non-rebreathing circuit, in the volume-limited, time-cycled, mode of operation. Recordings showing the effects of changes of lung characteristics.

Standard conditions: 'inflation pressure' maximum; fresh-gas flow 10·5 litres/min oxygen; volume control set to produce a tidal volume of 500 ml; 'rate of inflation' control set to produce an inspiratory time of 1 sec and 'expiratory pause' control set to produce an expiratory time of 2 sec, giving a respiratory frequency of 20/min and an inspiratory-expiratory ratio of 1 : 2; 'expiratory pressure' control set to produce a minimum alveolar pressure of -3 cmH_2O.

teristics alter the resultant flow into the patient and, in the Blease D.3, these alterations appreciably affect the rate of build-up of pressure in the ventilator; therefore the increasing-pressure-generator point of view cannot be rigorously maintained. However, if figs. 30.4 and 30.5 are studied, and if it is remembered that the mouth pressure follows the pressure in the main chamber only until the volume limit is reached, it can be seen that the variation of pressure waveform is little if any greater than the variation of flow waveform. Therefore it is probably just as helpful to regard the ventilator as an increasing-pressure generator as it is to consider it to be a flow generator.

When the tidal volume is very small, as with an infant, changes in the flow into the patient are so small as to have a negligible effect on the build-up of pressure in the ventilator. In these circumstances, therefore, the only tenable point of view is the increasing-pressure-generating one.

Change-over from inspiratory phase to expiratory phase

Fundamentally this change-over is pressure-cycled: it occurs when the pressure in the main chamber (40) has risen sufficiently to operate the ratchet mechanism. If the stroke-volume control (6) is fully unscrewed and the 'inflation pressure' control (30) set to a moderate level, the pressure in the main chamber is closely related to that at the patient's mouth and the change-over is indeed pressure-cycled. This is the situation in fig. 30.4 in which it can be seen that changing the lung characteristics has no effect on the peak mouth pressure at the end of the inspiratory phase although the tidal volume and inspiratory time are altered.

On the other hand, if the stroke-volume control is set to limit the excursion of the concertina bag, and the 'inflation pressure' control is set to a high level, the bag is always driven to its preset limit, expelling a preset volume, despite changes in lung characteristics. When this limit is reached, the pressure in the main chamber (40) continues to rise until the cycling pressure is reached. In most ventilators which operate in this way the pressure rise after the volume limit has been reached is rapid and the change-over can be regarded as effectively volume-cycled. In this ventilator, however, because of the large compliance on the driving-gas side of the concertina bag (4), the pressure rise is slow and there is a substantial delay between the attainment of the volume limit and the change-over. In fig. 30.5a, where a tidal volume of 500 ml is delivered to the 'standard' model lung and the cycling pressure is at its maximum, the delay is about half a second. This delay could be reduced by reducing the cycling pressure but, if it were made too small, a moderate decrease in compliance or increase in resistance would lead to pressure-cycling before the volume limit was reached. The delay is somewhat influenced by changes in lung characteristics since these affect the pressure in the main chamber at the moment the volume limit is reached. Therefore the change-over cannot even be said to occur at a fixed time after the volume limit is reached. However, if the inspiratory phase is considered as a whole it can be seen that, before the change-over can occur, a given volume must be delivered to the patient and a further given volume must be delivered to the main chamber to inflate its compliance to the cycling pressure. Gas is supplied at a constant flow by the compressor; therefore, if there is no leak through the needle valve (48), that is, if the 'rate of inflation' control is set at maximum, the sum of the two given volumes is delivered in a fixed time. That is, the change-over is time-cycled. If the 'rate of inflation' control is not at maximum the loss through the needle valve (48) varies with lung characteristics but the variation is not large and, at least for the range of lung characteristics used in fig. 30.5, it is a good approximation to regard the change-over as time-cycled.

Thus the two modes of operation for the end of the inspiratory phase are (a) pressure-cycled and (b) volume-limited, time-cycled.

Expiratory phase

During the expiratory phase the lungs are connected to the injector (51). The characteristics of this are such that it behaves as a constant-pressure generator (either negative or positive) but with some series resistance. The consequence of this is that the pressure at the mouth does not immediately fall to the generated pressure at the beginning of the phase but approaches it gradually as the flow declines. However, it is clear from both figs. 30.4 and 30.5 that the flow pattern is considerably affected by changes of lung characteristics particularly by halving the compliance.

The ripple on the flow and mouth-pressure waveforms in the expiratory phase arises from the fact that the output from the compressor (which drives the injector) is pulsatile. No ripple is seen in the inspiratory phase because there it is smoothed out by the compliance of the main chamber (40).

Change-over from expiratory phase to inspiratory phase

This change-over is time-cycled or patient-cycled whichever mode of cycling occurs first: the change-over occurs when the pressure in chamber (32) has risen to a preset level either (a) at a preset rate, through the needle valve (33) of the 'expiratory pause' control, and therefore in a preset time, or else (b) suddenly, when an inspiratory effort by the patient acts on the diaphragm (13) to open the valve (17). In figs. 30.4 and 30.5 the ventilator is purely time-cycled and it can be seen that, in the face of changes in lung characteristics, the expiratory phase ends at a fixed time after it starts; it does not end immediately some fixed volume has come out of the lungs nor immediately some critical pressure has been reached at the mouth. The only deviation from this is as follows. The short delay after the operation of the ratchet mechanism, during which the pressure in the pressure chamber builds up to overcome the weight in the concertina bag, normally forms an extension of the expiratory phase. This is the case in all tracings in fig. 30.5 and also in fig. 30.4a. But when the fresh-gas flow exceeds the total ventilation, as in fig. 30.4b and c, the fresh gas produces some inspiratory flow during this delay which then forms part of the inspiratory phase.

Closed circuit

Some brief notes on the effect of using the closed circuit are given on p. 431.

CONTROLS

Non-rebreathing circuit—pressure-cycled mode of operation—fig. 30.6

Total ventilation

This cannot be directly controlled but is equal to the product of tidal volume and respiratory frequency.

Tidal volume

This is indirectly controlled by adjustment of the cycling pressure by means of the 'inflation pressure' control (fig. 30.6b). It is reduced by a reduced compliance (fig. 30.4b) and by an increased resistance (fig. 30.4c). It is also influenced by almost every other control. Setting the 'expiratory pressure' control more negative (fig. 30.6e) increased the pressure range in the alveoli and hence the tidal volume. Decreasing the 'expiratory pause' setting may prevent the alveolar pressure from falling fully to the pressure generated in the expiratory phase (as in fig. 30.6c) and so reduce the tidal volume a little. Increasing the 'rate of inflation' increases the pressure drop across the airway resistance and hence leads to cycling at a lower alveolar pressure and to a reduced tidal volume (fig. 30.6d).

Increasing the tidal volume by means of the 'inflation pressure' control increases the inspiratory time (fig. 30.6b). It also decreases the expiratory time (fig. 30.6b) because it increases the restoring force on the diaphragm (34) whose return governs the end of the expiratory phase. Therefore when the tidal volume is changed by means of the 'inflation pressure' control the inspiratory-expiratory ratio is considerably altered and the respiratory frequency is also, in general, changed to some extent, although the direction of the change may depend on the exact circumstances.

Respiratory frequency and inspiratory-expiratory ratio

Neither of these parameters can be directly controlled but both are determined by the separately-variable inspiratory and expiratory times.

The inspiratory time is the time taken to raise the pressure in the main chamber (40) to the cycling pressure. It can therefore be reduced by reducing the leakage from the chamber through the needle valve (48), that is by increasing the 'rate of inflation' setting (fig. 30.6d). However, if this is done, the pressure drop across the airway resistance will be increased and the tidal volume will be decreased. If this drop in tidal volume is to be avoided it will be necessary to increase the cycling pressure. This increase in 'inflation pressure' will, in turn, shorten the expiratory time because of the increased restoring force on the diaphragm (34) and, if this is to be corrected, it will be necessary to decrease the leak past the needle valve (33) by increasing the 'expiratory pause' setting.

The inspiratory time is also influenced by any change in tidal volume resulting either from changes of control settings (fig. 30.6b, c and e) or from changes of lung characteristics (fig. 30.4b and c).

The expiratory time is directly controlled (fig. 30.6c) by the 'expiratory pause' control (33) which regulates the return of the diaphragm (34). However the expiratory time is also decreased by an increase in the 'inflation pressure' setting because this increases the restoring force on the diaphragm (34). The only other way in which the expiratory time is altered concerns the delay between the operation of the ratchet mechanism, closing the exhaust valve (49), and the start of the upward movement of the concertina bag (4). Normally there is no flow into the lungs in this period which therefore forms part of the expiratory phase. However, if the fresh-gas flow is much more than the total ventilation, fresh gas does flow into the lungs in this period which therefore becomes part of the inspiratory time: inspiratory time is increased and expiratory time is decreased. This can be seen to some extent in fig. 30.4b and c, where changes of lung characteristics have reduced the ventilation to less than the fresh-gas flow and, to a greater extent, in fig. 30.6f where the fresh-gas flow has been increased to about twice the total ventilation.

Thus the respiratory frequency and the inspiratory-expiratory ratio are both dependent on four controls: 'expiratory pause', 'rate of inflation', 'inflation pressure', and stroke-volume. In addition, the inspiratory-expiratory ratio, but not the respiratory frequency, may also be influenced by the fresh-gas flow. This is because, as explained at the end of the functional analysis, the delay between the operation of the ratchet mechanism and the start of the upward movement of the concertina bag forms part of the expiratory phase when the fresh-gas flow is low, but part of the inspiratory phase when the fresh-gas flow exceeds the total ventilation. If the respiratory frequency and inspiratory-expiratory ratio are to be set to specific values, both the 'rate of inflation' and the 'expiratory pause' controls must be adjusted, perhaps more than once each, because of their mutual interaction. Both frequency and inspiratory-expiratory ratio are affected by changes of lung characteristics.

Inspiratory waveforms

In this mode of operation there is no true choice of inspiratory waveforms. Increasing the setting of the 'rate of inflation' control (48) will increase the inspiratory flow and increase the rate of increase of mouth pressure, but a particular setting of the control may well have been chosen in order to deliver a given tidal volume in a given inspiratory time.

Expiratory waveforms

In the expiratory phase it is primarily the pressure waveform which is determined by the ventilator while the flow waveform depends on the effect of the pressure on the lungs. The generated pressure is constant throughout the phase although, as explained in the functional analysis, effective series resistance in the injector prevents the generated pressure showing immediately at the mouth. The magnitude of the pressure, positive or negative, can be varied by means of the 'expiratory pressure' control (fig. 30.6e) but not its form.

Pressure limits
The peak inspiratory pressure at the mouth is equal to the cycling pressure; the peak alveolar pressure is less than this by an amount equal to the airway resistance multiplied by the inspiratory flow. During the expiratory phase the alveolar pressure normally falls to equal the generated pressure unless the expiratory time is too short (fig. 30.6c) or the resistance is too high.

Mean pressure
This can be reduced by setting the 'expiratory pressure' control more negative but this results in an increased tidal volume (fig. 30.6e). If the tidal volume is to be restored to its original value the cycling pressure must be reduced by means of the 'inflation pressure' control and then the 'expiratory pause' setting must be decreased to compensate for the decreased restoring force on diaphragm (34). The mean pressure can also be reduced by reducing the inspiratory time in relation to the expiratory time.

Non-rebreathing circuit—volume-limited, time-cycled mode of operation—fig. 30.7

Total ventilation
This cannot be directly controlled but is equal to the product of tidal volume and respiratory frequency.

Tidal volume
This is directly controlled by the setting of the stroke-volume control (6) which limits the excursion of the concertina bag. It is therefore unaffected by changes in lung characteristics (see fig. 30.5). The tidal volume is however increased if the fresh-gas flow is increased to well above the total ventilation. Then the storage bag (12) becomes taut towards the end of the expiratory phase and some fresh gas enters the patient circuit during the delay between the operation of the ratchet mechanism, closing valve (49), and the start of the upward movement of the concertina bag. In the present tests, increasing the fresh-gas flow, from equal to the total ventilation to double the total ventilation, increased the tidal volume from 500 ml to 600 ml (not shown in fig. 30.7).

Fig. 30.6. Blease 'Pulmoflator' D.3, with non-rebreathing circuit, in the pressure-cycled mode of operation. Recordings showing the effects of changes in the settings of the controls.

(a) Standard conditions as in fig. 30.4.
(b) 'Inflation pressure' control increased $2\frac{1}{2}$ turns to produce a tidal volume of 750 ml.
(c) 'Expiratory pause' decreased 5 turns to produce a respiratory frequency of 30/min.
(d) 'Rate of inflation' increased 2 turns.
(e) 'Expiratory pressure' control turned, through 20°, to the maximum negative position.
(f) Fresh-gas flow increased to 20 litres/min.

For recordings (b), (c), and (e) the fresh-gas flow was increased just enough to keep the storage bag (12, fig. 30.3) taut at the end of the inspiratory phase.

Increasing the tidal volume, by means of the stroke-volume control (6) (fig. 30.7b) increases the inspiratory time and therefore decreases the frequency and alters the inspiratory-expiratory ratio.

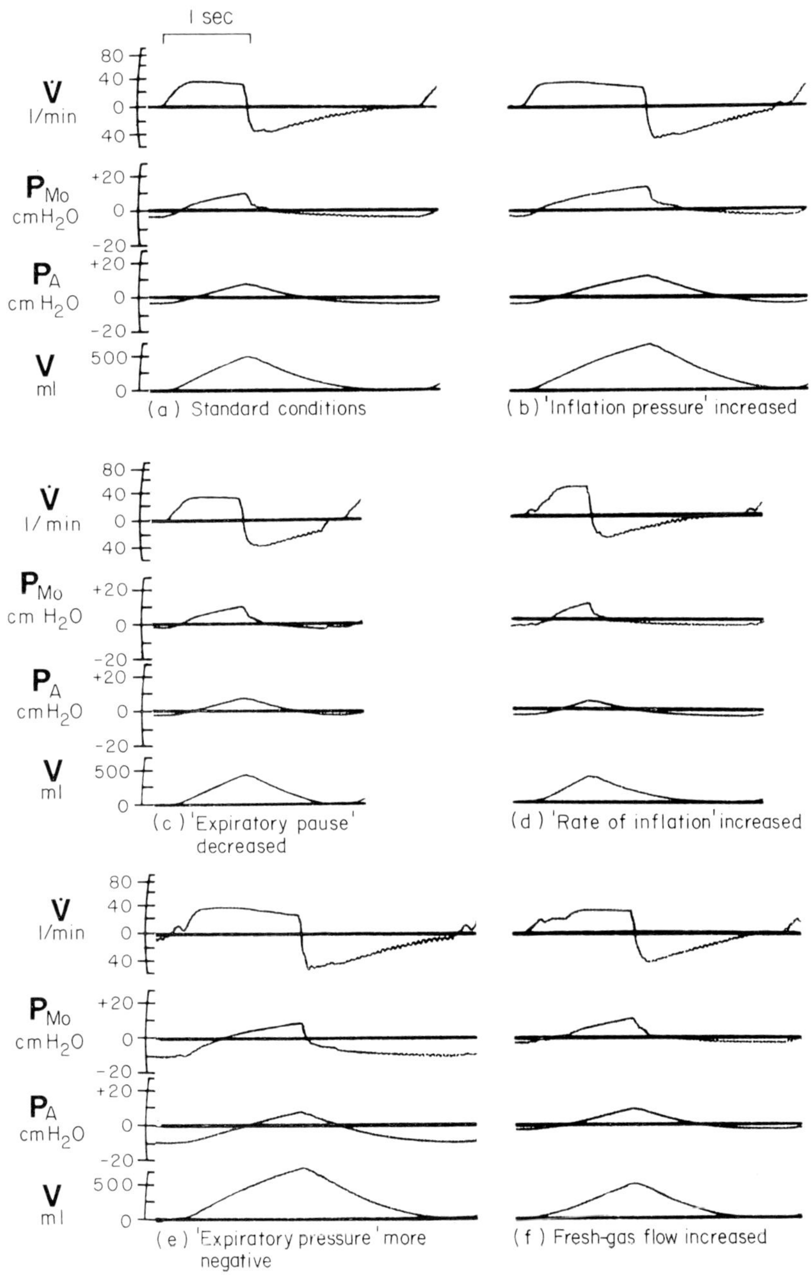

Respiratory frequency and inspiratory-expiratory ratio

Neither of these parameters can be directly controlled but both are determined by the separately-variable inspiratory and expiratory times.

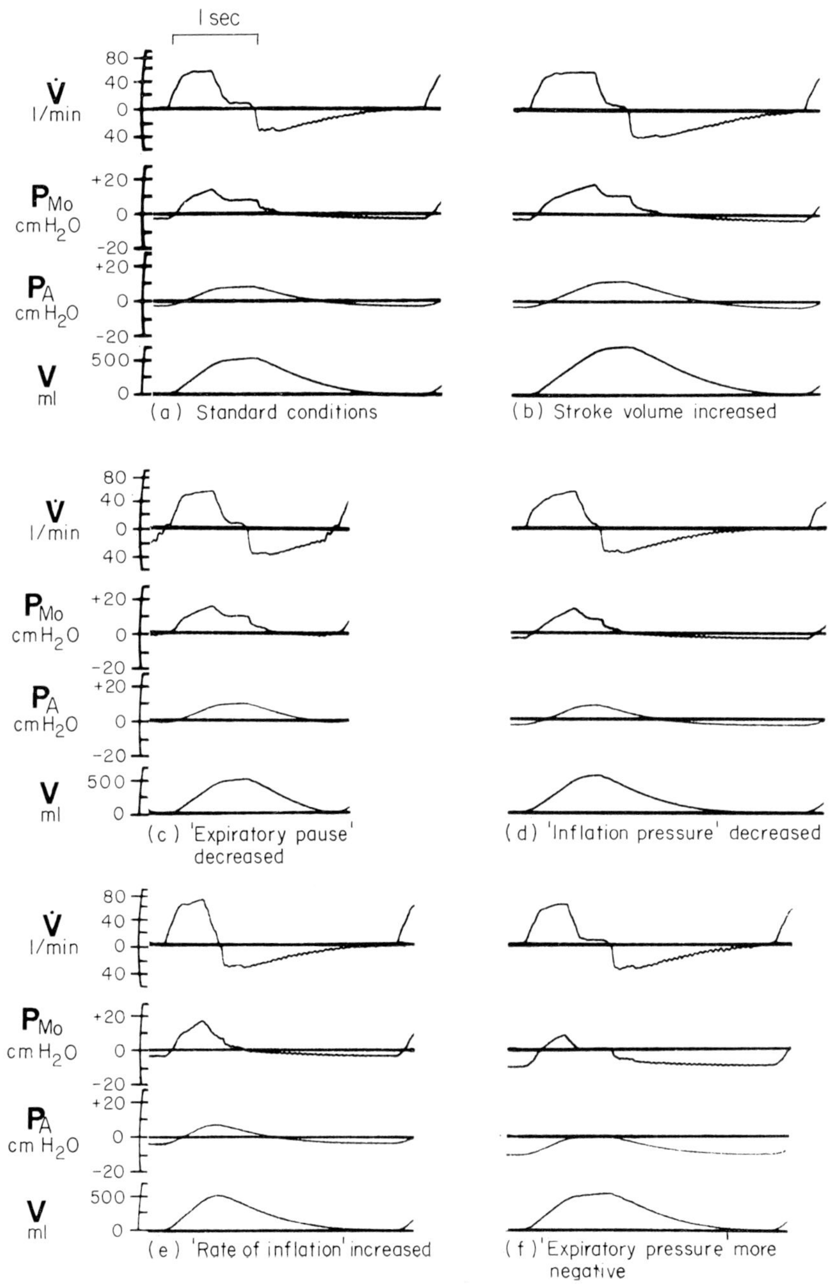

The inspiratory time is not directly controlled but is equal to the time taken for the constant flow from the compressor to supply the sum of three volumes: the tidal volume, the volume required to 'inflate' the compliance of the main chamber (40) to the cycling pressure, and the volume of any gas spilt through the needle valve (48) of the 'rate of inflation' control. Therefore changes in any of these three factors affect the inspiratory time. For deliberate control of the inspiratory time the 'rate of inflation' control can be adjusted to vary the amount of gas spilt through the leak: fig. 30.7e shows that increasing the 'rate of inflation' to maximum (eliminating the leak) decreases the inspiratory time considerably. If the tidal volume is changed this also changes the inspiratory time although not, as in some ventilators, in proportion to the tidal volume: in fig. 30.7b increasing the tidal volume by 50% increases the inspiratory time by only 15%. Finally, if the 'inflation pressure' (30) is reduced this reduces the volume of gas required to inflate the main-chamber compliance to the cycling pressure and therefore reduces the inspiratory time (fig. 30.7d): in this case the reduction in inspiratory time takes the form of a reduction of the period in which the lungs are held inflated, while the pressure in the main chamber builds up to the cycling pressure. As was shown in the functional analysis the inspiratory time is little affected by changes in lung characteristics; the change-over is approximately time-cycled.

The expiratory time is directly controlled by the 'expiratory pause' control (33). Since the change-over from the expiratory phase to the inspiratory phase is time-cycled (see the functional analysis) expiratory time is not affected by changes in lung characteristics. However, if the 'inflation pressure' control (30) is adjusted the force restoring the diaphragm (34) is altered and thereby the expiratory time is changed: in fig. 30.7d decreasing the 'inflation pressure' by five complete revolutions of the control has increased the expiratory time by 20%.

Thus, as in the pressure-cycled mode, the respiratory frequency and the inspiratory-expiratory ratio are both dependent on four controls: 'expiratory pause', 'rate of inflation', 'inflation pressure', and stroke volume. In addition, the inspiratory-expiratory ratio, but not the respiratory frequency, may be affected by the fresh-gas flow. This is because, as explained at the end of the functional analysis, the delay between the

---

Fig. 30.7. Blease 'Pulmoflator' D.3, with non-rebreathing circuit, in the volume-limited time-cycled mode of operation. Recordings showing the effects of changes in the settings of the controls.

(a) Standard conditions as in fig. 30.5.
(b) Stroke-volume control setting increased to produce a tidal volume of 750 ml.
(c) 'Expiratory pause' decreased to produce a respiratory frequency of 30/min.
(d) 'Inflation pressure' decreased 5 turns.
(e) 'Rate of inflation' increased to maximum.
(f) 'Expiratory pressure' set to maximum negative pressure.

For recordings (b), (c), and (d) the fresh-gas flow was increased just enough to keep the storage bag (12, fig. 30.3) taut at the end of the inspiratory phase.

operation of the ratchet mechanism and the start of the upward movement of the concertina bag forms part of the expiratory phase when the fresh-gas flow is low, but part of the inspiratory phase when the fresh-gas flow exceeds the total ventilation. If the respiratory frequency is to be altered the obvious control to use is the 'expiratory pause', but this will also alter the inspiratory-expiratory ratio. If this is to be restored to its original value an adjustment to the 'rate of inflation' control must be made. But this in turn will slightly alter the respiratory frequency and further adjustment of both controls may be necessary to achieve a given pattern precisely. If the inspiratory-expiratory ratio is to be altered without change of frequency the same two controls should be used but starting with the 'rate of inflation' control.

Since both change-overs are truly or very-nearly time-cycled neither the frequency nor the inspiratory-expiratory ratio is much affected by changes in lung characteristics (fig. 30.5).

Inspiratory waveforms

In this mode of operation some real choice of waveform is possible without altering the respiratory frequency or the inspiratory-expiratory ratio. To achieve this, however, requires matched adjustments to three controls. Thus, if the 'inflation pressure' is reduced from the maximum (fig. 30.7d) the period in which the lungs are held inflated after active inflation has almost stopped is decreased; but thereby the total inspiratory time is decreased. However, if the 'rate of inflation' control is also decreased the inspiratory time can be restored to its original value. Then the inspiratory waveform of flow will be nearer to a steady flow throughout the inspiratory phase than in fig. 30.7a. However, in reducing the 'inflation pressure' the expiratory time will have been increased and it will be necessary to decrease the 'expiratory pause' setting to restore the original timing completely.

Expiratory waveforms

In the expiratory phase it is primarily the pressure waveform which is determined by the ventilator while the flow waveform depends on the interaction of the pressure waveform with the lung characteristics. The generated pressure is constant throughout the phase although, as explained in the functional analysis, effective series resistance in the injector prevents this pressure showing immediately at the mouth. The magnitude of the pressure, positive or negative, but not its form, can be varied by means of the 'expiratory pressure' control (26) (fig. 30.7f).

Pressure limits

Since the ventilator operates as a constant-pressure generator during the expiratory phase the alveolar pressure, at the end of the phase, usually falls to this pressure unless the expiratory time is too short (as in fig. 30.7c) or the expiratory resistance is too high. The level to which the alveolar pressure usually falls can be adjusted by the 'expiratory pressure' control (fig. 30.7f). The peak alveolar pressure, in the inspiratory phase, is not directly controlled but is determined by the fact that it exceeds the minimum by an amount equal to the tidal volume divided by the compliance.

Mean pressure

This can be directly controlled by the 'expiratory pressure' control: setting this more negative (fig. 30.7f) moves the pressure waveforms (at the mouth and in the alveoli) downward without altering their shape and without affecting other parameters appreciably. The mean pressure can also be reduced by (a) reducing the period of held inflation at the end of the inspiratory phase, (b) reducing the inspiratory time in relation to the expiratory time.

Closed circuit

Complete tests have not been made with the closed-circuit system but it seems likely that the following will be the main points of difference.

Excess fresh gas spills past one-way valve (19) during the later part of the expiratory phase, as soon as the bag (3) is taut. The pressure drop across this valve is small so that negative pressures can still be developed in the alveoli even if not quite such large ones as with the non-rebreathing circuit. The presence of the additional bag-in-bottle should have little effect on the inspiratory phase or on the change-over mechanisms, except that now fresh gas enters the patient circuit continuously. Therefore the tidal volume exceeds the excursion of the concertina bag by the volume of fresh gas entering during the inspiratory phase. Therefore, in the volume-limited, time-cycled, mode of operation the tidal volume varies with the fresh-gas flow. In the pressure-cycled mode of operation it is the concertina-bag excursion which varies with fresh-gas flow, the tidal volume being unaffected. There will also be a tendency for the tidal volume to be less than expected from the concertina-bag excursion because some of the volume displaced from the concertina bag is absorbed in compressing the gas in the extra pressure chamber (2).

REFERENCE

1 Musgrove A.H. (1952) Controlled respiration in thoracic surgery. A new mechanical respirator. *Anaesthesia*, 7, 77.

CHAPTER 31

The Blease 'Open Circuit Paediatric Ventilator'

DESCRIPTION

This ventilator attachment (fig. 31.1) is designed primarily for use with the Blease 'Pulmoflator', but is suitable for use with certain other ventilators.

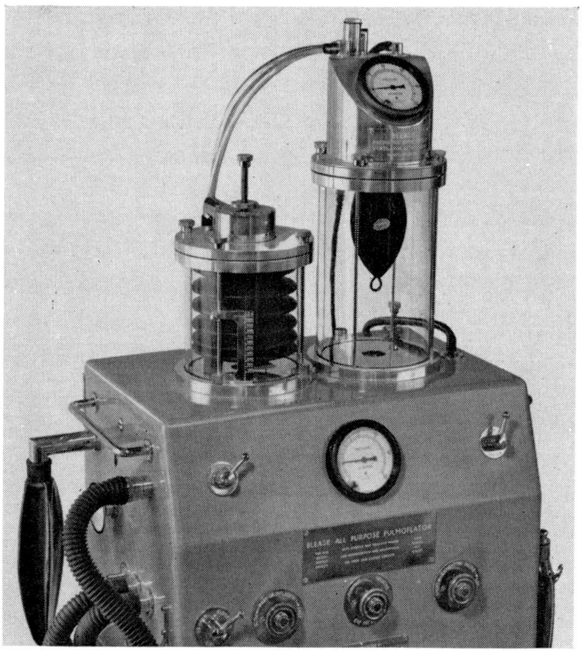

Fig. 31.1. The Blease 'Open Circuit Paediatric Ventilator'.
Courtesy of Blease Medical Equipment Ltd.

It consists of a non-rebreathing 'bag-in-bottle' arrangement to which fresh gas should be supplied at a flow equal to the desired total minute-volume ventilation. The reservoir bag (4) (fig. 31.2) which is enclosed in a rigid plastic pressure chamber (5) has a very small volume. During the inspiratory phase the reservoir bag (4) is compressed and the

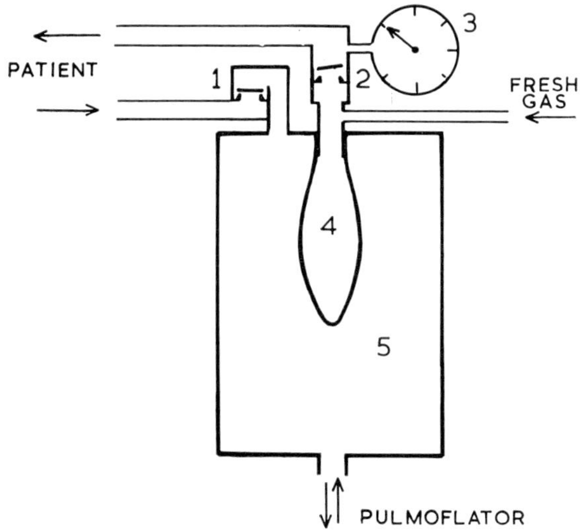

Fig. 31.2. Diagram of the Blease 'Open Circuit Paediatric Ventilator'.

1. One-way expiratory valve
2. One-way inspiratory valve
3. Manometer
4. Reservoir bag
5. Rigid plastic pressure chamber

gas within it, together with fresh gas entering the circuit during the phase, is forced past the one-way valve (2) to the infant, the one-way valve (1) being held closed by the higher pressure in the chamber (5). The pressure in the patient circuit is shown on the manometer (3). During the expiratory phase the pressure in the chamber (5) and the bag (4) falls, the one-way valve (2) closes, and the one-way valve (1) opens. Fresh gas flows steadily into the reservoir bag (4) and expired gas flows into the pressure chamber.

The duration of the inspiratory phase depends on the time taken to reach the cycling pressure set on the 'Pulmoflator'; it is therefore determined by the settings of the 'inflation pressure' and 'rate of inflation' controls of the 'Pulmoflator', and the combined compliance of the infant, the rigid plastic pressure chamber (5), and the main chamber of the 'Pulmoflator'. The duration of the expiratory phase is set by the 'expiratory pause' control of the 'Pulmoflator'. The sum of the inspiratory and expiratory times determines the respiratory period and hence the respiratory frequency.

The tidal volume depends on the respiratory frequency and the fresh-gas flow. So long as the 'inflation pressure' set on the 'Pulmoflator' is high enough and the inspiratory phase long enough for the reservoir bag (4) to be emptied during each inspiratory phase, the total minute-volume ventilation and fresh-gas flow are equal. That is, the ventilator operates as a minute-volume divider. The tidal volume is then equal to the fresh-gas flow divided by the respiratory frequency. If the fresh-gas flow is excessive the reservoir bag (4) will not be emptied by the time that the cycling pressure is reached in the 'Pulmoflator'. The reservoir bag (4) will therefore be progressively distended until it begins to become taut towards the end of each expiratory phase, and excess gas spills through the breathing tubes into the chamber (5), during the expiratory phase. Then, the total minute-volume ventilation is less than the fresh-gas flow.

FUNCTIONAL ANALYSIS

Inspiratory phase

When an infant or small child is inflated the flow to the patient is so small as to have a negligible effect on the way in which the 'Pulmoflator' inflates its own large compliance. Therefore the system must be regarded as an increasing-pressure generator (see the functional analysis of the Blease 'Pulmoflator'). If the increasing pressure outside the reservoir bag (4) causes the volume limit (set by the volume of gas in the bag at the start of the phase) to be reached before the end of the phase, the ventilator then operates for the remainder of the phase as a constant-flow generator due to the fresh-gas flow.

Change-over from inspiratory phase to expiratory phase

Although this change-over is fundamentally pressure-cycled, when ventilating small children the build-up of pressure is virtually uninfluenced by lung characteristics and determined almost entirely by ventilator characteristics. Therefore the change-over is better considered to be time-cycled.

Expiratory phase

In this phase the ventilator operates as a constant-pressure generator, positive, atmospheric, or negative, owing to the characteristics of the injector system in the Blease 'Pulmoflator'.

Change-over from expiratory phase to inspiratory phase

This change-over is time-cycled; it occurs when the pressure in a chamber in the Blease 'Pulmoflator' has risen to a preset level at a rate which is preset and is uninfluenced by the patient.

CHAPTER 32

The Bourns 'Pediatric Respirator' Model LS–104

DESCRIPTION

This ventilator (figs. 32.1, 32.3) is designed for use in the treatment of neonates suffering from the respiratory distress syndrome. It is powered by a.c. mains electricity. Air, or a mixture of air and oxygen, is drawn into the ventilator and delivered to the baby either through an endotracheal or tracheostomy tube or through a nasal mask which may be sealed to the face with surgical cement.

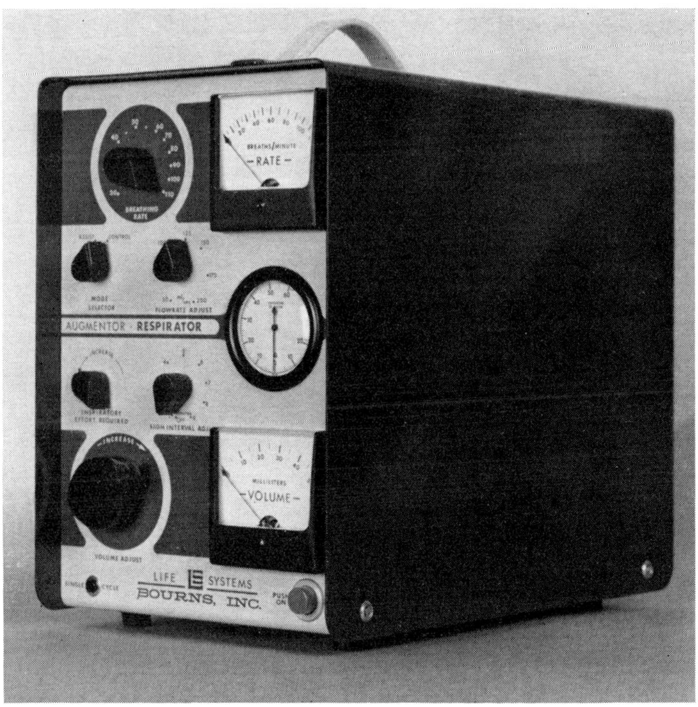

Fig. 32.1. The Bourns 'Pediatric Respirator' Model LS–104.

Courtesy of Bourns, Inc.

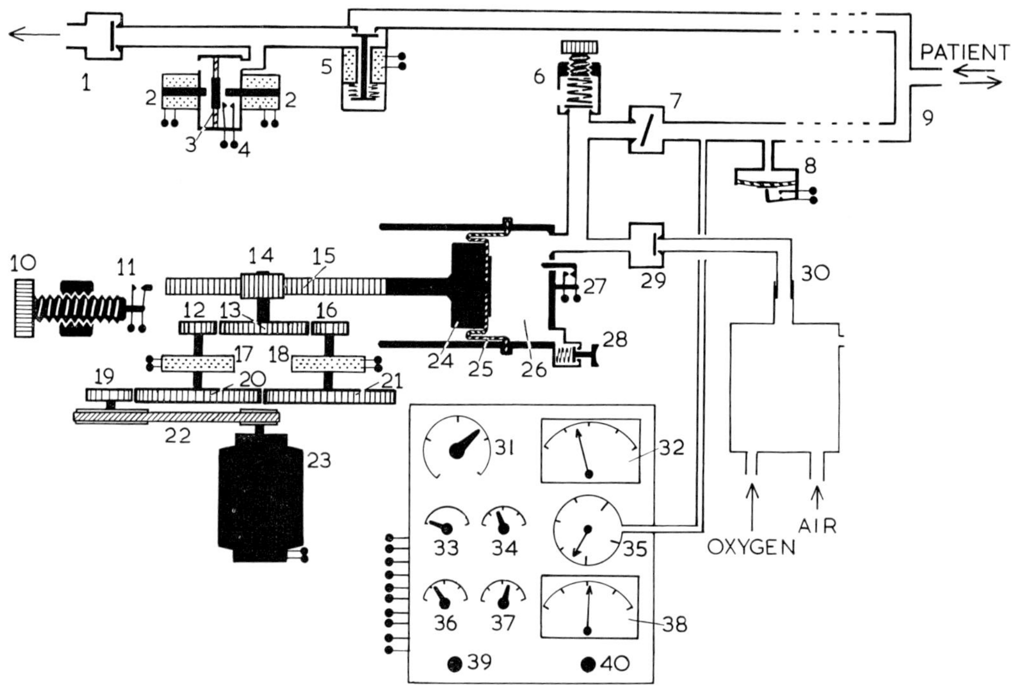

Fig. 32.2. Diagram of the Bourns 'Pediatric Respirator' Model LS–104.

1. One-way valve
2. Electro-magnets
3. Diaphragm
4. Patient-trigger contacts
5. Solenoid-operated valve
6. Pressure-limiting valve
7. One-way valve
8. Low-inflation-pressure alarm
9. Patient outlet
10. 'Volume adjust' control
11. Contacts
12. Gear-wheel
13. Gear-wheel
14. Pinion
15. Rack
16. Gear-wheel
17. Magnetic clutch
18. Magnetic clutch
19. Gear-wheel
20. Gear-wheel
21. Gear-wheel
22. Pulley drive
23. Electric motor
24. Piston
25. 'Rolling diaphragm'
26. Cylinder
27. Contacts
28. Drain
29. One-way valve
30. Fresh-gas inlet
31. 'Breathing rate' control
32. 'Breaths/minute rate' meter
33. 'Mode selector' control
34. 'Flowrate adjust' control
35. Manometer
36. 'Respiratory effort' control
37. 'Sigh interval adjust' control
38. Stroke-volume meter
39. 'Single cycle' button
40. On/off button

When the ventilator is turned on by the 'on/off' switch (40) (fig. 32.2), the electric motor (23) runs continuously, turning the meshing gear-wheels (20, 21) through the reduction pulley drive (22) and the gear-wheel (19). However, no motion is imparted to either of the gear-wheels (12) or (16) until the magnetic clutches (17) or (18) respectively are energized. At the start of the inspiratory phase the clutch (18) is energized and the gear-wheel (16) is rotated. Immediately before this, the solenoid-operated valve (5) is energized, closing the expiratory pathway.

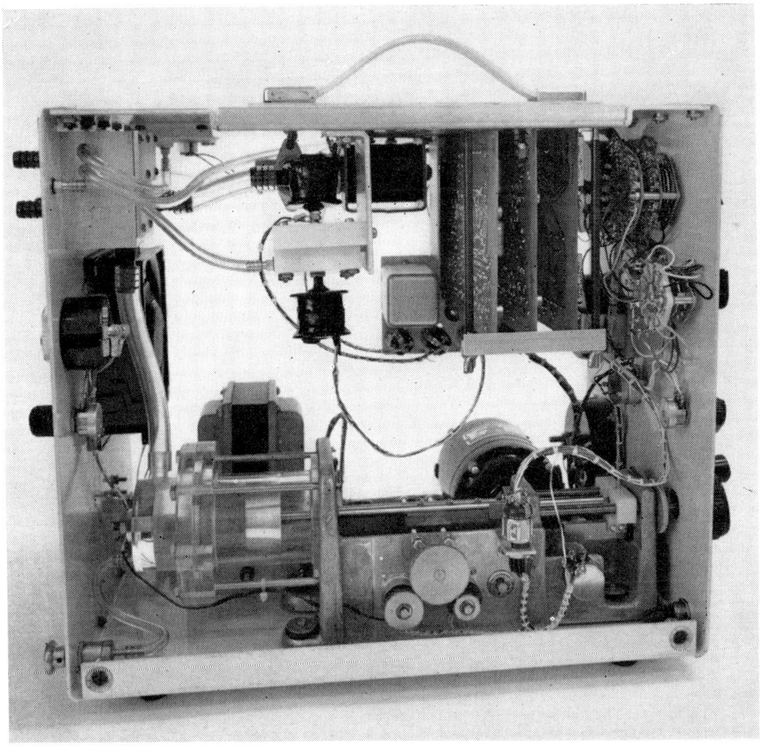

Fig. 32.3. The mechanism of the Bourns 'Pediatric Respirator' Model LS–104.
Courtesy of Bourns, Inc.

The gear-wheel (13), driven by the gear-wheel (16), turns the pinion (14), driving the rack (15) to the right and forcing the piston (24) into the cylinder (26). Gas contained in the cylinder (26) is forced, past the one-way valve (7), to the patient. It may be noted that the seal between the piston and the cylinder is obtained not by oil, which might contaminate the inspired gas, but by a 'rolling diaphragm' (25).

As the piston (24) completes its forward stroke, it opens the electrical contacts (27), and the inspiratory phase ends. The supply of electrical current to the solenoid-operated valve (5) is cut off and the valve opens. Expired gas now flows, through the valve (5) and the one-way valve (1), to atmosphere. At the same time the electrical supply to the magnetic clutch (18) is cut off, and a moment later the clutch (17) is energized. The pinion (14) is now driven by the gear-wheels (12) and (13) and so drives the rack (15) to the left, drawing back the piston (24). The one-way valve (7) now closes, the one-way valve (29) opens, and fresh gas is drawn into the cylinder (26) through the inlet (30). When the rack (15) has moved back far enough it closes the electrical contacts (11), and the electrical supply to the clutch (17) is cut off. The ventilator is then ready to start the next inspiratory phase but will not normally do so immediately.

If the 'mode selector' (33) is in the 'control' position the ventilator normally remains in the 'ready' condition, just described, until a preset time from the start of the previous inspiratory phase has elapsed. This time is determined by an electronic circuit and can be adjusted by means of the 'breathing rate selector' (31). When this time has elapsed, the solenoid-operated valve (5) is closed, the magnetic clutch (18) is energized, and a new inspiratory phase begins.

If the 'mode selector' (33) is in the 'assist' position, the ventilator remains in the 'ready' condition until an inspiratory effort by the patient draws the diaphragm (3) of the patient-trigger mechanism to the right, thereby closing the contacts (4); then a new inspiratory phase begins. The negative pressure required to trigger the ventilator in this way depends on the distance between the diaphragm (3) when at rest and the contacts (4). The diaphragm (3) has a soft-iron disc in its centre which lies between two electro-magnets (2, 2). The resting distance between the diaphragm (3) and the contacts (4) may therefore be varied by altering the currents flowing to the magnets (2, 2). These are determined by the setting of the 'inspiratory effort required' control (36). The minimum pressure is less than $-0{\cdot}075$ cmH_2O. When the 'mode selector' (33) is set to 'assist', the setting of the 'breathing rate' control (31) is still of relevance. Should the patient's respiratory frequency fall below 60 per cent of the value set on the 'breathing rate' control (31) for longer than 12 seconds, the ventilator will automatically inflate the patient at the rate set on the 'breathing rate' control (31) for approximately 7 seconds during which a continuous alarm will sound. After such a 7-second period of automatic inflation, the ventilator will revert to normal patient-triggered operation. However, if the patient-triggered frequency is still less than 60 per cent of the set value for 12 seconds, another 7-second period of automatic inflation and alarm sounding will follow. This sequence will be repeated, either until the patient's spontaneous efforts become adequate again, or until suitable corrective action is taken.

The tidal volume delivered is set by the 'volume adjust' control (10). The setting of this control determines the position of the contacts (11), and hence the traverse of the rack (15) and the piston (24). The maximum tidal volume is 50 ml. The meter (38) indicates the stroke volume of the piston (24). The speed of the motor (23) can be altered by the 'flowrate adjust' control (34) to deliver flows of 50 to 200 ml/sec (3 to 12 litres/min).

For the proper working of the ventilator it is essential that the settings of the 'volume adjust' (10), 'flowrate adjust' (34), and 'breathing rate' (31) controls should be compatible. For instance, if the volume is set to 50 ml and the flow rate to 100 ml/sec the forward (inspiratory) and return strokes of the piston will each take 0·5 sec, total 1 sec. In these circumstances, therefore, the 'breathing rate' must not be set for more than 60 breaths/min. If, in the 'controlled' mode, it is set for exactly 60 breaths/min the inspiratory-expiratory ratio will be 1 : 1. Smaller ratios can be obtained by increasing the 'flowrate adjust' setting. Thus if, in the above circumstances, the flow rate were increased to

200 ml/sec the inspiratory phase would last 0·25 sec and the inspiratory-expiratory ratio would be 1 : 3.

The breathing frequency in either the 'controlled' or 'assist' modes is shown on the 'rate' meter (32) and may be varied from 20 to 110 breaths/min in the controlled mode as set by the 'breathing rate' control (31). In the 'assist' mode the ventilator may be patient-triggered at up to 200 breaths/min.

A 'sigh interval adjust' control (37) is incorporated. When this is switched on, the valve (5) does not open at the end of an inspiratory phase, and a second tidal volume is delivered. The interval at which this 'sigh' occurs is variable between 1 and 9 minutes.

An alarm system (8), in the inspiratory pathway, sounds a 'beep' at the end of each inspiratory phase if the pressure in the circuit fails to reach at least 5–7 cmH_2O. The pressure in the circuit is shown on the manometer (35). The pressure-limiting valve (6) can be set to limit the maximum inflating pressure to any level between 15 and 70 cmH_2O.

A 'single cycle' button (39) can be pushed to initiate a respiratory cycle at any time, provided the 'mode selector' (33) is set to 'assist'.

A mixing box is available for attachment to the inlet port (30), to allow for controlled enrichment of air with oxygen. If humidification is desired, an ultrasonic nebulizer with variable output is available for attachment between the ventilator and the patient. Alternatively, humidification may be provided through the mixing box. A 'push-button' drain (28) allows condensed water to be drained from the cylinder (26).

FUNCTIONAL ANALYSIS

Inspiratory phase

In this phase, assuming that the speed of the motor (23) is uninfluenced by the pressure developed in the patient circuit, the ventilator operates as a constant-flow generator owing to the steady expulsion of gas from the cylinder (26).

If the pressure in the patient circuit rises high enough it is possible to set the positive-pressure-limiting valve (6) to open in every inspiratory phase. Then the mode of operation for the remainder of the phase is that of a constant-pressure generator. In these circumstances, however, the tidal volume is less than the volume delivered from the cylinder to an unknown extent.

Change-over from inspiratory phase to expiratory phase

This change-over is both volume-cycled and time-cycled: it occurs when the contacts (27) are opened after a preset volume has been delivered from the cylinder (26) at a preset flow determined by the speed of the motor (23).

Expiratory phase

In this phase the ventilator operates as a constant, atmospheric, pressure generator: the patient's expired gas passes to atmosphere through the one-way valve (1).

Change-over from expiratory phase to inspiratory phase

With the 'mode selector' switch (33) set to 'control' this change-over is time-cycled: it occurs at a preset time after the start of the previous inspiratory phase, provided that the piston (24) has by then completed its return stroke and closed the contacts (11). The preset time is determined by an electronic circuit and can be adjusted by the 'breathing rate' control (31).

With the 'mode selector' switch set to 'assist' the change-over is patient-cycled: it occurs when an inspiratory effort by the patient closes the contacts (4), provided the piston has by then completed its return stroke. If the resultant respiratory frequency falls below a preset level for a preset time the ventilator automatically changes to time-cycling for a period.

CHAPTER 33

The Cape-Waine 'Anaesthetic' and Cape Ventilators

DESCRIPTION

The Cape-Waine ventilator[1] is intended for anaesthetic use and the Cape ventilator for ward use. Both were developed from the original Smith-Clarke ventilator.[2,3] In all three the basic mechanism is the same. The Cape-Waine 'Anaesthetic' ventilator (figs. 33.1 and 33.2), which incorporates a complete anaesthetic apparatus, is described in detail here, and the points of difference to be found in the Cape ventilator are described on p. 444.

A spark-proof a.c. mains electric motor (25) (fig. 33.3), driving through an oil variator ('respiratory frequency' control) (27) and gear-box (28), is connected, by a chain drive, to a sprag clutch (30) on the main shaft (31). On this shaft are mounted two cams (16, 17) and two cranks (6, 15), together with a tachometer (29) which indicates respiratory frequency. The crank (6) drives the positive-pressure concertina bag (2), and the crank (15) drives the negative-pressure concertina bag (13). The cams (16, 17) actuate the inspiratory and expiratory poppet valves (18, 19), which are otherwise held closed by their springs. After the inspiratory valve (18) has been held open for the first one-third of the complete respiratory cycle, the expiratory valve (19) is held open for the other two-thirds of the cycle. The inspiratory-expiratory ratio is therefore fixed at 1 : 2. However, since the concertina bags (2, 13) are driven by the cranks (6, 15) they are compressed for one half of the respiratory cycle and expanded for the other half. The relationship beween the cranks (6, 15) and the cams (16, 17) is such that compression of both the bags (2, 13) starts at a time equal to one-sixth of a complete respiratory cycle before the cam (17) closes the expiratory valve (19) and the cam (16) opens the inspiratory valve (18). In this way pressure is built up in the bag (2) during the first one-third of the compression stroke before the inspiratory phase commences, and thus the inflating flow at the start of the inspiratory phase commences sharply. After the inspiratory valve (18) has opened, the continued compression of the bag (2) forces the gas within it, through the inspiratory valve (18) and the inspiratory tube (21), to the patient.

On the other hand the relationship between the cam (17) and the cranks (6, 15) is such that the expiratory valve (19) is opened at the same time as the expansion of the bags (2, 13) commences, but is closed at a time equal to one-sixth of a respiratory cycle after

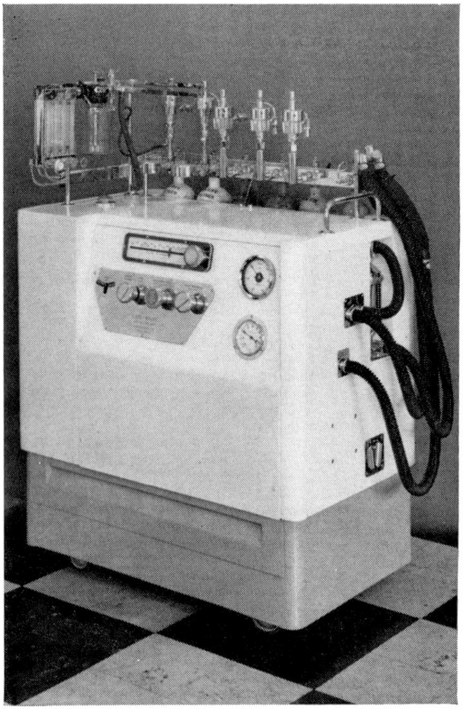

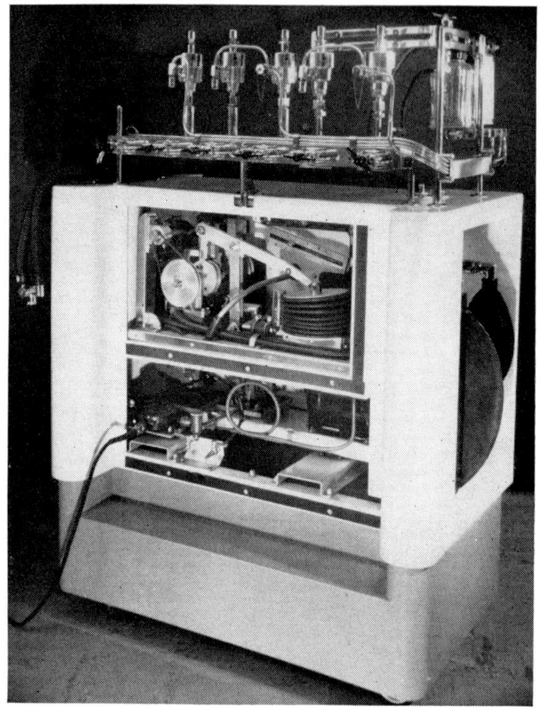

Fig. 33.1. Fig. 33.2.

Fig. 33.1. The Cape-Waine 'Anaesthetic' ventilator.

Courtesy of Cape Engineering Company Limited.

Fig. 33.2. The mechanism of the Cape-Waine 'Anaesthetic' ventilator.

Courtesy of Department of Medical Illustration, Cardiff Royal Infirmary.

the compression of the bags has commenced. The one-way valve (14) prevents any back flow to the patient occurring from the bag (13) while the expiratory valve (19) is still open.

The stroke of the positive-pressure bag (2) is varied by altering the fulcrum point of the connecting rod (3) by means of the stroke-volume control (5). A dead-weight safety-valve (4) limits the maximum inflating pressure. The valve normally fitted opens at 40 cmH_2O, but a valve opening at 70 cmH_2O is available. This valve is not in circuit when manual ventilation is performed.

The expansion of the concertina bag (13) during the expiratory phase produces a negative pressure within it. The maximum negative pressure thus produced is limited to -15 cmH_2O by the dead-weight valve (26). The negative-pressure control (24) allows a variable amount of gas to be drawn from the expired-gas storage bag (23), into the concertina bag (13). The capacity of the bag (23) greatly exceeds that of the bag (13), and therefore the negative pressure produced may be adjusted to any level between 0 and

−15 cmH_2O. The respiratory frequency is variable between 10 and 40 per minute and the tidal volume between 200 and 1,500 ml.

In the Cape-Waine 'Anaesthetic' ventilator the fresh gas enters continuously at the inlet (7) and passes through the 'manual/mechanical' tap (33) to the fresh-gas storage bag (8). During the expiratory phase gas is drawn from this storage bag (8), through the one-way valve (1), into the positive-pressure concertina bag (2). At the same time expired gas from the patient flows, through the expiratory tube (22), the 'manual/mechanical' tap (33), the expiratory valve (19), and the one-way valve (14), to the negative-pressure concertina bag (13).

If the negative expiratory pressure is limited by the 'negative phase' control (24) being partially opened, then some of the gas drawn into the bag (13) will come from the expired-gas storage bag (23). In any case, the expired gas stored in the concertina bag (13) is forced, through the one-way valve (12), into the storage bag (23), during the next inspiratory phase. During the expiratory phase the fresh-gas storage bag (8) is emptied first, and any further gas needed to fill the concertina bag (2) is drawn from the bag (23) through the one-way valve (9). Any excess gas in the bag (8) is spilled during the inspiratory phase through the Heidbrink valve (10) and excess gas in the bag (23) is spilled through the Heidbrink valve (11).

If a fully-closed circuit is required, the valves (10) and (11) must be completely shut, and the Waters soda-lime canister provided must be connected to the expiratory port (22). With this circuit only basal gas flow is needed. If this flow is exceeded, the bags (8) and (23) become progressively more distended. Should the flow of fresh gas be inadequate then the storage bags (8) and (23) gradually empty and ultimately air is drawn in through the dead-weight valve (26) during the expiratory phase. In this event the one-way valve (9), which is situated on the top of the ventilator, will be seen to open during the expiratory phase.

To obtain a semi-closed circuit, the fresh-gas flow is increased. The valves (10) and (11) are opened so that, when the bags (8) and (23) become distended, excess gas can be spilled through them.

To obtain a non-rebreathing circuit the fresh-gas flow is further increased until it equals or exceeds the total minute-volume ventilation. The Waters canister can now be dispensed with. Free escape of expired gas to atmosphere is assured by removing the large expired-gas storage bag (23). If the fresh-gas flow is less than the minute-volume ventilation, the one-way valve (9) opens during the expiratory phase as air is drawn in through it. Should the fresh-gas flow exceed the total minute-volume ventilation the excess is spilled through the valve (10).

In the 'manual' position of the tap (33) the motor is automatically switched off and there is no longer a connexion between the patient and the inspiratory and expiratory valves (18, 19). The reservoir bag (32), together with its one-way valves, is used for manual inflation. Any excess gas must be spilled through an expiratory valve near the patient. The fresh gas flows directly into the inspiratory tube (21).

To ventilate with air alone, thus dispensing with the need for any compressed gas, both storage bags (8) and (23) are removed, but if this air is to be enriched with oxygen, the storage bag (8) is retained, as in the non-rebreathing circuit, and oxygen is supplied through the fresh-gas inlet (7).

The manometer (20) indicates pressure at the inspiratory port of the ventilator. The ventilator can be supplied with a Wright respirometer fitted into the front panel. An electric humidifier, supplied by the manufacturers, which it should be noted is not flame-proof, can be attached to the ventilator.

The Cape ventilator

This ventilator is designed for ward use and therefore does not incorporate an anaesthetic apparatus. The other points of difference from the Cape-Waine ventilator are as follows. Both the storage bags (8) and (23), the valves (10) and (11), and the tap (33) are omitted, and therefore air can be drawn freely, through a filter, into the concertina bag (2), during the expansion stroke. If this inflating air is to be enriched with oxygen an assembly supplied with the ventilator is attached to the inlet to the valve (1). This assembly incorporates an air-inlet valve which opens at -7 cmH_2O and an oxygen-supply inlet. The expired gas stored in the concertina bag (13) is vented to atmosphere during the inspiratory phase. The 'manual/mechanical' tap (33) and the reservoir bag (32) are not included. The ventilator may however be operated manually by turning a handle which directly rotates the driving shaft (31). Manual rotation of the shaft in this way automatically disengages the sprag clutch (30). A positive-pressure-limiting valve allows the inflating pressure to be limited to any level below that imposed by the dead-weight valve (4), which, in this ventilator, is set to open at 70 cmH_2O. A 'Nordgas' spirometer may be fitted instead of a Wright respirometer. An alarm unit, which gives audible and visible warning of the absence of positive pressure and/or mains failure, is available.

FUNCTIONAL ANALYSIS

Inspiratory phase

Fundamentally this ventilator is a near-sine-wave-flow generator during the inspiratory phase because the positive-pressure concertina bag (2) is driven, by the constant-speed motor (25), through a pattern of movement which is uninfluenced by the build-up of pressure within the bag and which approximates to a sine wave. In the early part of the phase the fundamental action is modified, but in the later part, as can be seen in fig. 33.5, the flow waveform does indeed follow the course of the second half of the positive part of a sine wave and is unaltered by changes of lung characteristics. On the other hand the pressure at the mouth, in the later part of the phase, is considerably altered.

In the early part of the phase the action is considerably modified by the fact that the

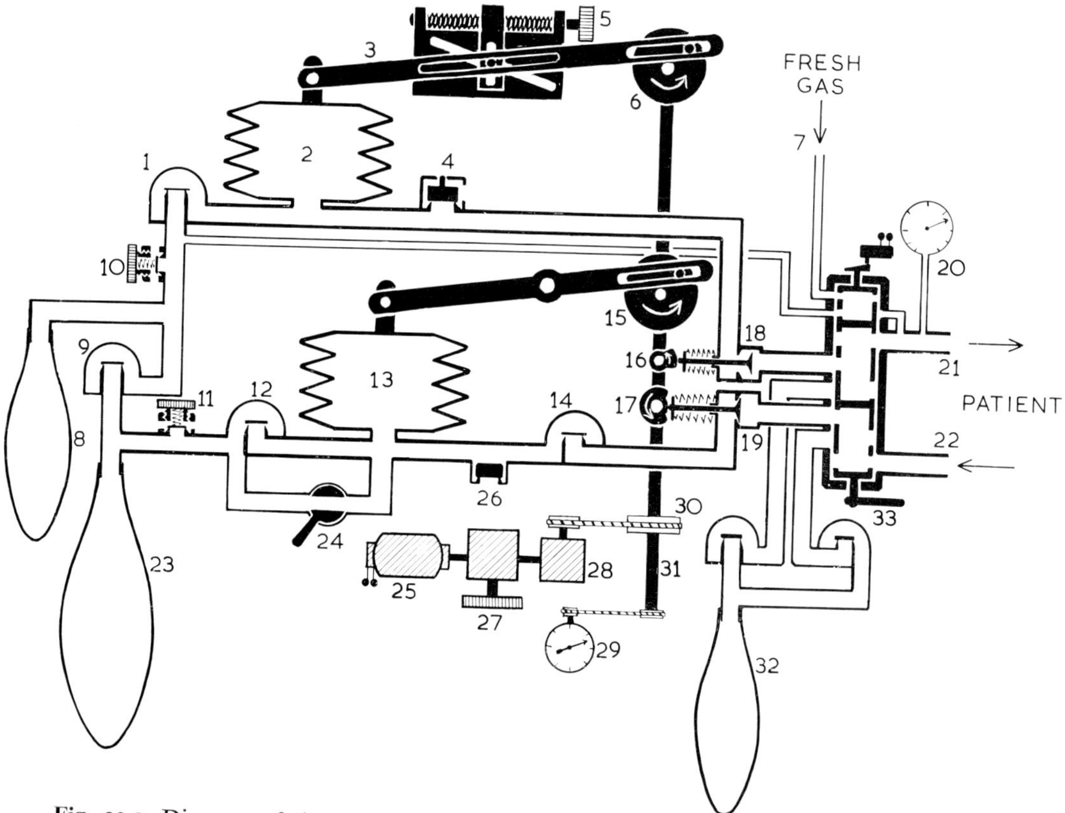

Fig. 33.3. Diagram of the Cape-Waine 'Anaesthetic' ventilator.

1. One-way valve
2. Positive-pressure concertina reservoir bag
3. Connecting rod
4. Positive-pressure safety-valve
5. Stroke-volume control
6. Crank
7. Fresh-gas inlet
8. Fresh-gas storage bag
9. One-way valve
10. Spring-loaded valve
11. Spring-loaded valve
12. One-way valve
13. Negative-pressure concertina bag
14. One-way valve
15. Crank
16. Inspiratory-valve cam
17. Expiratory-valve cam
18. Inspiratory valve
19. Expiratory valve
20. Manometer
21. Inspiratory tube
22. Expiratory tube
23. Expired-gas storage bag
24. 'Negative phase' control
25. Electric motor
26. Negative-pressure safety-valve
27. Oil variator ('respiratory frequency' control)
28. Gear-box
29. Tachometer
30. Sprag clutch
31. Main shaft
32. Reservoir bag for manual inflation
33. 'Manual/mechanical' control

concertina bag (2) performs one-third of its compression stroke before the inspiratory valve opens. This compresses the gas in the bag, perhaps even to the point at which some gas is blown off through the safety-valve (4). Therefore, when the inspiratory valve is opened, the generated sine wave of flow is supplemented for a short time by a further

lung characteristics and neither immediately a given pressure has been achieved at the mouth nor immediately a given volume has come out of the lungs.

CONTROLS

Total ventilation

This is not directly controlled but is equal to the product of tidal volume and respiratory frequency both of which can be directly controlled.

Tidal volume

This is directly controlled by the setting of the stroke-volume control (5). It is uninfluenced by changes of lung characteristics (fig. 33.5) except that at extreme values some of the stroke volume of the positive-pressure bag (2) may be lost in the compliance of the tubing and, at high tidal volumes, through the positive-pressure safety-valve (4).

The tidal volume is also uninfluenced by the settings of other controls (fig. 33.6). The only exception here is if the pressure in the fresh-gas storage bag (8) is greater than the mouth pressure at any time during the inspiratory phase. This can arise only if either the storage bag becomes distended (by setting the relief valve (10) too tight for the fresh-gas flow in use) or if so much negative pressure is used that the mouth pressure is still negative for part of the inspiratory phase. In either of these circumstances there could be a flow of gas from the fresh-gas storage bag (8) past the one-way valve (1) to the patient, thereby supplementing the stroke volume of the positive-pressure bag.

Respiratory frequency

This is directly controlled by the respiratory-frequency control and is quite uninfluenced by changes of lung characteristics (fig. 33.5) or by changes in the settings of the other controls (fig. 33.6).

Inspiratory-expiratory ratio

This is fixed at 1 : 2 and cannot be altered in any way.

Inspiratory waveforms

For a given tidal volume, frequency, compliance, and resistance these cannot be altered. The sine-wave-flow-generating characteristics of the ventilator determine the basic flow pattern, although this is supplemented at the start of the phase by the 'discharge' of the 'pressurized' compliance of the positive-pressure reservoir bag (2) into the compliance of the lungs. All other inspiratory waveforms are the results of the interactions of these fundamental mechanisms with the lung characteristics.

Expiratory waveforms

These waveforms are influenced by the setting of the 'negative phase' control but this setting will normally be determined by a requirement for a particular mean pressure. With the 'negative phase' control set to 'zero' (tap (24) open) atmospheric pressure is generated in the expiratory storage bag (23) and the flow waveform results from the effect of this generated pressure on the lungs. With tap (24) partly or wholly closed, it is the flow which is controlled by the ventilator for some parts of the phase and the pressure for others—in the manner described in the functional analysis above.

Pressure limits

The minimum alveolar pressure at the end of the expiratory phase can be controlled by the setting of the 'negative phase' control (24). When this is set to zero the alveolar pressure will always closely approach the generated, atmospheric, pressure at the end of the phase unless the airway resistance is very high or the expiratory time is very short (frequency very high). When the 'negative phase' control is adjusted so that the tap (24) is partly or wholly closed the (negative) end-expiratory alveolar pressure depends on the lung characteristics (fig. 33.5) and on the tidal volume (fig. 33.6b).

Whatever the minimum alveolar pressure happens to be, the peak alveolar pressure during the inspiratory phase is determined by the fact that it exceeds the minimum by an amount equal to the tidal volume divided by the compliance.

REFERENCES

1 WAINE T.E. and FOX D.E.R. (1962) A new and versatile closed circuit anaesthetic machine with automatic and manual ventilation. *Br. J. Anaesth.* **34**, 410.

2 SMITH-CLARKE G.T. and GALPINE J.F. (1955) A positive-negative pressure respirator. *Lancet*, **I**, 1299.

3 SMITH-CLARKE G.T. (1957) Mechanical breathing machines. *Proc. I. Mech. E.*, **171**, 52.

CHAPTER 34

The 'Clevedon' Ventilator[1, 2]

DESCRIPTION

The 'Clevedon' ventilator (fig. 34.1) is a modification of the Bang ventilator.

A supply of compressed gas enters at (4) (fig. 34.2) and distends the reservoir bag (9). When the solenoid-operated inspiratory-expiratory valve (2) is in the inflating position (as it is in fig. 34.2) the gas inflates the patient. The resultant pressure is transmitted to the chamber (6). As the pressure within this chamber rises the water level in the tube (14) is depressed, and the level in the tube (17), which is open to the atmosphere, rises. At a certain level the liquid reaches the float which is lifted until its push rod (12) tilts the mercury switch (11). This completes the circuit to the solenoid (1) and the slide valve (2) is pulled over. The expiratory phase now begins and expired gas escapes freely to atmosphere through the tube (3).

As the level of the water in the tube (14) returns to its former level it reaches the float (15) which is raised until the mercury switch (7) is tilted, completing the circuit to the

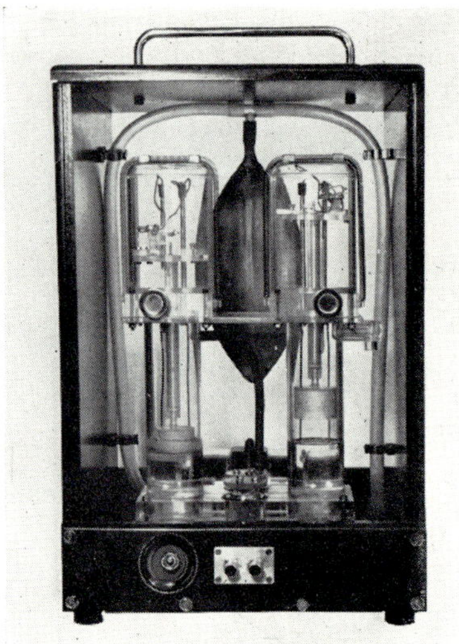

Fig. 34.1. The 'Clevedon' ventilator.

Courtesy of Messrs. Willcocks (Clevedon) Ltd.

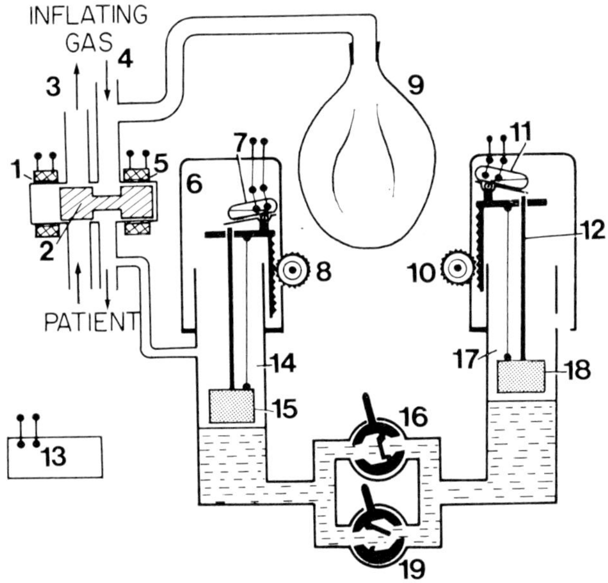

Fig. 34.2. Diagram of the 'Clevedon' ventilator.

1. Solenoid
2. Solenoid-operated inspiratory-expiratory valve
3. Expiratory tube
4. Inflating-gas inlet
5. Solenoid
6. Closed chamber
7. Tilting mercury switch
8. Rack and pinion
9. Reservoir bag
10. Rack and pinion
11. Tilting mercury switch
12. Push rod
13. 12-volt battery
14. Left-hand limb of U-tube
15. Float
16. Adjustable one-way valve controlling duration of expiratory phase
17. Right-hand limb of U-tube
18. Float
19. Adjustable one-way valve controlling duration of inspiratory phase

solenoid (5). The position of the sliding valve is reversed and the next inspiratory phase begins.

The electrical power for operating this ventilator is supplied by a 12-volt accumulator (13). As either push rod descends clear of its mercury switch, the switch automatically falls into the 'off' position under the effect of its own weight. Control 'strings' prevent the push rods falling free of their guides.

Provided the reservoir bag is not allowed to become indefinitely distended the ventilator operates as a minute-volume divider (see p. 140): the total ventilation is equal to the inflating-gas flow rate.

The rate at which water can pass from one tube to another is controlled by the two one-way taps (16 and 19). The valve (19) controls the length of the inspiratory phase and valve (16) the length of the expiratory phase. The volume delivered to the patient depends on the fresh-gas flow, the height of the float in the tube (17), and on the setting of the one-way valve (19). The height of the float in the tube (14) may also be varied to compensate for any evaporation of the water in the apparatus. The adjustment of the height of the floats is made with the rack-and-pinion mechanisms (8, 10).

The reservoir bag (9) accumulates gas during the expiratory phase and provides an adequate volume of inflating gas under pressure for rapid inflation in the inspiratory phase.

FUNCTIONAL ANALYSIS

Inspiratory phase

The mode of operation in this phase depends upon the average degree of inflation of the reservoir bag (9). If it is inflated only to a moderate degree, so that it operates within the range of the steep part of its pressure-volume characteristic (see fig. 3.12) it will behave as a discharging compliance (see p. 98). On the other hand, if the bag is inflated to a higher pressure, it may reach the plateau of its pressure-volume characteristic. In that case it will behave as a constant-pressure generator.

Change-over from inspiratory phase to expiratory phase

This change-over is a hybrid mixture of time-cycled and pressure-cycled (see p. 108). Cycling occurs when the pressure in the chamber (6) (fig. 34.2), which is the pressure applied to the patient, has driven enough water through the control tap (19) to operate the switch (11). If the pressure in the chamber (6) increases more rapidly, due to a change in the inflating-gas supply or to a change in the lung characteristics, cycling occurs after a shorter time, but at a higher mouth pressure, than before.

Expiratory phase

In this phase the ventilator operates as a constant, atmospheric, pressure generator: the patient's expired gas passes freely to atmosphere at the outlet (3).

Change-over from expiratory phase to inspiratory phase

This change-over is time-cycled: it occurs when switch (7) is operated, by enough water having leaked through the control tap (16) at a rate, and therefore in a time, which is determined by the ventilator, and is uninfluenced by the patient.

REFERENCES

1 MACRAE J., MCKENDRICK G.D.W., CLAREMONT J.M., SEFTON E.M. and WALLEY R.V. (1953) The Clevedon positive-pressure respirator. *Lancet*, **2**, 971.

2 MACRAE J., MCKENDRICK, G.D.W., SEFTON E.M. and WALLEY R.V. (1954) Positive-pressure respiration: management of patients treated with Clevedon respirator. *Lancet*, **2**, 21.

CHAPTER 35

The Clutton-Brock Ventilator[1]

DESCRIPTION

The concertina reservoir bag (3) (fig. 35.2) is compressed and expanded alternately by a lever system and gear-box (15), driven by an electric motor (10) whose speed is controlled electronically.

The electric motor (10) drives the gear-box (15) through a belt and pulley (13). A crank (12) on the output shaft of the gear-box drives the block (4) up and down over a fixed stroke. The stroke of the bag (3), and hence the volume delivered to the patient, is altered by adjusting the pivot point (5) of the lever (6) by means of the screw (7).

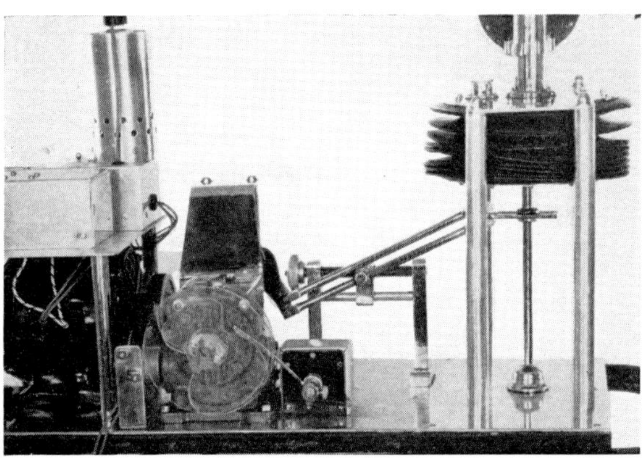

Fig. 35.1. The Clutton-Brock ventilator.
Courtesy of *British Journal of Anaesthesia*.[1]

On the opposite end of the output shaft of the gear-box (15) is a row of cams (16) of various shapes. A rod (17) bears on one of these cams and is connected to the controller (18) of a variable electrical resistance. As the cam rotates, the rod (17) follows its contour and the movement is transmitted to the controller (18). In this way the electrical resistance is varied as the output shaft of the gear-box rotates. This resistance is in an electronic circuit which controls the speed of the motor (10). The speed of the motor varies, therefore, in accordance with the shape of the cam, and almost any pattern of respiratory flow can be obtained by the use of a suitable cam. If the lock screw (19) is loosened, the rod

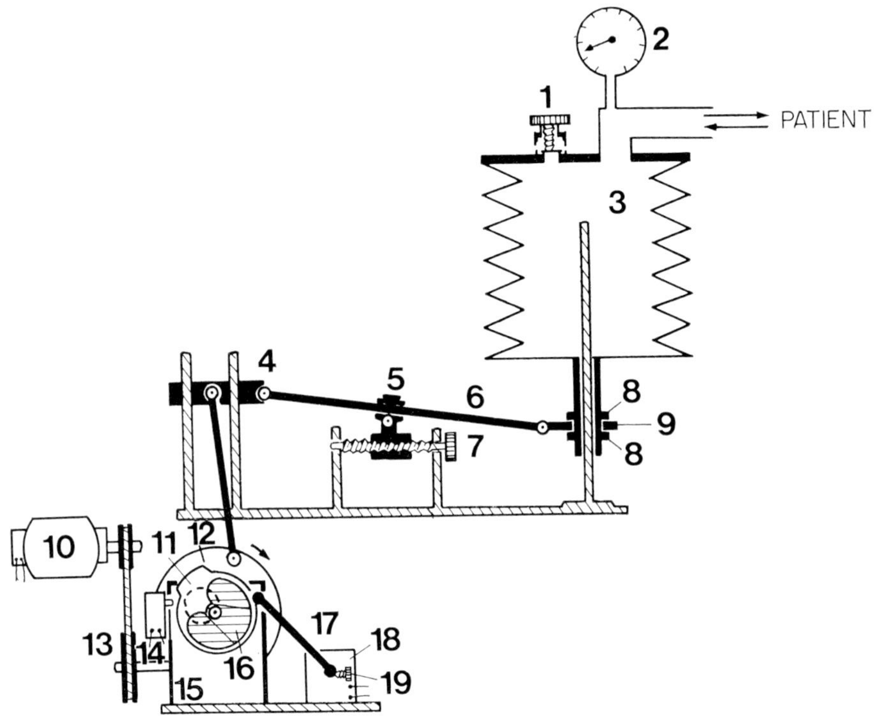

Fig. 35.2. Diagram of the Clutton-Brock ventilator.

1. Blow-off valve
2. Manometer
3. Concertina reservoir bag
4. Sliding block
5. Pivot point of lever (6)
6. Lever
7. Screw
8. Double washers
9. Fork
10. Electric motor
11. Cam
12. Crank
13. Belt-and-pulley drive
14. Microswitch
15. Gear-box
16. Cams of various shapes
17. Rod
18. Electronic controller
19. Lock screw

(17) may be moved so as to make contact with any one of the cams (16) on the gear-box shaft. A blow-off valve (1) can be set to spill excess gas. The pressure can be read on a manometer (2).

Since both the inspiratory and expiratory phases are power-driven, negative pressure can be developed during the expiratory phase. The peak positive pressure in the alveoli is largely governed by the setting of the blow-off valve (1); the minimum alveolar pressure at the end of the expiratory phase is determined by the fact that it must be less than the peak pressure, by an amount equal to the tidal volume divided by the compliance.

If the fork (9) is placed below, instead of between, the double washers (8, 8) the bag (3) is no longer pulled down during the expiratory phase, but falls freely.

A microswitch (14), operated by the cam (11), can be used to control a solenoid-operated valve in circuit with a sampling pump and carbon-dioxide analyser. By rotating the cam (11) on the shaft samples may be withdrawn at any point in the respiratory cycle.

The ratio of the inspiratory to expiratory times may be varied widely, depending on the shape of the cam (16).

FUNCTIONAL ANALYSIS

Inspiratory phase

In this phase the ventilator operates as a non-constant-flow generator; the pattern of flow depends on the shape of the cam (16) (fig. 35.2) which determines the motor speed. A pressure limit, due to the blow-off valve, comes into operation during the phase. Until then, the fresh-gas supply to the patient circuit acts as a small-constant-flow generator, supplementing the main flow generator.

Change-over from inspiratory phase to expiratory phase

This change-over is both volume-cycled and time-cycled: the controlled-speed motor expels a preset volume of gas from the concertina bag in a preset time. Since the supply of anaesthetic gas is continuous but its escape, through the blow-off valve, is restricted to the inspiratory phase, the patient's tidal volume is less than that of the concertina bag, by an amount equal to the volume of fresh gas supplied during the expiratory phase.

Expiratory phase

In this phase, with positive drive to the concertina bag the ventilator operates as a non-constant-flow generator just as in the inspiratory phase—except that the fresh-gas flow is now subtracted from instead of added to the main flow pattern.

If the fork (9) is placed below the double washers (8), and if a cam is used such that the fork falls rapidly, leaving the bag 'free', the ventilator will operate as a constant-pressure generator. The generated pressure will be atmospheric, or perhaps a little negative owing to the weight of the bag.

Change-over from expiratory phase to inspiratory phase

This change-over is both volume-cycled and time-cycled: the controlled-speed electric motor draws a preset volume of gas into the bag in a preset time (provided the fork (9) is engaged between the washers (8)). The volume leaving the patient's lungs is less than this, by an amount equal to the volume of fresh gas which enters the patient circuit during the expiratory phase.

REFERENCE

1 CLUTTON-BROCK J. (1957) A variable pattern respirator with phased sampling device. *Br. J. Anaesth.* **29**, 517.

CHAPTER 36

The 'Cyclator'

DESCRIPTION

Mark I

This description applies equally to the Mark II 'Cyclator' except for certain minor details noted on p. 463.

This compact ventilator (figs. 36.1 and 36.2) is driven by oxygen or air which must be supplied at a pressure between 45 and 60 lb/in^2. This driving gas flows through a sintered-bronze filter (1) (fig. 36.3) and a simple on/off control (2) into a small chamber (13), the only outlet from which is a small orifice (20).

This orifice (20) leads to the jet of an injector, which is of such a size that, when the

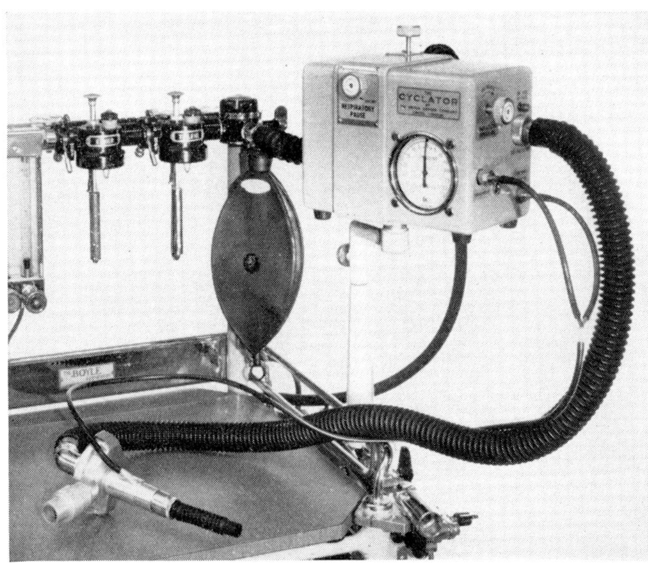

Fig. 36.1. The 'Cyclator' Mark I complete with Beaver inflating valve fitted to a Boyle anaesthetic apparatus.

Courtesy of Department of Medical Illustration, Cardiff Royal Infirmary.

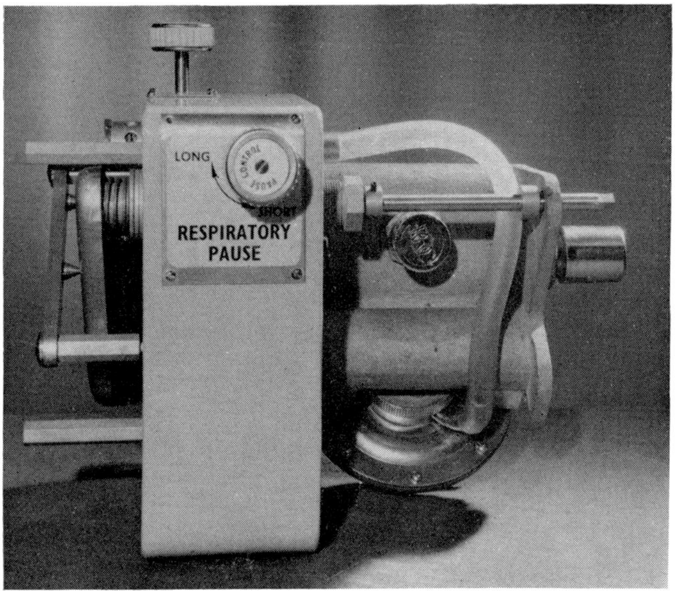

Fig. 36.2. The 'Cyclator' Mark II with outer case removed.
Courtesy of Department of Medical Illustration, Cardiff Royal Infirmary.

pressure drop across it is 60 lb/in², the gas flows through it at a rate of 12·5 litres/min, and when it is 45 lb/in² the flow is 10·0 litres/min. A second sintered-bronze filter (not shown in fig. 36.3) is fitted in the jet of the injector.

The pressure of the gas in the chamber (13) at once pushes over the piston (6) against the force exerted by the spring (10) thus forcing the valve (7) onto its seating and at the same time pushing the rod (12) outwards. The end of the rod (12) protrudes from the casing of the ventilator as a red knob and its outward movement indicates the presence of driving gas in the chamber (13).

The characteristics of the injector, when it is new, are such that gas is entrained in a ratio of approximately 3·5 volumes of entrained gas to 1 of driving gas, thus making the total flow from the injector about 56 litres/min when the driving gas is supplied at 60 lb/in². The rate of flow of driving gas through the injector tends to fall gradually with continued use, due to accumulation of dust in the sintered-bronze filters; this causes a reduction in the efficiency of the injector. The entrained gas, which enters through the port (3), consists of atmospheric air if the inlet (3) is left open to the atmosphere, or oxygen or anaesthetic gases if the inlet is connected to a reservoir.

The gas mixture flowing through the diffuser tube of the injector opens a lightly-loaded dual-action valve (18) and passes along the delivery tube (19), to a Beaver inflating valve (see p. 778), and then to the patient. As the pressure in the lungs rises there is a corresponding increase in the pressure in the delivery tube (19), in the main chamber (26),

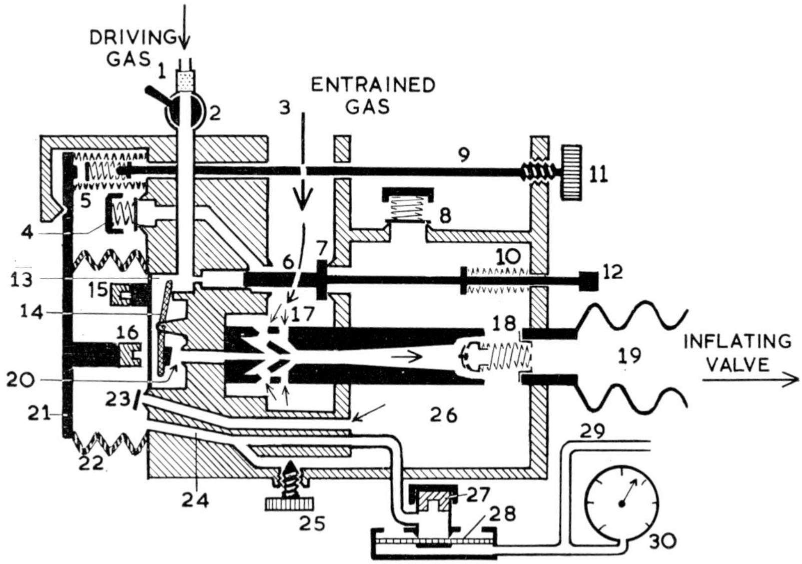

Fig. 36.3. Diagram of the 'Cyclator' Mark I.

1. Sintered-bronze filter
2. On/off control
3. Entrainment port
4. Spring-loaded one-way valve
5. Compression springs
6. Piston
7. Valve between main chamber and entrainment port
8. Safety-valve
9. Pressure-control rod
10. Compression spring
11. 'Inflation pressure' control
12. Indicator rod
13. High-pressure chamber
14. Rocking arm
15. Fixed magnet
16. Moving magnet
17. Entrainment orifices of injector
18. Dual-action valve
19. Delivery tube
20. Valve controlling flow to injector
21. Movable base-plate of concertina bag
22. Concertina bag
23. One-way valve
24. Channel from concertina bag
25. 'Respiratory pause' needle valve controlling duration of expiratory phase
26. Main chamber
27. Magnet
28. Diaphragm of patient-triggering mechanism
29. Manometer tube
30. Manometer

and, by way of the one-way valve (23), in the small rubber concertina bag (22). Within this bag there are two magnets (15, 16), so placed that they exert a pull on opposite ends of the rocking arm (14) which is inside the chamber (13). When the concertina bag is collapsed the magnet (16), attached to the movable base-plate (21), exerts the greater pull on the rocking arm (14), thereby holding open the valve connecting the chamber (13) with the injector. When the bag expands, the magnet (16) moves away and its pull on the arm (14) decreases until a point is reached at which it is less than the pull of the fixed magnet (15) on the other end of the arm. The position of the arm is therefore reversed, the jet of the injector is closed, and the flow of gas into the injector is cut off; inflation ceases.

The movable base-plate (21) is pivoted so that the pressure of the springs (5) opposes expansion of the concertina bag. In most positions of the base-plate only the outer spring, bearing against the main casing, is effective, but towards the end of the expansion movement of the base-plate the inner spring, bearing against the end of the rod (9), comes into contact with the plate. The pressure required in the bag to expand it to the position at which the rocking arm flicks over, i.e. the cycling pressure, depends on the tension of the inner of the two springs (5) which can be adjusted by the 'inflation pressure' control (11). The arrangement of the springs (5) ensures that, since only the outer fixed spring is effective for the greater part of the excursion of the bag, the duration of the expiratory phase is virtually unaffected by the setting of the pressure control (11).

The flow of gas to the injector has now been stopped; the pressure within the injector falls to atmospheric and the dual-action valve (18) is pushed by a light spring onto its seating in the diffuser of the injector. The pressure in the main chamber (26) and in the delivery tube (19) is released by the leak back of a small volume of gas past the one-way rubber mushroom valve in the centre channel of the dual-action valve (18), through the entrainment orifices (17) of the injector, and the entrainment port (3). The pressure in the delivery tube is now lower than that in the patient's lungs; the action of the inflating valve is therefore reversed, providing a free expiratory pathway through the valve to atmosphere.

At the same time gas in the concertina bag (22) escapes through the channel (24) back into the main chamber (26) and hence through the entrainment port (3). A needle valve (25), the 'respiratory pause' control, regulates the rate of this escape, and hence the time taken for the concertina bag (22) to collapse and for the magnet (16) to reach a point at which its pull on the rocking arm (14) overcomes that of the fixed magnet (15). When this point is reached, the valve (20) between the chamber (13) and the injector is re-opened and the next inspiratory phase commences.

Free connexion may be established between the entrainment port (3), the main chamber (26), and the patient, by pushing the rod (12) which opens the valve (7).

A narrow tube (29) is connected to the patient's side of the inflating valve so that the pressure at that point is registered on the manometer (30). The inflating pressure is limited to 35 cmH_2O by a preset safety-valve (8).

The patient-triggering mechanism allows the concertina bag (22) to collapse rapidly by providing an escape to atmosphere for its contained gas, by-passing the 'respiratory pause' needle valve (25), which controls the duration of the expiratory phase. A diaphragm (28) is normally held on its seat by the pull of a magnet (27). The chamber below the diaphragm is connected to the manometer tube (29). Negative pressure below the diaphragm, produced by any attempt at inspiration, overcomes the pull of the magnet, and the diaphragm moves down, thus opening the free pathway between the concertina bag (22) and atmosphere; the cycling mechanism is immediately tripped and inflation begins. In order to prevent the patient drawing gas through the injector, the dual-action valve (18) has a spring-loading on it slightly greater than the pressure difference required to operate the trigger mechanism. In order to prevent the patient inspiring directly from atmosphere, the expiratory port of the Beaver inflating valve must be fitted with a one-way valve. It is then only necessary for the patient to inhale a few millilitres of gas from the breathing circuit in order to produce the slight negative pressure needed to trigger the ventilator.

Ward use

In ward use the entrainment port (3) is normally open to atmosphere and the gas delivered to the patient is a mixture of driving gas and air in the proportion of 2 to 7. If the driving gas is compressed air, only air is delivered to the patient; if it is oxygen the final mixture has an oxygen content of nearly 40%. To increase this oxygen percentage still more the oxygen content of the entrained gas must be increased. This may be done either (a) by connecting to the entrainment port a wide-bore tube, open at its far end to atmosphere, and supplying oxygen close to the connexion; the capacity of this tube should at least equal $\frac{7}{9}$ of one tidal volume (since $\frac{2}{9}$ of the tidal volume is driving gas), so that the oxygen percentage delivered to the patient can be accurately set by regulating the flow of additional oxygen, or (b) by connecting to the entrainment port a reservoir bag with an oxygen supply. If the oxygen supply is less than $\frac{7}{9}$ of the minute-volume ventilation, an air-inlet valve is required. A reservoir bag, incorporating such a valve, can now be obtained. This valve, by enabling the patient to breathe air, also provides for any accidental failure of the oxygen supply.

Anaesthetic use

Anaesthetic gases are supplied to a reservoir bag connected to the entrainment port (3). A lightly-spring-loaded one-way valve (4) inside the ventilator ensures that the pressure of this gas mixture does not appreciably exceed atmospheric. The reservoir bag must be at least large enough to contain most of the tidal volume, and the total flow into it must be at least $\frac{7}{9}$ of the total minute-volume ventilation of the patient. If the fresh-gas flow is more than this, the reservoir bag, after a number of cycles, becomes fully distended during the expiratory phase and the excess then spills through the valve (4). If the fresh-gas flow is less than this, the reservoir bag collapses before the end of the inspiratory phase; the entrained flow is now limited to the fresh-gas flow, and the inspiratory time is therefore prolonged. An air-inlet valve on the reservoir bag, seen in fig. 36.1, prevents this. It is now supplied as standard.

If the driving gas is turned off at tap (2), the spring (10) restores the rod (12) to its resting position in which the valve (7) rests on its other seating and the pathway to the valve (4) is closed. A free pathway is thereby established between the patient and the reservoir bag connected to the entrainment port (3). This allows the patient's lungs to be inflated by the anaesthetist squeezing the reservoir bag, or the patient to inspire freely from the bag if he is breathing spontaneously. When the machine is shut off in this way there is no longer a supply of driving gas and the oxygen content of the mixture supplied to the patient is the same as that in the reservoir bag.

When the ventilator is used during anaesthesia, the driving gas is always oxygen and the content of the anaesthetic mixture must therefore be adjusted to allow for its enrichment by the driving gas. If the driving gas is subsequently turned off, to permit spontaneous respiration or manual inflation, extra oxygen must be added to the anaesthetic mixture if the same inspired oxygen concentration as before is to be maintained. With any injector, the rate at which gases are entrained decreases as the downstream pressure, i.e. the pressure on the delivery side of the injector, rises. This pressure builds up during inflation and the injector has therefore been designed so that the fall in entrainment, and hence the fall in the total flow over the range of inflation pressures, is small (fig. 36.4). The characteristics of the 'type A' injector fitted to the 'Cyclator' Mk. I are such that the flow of driving gas, supplied at 60 lb/in², is 12·5 litres/min. The total inflating flow, i.e. driving gas plus entrained gas, is now 63 litres/min and this falls to 48 litres/min when the downstream pressure in the delivery tube reaches 35 cmH_2O. There is thus an average flow of 56 litres/min over the range of 0 to 35 cmH_2O back pressure. In the final mixture, the concentration of oxygen derived from the driving gas is therefore approximately

$$\frac{12\cdot5}{56} \times 100 = 22\%.$$

If the anaesthetic mixture contains $x\%$ oxygen the final oxygen percentage will be increased by

$$\frac{56-12\cdot5}{56} \text{ of } x, \quad \text{i.e. approx. } \frac{4}{5}x.$$

The final total concentration is therefore

$$(22+\tfrac{4}{5}x)\%.$$

Naturally, if the inflating-pressure range is 0 to 20 cmH_2O, the final concentrations are higher. These figures are summarized in Table 36.1. As already mentioned these figures apply to a new ventilator. If for any reason the driving-gas flow falls off, the oxygen concentration in the inflating gas mixture will be higher.

Since driving gas flows during the inspiratory phase and not during the expiratory phase, the total driving gas used depends on the inspiratory-expiratory ratio. If this ratio is 1 : 3 and the flow during the inspiratory phase is 12·5 litres/min then the amount used is one quarter of this, i.e. 3·1 litres/min.

Mark II

In this development of the 'Cyclator' Mk. I the cycling pressure can be set up to a maximum of 45 cmH_2O and the setting of the safety-valve has been raised to this pressure.

Table 36.1. Calculated percentage of oxygen in gas mixture delivered to the patient for various percentages of oxygen in the entrained gas mixture. Injector rated at 12·5 litres/min; average total inflating flow 56 litres/min.

ENTRAINED GAS		GAS DELIVERED TO PATIENT
% OXYGEN	% NITROUS OXIDE	% OXYGEN
0	100	22
10	90	30
15	85	34
20	80	38
25	75	42
30	70	46
40	60	54
50	50	62
100	0	100

Interchangeable injectors, allowing a choice of inspiratory flow rates, are now available. The characteristics of types B, C, and D are shown in fig. 36.4.

A variable restrictor is available which can be plugged into the entrainment port (3). This permits further reduction of the inspiratory flow. Its use alters the proportions of driving gas and entrained gas in the inflating mixture.

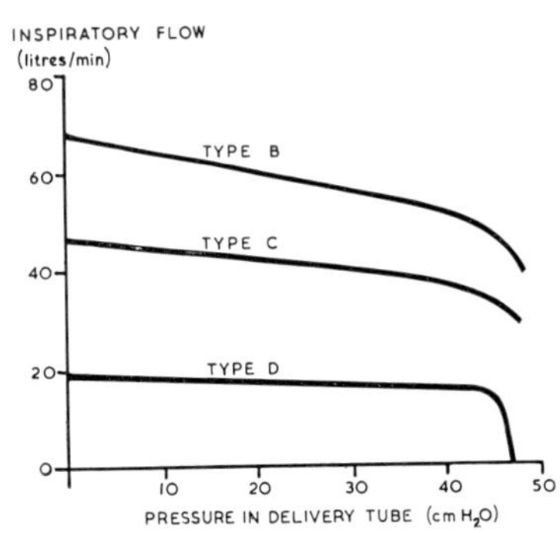

Fig. 36.4. 'Cyclator' Mark II. Flow-pressure characteristics of new injectors driven by oxygen at 60 lb/in².

FUNCTIONAL ANALYSIS

This analysis is applicable to both the Mark I and the Mark II 'Cyclators'. The recordings (figs. 36.5 and 36.6) however were derived from a Mark II 'Cyclator'.

Inspiratory phase

In this phase the 'Cyclator' approximates very closely to a constant-flow generator because the injector characteristics (fig. 36.4) are such that flow falls off only slightly with increasing back pressure. Fig. 36.5 shows that halving the compliance or doubling the airway resistance of the model lung has no effect upon the flow, except to shorten its duration. On the other hand, the rise of pressure at the mouth is made considerably steeper than in the standard conditions. The flow, which is recorded at the mouth, is in all conditions a little slow in reaching its full level—indeed, with the airway resistance doubled, it barely does so before the end of the phase. This is because, initially, some of the flow from the injector is absorbed in the compliance of the corrugated delivery tube.

Change-over from inspiratory phase to expiratory phase

This is pressure-cycled; it occurs when a preset pressure has been attained in the con-

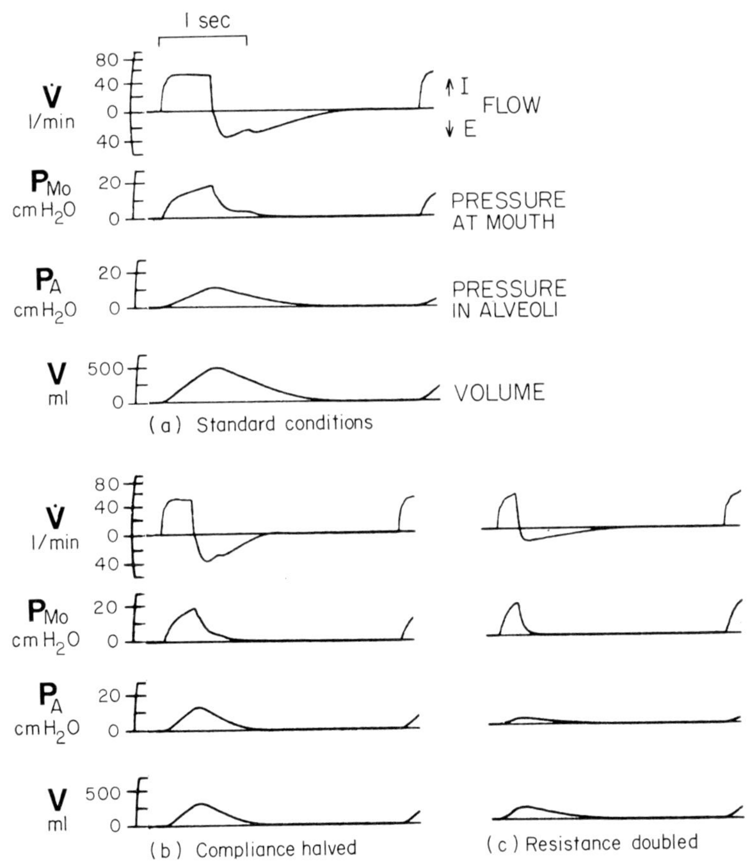

Fig. 36.5. 'Cyclator' Mark II. Recordings showing the effects of changes of lung characteristics.

Standard conditions: driving gas, oxygen at 60 lb/in^2; entrained gas, air; injector, 'type B'; 'inflation pressure' set to produce a tidal volume of 500 ml; 'respiratory pause' set to produce a respiratory frequency of 20/min.

certina bag (22). This pressure is very close to the mouth pressure and it can be seen from fig. 36.5 that halving the compliance or doubling the airway resistance has no effect on the mouth pressure at the end of the inspiratory phase. On the other hand these changes greatly reduce the tidal volume and the inspiratory time.

Expiratory phase

In this phase the 'Cyclator' is fundamentally a constant, atmospheric, pressure generator; the patient is connected to atmosphere through the inflating valve. The pressure at the mouth is slow to fall at the beginning of the phase because of the sluggish movement of the valve but, for the later part of the phase, the mouth pressure is zero for all three conditions in fig. 36.5. On the other hand the pattern of flow is considerably altered by changes in lung characteristics: with the compliance halved the decay of flow is more rapid; with the airway resistance doubled the decay is slower.

Change-over from expiratory phase to inspiratory phase

This change-over is time-cycled or patient-cycled whichever mode of cycling occurs first: the change-over occurs when the pressure in the concertina bag (22) has fallen to a preset level, either (a) at a preset rate through the 'respiratory pause' needle valve (25), and therefore in a preset time, or (b) suddenly, when an inspiratory effort by the patient lifts the diaphragm (28) from its seat. In fig. 36.5 the ventilator is purely time-cycled and it can be seen that, in the face of changes of lung characteristics, the expiratory phase ends at a fixed time after it starts; it does not end when some fixed volume has come out of the lungs nor does it end immediately some critical pressure has been reached at the mouth.

CONTROLS

This discussion of the controls of the 'Cyclator' is largely applicable to both the Mark I and the Mark II although the recordings (figs. 36.5 and 36.6) were derived from a Mark II.

Total ventilation

This cannot be directly controlled but is equal to the product of tidal volume and frequency.

Tidal volume

This is indirectly controlled by adjustment of the cycling pressure by means of the 'inflation pressure' control (11) (fig. 36.6b). It is reduced by a reduced compliance (fig. 36.5b) and by an increased airway resistance (fig. 36.5c). Since the inspiratory flow rate is constant, any increase in tidal volume results in an increase in inspiratory time, and hence in a change in the inspiratory-expiratory ratio and a decreased respiratory

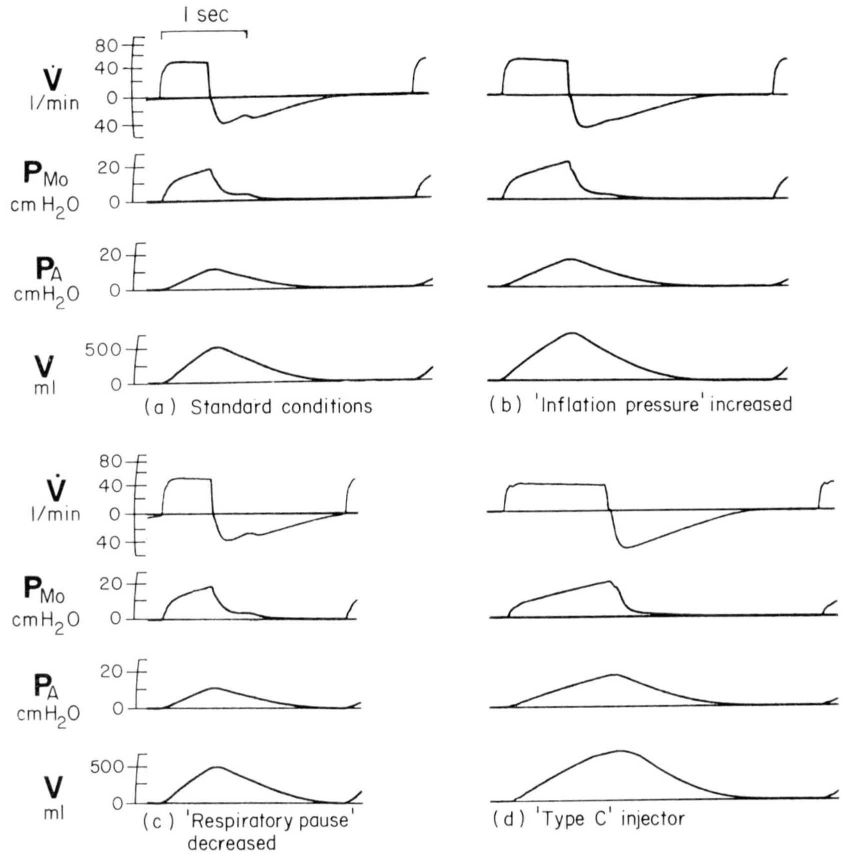

Fig. 36.6. 'Cyclator' Mark II. Recordings showing the effects of changes in the settings of the controls.

(a) Standard conditions as in fig. 36.5.
(b) 'Inflation pressure' increased $\frac{3}{8}$ of a turn to produce a tidal volume of 750 ml.
(c) 'Respiratory pause' decreased $\frac{1}{4}$ of a turn to produce a frequency of 25/min.
(d) 'Type C' injector.

frequency. Therefore the increase in the total ventilation is less than if it were in proportion to the increase in the tidal volume.

Respiratory frequency and inspiratory-expiratory ratio

Neither of these parameters can be directly controlled but both are determined by the separately-variable inspiratory and expiratory times.

The inspiratory time is the time taken to deliver the tidal volume at the nearly-constant generated flow. It therefore varies with lung characteristics in the same way as does the tidal volume. Once the tidal volume has been set (in so far as it can be set) the inspiratory time can be deliberately altered by changing the generated flow by changing to a different injector. However, if this is the only change that is made, and the new injector gives a lower generated flow, then (fig. 36.6d) there will be a reduced pressure difference between the mouth and the alveoli throughout the phase. Therefore, when the unaltered cycling pressure is reached at the mouth, the alveolar pressure is higher than with the previous injector, and so a larger tidal volume is delivered. Therefore, if the original tidal volume is to be restored, the cycling pressure must be reduced. Then the same tidal volume will be delivered over a longer inspiratory phase. The same considerations apply if the inspiratory flow is reduced by inserting the variable restrictor in the entrainment port (3).

The expiratory time is directly controlled by the 'respiratory pause' control (25) (fig. 36.6c). It is not affected by changes in lung characteristics (fig. 36.5), nor by changes, in the cycling pressure (fig. 36.6b), nor by changing the injector (fig. 36.6d). In many ventilators in which the distending and shrinking of a small bag ((22) in fig. 36.3) or of a diaphragm controls both change-over mechanisms, increasing the cycling pressure at the end of the inspiratory phase decreases the duration of the expiratory phase. This is because increasing the cycling pressure increases the force emptying the bag. This effect is largely eliminated in the 'Cyclator' by arranging that the spring which sets the cycling pressure is operative only when the concertina bag is nearly full; for most of the period of emptying the emptying force is provided solely by the outer spring (5) which is not affected by changing the cycling pressure.

In summary: the respiratory frequency is primarily controlled by the 'respiratory pause' control (25), although it is also influenced by choice of injector, by the use and setting of the variable restrictor, by cycling pressure, and by lung characteristics. Having set the 'respiratory pause' control the three injectors provide a choice of three basic inspiratory-expiratory ratios, which can be further modified by the use of the variable restrictor. The exact values of the ratios depend on and vary with the cycling pressure and the lung characteristics.

Inspiratory waveforms

In the inspiratory phase the flow waveform is determined by the constant-flow-generating characteristics of the injector, while the pressure waveforms result from the interaction of the flow waveform with the lung characteristics. The magnitude of the flow can be altered by changing the injector. This choice cannot be exercised if an injector has already been chosen on the basis of a desired inspiratory-expiratory ratio (see above).

Expiratory waveforms

In the expiratory phase atmospheric pressure is applied, by way of the inflating valve, to the lungs. It cannot be varied in any way. The expiratory flow which results depends on the effect of this pressure on the lungs.

Pressure limits

The peak inspiratory pressure at the mouth is equal to the cycling pressure; the peak alveolar pressure is less than this by an amount equal to the airway resistance multiplied by the generated flow. During the expiratory phase the alveolar pressure normally falls to equal the applied, atmospheric, pressure. It does so in all the tracings in figs. 36.5 and 36.6. It will fail to do so only when the airway resistance is very high or when the expiratory time is very short.

CHAPTER 37

The 'Cyclator Combined Automatic Ventilator Unit'

DESCRIPTION

This ventilator (fig. 37.1) comprises a 'bag-in-bottle' apparatus driven by a Mark II 'Cyclator'. It incorporates a closed anaesthetic circuit complete with soda-lime canister. For brevity the unit is referred to elsewhere in this book as the 'Cyclator CAV'.

The delivery tube of the 'Cyclator' is connected to the inlet port (7) (fig. 37.2) of the diaphragm valve (9, 10) on the top of the rigid plastic pressure chamber (17) into which it opens. The action of this valve is comparable to that of the Beaver inflating valve (see p. 778). During the inspiratory phase the gas delivered by the 'Cyclator' flows past the flexible diaphragm (10) into the chamber (17), the valve (9) being held closed by its light spring and the pressure of the delivered gas. As the pressure rises in the chamber (17) the concertina reservoir bag (15) is compressed and the anaesthetic gas mixture within it is forced, past the one-way valve (2), through the inspiratory tube (5), to the patient. When the pressure in the chamber (17) has risen to the cycling pressure set on the 'Cyclator', the latter changes from inspiration to expiration and pressure at the inlet port (7) falls rapidly to atmospheric. The pressure in the chamber (17) now pushes up the diaphragm (10), which takes with it the valve (9), and thereby allows the gas stored in the chamber (17) to escape to atmosphere through the outlet (6). As pressure within the bag (15) falls the inspiratory valve (2) closes and expired gas from the patient can flow freely past the one-way expiratory valve (14) into the bag. The tap (13) allows the expired gas to be directed through, or to by-pass, the large transparent reversible soda-lime canister (18).

The expansion of the reservoir bag (15) during the expiratory phase is assisted by a weight (16) in its base, and opposed by the adjustable pressure difference across the diaphragm valve (9, 10). If this pressure difference is less than the pressure difference produced by the weight, then a negative pressure will exist in the bag so long as it is still falling. With this method of generating negative pressure, there are two possible modes of operation.

Mode A. The cycling pressure on the 'Cyclator' is set to maximum and the graduated, spring-loaded, blow-off valve (1) ('positive pressure' valve) is set to some lower pressure, chosen to achieve the desired tidal volume.

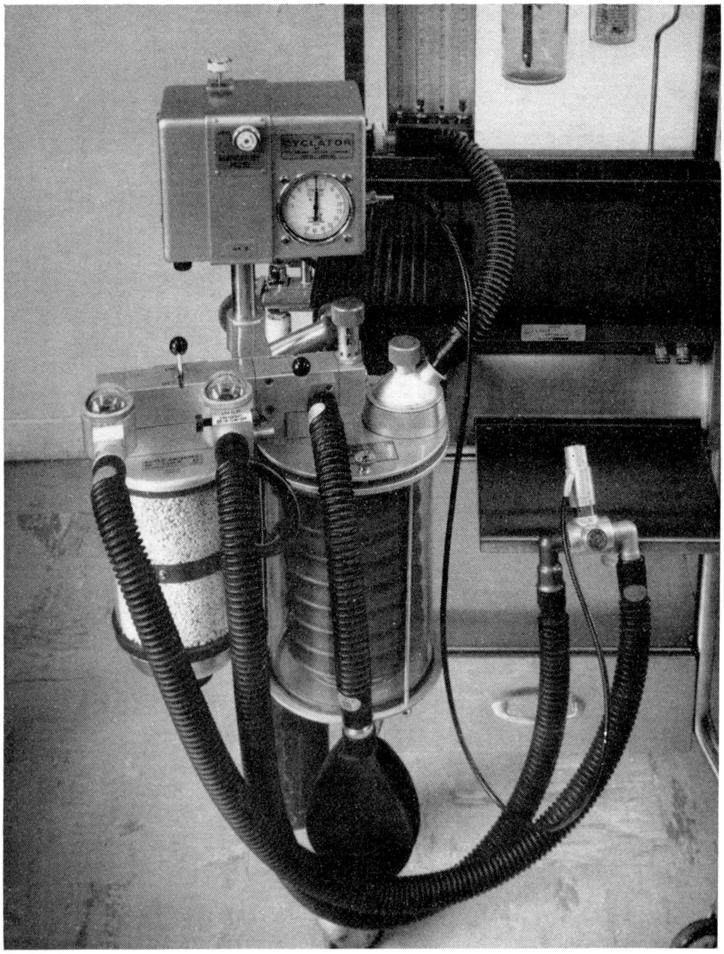

Fig. 37.1. The 'Cyclator Combined Automatic Ventilator Unit' fitted to a Boyle anaesthetic apparatus.

Courtesy of Department of Medical Illustration, Cardiff Royal Infirmary.

In these circumstances the concertina bag (15) must empty completely during the inspiratory phase before the cycling pressure is reached in chamber (17). Therefore, during the expiratory phase the bag will receive the tidal volume of gas from the patient's lungs together with the volume of fresh gas entering the patient circuit during this phase. This total volume is normally less than the capacity of the bag. Therefore the weight will still be acting on the contents of the bag at the end of the expiratory phase, maintaining negative pressure throughout the phase. Also, the spill valve (11) will not open during the phase. As a result of this, excess gas must spill through the 'positive pressure' valve (1) during the inspiratory phase. During this phase the gas in the bag is delivered to the

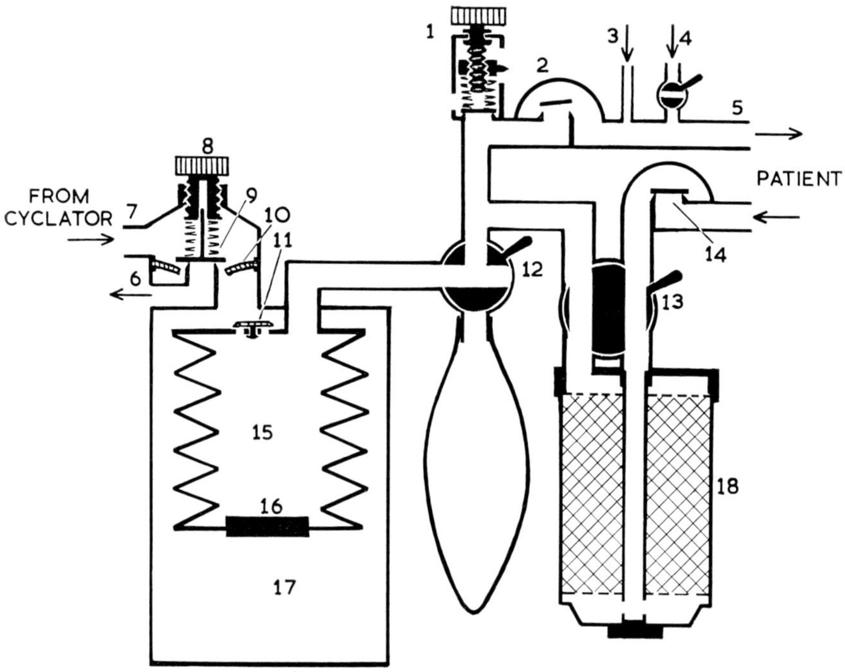

Fig. 37.2. Diagram of the 'Cyclator Combined Automatic Ventilator Unit'.

1. Adjustable spring-loaded valve acting as safety-valve or blow-off valve ('positive pressure' control)
2. One-way inspiratory valve
3. Fresh-gas inlet
4. Emergency oxygen inlet
5. Inspiratory tube
6. Outlet port
7. Inlet port, connected to delivery tube of 'Cyclator'
8. 'Negative pressure' control
9. Spring-loaded valve
10. Flexible diaphragm
11. Spill valve
12. 'Automatic/manual' tap
13. On/off tap for soda-lime canister
14. One-way expiratory valve
15. Concertina reservoir bag
16. Weight
17. Rigid plastic pressure chamber
18. Transparent reversible soda-lime canister

patient until the pressure in the inspiratory pathway is high enough to open the 'positive pressure' valve (1). From this moment the flow from the bag is divided between the patient and atmosphere until all the remaining contents of the bag have been discharged. Once the bag is fully compressed, the pressure in the chamber (17) rises rapidly and the 'Cyclator' cycles from inspiration to expiration.

Mode B. The 'positive pressure' valve (1) is set to maximum and the tidal volume is controlled by setting the cycling pressure of the 'Cyclator' to some lower value.

In these circumstances the valve (1) cannot open during the inspiratory phase and therefore excess gas must escape through the spill valve (11) during the expiratory phase. This cannot occur unless the pressure inside the reservoir bag (15) exceeds that in the chamber (17), i.e. unless the bag has fully expanded so that the weight rests on the bottom of the chamber. Therefore, in these circumstances, negative pressure is applied to the patient's respiratory tract only during the first part of the expiratory phase. At the end of the phase pressure must rise slightly above atmospheric. During the inspiratory phase pressure in the bag rises to a value equal to the cycling pressure minus the pressure drop across the bag wall due to the weight. The valve (1) acts only as a safety-valve.

In either set of circumstances the duration of the inspiratory phase is the time taken for the pressure in the chamber (17) to reach the cycling pressure set on the 'Cyclator'. When excess gas is spilled through the valve (11) during the expiratory phase (mode B), the pressure increases steadily throughout the inspiratory phase. However, if excess gas is spilled through the 'positive pressure' valve (1) during the inspiratory phase (mode A), the pressure in the chamber (17) increases steadily only until the pressure within the bag reaches the blow-off pressure, whereupon both pressures remain constant until the concertina bag has emptied, partly into the patient's lungs and partly to atmosphere through the valve (1). Then the pressure in the chamber (17) rises rapidly to the cycling pressure. In these circumstances, therefore, with excess gas escaping through the blow-off valve (1), the duration of the inspiratory phase, is slightly more than the time taken for the bag (15) to empty. With both methods of excess-gas escape the duration of the expiratory phase depends entirely on the setting of the 'respiratory pause' control on the 'Cyclator'.

The control (8) can be set to impede the escape of gas from the chamber (17) during the expiratory phase. In this way it opposes the influence of the weight (16) on the expansion of the bag, and thereby controls the negative pressure attained.

Fresh gas enters the inspiratory pathway at the inlet (3) and emergency oxygen may be added at the inlet (4). The tap (12) may be turned to allow manual ventilation.

FUNCTIONAL ANALYSIS

This functional analysis is made on the assumption that the ventilator is used in the manner recommended by the manufacturers (mode A above), i.e. with the cycling pressure on the 'Cyclator' set at maximum and with the tidal volume controlled by the settings of the 'positive pressure' valve (1) and the 'negative pressure' valve (8) so that excess gas escapes through the blow-off valve (1) during the inspiratory phase.

Inspiratory phase

The functioning of this ventilator during the inspiratory phase is somewhat different from that of the 'Cyclator' alone. In the first part of the phase the ventilator still approximates to a constant-flow generator. But when the pressure in the patient circuit has risen high enough to open the 'positive pressure' valve (1) it changes to a constant-pressure generator. This is because the characteristics of this valve are such (fig. 37.3) that, once it is open, the pressure below the valve seating is held nearly constant irrespective of the flow through it. Finally, when the concertina reservoir bag (15) is fully compressed, there is a short delay during which the pressure around the bag builds up to the cycling pressure. During this period fresh gas continues to enter the patient circuit and gas may also continue to escape through the 'positive pressure' valve (1); in any event the net flow during this period is small, and the whole unit approximates to a zero-flow generator, i.e. no flow occurs into the patient's lungs, irrespective of the pressure within them.

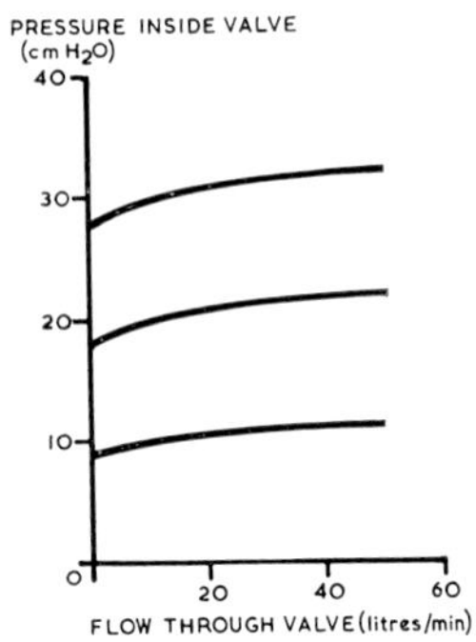

Fig. 37.3. 'Cyclator Combined Automatic Ventilator Unit'. Pressure-flow characteristics of the 'positive pressure' valve at three different settings.

Thus there are three periods in the inspiratory phase in which the ventilator functions successively as a constant-flow generator, a constant-pressure generator, and then a zero-flow generator. The period of constant-pressure generation occurs while gas is escaping through the 'positive pressure' valve (1); the volume of gas which so escapes is equal to the volume of fresh gas which enters the patient circuit in one complete respiratory cycle; therefore this volume, and hence the duration of the period of constant-pressure generation, increases as the fresh-gas flow is increased.

In fig. 37.4 the fresh-gas flow is only 0·5 litre/min and the period of pressure generation is so short as to be barely detectable, but the initial period of flow generation shows clearly. Admittedly the waveform of flow differs from the ideal of fig. 3.6 (see p. 81) rather more than is the case with the 'Cyclator' alone (fig. 36.5), but this can be attributed to the additional compliance of the pressure chamber (17) and to the additional pressure drop across the concertina reservoir bag (15). Even so, the flow rises rapidly to some level, which is not greatly affected by changes in lung characteristics, and then stays nearly constant until near the end of the phase. On the other hand, the rate of rise of pressure at the mouth is considerably modified by changes in lung characteristics. The short period of constant-pressure generation which follows the period of constant-flow generation is difficult to detect, but the final period of near-zero-flow generation is quite clear.

In fig. 37.5 the fresh-gas flow is much larger, 4 litres/min. Here the initial period of flow generation is shortened and the period of constant-pressure generation occupies the greater part of the phase. It can be seen that, after a short period, the pressure at the

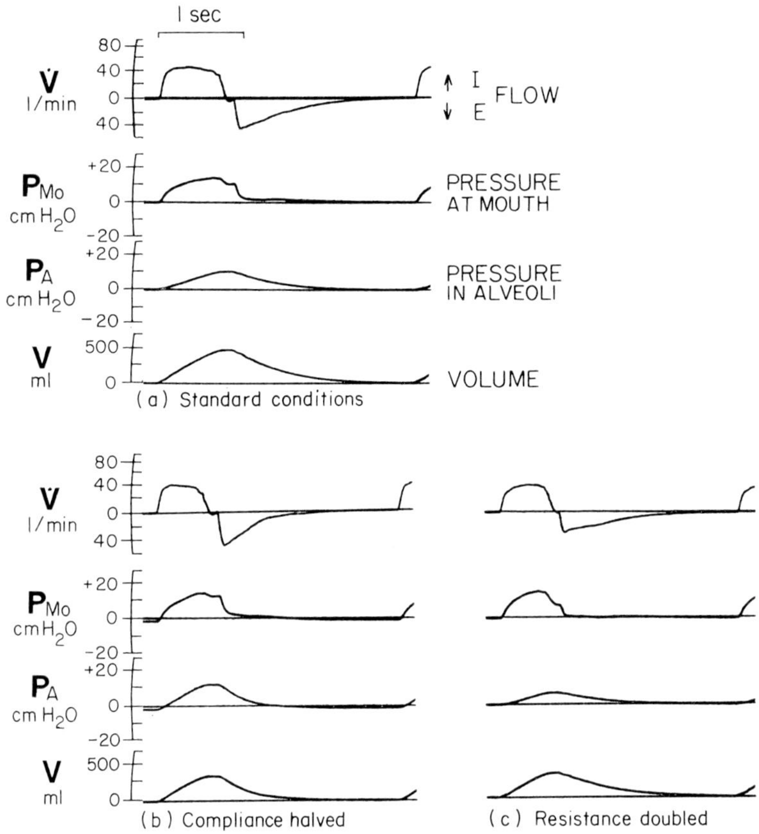

Fig. 37.4. 'Cyclator Combined Automatic Ventilator Unit'. Recordings, with a fresh-gas flow into the closed circuit of 0·5 litre/min, showing the effects of changes of lung characteristics. Standard conditions: driving gas, oxygen at 60 lb/in^2; entrained gas, air; fresh gas (to closed circuit), oxygen; soda-lime, 'on'; injector, 'type B'; 'inflation pressure', maximum; 'positive pressure', 'negative pressure', and 'respiratory pause', set for a tidal volume of 500 ml at a frequency of 20/min with a minimum alveolar pressure of 0 cmH_2O.

mouth stays nearly constant, at a level which is unaffected by changes in lung characteristics, until the final period of near-zero-flow generation commences. On the other hand the flow during the pressure-generation period falls off with time in a manner which varies markedly with changes in lung characteristics.

Change-over from inspiratory phase to expiratory phase

In this ventilator, this change-over still occurs when some critical pressure has been attained in the small concertina bag (22, fig. 36.3) in the 'Cyclator', but this pressure is now related to the pressure at the patient's mouth only in a very indirect way. With the cycling pressure set at maximum, the critical pressure is normally reached shortly after the concertina bag (15) has reached its upper limit. The delay arises from the time taken to compress the gas in the chamber (17) to the cycling pressure. Therefore the change-over occurs a short time after a particular volume has been expelled from the bag.

It is tempting, therefore, to regard the change-over as approximately volume-cycled. However, the volume expelled from the reservoir bag (15) during the inspiratory phase is the sum of the previous expired tidal volume and the volume of fresh gas which entered the circuit during the expiratory phase. This volume of fresh gas is unaffected by lung characteristics but the tidal volume is very much dependent on them (figs. 37.4 and 37.5). Therefore the change-over cannot be said to be volume-cycled in the conventional sense of the term.

By the same argument the time taken to empty the bag depends on lung characteristics (see figs. 37.4 and 37.5) so that the change-over cannot be said to be time-cycled either.

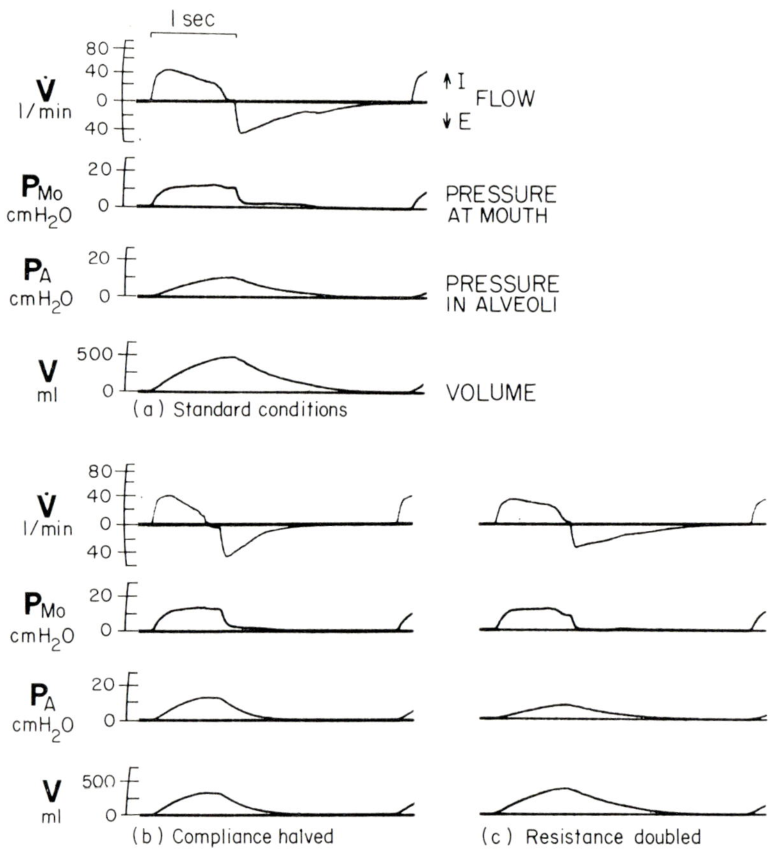

Fig. 37.5. 'Cyclator Combined Automatic Ventilator Unit'. Recordings, with a fresh-gas flow into the closed circuit of 4 litres/min, showing the effects of changes of lung characteristics. Standard conditions otherwise as for fig. 37.4.

Nor can the change-over be said to be flow-cycled: although the flow is always virtually zero at the end of the phase in figs. 37.4 and 37.5, this is simply because the bag (15) has ceased to be compressed shortly before. The flow into the patient at the moment the bag empties depends in a complex way on lung characteristics and ventilator control settings and it is clear from fig. 37.5 that the flow at this moment has not just reached some critical level.

When the fresh-gas flow is small (fig. 37.4) the change-over can be said to be approximately pressure-cycled. In these circumstances, only a small volume of excess gas has to be blown off at the end of the inspiratory phase; therefore the pressure within the reservoir bag (15) reaches the opening pressure of the 'positive pressure' valve (1) only a short time before the bag empties and therefore not long before the phase ends. Since the mouth pressure is nearly the same as the bag pressure the change-over is very nearly pressure-cycled in the conventional sense of the term. However, this does not apply to the case when the fresh-gas flow is high (fig. 37.5) because then the 'positive pressure' valve opens early in the phase, which then continues for a long and variable time during which the pressure in the bag and at the mouth is virtually constant.

Thus this change-over cannot be confidently assigned to any of the conventional cycling mechanism categories. The most general statement that can be made about it is that it occurs when a certain volume has been delivered from the 'Cyclator' but that this volume includes the tidal volume which happened to be expired by the patient in the previous respiratory cycle.

Expiratory phase

In this phase the ventilator approximates to a constant-pressure generator: the negative pressure due to the weight (16) in the concertina bag (15) is offset to a preset extent by the loading of the 'negative pressure' valve (9, 10). In fact, due to the elasticity of the bag material, the negative pressure declines as the bag expands (fig. 37.6). In addition, due to the characteristics of the 'negative pressure' valve (9, 10), the degree of offset it produces declines somewhat as the flow decreases. These complications are sufficient to explain the slight differences in mouth-pressure waveforms in the different sets of tracings in figs. 37.4 and 37.5. These figures also show the effect of lung characteristics on flow waveforms: halving the compliance makes the flow decay more rapidly; doubling the airway resistance makes it decay more slowly.

Change-over from expiratory phase to inspiratory phase

In this ventilator the patient-triggering mechanism of the 'Cyclator' cannot be used: if it were connected to the inside of the bag (15) the negative pressure which may be developed during the expiratory phase would cycle the ventilator prematurely; on the other hand, if the trigger mechanism were connected to the outside of the bag (15) the patient would have to produce a large inspiratory effort, sufficient to lift the weight (16), before any negative pressure was applied to the trigger mechanism. However, the time-cycling mechanism operates exactly as in the 'Cyclator' on its own. It can be seen from figs. 37.4 and 37.5 that the expiratory phase ends after a fixed time, not when a fixed volume has come out of the lungs nor when a fixed mouth pressure is first achieved.

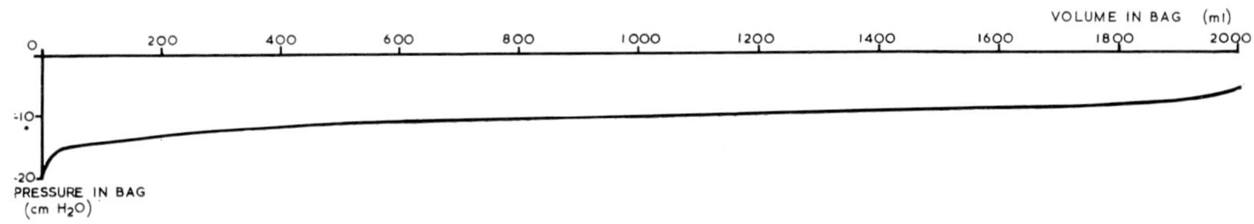

Fig. 37.6. 'Cyclator Combined Automatic Ventilator Unit'. Pressure-volume characteristic of the concertina reservoir bag. The 'negative pressure' control was set to maximum so that it did not oppose the expansion of the reservoir bag.

CONTROLS

Like the functional analysis this section is written on the assumption that the ventilator is used in 'mode A' (see p. 470), that is, with excess gas blown off through the 'positive pressure' valve (1) during the inspiratory phase.

Total ventilation

This cannot be directly controlled but is equal to the product of tidal volume and respiratory frequency.

Tidal volume

This is indirectly controlled by the settings of both the 'positive pressure' and the 'negative pressure' controls (1 and 8). Increasing the setting of either of these controls (fig. 37.7b, c) increases the range of pressure applied to the lungs and hence the tidal volume. The magnitude of the tidal volume depends also on the lung characteristics and decreases with any decrease in compliance (figs. 37.4b and 37.5b) or increase in airway resistance (figs. 37.4c and 37.5c).

The tidal volume is also somewhat influenced by the fresh-gas flow. Increasing this (fig. 37.7e) increases the volume of gas to be blown off through the 'positive pressure' valve during each inspiratory phase. Therefore the inspiratory phase is prolonged and, during the prolongation, the pressure limit set by the 'positive pressure' valve is maintained at the mouth. This allows the alveolar pressure to approach the pressure limit more closely than with a low fresh-gas flow (compare fig. 37.7e with 37.7a) and so gives a larger tidal volume.

When the tidal volume is deliberately increased by adjusting the 'positive pressure' or 'negative pressure' valves a number of other parameters are changed. Since the ventilator operates as a constant-flow generator for part of the phase, the increased tidal volume takes longer to deliver and the inspiratory phase is lengthened; but the expiratory phase, the end of which is time-cycled, is unaffected. Therefore, the frequency is decreased and the inspiratory-expiratory ratio is altered. The total ventilation is increased but less than in proportion to the tidal volume.

Respiratory frequency and inspiratory-expiratory ratio

As with the 'Cyclator' alone, neither of these parameters can be directly controlled but both are determined by the separately-variable inspiratory and expiratory times.

The inspiratory time is a little longer than the time taken to empty the concertina bag (15) at the nearly-constant flow from the injector of the 'Cyclator'. At the start of the inspiratory phase the bag contains not only the tidal volume of gas, but also the volume of fresh gas which entered the patient circuit during the previous expiratory phase. Therefore the inspiratory time will be influenced, firstly, by changes of tidal volume, either deliberate, (fig. 37.7b, c) or incidental, (figs. 37.4b, c and 37.5b, c); secondly, by changes in fresh-gas flow, (fig. 37.7e) both directly and via the effect of fresh-gas flow on the tidal volume; and finally, to a small degree, by changes in the expiratory time (fig. 37.7d). This last is because a change in the expiratory time produces a change in the amount of fresh gas entering the concertina bag during the expiratory phase. As with the 'Cyclator' alone, the inspiratory time can be deliberately altered by changing the generated flow by means of changing to a different injector or using the variable restrictor at the entrainment port. If the flow is reduced (fig. 37.7f) then, at least during that part of the inspiratory phase in which the ventilator is operating as a flow generator, the pressure difference between the mouth and the alveoli is reduced. Therefore, at least when the fresh-gas flow is low (and there is no prolonged subsequent period of pressure generation), reducing the generated flow allows the alveolar pressure to approach more closely the pressure limit set by the 'positive pressure' valve. This leads to the delivery of a larger tidal volume (fig. 37.7f). Therefore, if the original tidal volume is to be restored, the 'positive pressure' valve must be adjusted after changing the injector. Then the same tidal volume will be delivered over a longer inspiratory phase.

As with the 'Cyclator' alone, the expiratory time is directly controlled by the 'respiratory pause' control (25 in fig. 36.3) (fig. 37.7d). It is not affected by changes in lung characteristics (figs. 37.4 and 37.5) nor by changes in any of the other ventilator controls (fig. 37.7).

In summary then, as with the 'Cyclator' alone, the respiratory frequency is primarily controlled by the 'respiratory pause' control, but it is also affected by the settings of all the other controls and by the lung characteristics.

Having decided the respiratory frequency required, the other injectors and the restrictor allow variation of the inspiratory-expiratory ratio, although the exact value of the ratio will depend on and vary with the settings of all the other controls and with the lung characteristics.

Inspiratory waveforms

During the initial, flow-generating, period of the inspiratory phase the flow waveform is largely determined by the characteristics of the injector while the pressure waveforms result from the interaction of the flow waveform with the lung characteristics. Although the magnitude of the flow can be altered by changing the injector or using the variable restrictor, a particular flow may already have been chosen in order to deliver a given tidal volume in a given inspiratory time.

During the subsequent, pressure-generating, period the pressure at the mouth is maintained constant, while the flow decays as a result of the effect of this pressure on the lung characteristics. The magnitude of the pressure can be altered by adjusting the 'positive pressure' valve but this will usually have been set in accordance with the tidal volume required.

The relative durations of the flow-generating and pressure-generating periods can be adjusted by altering the fresh-gas flow. Furthermore, the adjustment can be made without alteration of the tidal volume if a compensatory adjustment of the 'positive pressure' valve is made. However, increasing the fresh-gas flow necessarily involves some increase in the duration of the inspiratory phase and, in any event, its magnitude may be dictated by other factors common to the use of any closed-circuit apparatus.

Expiratory waveforms

Throughout the expiratory phase the pressure at the mouth is held nearly constant by the constant-pressure-generating characteristics of the ventilator, while the flow waveform results from the application of this constant pressure to the lungs. The magnitude of the pressure and its sense (positive or negative) can be adjusted, but the setting used may be dictated by a requirement for a particular mean pressure.

Pressure limits

The pressure limits at the mouth are both directly controlled by the 'positive pressure' and 'negative pressure' valves, although both limits are slightly dependent on the flow through the valves, and the negative-pressure limit is also slightly dependent on the degree of expansion of the concertina reservoir bag. The maximum alveolar pressure is

---

Fig. 37.7. 'Cyclator Combined Automatic Ventilator Unit'. Recordings showing the effects of changes in the settings of the controls.

(a) Standard conditions as in fig. 37.4 with the fresh-gas flow into the closed circuit set at 0·5 litre/min.

(b) 'Positive pressure' increased to produce a tidal volume of 750 ml.

(c) 'Negative pressure' increased to give an end-expiratory alveolar pressure of -5 cmH_2O.

(d) 'Respiratory pause' decreased to give a respiratory frequency of 24/min.

(e) Fresh-gas flow increased to 4 litres/min.

(f) 'Type C' injector.

less than the maximum mouth pressure by the pressure drop across the airway resistance. This pressure drop is smaller when a low generated flow is used or when a high fresh-gas flow leads to a prolonged period of constant-pressure generation during the later part of the inspiratory phase. During the expiratory phase the alveolar pressure normally falls to

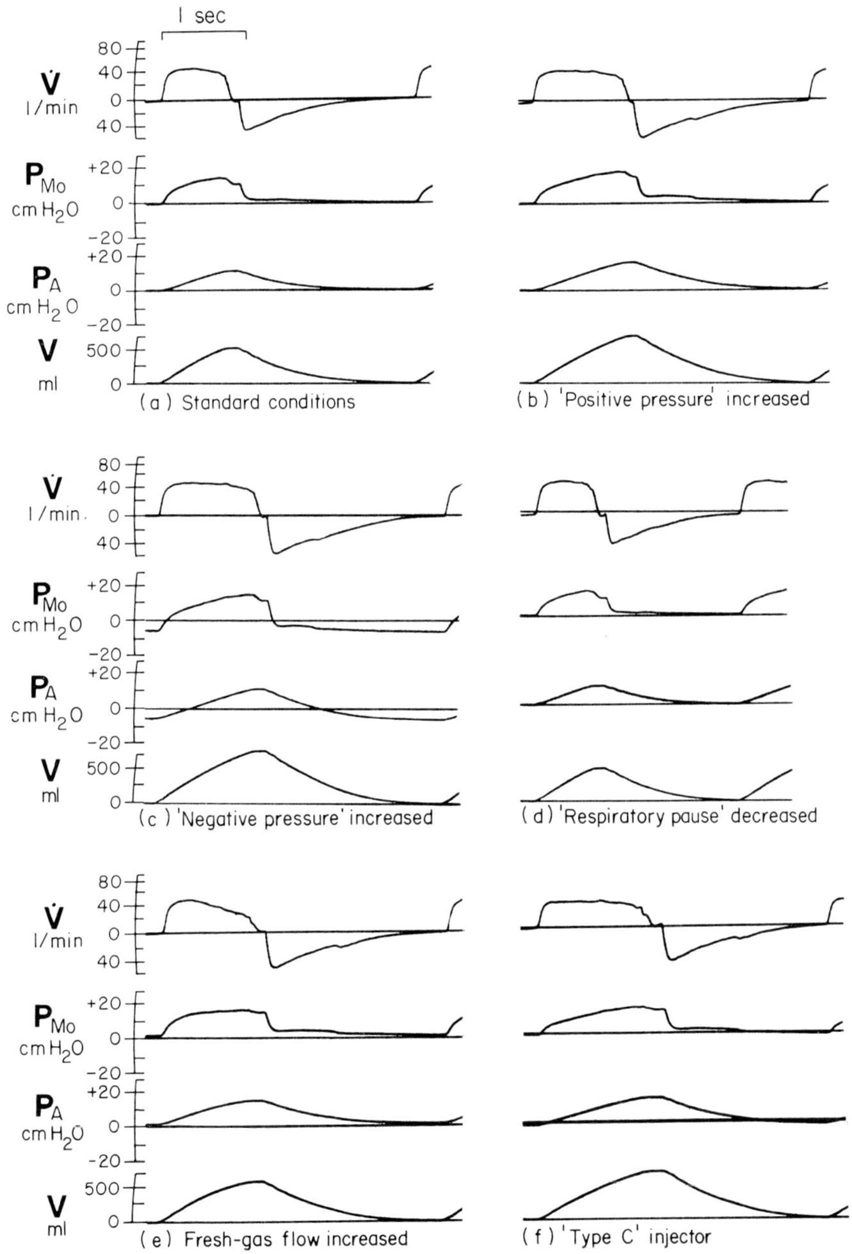

equal the generated pressure at the mouth. It does so in all the tracings in figs. 37.4, 37.5 and 37.7. It will fail to do so only when the airway resistance is very high or when the expiratory time is very short.

By balanced adjustments of both the 'positive pressure' and the 'negative pressure' valves the mean pressure may be altered without making any change in the tidal volume, respiratory frequency, inspiratory-expiratory ratio, or the general pattern of the waveforms.

CHAPTER 38

The Dennis Ventilator[1, 2]

DESCRIPTION

This ventilator, like several others, incorporates a toggle mechanism similar to that used in the 'Pulmotor' of 1911 (see p. 198) and in the Janeway ventilator of 1913 (see p. 197).

During the inspiratory phase (fig. 38.1) driving gas enters the valve chamber at (1) and

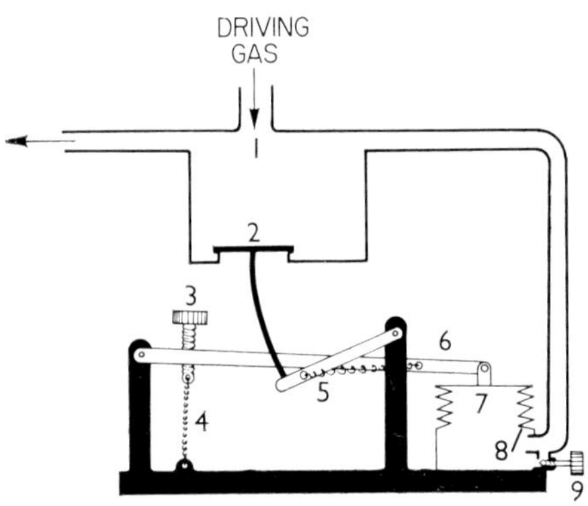

Fig. 38.1. Diagram of the Dennis ventilator —inspiratory phase.

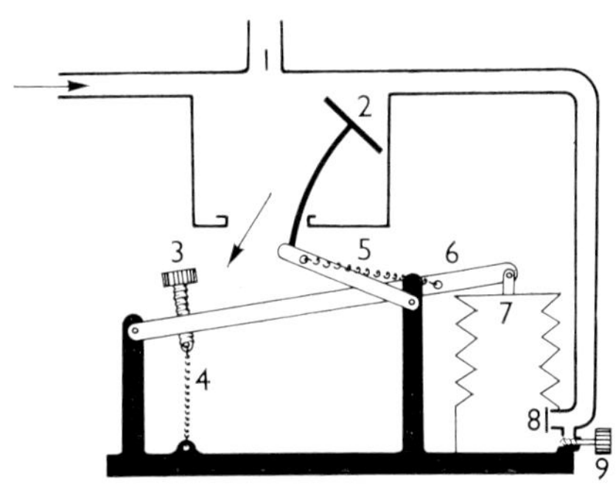

Fig. 38.2. Diagram of the Dennis ventilator —expiratory phase.

1. Driving-gas inlet
2. Exhaust valve
3. Cycling-pressure control
4. Spring
5. Toggle mechanism
6. Arm
7. Concertina bag
8. One-way valve
9. Needle valve

After Mörch E.T. and Benson D.W.,[2] by courtesy of the Scandinavian Society of Anaesthesiologists.

passes into one half of a partitioned reservoir bag (fig. 38.3). The small rubber concertina bag (7) is inflated against the pull of the spring (4) attached to the arm (6). When the pressure in the apparatus reaches the cycling pressure determined by the control (3) the expansion of the bag (7) carries the arm (6), and with it the toggle mechanism (5), past its critical point. The toggle flicks over suddenly, opening wide the exhaust valve (2) and allowing expiration to take place freely. Air is prevented from escaping rapidly from the bag (7) by the one-way valve (8), and is compelled to pass out through the needle valve (9) which therefore controls the duration of the expiratory phase.

During expiration (fig. 38.2) the escape of driving gas is prevented, by a device not shown in the figure, thus economizing in the amount of compressed air used. When the concertina bag (7) collapses, the arm (6) carries the toggle mechanism (5) back past its critical point, the exhaust valve (2) closes, driving gas flows into the apparatus once more, and the next inspiratory phase begins.

For use with this apparatus, Dennis and his co-workers designed a partitioned reservoir bag (fig. 38.3), made of polyvinyl film, to fit on the Heidbrink anaesthetic

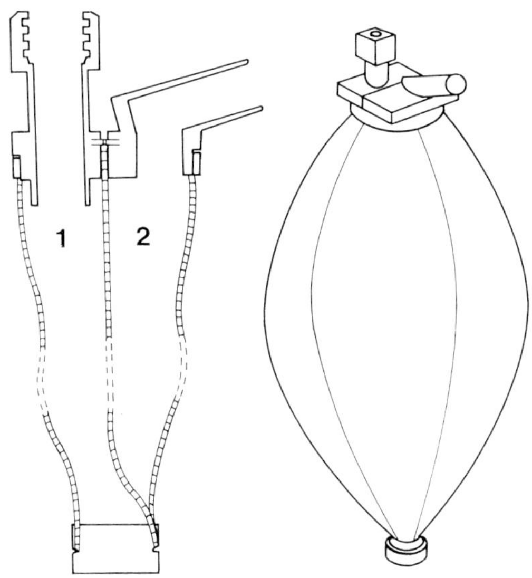

Fig. 38.3. Diagram of the Dennis ventilator reservoir bag.

1. Connexion to anaesthetic apparatus 2. Connexion to ventilator

Courtesy of *Surgical Forum*.[1]

apparatus. The capacity of the bag is 5·7 litres. Inside is a hemispherical partition which divides the interior into two compartments. This is sufficiently loose to be able to adapt itself to either wall of the bag. The top of the bag is attached to a plastic holder with two openings, one of which (1) is connected to the anaesthetic apparatus and the other (2) to the ventilator. Owing to the bag's inelasticity, driving gas passing into one half of the bag forces the anaesthetic mixture out of the other into the lungs. The bag takes the place of the reservoir bag and pressure chamber common on many ventilators to transmit the variations in pressure in the ventilator to the reservoir bag of the anaesthetic apparatus. The undesirable electrostatic properties of the polyvinyl chloride are overcome by coating its surface with aluminium powder suspended in ethylene chloride. Manual control of respiration can be carried out by squeezing the partitioned reservoir bag in the usual way. No spill valve is fitted and the expiratory valve on the anaesthetic apparatus should be adjusted so that excess gas does not accumulate in the patient circuit. Increasing the cycling pressure in the driving circuit will therefore not increase the tidal volume unless the blow-off pressure on the expiratory valve is correspondingly increased.

FUNCTIONAL ANALYSIS

Inspiratory phase

The mode of operation during this phase depends largely on the source of compressed gas, but is likely to be that of a high-constant-pressure generator with substantial series resistance, or that of a constant-flow generator. In all events, there is a pressure limit, due to the blow-off valve which must be provided in the patient circuit, which comes into operation during the phase. Until then, the fresh-gas supply to the patient circuit acts as a small-constant-flow generator, supplementing the action of the main compressed-gas source.

Change-over from inspiratory phase to expiratory phase

Superficially this change-over appears to be pressure-cycled: the pressure in the control concertina bag (7) which produces cycling is that applied to the patient via the double bag. However, the blow-off valve in the patient circuit must open at less than the cycling pressure in order to vent excess anaesthetic gas. Therefore the pressure in the patient circuit can never rise to the cycling pressure. However, the pressure in the driving circuit does rise to the cycling pressure, and therefore produces the change-over, but only shortly after the patient-half of the double reservoir bag has been emptied. From this it might appear that the change-over is effectively volume-cycled, but even this is not true in the conventional sense of the term. A precisely similar situation arises in the 'Cyclator CAV' and in the functional analysis of that ventilator it is shown that the change-over can best be described in the following way.

If the fresh-gas flow is large, the only way of describing the change-over is to say that it is volume-cycled but that the volume involved (that in the patient-half of the double reservoir bag at the beginning of the inspiratory phase) includes the tidal volume which happened to be expired by the patient in the previous respiratory cycle and which is dependent upon lung characteristics. If the fresh-gas flow is small, the above statement is still true, but there is now so little excess gas to be vented through the blow-off valve that the change-over occurs almost immediately the blow-off valve opens. Therefore the change-over is effectively pressure-cycled at the opening pressure of the blow-off valve.

Expiratory phase

In this phase the ventilator operates as a constant, atmospheric, pressure generator: the patient's expired gas effectively has free passage to the atmosphere at the exhaust valve.

Change-over from expiratory phase to inspiratory phase

This change-over is time-cycled: the expiratory time is equal to the time in which enough gas leaks out of the control concertina bag (7) for cycling to occur. This time is uninfluenced by the patient but depends on the force of the spring (4), as well as the setting of the needle valve (9). Therefore raising the cycling pressure at the end of the inspiratory phase, by means of extending this spring further, shortens the expiratory phase.

REFERENCES

1 Dennis C., Karlson K.E., Eder W.P., Nelson R.M., Spreng D.S., Thomas J.V. and Nelson G.E. (1950) *Surg. Forum*, p. 583.

2 Mörch E.T. and Benson D.W. (1955) Proceedings of the Third Congress of the Scandinavian Society of Anaesthesiologists, Copenhagen, 1954, p. 30.

CHAPTER 39

The Donald Ventilator[1]

DESCRIPTION

This ventilator was designed to assist the weak inspiratory efforts of the new-born baby suffering from asphyxia neonatorum. Because the ventilator only operates in response to spontaneous inspiratory efforts, when the diaphragm is contracting and closing the lower end of the oesophagus, inflation of the stomach, a bugbear during ventilation of the apnoeic baby, is said not to occur.

The mechanism is electrically-operated by the 24-volt battery (14) (fig. 39.1). A

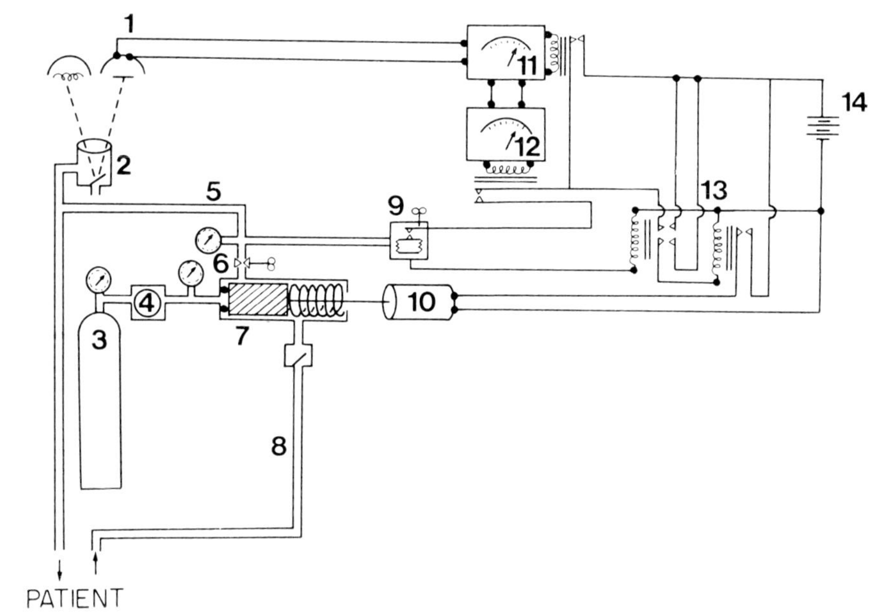

Fig. 39.1. Diagram of the Donald ventilator.[1]

1. Photo-electric cell
2. Silvered inspiratory valve
3. Cylinder
4. Reducing valve
5. Inspiratory tube
6. Tap
7. Piston valve
8. Expiratory tube
9. Pressure-sensitive switch
10. Solenoid
11. Amplifier
12. Time switch
13. Relay system
14. 24-volt battery

Courtesy of *The Lancet*.

beam of light shines onto the silvered inspiratory valve (2), and is reflected onto the photo-electric cell (1) so that the slightest movement of the valve caused by the baby's inspiratory effort deflects light from the cell. The commencement of an inspiration therefore causes a change of voltage which, when amplified at (11), operates the relay system (13) and the solenoid (10). The latter pulls the piston (7) back, closing the expiratory pathway (8) and allowing oxygen mixture from the cylinder (3) to flow through the inspiratory tube (5) to the patient. The gas flow is controlled by the tap (6). The pressure-sensitive switch (9) can be adjusted to open when a certain pressure is reached. Cycling occurs and the inspiratory phase ends.

The amplifier (11) is so designed that it will pass only the first impulse from the photo-electric cell (1) rejecting all others over a variable and adjustable period of time, usually one second. Repetitive triggering is thus prevented. The time switch (12) is connected in series with the pressure-sensitive switch (9) so that if the maximum pressure set by (9) is not reached within the time interval set by (12) the opening of the contacts on (12) puts the solenoid (10) out of action and brings the inspiratory phase to an end.

The reducing valve (4) maintains a pressure of just under 2 lb/in^2 (130 cmH_2O). The manometer indicates the pressure in the inspiratory tube. In practice, the tap (6) is adjusted so that a peak pressure of about 15 cmH_2O is reached by the end of the inspiratory phase. The gas mixture used by Donald with this apparatus was 50 per cent oxygen in nitrogen, supplied ready-mixed in cylinders.

FUNCTIONAL ANALYSIS

Inspiratory phase

In this phase the ventilator makes a good approximation to a constant-flow generator owing to the constant pressure of 130 cmH_2O from the reducing valve (4) (fig. 39.1) applied to the resistance of the tap (6).

Change-over from inspiratory phase to expiratory phase

This change-over is either time-cycled or pressure-cycled, whichever limit is reached first: cycling occurs when the solenoid (10) is de-energized. This may result either from the opening of the timing-circuit contacts, after a preset time; or by the opening of the pressure-sensitive-switch contacts (9), when a preset pressure is reached in the patient circuit.

Expiratory phase

In this phase the ventilator operates as a constant, atmospheric, pressure generator: the patient's expired gas passes freely to atmosphere at the expiratory outlet.

Change-over from expiratory phase to inspiratory phase

This change-over is patient-cycled: cycling occurs only when an inspiratory effort by the patient produces a negative pressure at the inspiratory valve (2) sufficient to actuate the triggering mechanism.

REFERENCE

1 DONALD I. (1954) Augmented respiration; an emergency positive-pressure patient-cycled respirator. *Lancet*, **1**, 895.

CHAPTER 40

The Dräger 'Assistor 640'

DESCRIPTION

This compact ventilator (fig. 40.1) is designed for ward use. It can normally only be patient-triggered.

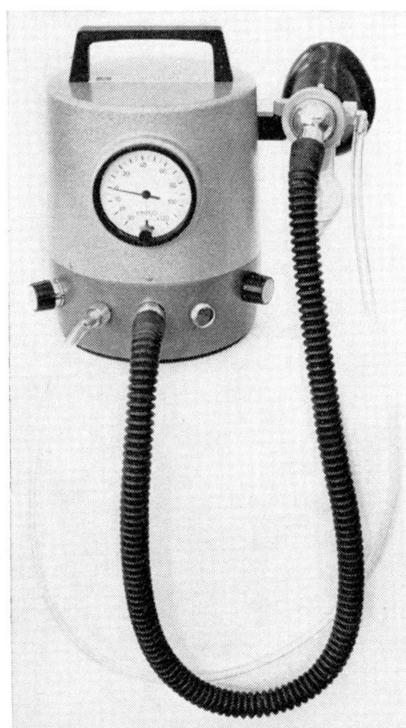

Fig. 40.1. The Dräger 'Assistor 640'.
Courtesy of Drägerwerk (Heinr. & Bernh. Dräger), Lubeck.

Compressed air or oxygen at a pressure of 28–140 lb/in² is supplied at the inlet (8) (fig. 40.2), and flows through the on/off tap (7) to the reducing valve (6).

When the patient makes an inspiratory effort, the expiratory port of the inflating valve (12) is closed and the one-way valve (11) in the centre of the diaphragm is opened.

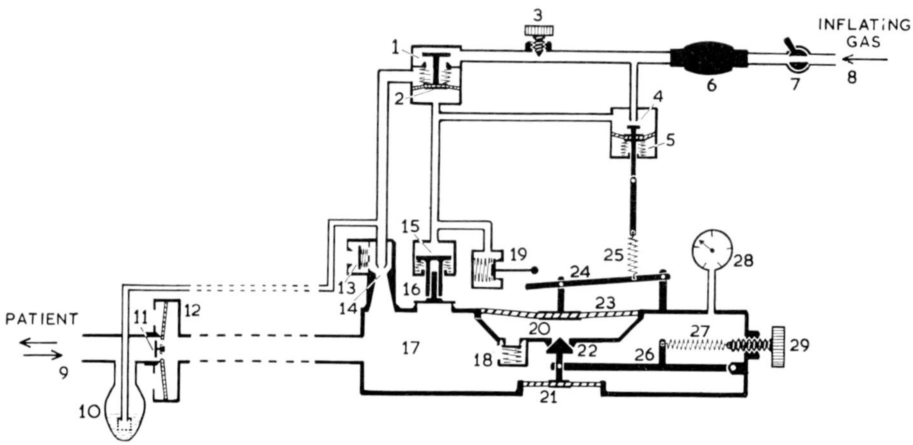

Fig. 40.2. Diagram of the Dräger 'Assistor 640'.

1. Relay valve
2. Diaphragm
3. Inspiratory-flow control
4. Valve
5. Spring
6. Pressure-reducing valve
7. On/off tap
8. Gas inlet
9. Patient port
10. Nebulizer
11. One-way valve
12. Inflating valve
13. One-way valve
14. Injector
15. Piston
16. Pressure-relief valve
17. Main chamber
18. One-way valve
19. Tilt valve
20. Small chamber
21. Diaphragm
22. Valve
23. Diaphragm
24. Pivoted lever
25. Spring
26. Pivoted lever
27. Spring
28. Manometer
29. Inflating-pressure control

The negative pressure produced in the main chamber (17) opens the one-way valve (18), which is only very-lightly loaded, the negative pressure is transmitted to the small chamber (20), and the diaphragm (23) moves down. This diaphragm (23) is connected by a rod to a pivoted lever (24) which is moved downwards, expanding the spring (25) until the pull exerted through a second connecting rod is sufficient to overcome the force of the compression spring (5) and thereby open the valve (4). The negative pressure required to operate this mechanism is -1 cmH_2O.

Gas from the reducing valve (6) can now flow through the valve (4) to the chamber below the diaphragm (2) of the relay valve and the chamber (15) above the piston of the pressure-relief valve (16). The upward movement of the diaphragm (2) opens the relay valve (1) and the inspiratory phase begins. Compressed gas flows, at a rate controlled by the needle valve (3), to the injector (14) where it entrains atmospheric air through the one-way valve (13). The gas mixture passes, through the main chamber (17) and the inflating valve (12), to the patient. A nebulizer (10) between the inflating valve and the patient is connected to the compressed-gas supply to the injector and is actuated throughout the inspiratory phase. If the compressed-gas supply is oxygen, the oxygen concentration in the mixture delivered to the patient is approximately 50%. As soon as the pressure in the main chamber (17) begins to rise, the valve (18) is closed. As this pressure, which is indicated on the manometer (28), rises further, the force exerted on the diaphragm (21) increases until it is sufficient to move the diaphragm outwards against the pull exerted by the spring (27) through the lever (26). The valve (22) is opened, connecting the main chamber (17) and the small chamber (20). The diaphragm (23) is immediately moved upwards by the positive pressure below it and the tension of the spring (25) is reduced sufficiently to allow the spring (5) to close the valve (4). Further upward movement of the diaphragm (23), and with it the lever (24), causes the end of the lever (24) to strike the stem of the valve (19) and tilt the valve (19) open.

The chamber of the relay valve (1, 2) and the cylinder (15) of the pressure-relief valve, are now connected with the atmosphere and the pressure within them falls. The valve (1) closes and inflation ceases. At the same time the piston of the pressure-relief valve is moved upwards by its spring, allowing the one-way valve (16) to be opened by the pressure within the main chamber (17). Pressure in the main chamber (17), the small chamber (20), and behind the diaphragm of the inflating valve (12), falls to atmospheric. The higher pressure on the patient side of the inflating valve closes the one-way valve (11) and moves the diaphragm to its expiratory position. The expiratory phase begins and expired gas flows to atmosphere through the ports of the inflating valve (12).

Meanwhile the fall in pressure in the small chamber (20) has allowed the diaphragm (23) to return to its resting position, and the tilt valve (19) to be closed by its spring. At the same time the fall in pressure in the main chamber (17) has allowed the spring (27) to close the valve (22). The ventilator remains in this resting position until triggered by the patient's next inspiratory effort.

The control (3) allows the inspiratory flow to be adjusted between 5 and 50 litres per minute. The pressure at which the ventilator cycles from the inspiratory phase to the expiratory phase depends on the setting of the control (29) and may be varied between +10 and +80 cmH_2O.

For any particular patient, the duration of the inspiratory phase depends on the settings of these two controls. The duration of the expiratory phase is the time between the end of the inspiratory phase and the patient's next inspiratory effort.

An electronic 'timer' is now available for connexion to this ventilator if fully-automatic functioning is desired. Alternatively, a version known as the '641' is available which incorporates a pneumatic timer.

FUNCTIONAL ANALYSIS

Inspiratory phase

In this phase the ventilator operates fundamentally as a constant-pressure generator due to the injector (14).

Change-over from inspiratory phase to expiratory phase
This change-over is pressure-cycled: it occurs when the pressure on the diaphragm (21), which is similar to the pressure at the mouth, is sufficient to overcome the force of the spring (27).

Expiratory phase
In this phase the ventilator operates as a constant, atmospheric, pressure generator: the patient's expired gas passes to atmosphere through the expiratory ports of the inflating valve (12).

Change-over from expiratory phase to inspiratory phase
This change-over is patient-cycled: it occurs when an inspiratory effort by the patient produces enough negative pressure below the diaphragm (23) to open the valve (4).

CHAPTER 41

The Dräger 'Narkose Spiromat 650' and 'Spiromat 661'

DESCRIPTION

In the 'Narkose Spiromat 650' the ventilator mechanism is combined with an anaesthetic apparatus (fig. 41.1). It is intended for ward or theatre use. The basic ventilator mechan-

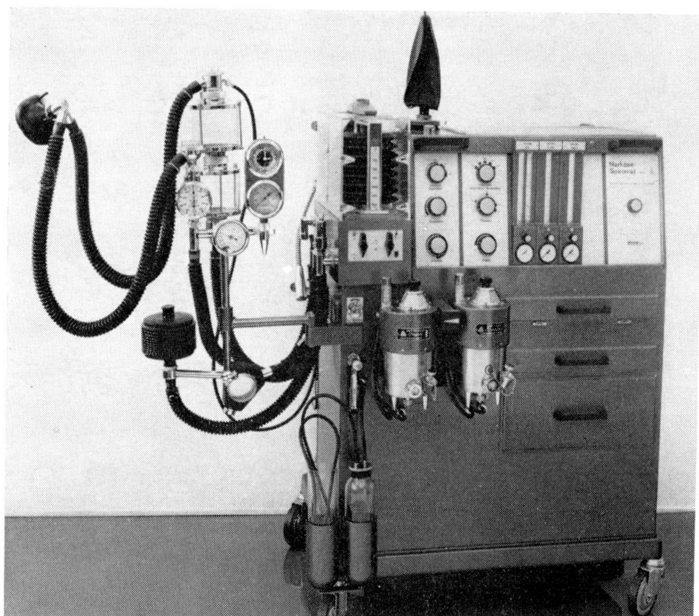

Fig. 41.1. The Dräger 'Narkose Spiromat 650'.
Courtesy of Drägerwerk (Heinr. & Bernh. Dräger), Lubeck.

ism with minor modifications (see p. 498) is available as the Dräger 'Spiromat 661' (fig. 41.2) which is intended for ward use only.

An electronic timing mechanism controls the flow of air from the blower (41) (fig. 41.3) to the rigid plastic pressure chamber (17). This chamber contains a concertina

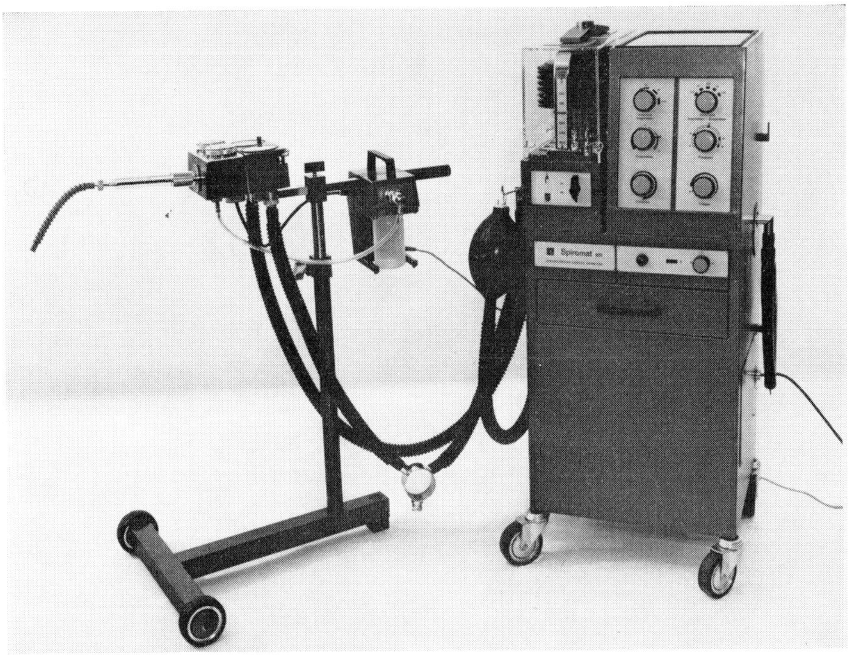

Fig. 41.2. The Dräger 'Spiromat 661'.
Courtesy of Drägerwerk (Heinr. & Bernh. Dräger), Lubeck.

reservoir bag (19) which forms part of a non-rebreathing or of a closed anaesthetic circuit. Negative pressure is available during the expiratory phase. The ventilator may be patient-triggered.

The tidal volume can be adjusted continuously between 20 and 1500 ml, the frequency in steps between 12 and 40/min, and the inspiratory-expiratory ratio in steps between 1 : 1·5 and 1 : 3·5.

The maximum inspiratory pressure is limited to 100 cmH_2O by the characteristics of the blower (41). It can be further limited to 40 cmH_2O, or lower, by the control (40). During manual inflation it is limited by the safety-valve (13). Expiratory pressure may be varied between -20 cmH_2O, and $+20$ cmH_2O by the 'expiration' control (32).

A spark-proof and flame-proof a.c. mains electric motor (42) drives the blower (41) continuously. During the inspiratory phase the solenoid (39) is energized, the port (33) of the valve assembly is open, and the port (38) is closed.

Closed circuit

Air is drawn from the atmosphere through the port (33) by the blower which drives it past the 'working pressure' control (40), to the rigid plastic chamber (17). The concertina

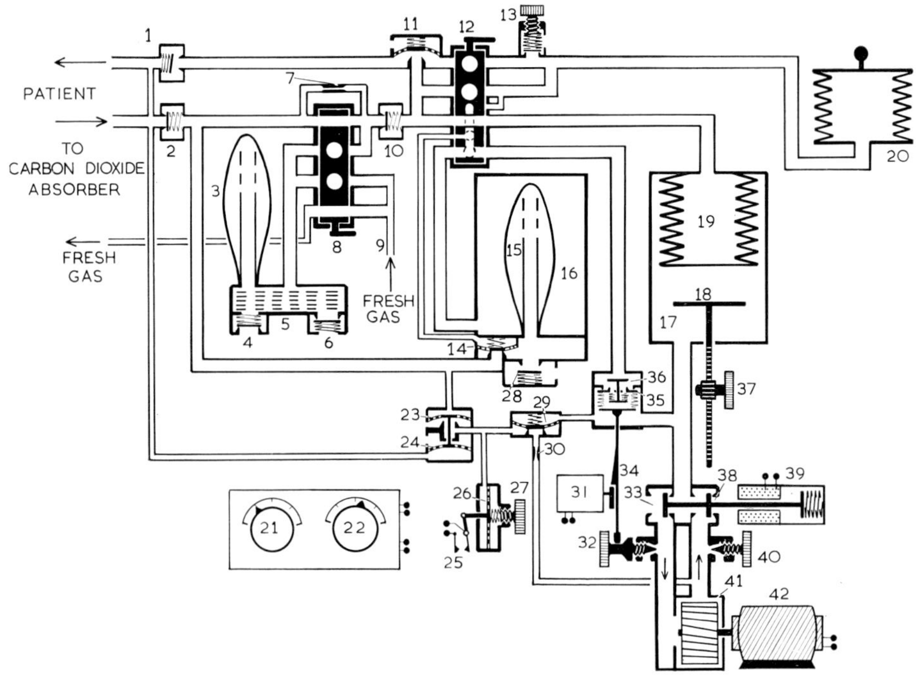

Fig. 41.3. Diagram of the Dräger 'Narkose Spiromat 650'.

1. One-way valve
2. One-way valve
3. Storage bag
4. One-way valve
5. Bacterial filter
6. One-way valve
7. Constriction
8. 'Open/closed circuit' tap
9. Fresh-gas inlet
10. One-way valve
11. Diaphragm valve
12. 'Automatic/manual' tap
13. Safety-valve operative during manual inflation
14. Diaphragm valve
15. Storage bag
16. Rigid plastic chamber
17. Rigid plastic chamber
18. Stop
19. Concertina bag
20. Concertina bag
21. 'Inspiration: expiration' ratio control
22. Respiratory 'frequency' control
23. Diaphragm
24. Diaphragm
25. Electrical contacts
26. Diaphragm
27. Patient 'trigger' control
28. One-way valve
29. Diaphragm
30. Constriction
31. Sigh activator ('Spiromat 661' only)
32. Negative-pressure 'expiration' control
33. Port
34. Rod
35. Double-action valve
36. One-way valve
37. 'Volume' control
38. Port
39. Solenoid
40. 'Working pressure, inspiration' control
41. Blower
42. Motor

reservoir bag (19) is compressed and the gas within it is forced, through the 'automatic/manual' control tap (12), the diaphragm valve (11), the one-way valve (1), and a soda-lime canister, to the patient. After a time set by the electronic timing unit (21, 22) the electrical supply to the solenoid (39) is cut off, the port (33) is closed and the port (38) is opened. Expired gas flows, through the one-way valve (2), the 'open/closed circuit' tap

(8), the one-way valve (10), and the 'automatic/manual' tap (12), to the concertina reservoir bag (19).

Fresh gas is supplied at the inlet (9) and flows through the 'open/closed circuit' tap (8) and enters the inspiratory pathway on the patient side of the soda-lime canister. During the expiratory phase the expansion of the concertina bag (19) is limited by the plate (18), the height of which is set by the 'volume' control (37). When the bag (19) has expanded to this limit any excess gas flows, through the diaphragm valve (14), into the storage bag (15) in the rigid plastic chamber (16). This chamber is connected, through the 'automatic/manual' tap (12) and the double-action valve (35, 36), to the intake of the blower. Therefore the outside of the bag (15) is normally subjected to the same pressure as the outside of the concertina bag (19). During the next inspiratory phase the compressed-air flow through the central port of the double-action valve (35, 36) closes the diaphragm valve (14) and compresses the storage bag (15). Excess gas stored in this bag is forced, through the loaded one-way valve (28), to atmosphere.

During the expiratory phase the port (38) is open and the port (33) is closed. The blower (41) therefore draws air from the pressure chamber (17), and from atmosphere through the 'expiration' control (32). The proportion of air thus drawn from the chamber (17), and hence the negative pressure produced inside the concertina reservoir bag (19), depends on the setting of the 'expiration' control (32). If desired this control may be set (in the manner described below) to restrict the outlet of gas from the chamber (16) and thereby maintain a positive pressure during the latter part of expiration when excess gas is entering the bag (15). If negative pressure is used during the expiratory phase the whole of the double-action valve (35, 36) is moved down away from the outer seating, and negative pressure exists in the chamber (16) as well as the chamber (17) since the blower draws air from both chambers. If the control (32) is set to provide a positive pressure during expiration, the expanded portion of the 'expiration' control (32) pushes up the rod (34), compresses the spring of the outer valve (35), and impedes the flow of air from the chamber (16) and hence the flow of expired gas into the storage bag (15).

Non-rebreathing circuit

The tap (8) is turned to the 'open circuit' position. During the inspiratory phase gas from the concertina reservoir bag (19) flows along the same pathway as during closed-circuit use. During the expiratory phase expired gas can flow only, through the one-way valve (2) and the diaphragm valve (14), to the storage bag (15), from which it is discharged to atmosphere during the next inspiratory phase.

Fresh gas supplied at the inlet (9) is stored in the storage bag (3) during the inspiratory phase. During the expiratory phase this gas, together with further fresh gas entering, is drawn, through the 'open/closed circuit' tap (8), the one-way valve (10), the 'automatic/manual' tap (12), into the concertina reservoir bag (19). If the fresh-gas flow is less than the total minute-volume ventilation, air is drawn in during the expiratory phase through the one-way valve (4) and the bacterial filter (5). If the fresh-gas flow is greater than the total minute-volume ventilation, the excess escapes through the one-way valve (6).

The operation of the ventilator is, in all other respects, identical to that during closed-circuit use, except that, since the whole of the expired gas flows into the bag (15), positive pressure can be maintained throughout the expiratory phase (by appropriate setting of control (32)) instead of only during the last part.

Patient-triggering

During the inspiratory phase the valve (29) is held closed by the positive pressure above the diaphragm. During the expiratory phase the negative pressure above this diaphragm opens the valve against its spring. There is now a flow of gas from the blower, past the constriction (30), through the valve (29), to the double-diaphragm valve (23, 24). The chamber beneath the lower diaphragm (24) is connected to the expiratory pathway on the patient side of the one-way valve (2). The chamber above the upper diaphragm (23) is connected to the expiratory pathway on the other side of the valve (2). Therefore, whatever the pressure existing in the expiratory pathway there is a pressure-balance across the double diaphragms. During the expiratory phase the flow of compressed air from the valve (29) forces the upper diaphragm away from its seating, taking with it the lower diaphragm, and the compressed air escapes to atmosphere through the valve.

Any attempt at inspiration by the patient produces a pressure drop from right to left across the one-way valve (2), thereby tending to push the double-diaphragm valve (23, 24) downward. This restricts the escape of gas from the valve (29) and raises the pressure behind the diaphragm (26) tending to close the contacts (25). The degree of inspiratory effort needed to complete this closure, and hence triggering of the ventilator to the next inspiratory phase, depends on the setting of the control (27) and can be varied from -1 to -5 cmH_2O.

Manual operation

For manual operation the tap (12) is turned and this brings the reservoir bag (20) into the breathing circuit whether this is closed or open.

Compression of the reservoir bag (20) not only inflates the patient but also discharges expired gas from the previous inflation stored in the bag (15). If the tap (8) is set to the non-rebreathing circuit, a complete tidal volume will be stored in the bag (15) and therefore twice the required tidal volume must be squeezed from the bag (20) at each inflation.

Dräger 'Spiromat 661'

This ventilator is designed for long-term use in the ward. It is not flame- and spark-proof like the 'Spiromat 650'. It does not incorporate an anaesthetic apparatus. There is no provision for use with a closed circuit and the 'open/closed circuit' tap (8) is omitted. An additional electronic mechanism (31) can be switched on if a 'sigh' is desired; this increases the expiratory resistance for 3 or 4 consecutive cycles in every 100, thereby producing an increase in the distension of the lungs during this period.

The manual concertina bag (20) is replaced by a self-inflating bag.

A nebulizer is supplied for use with either ventilator. In the model '661', the unidirectional-valve assembly close to the patient is electrically-heated (40°–45°C) to prevent condensation. This valve assembly (in both adult and infant forms) can also be supplied for use with the model '650' for long-term ventilation.

The '661' is also available in a version which includes a bank of nickel-cadmium gas-tight accumulators which automatically come into action if the mains supply falls below a preset level. They will run the ventilator for one hour. In this version the ventilator has two electric motors (220-volt a.c. and 24-volt d.c.). A third version of the '661' is almost independent of mains electricity. It is driven not by a blower but by an injector connected to a source of driving gas at high pressure. A small accumulator is included which is sufficient to power the electronic circuits in the event of a mains failure.

An attachment, the 'Dräger Respiratory Apparatus 7400 for Infants', which has a minimal dead-space, is available for use with infants.

FUNCTIONAL ANALYSIS

This functional analysis is written from the point of view of the 'Narkose Spiromat 650' but, apart from the references to the closed circuit, is equally applicable to the 'Spiromat 661'.

Inspiratory phase

Fundamentally this ventilator operates as a constant-pressure generator. The maximum generated pressure, of about 100 cmH_2O, is determined by the characteristics of the blower (41); lesser generated pressures can be set by means of the 'working pressure, inspiration' control (40) which adjusts the size of a leak to atmosphere.

There are a number of modifications of this basic action. One such modification arises from the 'diaphragm valve' (11). The resistance of this valve to inspiratory flow decreases as the mouth pressure increases. Except perhaps when the generated pressure is set very low indeed, the decrease in this resistance, as the mouth pressure rises, is greater than the concomitant decrease in the pressure drop across it (generated pressure minus mouth pressure). Therefore the flow normally increases in the course of the phase.

A second modification arises from the fact that the concertina bag (19) provides a volume limit which can be adjusted by the 'volume' control (37) and which will commonly be reached before the end of the phase. Once the volume limit is reached no further flow can pass the one-way valve (1). Therefore if there were only a short non-distensible tube from that valve to the patient the ventilator would immediately become a zero-flow generator. In fact, however, there is a considerable total length of corrugated tubing which constitutes a sizeable compliance and which, at the moment at which the volume limit is reached, is 'charged' to a mouth pressure appreciably in excess of the alveolar pressure. Therefore, after the volume limit has been reached, the compliance of the tubing has to 'discharge' into the lungs so that the flow takes some time to decay to zero.

A third, minor, modification arises from the fact that in the early part of the phase some of the flow from the blower is used in expelling gas from the storage bag (15).

The overall effect of these modifications on the basic mechanism is complex and results in waveforms of flow and mouth pressure both of which are influenced by lung characteristics and by the settings of many of the controls on the ventilator. The only fixed feature is that, providing the generated pressure and inspiratory time are sufficient, the volume limit will be reached during the phase.

Change-over from inspiratory phase to expiratory phase

This change-over is time-cycled: it is brought about by the de-energization of the solenoid (39) by the electronic timing mechanism (21, 22).

Expiratory phase

In this phase the inlet side of the blower (41), in combination with the adjustable leak (32), acts as a constant, negative, pressure generator. This negative pressure is applied to the outside of both the concertina bag (19) and the storage bag (15) and therefore operates throughout the expiratory phase no matter whether the tap (8) is set for non-rebreathing or closed circuit. The magnitude of the negative pressure is adjusted by the 'expiration' control (32). If this is opened far enough no negative pressure is developed and the ventilator operates as a constant, atmospheric, pressure generator.

If the control (32) is opened further, the spring loading of the valve (35) in series with the bag (15) is increased so that, whenever gas is flowing into the bag (15) the ventilator operates as a constant, positive, pressure generator. With the tap (8) set for a non-rebreathing circuit this occurs throughout the expiratory phase; with it set to closed circuit the ventilator first operates as a constant, atmospheric, pressure generator via the concertina bag (19) and then, when this bag reaches its adjustable stop (18), the ventilator operates as a constant, positive, pressure generator via the bag (15).

Change-over from expiratory phase to inspiratory phase

This change-over is either time-cycled or patient-cycled whichever occurs first: it is brought about by the energization of the solenoid (39), either after a preset time determined by the electronic timing mechanism (21, 22), or when an inspiratory effort by the patient closes the contacts (25).

CHAPTER 42

The Dräger 'Poliomat'

DESCRIPTION

The operating mechanism of both the Dräger 'Poliomat' and the 'Pulmomat' represents over 50 years of continuous development by this firm of the original 'Pulmotor', the modern version of which is still available for emergency resuscitation.

The 'Poliomat' is a compact ventilator (fig. 42.1), designed for ward use, and is driven

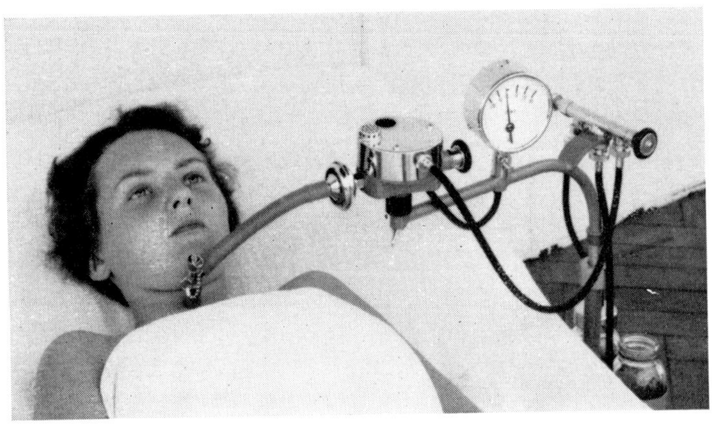

Fig. 42.1. The Dräger 'Poliomat'.
Courtesy of Drägerwerk (Heinr. & Bernh. Dräger), Lubeck.

by compressed air or oxygen. It is connected to the patient by two breathing tubes (7, 8) (fig. 42.2) fitted with one-way valves (4, 5). The driving gas, supplied at the inlet (6), enters the 'Pulmotor' unit through the jet of the injector (14). During the inspiratory phase the slider (18) is in its 'up' position, the inspiratory valve (17) is open, and the expiratory valve (16) is closed. Air is entrained through the spring-loaded valve (11), the inlet (12) of which can be fitted with a dust and bacterial filter. The gas mixture enters the chamber (19), from which it flows, along the inspiratory tube (7), past the one-way valve (4), to the patient. The pressure throughout the circuit rises and the diaphragm (22) is pushed up, taking with it the toggle mechanism (24) against the pull of the spring (23).

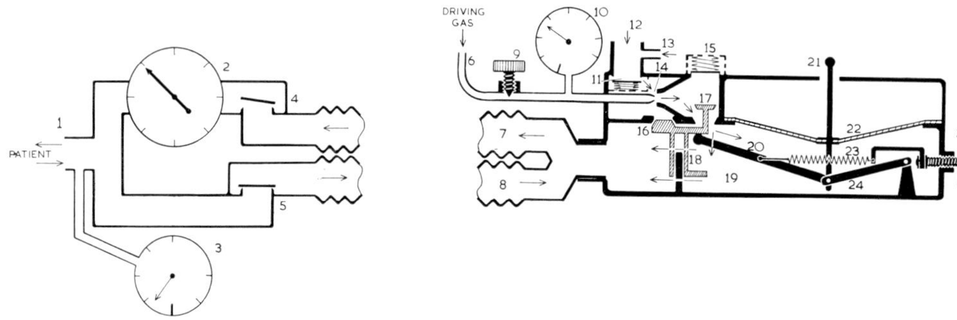

Fig. 42.2. Diagram of the Dräger 'Poliomat'.

1. Outlet port
2. 'Volumeter'
3. Manometer
4. One-way valve
5. One-way valve
6. Driving-gas inlet
7. Inspiratory tube
8. Expiratory tube
9. 'Ventilation' control
10. Pressure gauge calibrated in litres/min ventilation
11. Spring-loaded inlet valve
12. Entrainment port
13. Inlet for additional oxygen
14. Injector
15. Spring-loaded outlet valve
16. Expiratory valve
17. Inspiratory valve
18. Slider
19. Chamber
20. Lever
21. Rod for manual cycling
22. Diaphragm
23. Spring
24. Toggle mechanism
25. Cycling-pressures control

When the toggle passes its central position it is snapped over by the pull of the spring (23). The lever (20) of the toggle mechanism flicks the slider (18) downwards, closing the inspiratory valve (17) and opening the expiratory valve (16). Inflation ceases and the driving gas, flowing through the injector (14), now lifts the spring-loaded valve (15) and escapes to atmosphere. The flow through the injector now produces a negative pressure in the chamber (19). Expired gas flows, past the one-way valve (5) and along the expiratory tube (8), to the chamber (19), and is entrained by the injector. As the pressure in the chamber (19) is now negative, the diaphragm (22) moves down until the toggle mechanism (24) flicks over. The valve (16) is closed, the valve (17) is opened, and the next inspiratory phase commences.

The tidal volume delivered depends on the compliance of the patient and the pressures at which the ventilator cycles. The latter are determined by the tension of the spring (23) which may be adjusted by the control (25). Any change in the tension of the spring (23) will alter the cycling pressure for both phases of respiration. The toggle mechanism is so designed that the positive pressure at the end of the inspiratory phase, and the negative pressure which always exists at the end of the expiratory phase, are always in the ratio of 3 : 2. The characteristics of the injector (14) are such that, with this pressure ratio, the inspiratory-expiratory ratio is about 1 : 1·2.

The inspiratory and expiratory times depend on the times taken to reach the cycling pressures, and therefore, for any set cycling pressures (and hence tidal volume), on the gas flow through the injector, which is controlled by the needle valve (9). The ventilator may be cycled at any time by manual reversal of the toggle mechanism using the rod (21).

The injector characteristics are such that if the driving gas is oxygen, and air is entrained, the oxygen concentration in the inspired mixture is 40–50%. A higher concentration still may be attained by adding oxygen through the side inlet (13) of the entrainment orifice. If the driving gas is compressed air, and the additional oxygen for entrainment is supplied from the recommended Dräger flowmeter, then the final oxygen concentration is 30–50%.

A Dräger 'Volumeter' (2) (see p. 49) is incorporated in the inspiratory pathway. A Dräger condenser-humidifier may be screwed into the outlet port (1) of the valve unit.

A pressure gauge (10) is fitted to the driving-gas inlet. This is calibrated in litres/min ventilation. This calibration should be fairly accurate since driving gas is flowing at a more or less constant rate through the injector at all times, the air entrainment during the inspiratory phase is constant, and the inspiratory-expiratory ratio is almost constant. The minute-volume ventilation is controlled by adjusting the 'ventilation' needle valve (9). The tidal volume, and hence the frequency, depend on the setting of the cycling-pressures control (25).

The manometer (3) on the valve unit indicates pressure at the mouth.

FUNCTIONAL ANALYSIS

Inspiratory phase

In this phase the ventilator approximates very closely to a constant-flow generator because the injector characteristics (fig. 42.3) are such that flow falls off only very slightly

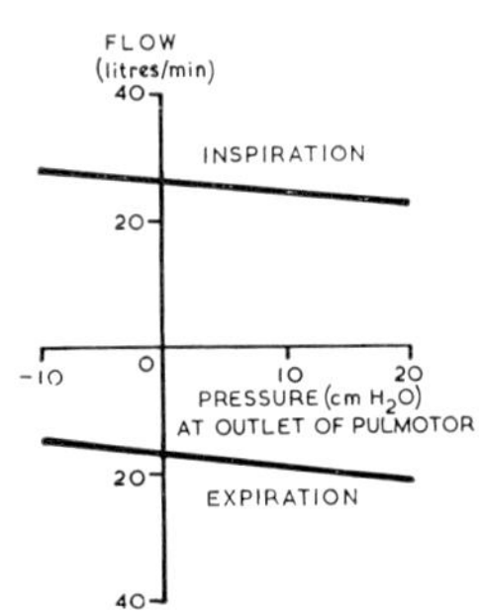

Fig. 42.3. Dräger 'Poliomat'. Flow-pressure characteristics of the injector. Driving gas, oxygen. Setting of the 'ventilation' control: such as would deliver a total ventilation of 10 litres/min to the model lung.

with increasing back pressure. This can be seen in fig. 42.4, where halving the compliance (b) or doubling the resistance (c) has no effect on the inspiratory flow rate, but considerably increases the slope of the waveform of pressure at the mouth.

Change-over from inspiratory phase to expiratory phase

This is pressure-cycled and occurs when a preset pressure has been attained in the chamber (19). This is very nearly the same as the pressure at the mouth and it can be seen

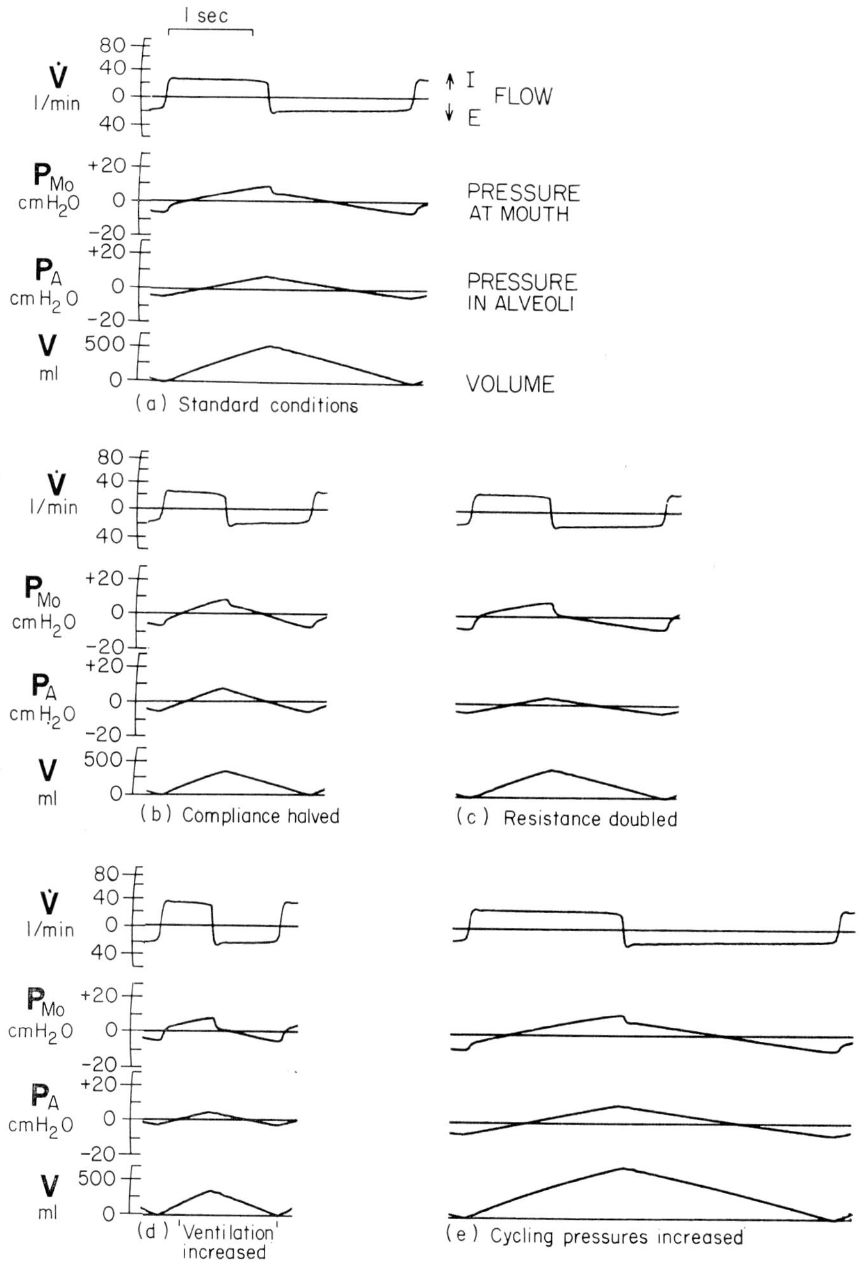

Fig. 42.4. Dräger 'Poliomat'. Recordings showing the effects of changes of lung characteristics and of changes in the settings of the controls.

Standard conditions: driving gas, oxygen at 60 lb/in^2; cycling-pressures and 'ventilation' controls, set for a tidal volume of 500 ml and a respiratory frequency of 20/min.

that halving the compliance (fig. 42.4b) or doubling the resistance (fig. 42.4c) has no effect on the peak pressure at the mouth at the end of the inspiratory phase. On the other hand the tidal volume and the inspiratory time are reduced by halving the compliance or doubling the airway resistance.

Expiratory phase

As in the inspiratory phase, the injector characteristics make the ventilator operate very nearly as a constant-flow generator. Therefore the flow waveform is unaffected by changes of lung characteristics, but the pressure waveforms are considerably modified.

Change-over from expiratory phase to inspiratory phase

Like the other change-over this is pressure-cycled, and the pressure at the mouth at the end of the expiratory phase is unaffected by changes of lung characteristics, although the tidal volume and the expiratory time are considerably modified.

CONTROLS

Total ventilation

This is directly controlled by adjusting the flow of driving gas to the injector by means of the 'ventilation' control (9) although the total ventilation is greater than the flow rate of driving gas. This arises because the flow to the injector, by virtue of the injector characteristics, determines the inspiratory and expiratory flow rates within very close limits, and at levels considerably greater than the driving-gas flow rate. The total ventilation is therefore also determined. An increase in airway resistance produces a very slight fall in total ventilation because it slightly reduces both the inspiratory and expiratory flows, but the effect is barely detectable in fig. 42.4c where the airway resistance has been doubled.

Increasing the total ventilation increases the frequency but decreases the tidal volume (fig. 42.4d). This is because the increased inspiratory and expiratory flows give larger pressure drops across the airway resistance, and so, although the range of pressure at the mouth (from the end of the inspiratory phase to the end of the expiratory phase) is little altered, the range of pressure in the alveoli, and hence the tidal volume, is reduced.

Tidal volume

This is indirectly controlled by adjustment of the cycling-pressures control (25) (fig. 42.4e). It is therefore reduced by a decrease in the compliance (fig. 42.4b) and by an increase in the airway resistance (fig. 42.4c). It is also reduced, as explained above, when the total ventilation is increased.

Changing the tidal volume does not alter the total ventilation and therefore results in a reciprocal change in respiratory frequency (fig. 42.4e).

Respiratory frequency

This is not directly controlled but is equal to the total ventilation divided by the tidal volume.

Inspiratory-expiratory ratio

This is primarily determined by the injector characteristics and therefore cannot be adjusted. It varies only slightly with lung characteristics and with the settings of the controls.

Waveforms

The flow waveform is virtually fixed, the flow being almost constant throughout each phase at levels which are determined by the setting of the 'ventilation' control (9). The pressure waveforms are determined entirely by the interaction of the flow waveforms with the lung characteristics.

Pressure limits

The pressure limits at the mouth are directly determined by the setting of the cycling-pressures control (25), but they cannot be varied independently of each other. The ratio of positive cycling pressure to negative cycling pressure is fixed at 3 : 2. A consequence of this, combined with the injector characteristics, is that the mean pressure is always slightly above atmospheric—by about one-tenth of the range between the positive and negative cycling pressures.

CHAPTER 43

The Dräger 'Pulmomat'

DESCRIPTION

In the 'Pulmomat' (fig. 43.1) the 'Pulmotor' unit is connected to a transparent rigid plastic pressure chamber (5) (fig. 43.2) which contains the concertina reservoir bag (4) of a closed anaesthetic circuit. In fig. 43.1 it is shown connected to a Dräger 'Octavian' anaesthetic apparatus.

The basic functioning of the 'Pulmotor' is the same as that described for the 'Polio-

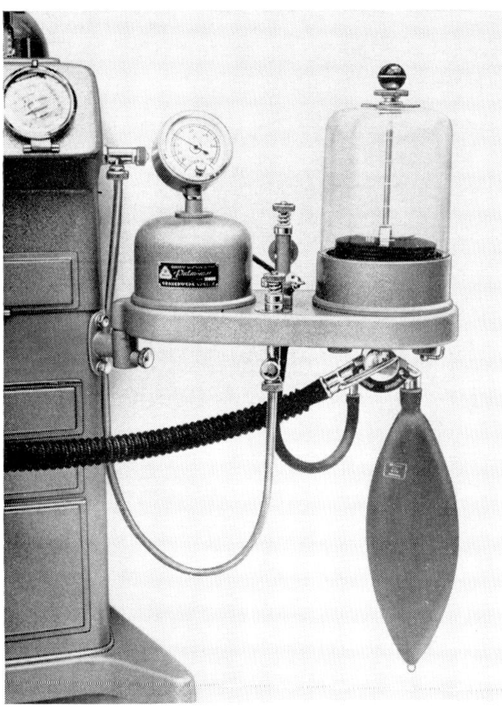

Fig. 43.1. The Dräger 'Pulmomat' connected to a Dräger 'Octavian' anaesthetic apparatus. Courtesy of Drägerwerk (Heinr. and Bernh. Dräger), Lubeck.

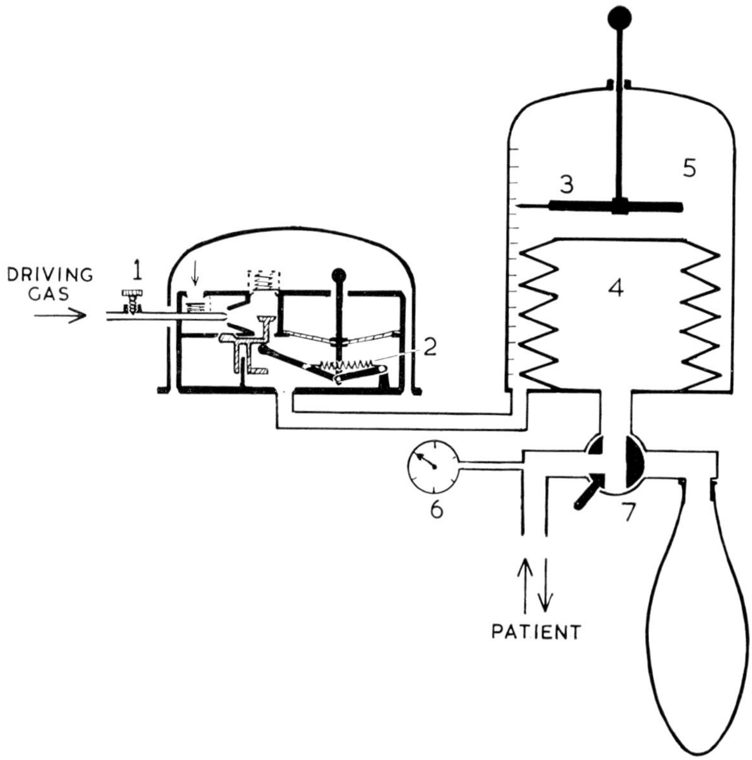

Fig. 43.2. Diagram of the Dräger 'Pulmomat'.

1. 'Ventilation' control
2. Spring
3. Stop
4. Concertina reservoir bag
5. Rigid plastic pressure chamber
6. Manometer
7. Tap

mat'. The total minute-volume ventilation is controlled by the needle valve (1). The tension of the spring (2) is fixed, and adjustment of the tidal volume is now effected by the setting of the stop (3), which limits the expansion of the concertina reservoir bag (4). The stroke volume of the bag is read from a scale.

The characteristics of the apparatus are such that the inspiratory-expiratory ratio is about 1 : 1·2. If the stroke volume is set too high, or if there is any respiratory obstruction, the apparatus cycles at a positive pressure of +20 cmH_2O and a negative pressure of −10 cmH_2O.

The frequency may be varied between 8/min and 30/min, and the tidal volume between 100 and 700 ml. The consumption of compressed gas to drive the apparatus is 6–10 litres/min.

The manometer (6) indicates the pressure in the patient circuit. The tap (7) allows manual inflation to be performed.

FUNCTIONAL ANALYSIS

Inspiratory phase

At the beginning of this phase the mode of operation is determined primarily by the injector characteristics and therefore, like the 'Poliomat', the 'Pulmomat' operates very nearly as a constant-flow generator. Later, when the blow-off valve on the anaesthetic apparatus opens, some of the generated flow escapes through the valve and the action of the complete system ('Pulmomat' plus blow-off valve) tends towards that of a constant-pressure generator. The approach to constant-pressure generation is not likely to be very close with the commonly-used Heidbrink-type expiratory valve. Until the blow-off valve opens the fresh-gas flow to the patient circuit acts as a small-constant-flow generator, supplementing the main flow generator.

Change-over from inspiratory phase to expiratory phase

Fundamentally this is pressure-cycled by the pressure in the 'Pulmotor' unit. However, this is usually modified to volume-cycling by the 'bag-in-bottle' arrangement, and the change-over occurs at a short delay after the concertina reservoir bag (4) has emptied. Nevertheless, if the lung characteristics are sufficiently abnormal, or if the blow-off valve is too tight, or if the fresh-gas flow is too high, the cycling pressure of +20 cmH_2O may be reached before the volume limit set by the reservoir bag. In this event the ventilator operates in its fundamental pressure-cycled mode.

Expiratory phase

Throughout this phase the action is governed by the characteristics of the injector; therefore, like the 'Poliomat', the 'Pulmomat' approximates closely to a constant-flow generator. The fresh-gas flow to the patient circuit acts as a small-constant-flow generator opposing the main flow generator.

Change-over from expiratory phase to inspiratory phase

This change-over is also fundamentally pressure-cycled but modified to volume-cycled by the 'bag-in-bottle' arrangement. In this change-over the conditions for volume-cycling are that the blow-off valve setting and the fresh-gas flow are not too low and, again, that the lung characteristics are not seriously abnormal. The change-over then occurs at a short delay after the bag has expanded to the limit set by the stop (3).

CONTROLS

This 'Controls' section, unlike all but one of the others (Ohio (Monaghan) 120), has been deduced purely theoretically from data supplied by the manufacturers and from our measurements on the Dräger 'Poliomat'.

Total ventilation

As in the 'Poliomat', this is controlled by adjusting the flow of driving gas to the injector by means of the 'ventilation' control (1). It is practically unaffected by changes in the lung characteristics or in any of the other controls, except for the fresh-gas flow (see below under 'tidal volume'). Increasing the ventilation increases the frequency and, in view of the volume-cycling, leaves the tidal volume and inspiratory-expiratory ratio almost unchanged.

Tidal volume

So long as the 'Pulmomat' is volume-cycled in both phases (see the functional analysis above) the tidal volume is directly controlled by adjustment of the volume limit (3). The tidal volume is less than the stroke volume of the bag (4) by the volume of fresh gas which enters the breathing circuit during the expiratory phase. Therefore a decrease in fresh-gas flow or an increase in the total ventilation (which increases the frequency and therefore decreases the expiratory time) leads to a small increase in the tidal volume.

The tidal volume is practically unaffected by changes of lung characteristics unless the changes are so severe as to produce pressure-cycling before the reservoir bag (4) has reached either of its volume limits.

When the tidal volume is changed by means of the adjustable stop (3) the total ventilation is unaltered and the respiratory frequency is therefore changed in a reciprocal fashion.

Respiratory frequency

This is not directly controlled but is equal to the total ventilation divided by the tidal volume. Therefore it is influenced by changes in these parameters but it is usually unaffected by changes of lung characteristics.

Inspiratory-expiratory ratio

As in the 'Poliomat', this is primarily determined by the injector characteristics and therefore cannot be adjusted. It varies only slightly with lung characteristics and with the settings of the controls.

Waveforms

As in the 'Poliomat', the flow waveform is virtually fixed, being almost constant throughout each phase at levels which are determined by the setting of the 'ventilation' control (1). The pressure waveforms are determined by the interaction of the flow waveform with the lung characteristics. The only exception to these remarks occurs in the later part of the inspiratory phase when, with gas escaping through the blow-off valve of the anaesthetic circuit, the functioning tends towards that of a pressure generator.

Pressure limits

The pressure range in the alveoli is equal to the tidal volume divided by the compliance. The pressure range at the mouth exceeds this by the sum of the pressure drops across the airway due to the inspiratory and expiratory flows. However, the upper and lower limits of mouth pressure are affected by the following factors. The upper limit cannot exceed +20 cmH_2O because this is the pressure at which the toggle mechanism cycles. Likewise the lower limit cannot be below −10 cmH_2O. Usually the pressure range at the mouth is less than this maximum of 30 cmH_2O and the range lies at a level, within the absolute limits of +20 and −10 cmH_2O set by the cycling mechanism, such that the loss through the blow-off valve in the anaesthetic circuit in one respiratory cycle is equal to the volume of fresh gas entering during the cycle. Therefore any increase of fresh-gas flow, or tightening of the blow-off valve, raises both the upper and lower extremes of the mouth-pressure waveform (and therefore raises the mean pressure) without altering the pressure range.

CHAPTER 44

The 'E.G.C. Paediatric' Ventilator

DESCRIPTION

This compact apparatus (fig. 44.1) is intended for the ventilation of infants in the ward or theatre. Gas is supplied continuously through a flowmeter to the inlet tube (10) (fig. 44.2). An electronic timing mechanism (4) intermittently energizes the solenoid (9) closing the expiratory valve (8) in the separate valve unit (8, 9). The inspiratory phase is the time during which the valve (8) is closed, allowing the gas supplied at the inlet (10) to flow to the patient. After a time set by the 'inspiratory time' control (2), the supply of current to the solenoid (9) is cut off, and the expiratory valve (8) is opened by its spring. The fresh gas entering the circuit, together with the expired gas, now flows to atmosphere through the expiratory valve (8). The expiratory phase continues until the time set by the 'expira-

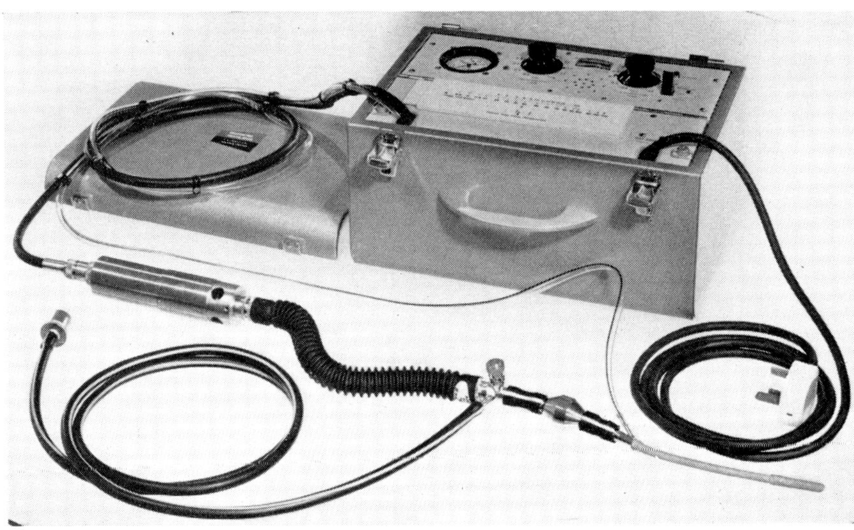

Fig. 44.1. The 'E.G.C. Paediatric' ventilator.

Courtesy of J.F. Eardley Limited, Sheffield.

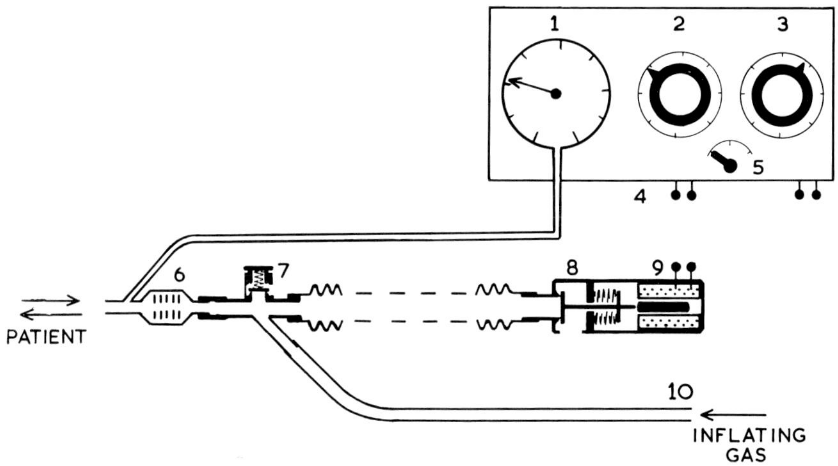

Fig. 44.2. Diagram of the 'E.G.C. Paediatric' ventilator.

1. Manometer
2. 'Inspiratory time' control
3. 'Expiratory time' control
4. Electronic timing mechanism
5. 'Manual-Off-Auto' switch
6. Condenser humidifier
7. Safety-valve
8. Expiratory valve
9. Solenoid
10. Inflating-gas inlet

tory time' control (3) has elapsed, whereupon the solenoid (9) is again energized, and the expiratory valve (8) is closed.

The inspiratory and expiratory time controls are graduated in intervals of 0·1 sec from 0·5 to 1·5 sec. An adjustable safety-valve (7) can be set to limit the inflating pressure at any level up to 35 cmH_2O. An alternative safety-valve can be fitted to allow inflating pressures up to 70 cmH_2O. The manometer (1) indicates the pressure at a point close to the patient.

The solenoid (9) is energized by current from low-voltage batteries in the timing unit. Normally the ventilator is connected to an a.c. mains supply and the batteries are recharged continuously by a charging unit incorporated in the ventilator. If the mains supply fails the batteries will maintain full operation of the ventilator for six hours.

A 'mains' indicator light shows when the mains supply is switched on. Another indicator shows the state of charge of the battery. An audible warning sounds if the mains supply fails at any time, or if either phase of respiration is prolonged over 5 sec.

The tidal volume delivered to the patient depends on the fresh-gas flow set by the flowmeter and the duration of the inspiratory phase set by the 'inspiratory time' control. A calculator which relates frequency, fresh-gas flow, and tidal volume, is fitted on the top panel of the ventilator.

A switch (5) has three positions 'Automatic', 'Off', and 'Manual'. This switch is spring-loaded to ensure that it cannot be left in the 'Manual' position. When the switch is held in the 'Manual' position the solenoid (9) is energized and the expiratory valve (8) is closed, thereby commencing an inspiratory phase which continues until the switch is released.

FUNCTIONAL ANALYSIS

Inspiratory phase
In this phase the ventilator operates as a constant-flow generator assuming that, as is usual, the inflating gas comes from a high-pressure high-resistance source.

Change-over from inspiratory phase to expiratory phase
This change-over is time-cycled: it occurs when the solenoid-operated expiratory valve (8) opens at a time determined by the electronic timer (4).

Expiratory phase
In this phase the ventilator operates as a constant, atmospheric, pressure generator: the patient's expired gas passes to atmosphere through the expiratory valve (8).

Change-over from expiratory phase to inspiratory phase
This change-over also is time-cycled: it occurs when the solenoid-operated expiratory valve (8) closes at a time determined by the electronic timer (4).

CHAPTER 45

The East-Freeman Ventilator

DESCRIPTION

This ventilator (fig. 45.1) is designed for long-term ventilation with a non-rebreathing circuit. It must be connected to an electrical mains supply. An electronic timer controls solenoid-operated inspiratory and expiratory valves which connect the patient alternately to a weighted concertina reservoir bag and to atmosphere.

A compressor, fitted in the base of the ventilator, supplies compressed air to a concertina storage bag (4) (fig. 45.2) at a rate in excess of any total minute-volume ventilation likely to be required. If desired, oxygen can be added through the inlet (1). Any flow of oxygen or compressed air in excess of the total minute-volume ventilation escapes to atmosphere through the valve (2) which is opened by the storage bag (4) when it is fully expanded. The weight (3) on top of the bag (4) ensures that the air contained in the bag is kept at a pressure of 70–80 cmH_2O.

During the expiratory phase, the inspiratory valve (14) is closed and the 'surge limit' valve (6) is open. Air, from the storage bag (4), therefore flows into the concertina reservoir bag (7) which expands against the force exerted by the moveable weight (11), until the arm (8) on the pivoted lever (12) makes contact with the switch (9). Then the 'surge limit' valve (6) is closed. Thus, before the end of the expiratory phase, the concertina reservoir bag (7) normally contains a volume of gas regulated by the volume control (10), at a pressure dependent upon the position of the sliding weight (11) on the arm (12), which position is regulated by the pressure control (13).

When the ventilator switches to the inspiratory phase, the electrical supply to the solenoid-operated expiratory valve (27) is cut off and the valve closes. If for any reason the 'surge limit' valve (6) has not already closed it now does so. At the same time the solenoid-operated inspiratory valve (14) is energized; the valve opens, and air contained in the reservoir bag (7) is forced through the breathing tube (16) to the patient. The pressure at the mouth is indicated on the manometer (15) which is connected to a Y-piece close to the patient.

After a time set by the inspiratory-time control (19) the inspiratory valve (14) is closed and the expiratory valve (27) and the 'surge limit' valve (6) are opened. Expired gas flows, through the breathing tube (29) and past the one-way valve (28), the expiratory

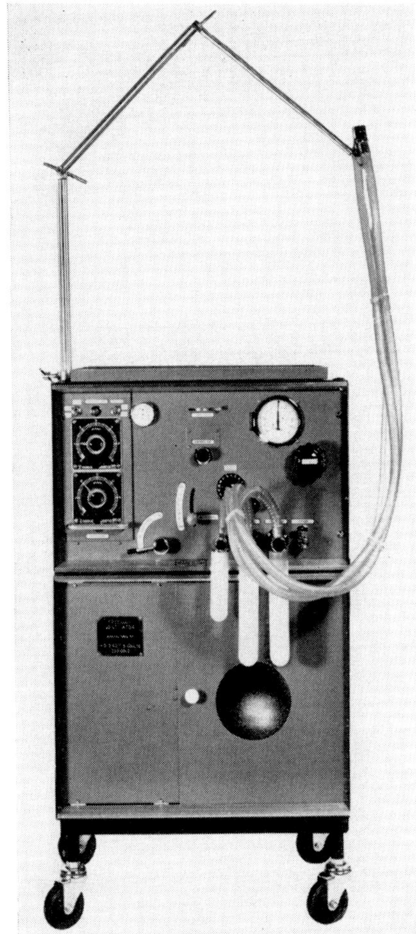

Fig. 45.1. The East-Freeman ventilator.

Courtesy of H.G.East & Co.Ltd.

valve (27), and the spirometer tap (22), to atmosphere. At the same time the reservoir bag (7) is refilled with air from the storage bag (4).

The next inspiratory phase is initiated either after a preset time determined by the setting of the expiratory-time control (20) or, if the switch (18) is set to patient-triggering, when the patient makes an adequate inspiratory effort. When the patient does make an inspiratory effort the one-way valve (28) closes and a negative pressure is produced above diaphragm (26) tending to lift the diaphragm and close the electrical contacts, thereby initiating the next inspiratory phase. The pressure needed to do this can be adjusted to between 0·5 and 5·0 cmH_2O by the sensitivity control (25).

There are three possible modes of operation of this ventilator.

The first mode occurs when the volume control (10) is set to maximum and the

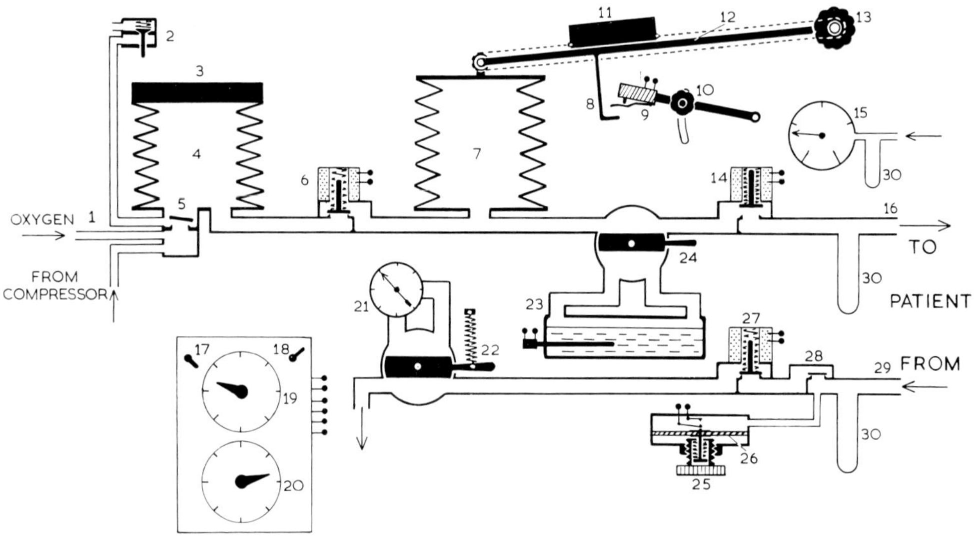

Fig. 45.2. Diagram of the East-Freeman ventilator.

1. Oxygen inlet
2. Release valve
3. Weight
4. Storage bag
5. One-way valve
6. Solenoid-operated 'surge limit' valve
7. Concertina reservoir bag
8. Arm
9. Electric switch
10. Volume control
11. Weight
12. Pivoted lever
13. Pressure control
14. Solenoid-operated inspiratory valve
15. Manometer
16. Inspiratory tube
17. On/off switch
18. Patient-triggering switch
19. Inspiratory-time control
20. Expiratory-time control
21. Wright respirometer
22. Spring-loaded tap
23. Heated humidifier
24. Tap
25. Patient-trigger sensitivity control
26. Diaphragm
27. Solenoid-operated expiratory valve
28. One-way valve
29. Expiratory tube
30. Water traps

pressure control (13) is set to some fairly-low value—such that the pressure in the concertina reservoir bag (7) is not sufficient to drive the whole of the contents into the patient's lungs. Then this pressure is applied throughout the inspiratory phase and the tidal volume depends on the setting of the pressure control (13) and on the effect of the resultant pressure on the lungs.

The second mode of operation occurs when the volume control (10) is set to a relatively-low value and the pressure control (13) to a relatively-high value, so that the bag (7) is always emptied into the lungs in every inspiratory phase. Then the tidal volume is controlled by the setting of the volume control (10).

The third mode of operation occurs when the compressor is switched off and the fresh gas is supplied at the inlet (1) at a flow equal to the desired total minute-volume ventilation. Then the storage bag (4) never fills very far, the release valve (2) never opens, and the ventilator operates as a minute-volume divider (see p. 140). Provided that the volume control (10) is set high enough, the volume contained in the reservoir bag (7) at the start of the inspiratory phase is the volume of fresh gas which entered the ventilator during the whole of the previous respiratory cycle, and provided the pressure control (13) is set high enough, the whole of this volume is delivered to the patient during the inspiratory phase and therefore constitutes the tidal volume. The magnitude of the tidal volume is equal to the product of the fresh-gas flow and the duration of the complete respiratory cycle, which duration is determined by the settings of the inspiratory-time (19) and expiratory-time (20) controls.

In all modes of operation a heated humidifier (23) may be switched into the inspiratory line by the tap (24), and the expired tidal volume can be measured with the fitted Wright respirometer (21) by holding open the spring-loaded tap (22).

FUNCTIONAL ANALYSIS

Inspiratory phase

In this phase the ventilator operates as a pressure generator due to the force exerted by the weight (11) on the contents of the concertina bag (7). The pressure probably decreases somewhat as the bag empties owing to the elasticity of the bag wall. The contents of the bag at the start of the phase constitute a volume limit. This limit will be reached in each inspiratory phase if the pressure control (13) is set high enough and the volume limit is low enough, either due to a low setting of the volume control (10) or to restriction of the inflow to the storage bag (4) (see the 'Description' above). Once the volume limit is reached, the ventilator operates as a zero-flow generator for the remainder of the phase.

Change-over from inspiratory phase to expiratory phase

This change-over is time-cycled: it occurs when the valve (14) closes and the valve (27) opens at a preset time after the start of the inspiratory phase determined by the setting of the inspiratory-time control (19).

Expiratory phase

In this phase, the ventilator operates as a constant, atmospheric, pressure generator: the, patient's expired gas passes to atmosphere at the expiratory port.

Change-over from expiratory phase to inspiratory phase

This change-over is either purely time-cycled or, if the switch (18) is set to patient-triggering, time-cycled or patient-cycled whichever occurs first. The change-over occurs when the valve (27) closes and the valve (14) opens, either at a preset time after the start of the expiratory phase determined by the setting of the expiratory-time control (20), or when an inspiratory effort by the patient exerts enough force on the diaphragm (26) to overcome the force of the spring and close the electrical contacts.

CHAPTER 46

The East-Radcliffe 'Positive Pressure Respirator'[1]

DESCRIPTION

The P3 and P3s (fig. 46.1) ventilators are designed for ward use, but with the necessary attachments (PA1 and PA1s) can be adapted for anaesthetic use. There are also other simplified models (B/2 and M/2) intended for portable use.

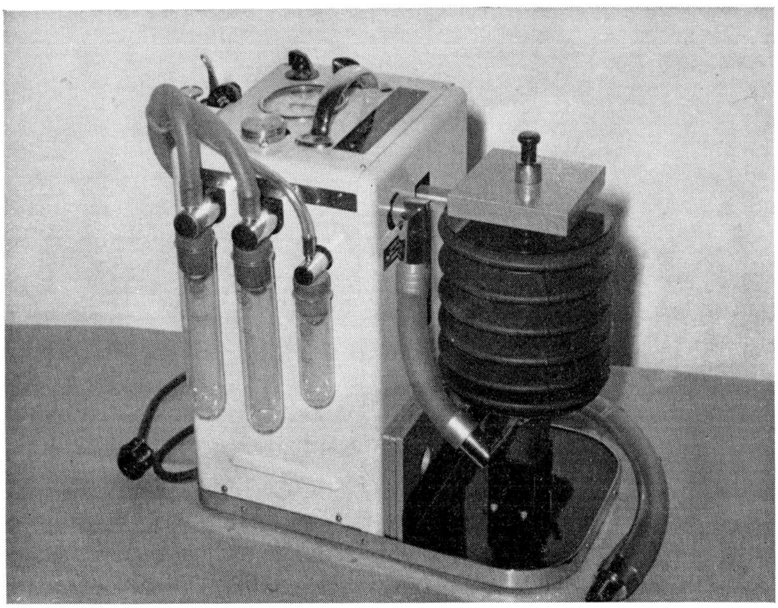

Fig. 46.1. The East-Radcliffe 'Positive Pressure Respirator, P3s'.
Courtesy of H.G. East & Co. Ltd.

There are two electric motors (7, 20) (fig. 46.2). One (20), for normal use, is an induction motor which runs off a 240-volt a.c. mains supply and is spark-proof. The other (7) runs off a 12-volt battery and is not spark-proof. One (15) of the two locking plugs is pushed on to the output shaft of the gear-box (6, 19) of the motor in use, thereby

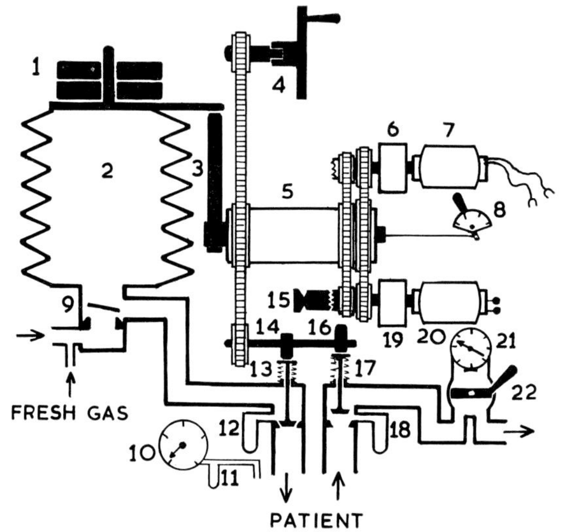

Fig. 46.2. Diagram of the East-Radcliffe 'Positive Pressure Respirator'.

1. Weights
2. Concertina reservoir bag
3. Cam
4. Handle for manual ventilation
5. 4-speed Sturmey-Archer bicycle hub
6. Gear-box
7. 12-volt motor
8. 'Respiration rate' control
9. One-way inlet valve
10. Manometer
11. Water trap
12. Water trap
13. Inspiratory valve
14. Cam
15. Locking plug
16. Cam
17. Expiratory valve
18. Water trap
19. Gear-box
20. a.c. mains motor
21. Wright respirometer
22. Tap

engaging one of the two chain-and-sprocket drives to the 4-speed Sturmey-Archer bicycle hub (5). The output shaft of this hub carries a large cam (3) and a sprocket which is connected by a chain to the shaft bearing the cams (14, 16).

During the expiratory phase, the expiratory valve (17) is held open by its spring and the inspiratory valve (13) is held closed by the cam (14). At the same time the large cam (3) lifts the top-plate of the concertina reservoir bag (2) and air is drawn into the bag past the one-way valve (9), together with any additional gas which may be supplied at the inlet. The cam (3) is so shaped that the top-plate can fall freely under the influence of the weights (1) as soon as the bag has been fully expanded. At the same time, the positions of the inspiratory and expiratory valves are reversed by their cams and the gas stored in the bag (2) is delivered to the patient.

The inspiratory phase ends when the positions of the inspiratory and expiratory valves (13, 17) are again reversed, and the patient's expired gas flows, past the expiratory valve (17), to atmosphere. The cams (14, 16) of these valves are shaped in such a way that the inspiratory phase occupies one-third of each respiratory cycle.

The 'respiration rate' control (8) allows any one of the four ratios of the hub gear (5) to be selected, and the choice of locking plug (15) allows either of the two chain-and-sprocket drives to be engaged. In fact, as one combination happens to be duplicated, there is an overall choice of seven respiratory frequencies (13, 16, 20, 23, 25, 30, and 37 per minute).

The pressure reached during the inspiratory phase can be adjusted between 5 and 30 cmH_2O by varying the weights (1) on the top-plate. This pressure, together with the compliance of the patient and the total resistance of the gas pathway between bag and alveoli, determines the tidal volume, and the proportion of the inspiratory phase during which gas flows to the patient. The pressure is indicated on the manometer (10). The maximum tidal volume is 1500 ml. Water traps (11, 12, 18) are included in the manometer, the inspiratory, and the expiratory tubes. A Wright respirometer (21) can be brought into the expiratory pathway by turning the tap (22). It is a standard fitting on the P3s.

In the event of motor failure, the ventilator may be operated by turning the handle (4).

FUNCTIONAL ANALYSIS

The mode of action of this ventilator is very similar to that of the 'East-Radcliffe Positive-Negative Respirator' except for the absence of negative pressure in the expiratory phase. A brief functional analysis is given here for the sake of completeness; if more information is required it may be helpful to read the more-detailed account, complete with recordings, of the 'Positive-Negative' ventilator provided that it is remembered that the 'Positive Pressure' ventilator always operates as a constant, atmospheric, pressure generator throughout the expiratory phase.

Inspiratory phase

During this phase the ventilator operates as a constant-pressure generator with low series resistance due to the action of the weights (1) on the concertina reservoir bag (2) and the wide-bore connexions from bag to patient.

Change-over from inspiratory phase to expiratory phase

This change-over is time-cycled: it occurs when the expiratory valve (17) opens at a preset time after the start of the inspiratory phase, determined by the constant speed of the motor, the shape of the cam (16), and the particular gear-train engaged.

Expiratory phase

During this phase the ventilator operates as a constant, atmospheric, pressure generator.

Change-over from expiratory phase to inspiratory phase

This change-over also is time-cycled: it occurs when the inspiratory valve (13) opens at a preset time after the start of the expiratory phase.

REFERENCE

1 RUSSELL W.R. and SCHUSTER E. (1953) Respiration pump for poliomyelitis. *Lancet*, **2**, 707.

CHAPTER 47

The East-Radcliffe 'Positive-Negative Respirator'

DESCRIPTION

There are three versions of this ventilator. The PNA1 (figs. 47.1 and 47.2) is designed for anaesthetic or ward use. The PN2 is for ward use only. The CAP Mk. II comprises a PNA1 and an anaesthetic apparatus. This description is primarily of the PNA1, and notes on the PN2 are added on p. 527.

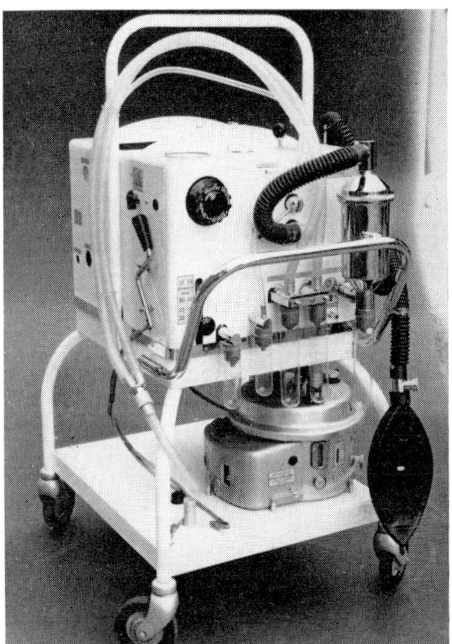

Fig. 47.1.

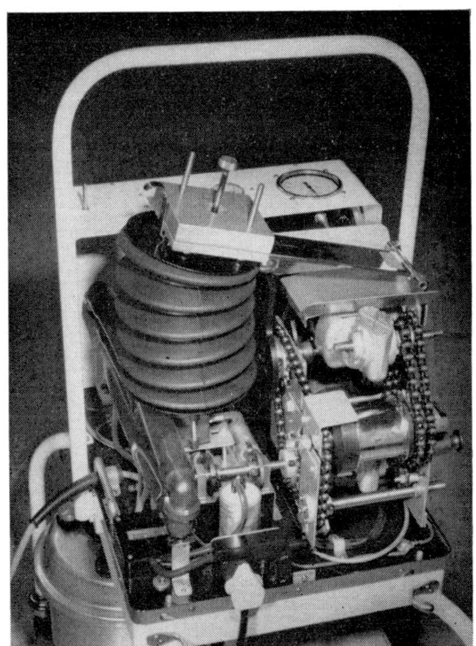

Fig. 47.2.

Fig. 47.1. The East-Radcliffe 'Positive-Negative (PNA1) Respirator'.
Courtesy of H.G.East & Co. Ltd.

Fig. 47.2. The mechanism of the East-Radcliffe 'Positive-Negative (PNA1) Respirator'.
Courtesy of Department of Medical Illustration, Cardiff Royal Infirmary.

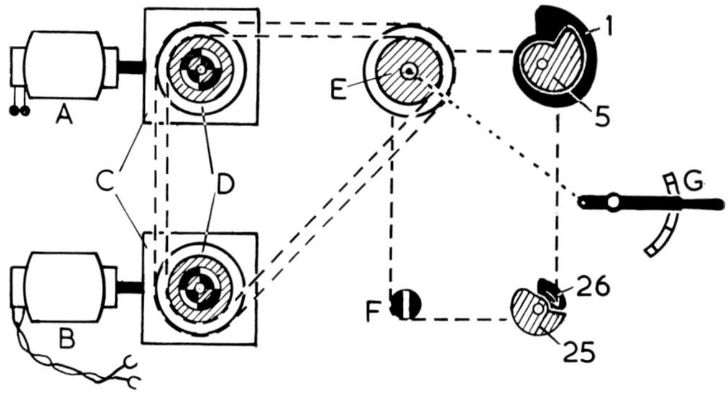

Fig. 47.3. Diagram of the driving mechanism of the East-Radcliffe 'Positive-Negative Respirator'.

A. 240-volt a.c. electric motor
B. 12-volt d.c. electric motor
C. Gear-boxes
D. Pairs of sprocket wheels
E. 4-speed bicycle hub
F. Idling shaft
G. 4-speed selector

1. Cam for expanding the positive-pressure concertina bag
5. Cam for compressing the negative-pressure concertina bag
25. Cam controlling the inspiratory valve
26. Cam controlling the expiratory valve

There are two electric motors (A and B) (fig. 47.3). One (A), for normal use, is a spark-proof 240-volt a.c. motor. The other (B), for emergency use, is a 12-volt d.c. motor, and is not spark-proof; its leads are fitted with crocodile clips for easy attachment to a car battery. Each motor drives its own gear-box (C). On the output shaft of each gear-box there is an identical pair of different-sized sprocket wheels (D). Two driving chains connect these sprockets with each other and with matching sprockets on the 4-speed bicycle hub (E). All four driving sprockets are free to idle independently on their shafts, unless mated with their shafts by the insertion of the appropriate locking plug. Normally the mains motor (A) is used and the locking plug is engaged on the shaft of this motor's gear-box; when the emergency 12-volt motor (B) is used, the plug is transferred to the driving shaft of the other gear-box. As either one of each pair of driving sprockets (D) may be combined with any of the four gear ratios of the bicycle hub, selected by the control (G), a range of eight speeds is available. In fact, as one combination happens to be duplicated, there is an overall choice of seven respiratory frequencies (13, 16, 20, 23, 25, 30, and 37 per minute). The output shaft of the bicycle hub is connected by another chain to three shafts; one (F) is an idling shaft, to which a handle can be fitted when manual operation of the ventilator is necessary; one carries the two cams (1, 5); and one carries the two cams (25, 26).

The cams (1, 5) (fig. 47.4) operate the inspiratory and expiratory concertina bags (4, 16). The cams (25, 26) operate the inspiratory and expiratory valves (27, 28).

When used in the ward, air is drawn into the bag (4) from the inlet tube (9) past a

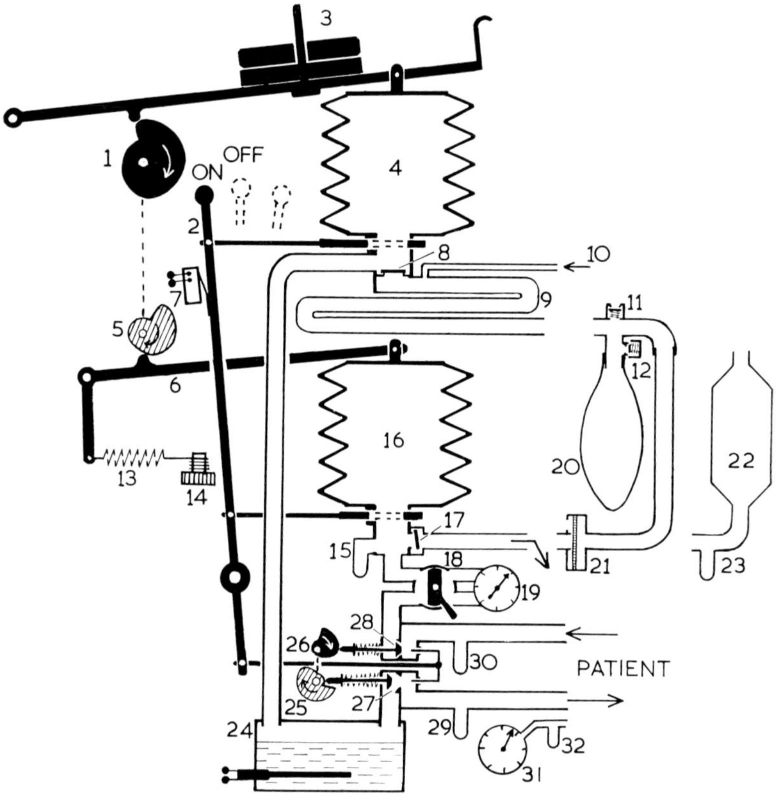

Fig. 47.4. Diagram of the East-Radcliffe 'Positive-Negative (PNA1) Respirator'.

1. Cam for expanding positive-pressure concertina bag
2. Control lever
3. Weights
4. Positive-pressure concertina reservoir bag
5. Cam for compressing the negative-pressure concertina bag
6. Lever
7. On/off switch for motor
8. One-way valve
9. Reservoir tube
10. Fresh-gas inlet
11. One-way air-inlet valve
12. Blow-off valve
13. Expansion spring
14. 'Negative pressure' control
15. Water trap
16. Negative-pressure concertina bag
17. One-way valve
18. Respirometer tap
19. Wright respirometer
20. Reservoir or storage bag
21. Diaphragm valve
22. Waters soda-lime canister
23. Water trap
24. Humidifier
25. Cam controlling the inspiratory valve
26. Cam controlling the expiratory valve
27. Inspiratory valve
28. Expiratory valve
29. Water trap
30. Water trap
31. Manometer
32. Water trap

one-way valve (8). Oxygen may be added at the inlet (10). The inlet tube (9) has a capacity of over 500 ml; therefore, when oxygen is being added, the amount present in the mixture delivered to the patient may be accurately controlled. When the cam (1) releases the top-plate of the concertina bag (4), the weights (3) force the gas within the bag, past the open inspiratory valve (27), to the patient. Flow continues until the pressure in the lungs is the same as the pressure in the bag, or until the inspiratory valve (27) is closed. When the cams (25, 26) close the inspiratory valve (27) and allow the expiratory valve (28) to open, expired gas flows, past the expiratory valve (28) and the one-way valve (17), to atmosphere. During the expiratory phase the bag (4) is expanded by the cam (1) and refilled with fresh gas until it is released by the cam and a new inspiratory phase commences.

The cams (25, 26) are shaped so that the inspiratory valve (27) is open for about one-third of a complete respiratory cycle, and the expiratory valve (28) is open for the other two-thirds of the cycle. The cam (1), which controls the bag (4), is shaped so that it lifts the top-plate of the bag during the two-thirds of the cycle for which the expiratory valve is open, and is free of the top-plate during the one-third of the cycle for which the inspiratory valve is open. Thus the inspiratory-expiratory ratio is fixed, nominally at 1 : 2. In the model tested (see figs. 47.7 and 47.8) it was about 1 : 1·7.

The negative-pressure concertina bag (16) is connected between the expiratory valve (28) and the one-way valve (17). Negative pressure can be applied by turning the 'negative pressure' control (14) so as to expand the spring (13). During the expiratory phase the lever (6) does not bear on the cam (5), and so the force exerted by the spring (13), and transmitted through the lever (6), can expand the bag (16). In this way a negative pressure is developed within the bag (16), and hence in the patient's expiratory pathway. During the inspiratory phase the cam (5) bears on the lever (6), the spring (13) is re-expanded, the bag (16) is compressed, and the gas contained in it is forced, past the one-way valve (17), to atmosphere.

The negative pressure developed within the bag (16) depends on the setting of the control (14), which determines the pull exerted on the bag by the spring (13). It may be varied between 0 and −15 cmH_2O. If the control (14) is so set that there is no tension exerted by the spring (13), then the bag (16) remains collapsed and no negative pressure is produced.

Positive pressure can be varied between 5 and 30 cmH_2O by adding or removing weights (3) on the top-plate of the concertina reservoir bag (4). The volume of the bag (4), and hence the maximum tidal volume, is 1200 ml.

Connexions are provided to allow the electrically-heated humidifier (24) to be incorporated in the inspiratory pathway if required. The pressure at the mouth is shown on a manometer (31), and a Wright respirometer (19), housed in the ventilator cabinet, can be brought into action by turning the tap (18). Water traps (15, 23, 29, 30, 32) are fitted to the inspiratory and expiratory tubes, the manometer tube, and the negative-pressure concertina bag.

When a non-rebreathing anaesthetic circuit is to be used, the fresh-gas flow, supplied at the inlet (10), must at least equal the minute-volume ventilation. To enable manual inflation to be performed with this circuit a reservoir bag (20) must be attached to the inlet tube (9), and a pressure-operated diaphragm valve (21) interposed between this reservoir bag and the expiratory port. The control lever (2) has three positions; two are simply 'On' and 'Off' for the switch (7) of the mains electric motor. For manual ventilation, the lever is put into its third position; this switches off the motor, shuts off the positive-pressure and negative-pressure concertina bags (4, 16), and holds open the inspiratory and expiratory valves (27, 28). The one-way valves (8, 17) in the inlet and outlet tubes prevent any rebreathing. When the reservoir bag (20) is squeezed, the diaphragm of the valve (21) occludes the expiratory port and the lungs are inflated; when it is released, expired gas escapes, through the valve (21), to atmosphere.

For closed-circuit anaesthesia, with either automatic or manual ventilation, the reservoir bag (20) must be connected to the inlet port, and connexion to the outlet port made through a Waters soda-lime canister (22) instead of through the diaphragm valve (21) used in the manual non-rebreathing circuit. Manual or automatic ventilation is selected in the same way as with the non-rebreathing circuit by adjusting the position of the lever (2). Only basal flows of fresh gas need to be supplied at the inlet (10).

Whichever circuit is used, the flow of fresh gas, supplied at the inlet (10), should be such as to prevent over-filling or emptying of the reservoir bag (20). If the flow is too big, the adjustable spring-loaded valve (12) on the reservoir bag (20) permits the excess gas to be blown off. If the flow is too small, the one-way valve (11) allows air to be drawn in during the expiratory phase.

The PN2, for ward use, is similar to the PNA1 except that the control lever (2) is not included. For this reason the valves (27) and (28) cannot be held open, and the reservoir bags (4) and (16) cannot be shut off. Manual ventilation therefore can be performed only by fitting the handle on the idling shaft of the driving mechanism.

FUNCTIONAL ANALYSIS

This functional analysis, the 'Controls' section which follows, and the measurements and recordings of figs. 47.5 to 47.8 refer to a PN2 ventilator. It seems unlikely that the addition of the anaesthetic circuits in the PNA1 model can have any appreciable effect on the functioning of the ventilator.

Inspiratory phase

The force exerted by the weights (3) on the positive-pressure concertina bag (4) make this ventilator operate as a pressure generator during the inspiratory phase. Because of the elasticity of the wall of the bag the generated pressure falls off a little as the bag empties (see the characteristics in fig. 47.5) but generally the fall-off is not sufficient to make it necessary to treat the system as a discharging compliance. Because there is some resistance between the bag (4) and the mouth, the waveform of pressure at the mouth (fig. 47.7) is intermediate between the falling generated pressure in the bag and the resultant rising

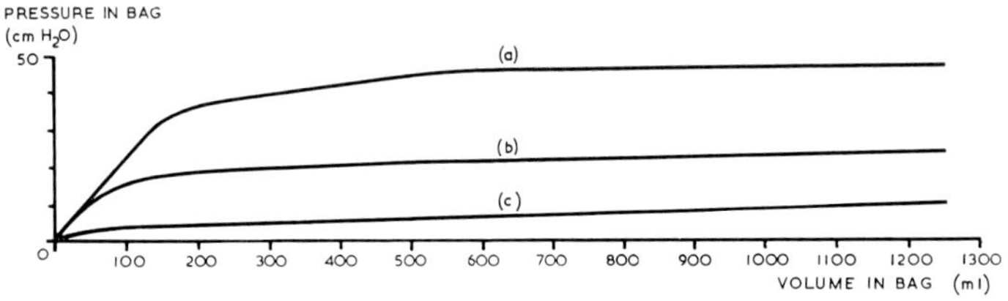

Fig. 47.5. East-Radcliffe 'Positive-Negative (PN2) Respirator'. Pressure-volume characteristics of the positive-pressure concertina bag.

(a) With three weights at the 'maximum' position, i.e. as far as possible in the 'increase positive pressure' direction.

(b) With no weights but with the weight carrier at the 'maximum' position.

(c) With no weights and with the weight carrier at the 'minimum' position.

pressure in the alveoli. Under the standard conditions (a) and with the compliance halved (b) this results in a waveform of mouth pressure which, after the rapid initial rise, increases slightly during the phase. However, when the airway resistance, between the mouth and the alveoli, is doubled (c) the mouth pressure approximates more closely to the generated pressure and happens to run at a steady level for the majority of the phase.

The pressure-generating action is also demonstrated by the very large changes of inspiratory flow waveform when the lung characteristics are changed. Since the inspiratory resistance of the ventilator is low (less than the standard airway resistance of the model lung) the time constant of the complete system, patient plus ventilator, is short enough when the compliance is halved for the flow to decay completely to zero well before the end of the phase (fig. 47.7b).

In other ventilators in which pressure is generated by a weight acting on a concertina bag (Manley, 'Vellore') substantial oscillations of flow and mouth pressure occur at the beginning of the phase, because of the inertia of the weight; yet such oscillations are barely perceptible in fig. 47.7. This is because the weights are set almost to the minimum for the tracings of fig. 47.7. When more weight was added (fig. 47.8b) to increase the generated pressure, oscillations of flow and pressure became apparent with this ventilator.

At the very end of the inspiratory phase there is a short period of zero-flow generation. This arises because the inspiratory valve (27) closes 1/30 of a cycle before the expiratory valve opens: in the tracings in fig. 47.7 it can be seen that for the last 1/10 sec of the inspiratory phase the flow is zero for all three conditions of the lungs although the mouth pressures are somewhat different.

Change-over from inspiratory phase to expiratory phase

This change-over is purely time-cycled; it occurs when the expiratory valve (28) opens at a preset time after the start of the inspiratory phase, determined by the constant speed of the driving motor, the shape of the cams (25, 26) and the particular gear-train engaged. Fig. 47.7 confirms that changes of lung characteristics have no effect on the inspiratory time.

Expiratory phase

During this phase the ventilator operates as a pressure generator. At the start of the phase the force exerted by the spring (13) on the negative-pressure concertina bag (16) generates a negative pressure within the bag. Therefore, all the expiratory flow enters the bag, allowing it to expand and the spring (13) to contract, so that the generated pressure becomes less negative. If the 'negative pressure' control (14) is set at minimum, a balance between the elasticity of the wall of the bag and the force of the spring is soon achieved and the negative pressure becomes zero; this occurs after only 120 ml of gas has entered the bag (curve (a) in fig. 47.6). The remainder of the tidal volume is expired directly to

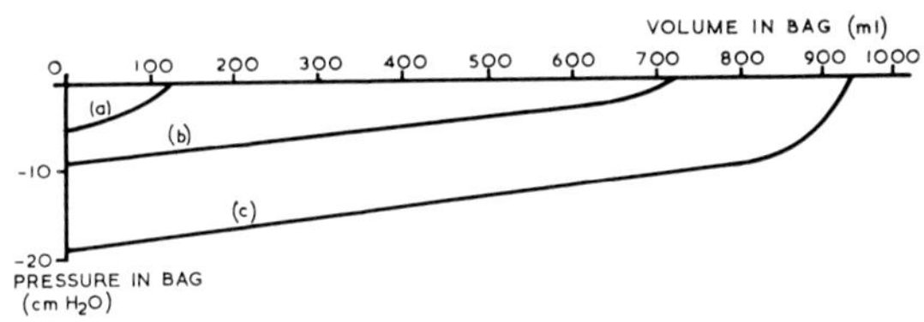

Fig. 47.6. East-Radcliffe 'Positive-Negative (PN2) Respirator'. Pressure-volume characteristics of the negative-pressure concertina bag. 'Zero' volume represents the condition of the bag when the expiratory valve first opens.

(a) With the 'negative pressure' control at minimum.

(b) With the 'negative pressure' control advanced about 90° from minimum as for the recording of fig. 47.7 and most of those in fig. 47.8.

(c) With the 'negative pressure' control at maximum.

Note that the pressure scale is more open than in the graph of the positive-pressure bag characteristics in fig. 47.5. The same open scale is used for all the other graphs of negative-pressure bag characteristics in this book.

atmosphere through the one-way valve (17) so that the ventilator operates as a constant, atmospheric, pressure generator for the greater part of the phase. At higher settings of the 'negative pressure' control (14) the initial negative pressure is greater, and larger volumes have to enter the bag before the negative pressure is reduced to zero (curves (b) and (c) in fig. 47.6). At these settings, therefore, negative pressure may well be generated throughout the phase although the magnitude gradually declines during the phase.

This is the case in the recordings of fig. 47.7 for which the setting of the 'negative pressure' control (14) was the same as for curve (b) in fig. 47.6. Because of the resistance between the bag, where the pressure is generated, and the mouth, the pressure at the mouth only approaches the generated pressure as the flow decays and actually becomes more negative during the phase. However, the flow waveforms show the typical changes for a pressure generator when the compliance is halved (fig. 47.7b) or the resistance doubled (fig. 47.7c).

Towards the end of the expiratory phase, when the flow has fallen to zero, the mouth pressure must be equal to the generated pressure in the bag and yet the end-expiratory mouth and alveolar pressures are slightly lower when the compliance is halved. This is because the waveform of generated pressure is preset in relation to expired volume (fig. 47.6) and not in relation to time. Thus, when the compliance is halved the tidal volume is decreased (fig. 47.7) and this smaller volume entering the negative-pressure concertina bag results in a more-negative pressure at the end of expiration (fig. 47.6 curve (b) and fig. 47.7b).

The negative-pressure concertina bag could be regarded as a 'charging compliance'—by analogy with the idea of the 'discharging compliance' (see p. 98) which we have used to explain the action of some ventilators during the inspiratory phase. The compliance of the patient can be thought of as 'discharging' into the negative-pressure bag, the compliance of which therefore gradually becomes charged. The pressure within the bag therefore gradually rises (becomes less negative) in accordance with its compliance and with the volume delivered to it by the patient.

Change-over from expiratory phase to inspiratory phase

This change-over like the other is purely time-cycled; it occurs when the inspiratory valve (27) opens at a preset time after the start of the expiratory phase. Fig. 47.7 confirms that changes of lung characteristics have no effect on the expiratory time.

CONTROLS

Total ventilation

This cannot be directly controlled but is equal to the product of tidal volume and respiratory frequency.

Tidal volume and pressure limits

The tidal volume cannot be directly controlled. It is determined by the product of compliance and the difference between the end-inspiratory and end-expiratory alveolar pressure limits. It is therefore convenient to consider these limits together with the tidal volume.

During the inspiratory phase the ventilator operates as a slowly-decreasing-pressure generator and therefore the alveolar pressure approaches the generated pressure in an approximately-exponential fashion. However, the time constant of the complete system (patient plus ventilator) is such that the alveolar pressure commonly does not reach the generated pressure by the end of the phase. Consequently, the 'positive pressure' control, that is, the position and number of the weights (3), is the primary means of controlling the peak alveolar pressure, and hence the tidal volume (fig. 47.8b). Other controls, and the lung characteristics, also influence these two parameters of ventilation. Thus, increasing the setting of the 'negative pressure' control increases the range of alveolar pressure and hence the tidal volume (fig. 47.8c). In addition, increasing the respiratory frequency (fig. 47.8d) decreases the inspiratory time so that the alveolar pressure cannot approach the generated pressure as closely as before; hence the peak alveolar pressure is reduced and therefore so is the tidal volume.

During the expiratory phase the ventilator again operates as a pressure generator but the time available for the alveolar pressure to approach the generated pressure is almost

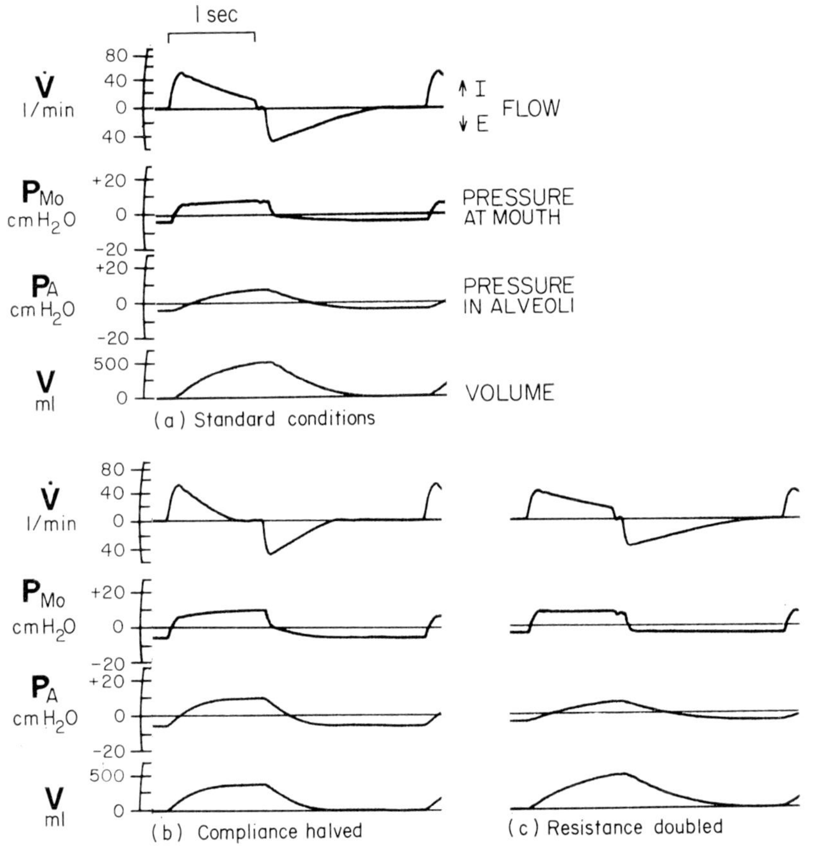

Fig. 47.7. East-Radcliffe 'Positive-Negative (PN2) Respirator'. Recordings showing the effects of changes of lung characteristics.

Standard conditions: mains motor in use; 'respiration rate', 20/min; 'positive pressure' and 'negative pressure' set to give a tidal volume of 500 ml with an end-expiratory alveolar pressure of -3 cmH_2O i.e. with the carrier (3), with no weights on it, near the minimum position, and with the 'negative pressure' control advanced about 90° from the minimum position.

doubled, while the time constant is almost the same as in the inspiratory phase. Therefore the approach to the generated pressure is much closer and, indeed, in all the tracings in figs. 47.7 and 47.8 the flow has fallen to zero and the alveolar pressure has become equal to the generated pressure by the end of the expiratory phase. Equalization will fail to

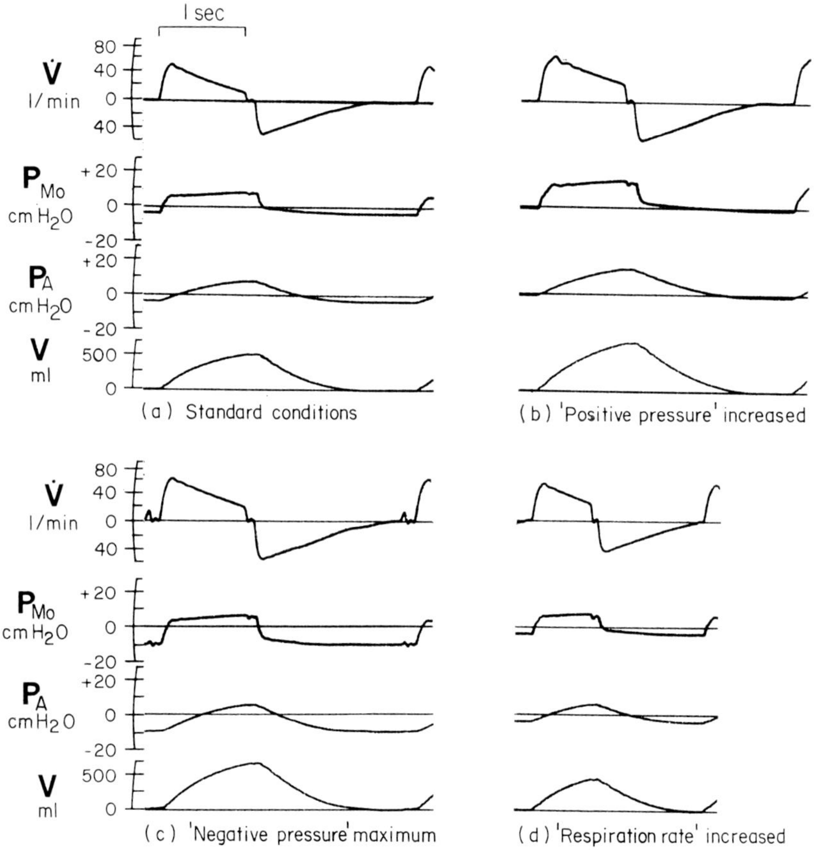

Fig. 47.8. East-Radcliffe 'Positive-Negative (PN2) Respirator'. Recordings showing the effects of changes in the settings of the controls.

(a) Standard conditions as in fig. 47.7.

(b) 'Positive pressure' increased by adding one weight to the carrier and moving the latter 5 cm towards the maximum position in order to increase the tidal volume to 750 ml.

(c) 'Negative pressure' increased to maximum.

(d) 'Respiration rate' increased to 30/min.

occur only with extreme combinations of high airway resistance, high respiratory frequency (short expiratory time) and large tidal volume. Therefore the 'negative pressure' control, which alters the magnitude of the negative pressure generated (fig. 47.6), provides a direct control of the lower limit of alveolar pressure (fig. 47.8c). However, it must be remembered that, as shown in the functional analysis above, the waveform of generated pressure is preset in relation to expired volume and not in relation to time, and that it declines appreciably as the expired volume increases (fig. 47.6)—except when the control is set to minimum. Therefore any change in tidal volume usually results in a change in the pressure generated at the end of the phase and hence in the end-expiratory alveolar pressure—no matter whether the change of tidal volume is deliberately produced by a change in the 'positive pressure' setting (fig. 47.8b), or is merely incidental to a change of the 'respiratory frequency' setting (fig. 47.8d) or to a change of lung characteristics (fig. 47.7b).

Changes of lung characteristics produce quite complex reactions. Thus, when the compliance is halved (fig. 47.7b) the time constant of the system is halved and, during the inspiratory phase, the alveolar pressure approaches the generated pressure more closely and the peak alveolar pressure is increased. In addition, since the tidal volume is reduced by the reduction in compliance the generated pressure at the end of the expiratory phase usually becomes more negative (fig. 47.6) and hence so does the end-expiratory alveolar pressure (fig. 47.7b). Therefore the pressure range in the alveoli is extended at both limits. Since the tidal volume is determined by the product of compliance and alveolar pressure range, halving the compliance reduces the tidal volume but not by as much as a half. In fig. 47.7b the reduction is only by about a quarter.

When the airway resistance is doubled (fig. 47.7c) the time constant is increased and the alveolar pressure does not rise so high during the inspiratory phase. This results in a drop in tidal volume which in turn makes the end-expiratory generated and alveolar pressures slightly more negative, so making the drop in tidal volume less than it would otherwise be. In fig. 47.7b doubling the airway resistance decreases the tidal volume by less than 10%.

In summary, the 'positive pressure' control is the primary means of adjusting tidal volume and the 'negative pressure' control is the primary means of setting the degree of negative pressure, but both controls have some effect on the parameter primarily controlled by the other. Therefore, to obtain a given tidal volume, together with a given negative pressure, will normally require more than one adjustment of each control. Furthermore, if the respiratory frequency is subsequently changed or if the lung characteristics alter, fresh adjustments of the 'positive pressure' and 'negative pressure' controls will be required to restore the original tidal volume and negative pressure.

Respiratory frequency

This is directly controlled by the 'respiration rate' selector lever and the use of the 'high speeds' locking plug or the 'low speeds' locking plug. The adjustment can be made only in discrete steps and not continuously. The characteristics of the motors are such that the respiratory frequency is practically uninfluenced by the settings of the other controls and quite uninfluenced by changes of lung characteristics.

When the respiratory frequency is deliberately increased (fig. 47.8d) the tidal volume is somewhat reduced, as explained above, although there is a net increase in total ventilation.

Inspiratory-expiratory ratio

This is fixed at 1 : 1·7 and cannot be altered in any way.

Waveforms

Since the ventilator is a pressure generator in both phases, the flow waveforms are determined by the effects of the generated-pressure waveforms on the lungs. The heights and durations of the pressure waveforms can be adjusted but not their slopes. Therefore the shapes of the flow waveforms cannot be deliberately influenced, although they are modified by changes of lung characteristics (fig. 47.7).

REFERENCE

1 Russell W.R., Schuster E., Smith A.C. and Spalding J.M.K. (1956) Radcliffe respiration pumps. *Lancet*, **1**, 539.

CHAPTER 48

The Emerson 'Assistor'[1]

DESCRIPTION

This ventilator (fig. 48.1) assists inadequate spontaneous inspiratory efforts of a patient. On the patient attempting to inspire, the reservoir bag (15) (fig. 48.2) begins to collapse and the pressure in the plastic pressure chamber (16) falls slightly. This fall in pressure is transmitted through the tubing to the pressure-sensitive valve (7), lifting the diaphragm and so permitting gas to flow through the valve (7). Compressed gas from the cylinder (1) flows through an injector (9) which is an integral part of the valve (7), and creates negative pressure which, by acting on the diaphragm, holds the valve open widely. The

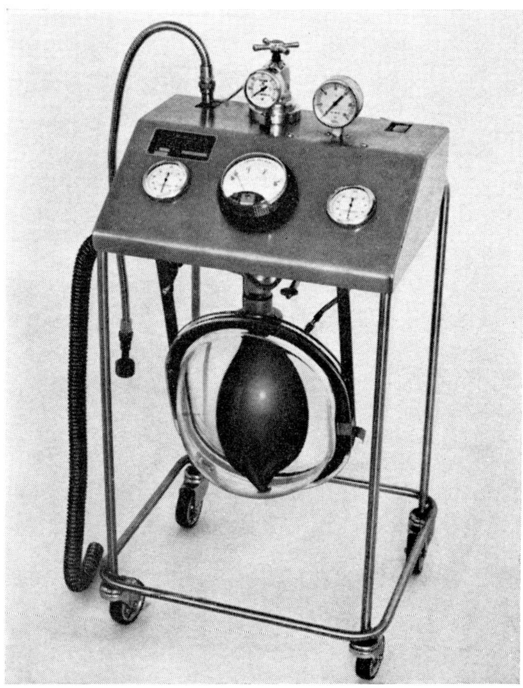

Fig. 48.1. The Emerson 'Assistor'.

Courtesy of J.H.Emerson Co.

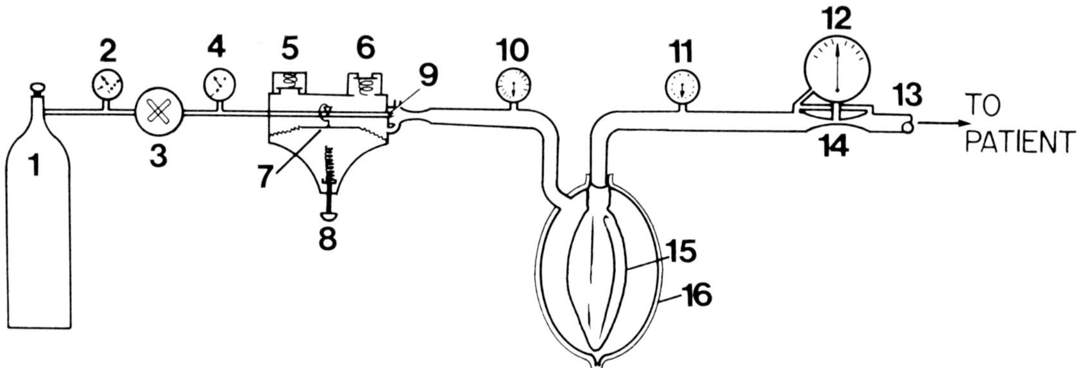

Fig. 48.2. Diagram of the Emerson 'Assistor'.

1. Cylinder of compressed gas
2. Pressure gauge
3. Regulator
4. Pressure gauge
5. Safety outlet
6. Safety inlet
7. Diaphragm valve
8. Manual trip
9. Injector
10. Pressure gauge
11. Pressure gauge
12. Ventigrator gauge
13. Delivery tube
14. Ventigrator
15. Reservoir bag
16. Rigid plastic pressure chamber

Courtesy of *Anesthesiology*.[1]

pressure in the pressure chamber (16) rises and compresses the reservoir bag (15), so assisting the inspiration of the patient. The flow of gas into the lungs is controlled by the setting of the regulator (3). The pressure changes in the pressure chamber (16) are shown on the gauge (10) and those in the patient circuit on the gauge (11). Once started by an inspiratory effort, the compressed gas continues to flow until the positive pressure in the pressure chamber (16) overcomes the negative pressure developed by the injector (9) to a sufficient extent to move the diaphragm down and close the valve (7). Once the flow of compressed gas falls off, the negative pressure from the injector (9) falls and the valve (7) snaps down. The pressure chamber (16) empties through the air inlet of the injector (9) and passive expiration begins. The sensitivity of the valve (7) (i.e. the small fall in pressure which starts the flow of compressed gas) is adjusted by a set screw. A lever (8) is provided to trip this valve manually if desired. The 'ventigrator'[2] (12, 14) is an integrating ventilation meter, which gives a continuous measure of pulmonary ventilation. The device is a specially-modified venturi tube which registers the average volume flow rate of breathing.

The pressure chamber (16) may be opened for manual compression of the reservoir bag (15). A blow-off valve is needed in the patient circuit for venting excess gas.

FUNCTIONAL ANALYSIS

Inspiratory phase

The mode of operation in this phase depends upon the characteristics of the injector, but is probably that of a high-constant-pressure generator with substantial series resistance. A pressure limit, due to the blow-off valve which must be incorporated in the patient circuit, comes into operation during the phase. Until then the fresh-gas supply to the patient circuit acts as a small-constant-flow generator, supplementing the action of the main pressure generator.

Change-over from inspiratory phase to expiratory phase

Superficially this change-over appears to be pressure-cycled: the pressure in the pressure chamber (16) (fig. 48.2) which is sufficient to overcome the negative pressure developed by the injector (9) and produce cycling is that applied to the patient via the reservoir bag (15). However, the blow-off valve in the patient circuit must open at less than the cycling pressure in order to vent excess gas. Therefore the pressure in the patient circuit can never rise to the cycling pressure. However, the pressure in the pressure chamber rises to the cycling pressure, and therefore produces the change-over, very shortly after the reservoir bag (15) has been emptied. From this it might appear that the change-over is volume-cycled, but even this is not true in the conventional sense of the term. A precisely-similar situation arises in the 'Cyclator CAV'; in the functional analysis of that ventilator it is shown that the change-over can best be described in the following way.

If the fresh-gas flow to the patient circuit is large, the only way of describing the change-over is to say that it is volume-cycled but that the volume involved (that in the reservoir bag at the beginning of the inspiratory phase) includes the tidal volume which happened to be expired by the patient in the previous respiratory cycle and which is dependent upon lung characteristics. If the fresh-gas flow is small, the above statement is still true, but there is now so little excess gas to be vented through the blow-off valve that the change-over occurs almost immediately the blow-off valve opens. Therefore the change-over is effectively pressure-cycled at the opening pressure of the blow-off valve.

Expiratory phase

In this phase the ventilator operates as a constant, atmospheric, pressure generator: the patient's expired gas effectively has free passage to the atmosphere at the entrainment port of the injector.

Change-over from expiratory phase to inspiratory phase

This change-over is patient-cycled: cycling occurs only when an inspiratory effort by the patient produces a negative pressure above the diaphragm, sufficient to open the inlet valve (7).

REFERENCES

1 Maloney J.V., Derrick W.S. and Whittenberger J.L. (1952) Device producing regulated assisted respiration; the prevention of hypoventilation and mediastinal motion during intra-thoracic surgery. *Anesthesiology*, **13**, 23.

2 Maloney J.V., Silverman L. and Whittenberger J.L. (1951) An integrating ventilation meter for clinical use. *J. Lab. clin. Med.* **37**, 828.

CHAPTER 49

The Emerson 'Controller-Assistor'

DESCRIPTION

This ventilator (fig. 49.1) was evolved from the earlier 'Assistor'. Driving gas at a pressure of 50 lb/in^2 enters at (9) (fig. 49.2). A reducing valve (10) drops this pressure to about 15 lb/in^2. The driving gas flows through the injector (16) producing a negative pressure in the chamber (13) behind the diaphragm (12). This allows the diaphragm to move to the right under the influence of the compression spring (11). This movement opens the valve (20) through a link mechanism. Driving gas can now flow through the injector (14) into the rigid plastic pressure chamber (3). The action of the injector (14) produces a further drop in pressure behind the diaphragm (12) thus increasing the movement of the diaphragm and further opening the valve (20). Air is entrained through the valve (2), economizing in the supply of driving gas. Pressure builds up in the pressure chamber (3), compressing the concertina reservoir bag and forcing its contents to the patient. As this pressure increases, so does the pressure in the chamber (18). The diaphragm (19) moves up against the pressure of the spring until the ball (17) seals off the injector (16). Pressure continues to rise in the pressure chamber (3) until it neutralizes the negative pressure from the injector (14). The diaphragm (12) is forced outwards against the spring (11). Through the link mechanism this partially closes the valve (20). This further reduces the negative pressure from the injector (14) rapidly producing complete closure of the valve (20) and cutting off the supply of driving gas to the pressure chamber (3).

The pressure in the pressure chamber (3) is now released through the exhaust valve (4) which until now was kept closed by the negative pressure from the injector (14). The concertina reservoir bag re-expands under the influence of adjustable weights and the expired gas flow. As the pressure in the chamber (18) falls, at a rate controlled by the leak-off screw (15), the diaphragm (19) returns, under the force of its spring, moving the ball valve (17) from its seating, and allowing the injector (16) to operate again and so start another inspiratory phase.

The speed of inflation is controlled by the setting of the adjustable reducing valve (10), which also influences the maximum positive pressure in the pressure chamber (3), as explained in the functional analysis. The frequency of respiration is governed also, and mainly, by the duration of the expiratory phase which is set by the needle valve (15).

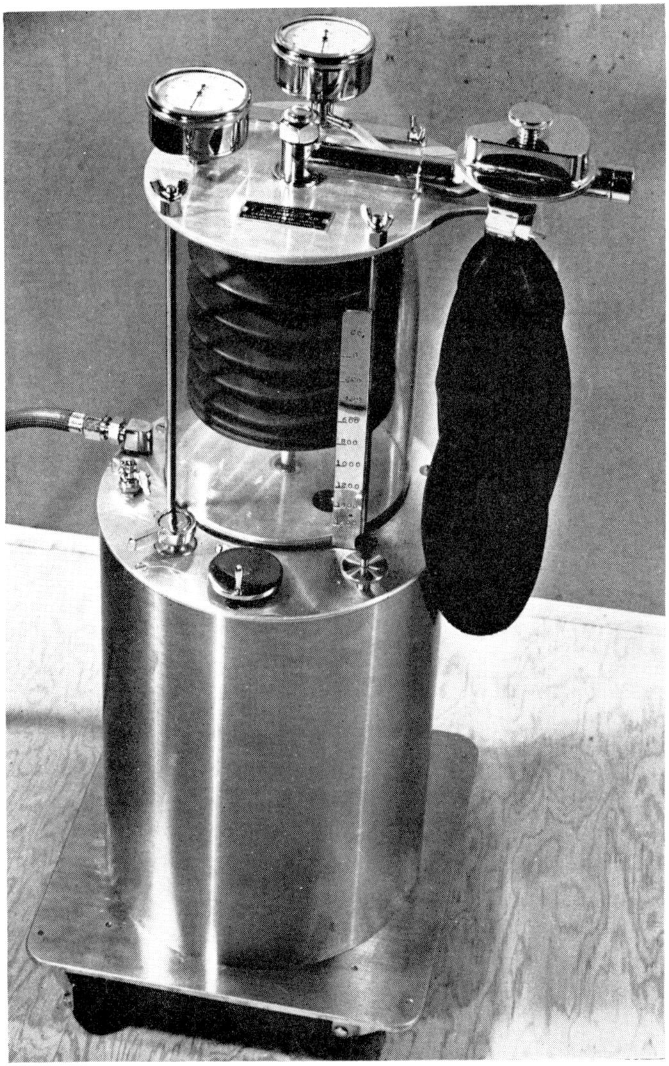

Fig. 49.1. The Emerson 'Controller-Assistor'.

Courtesy of J.H. Emerson Co.

Negative pressure during the expiratory phase can be obtained and varied by inserting the rod (6) and placing weights (7) of various sizes on its end. A manometer indicates the pressure in the patient circuit. The volume delivered to the patient can be set by positioning the stop (8) by means of the screw-thread control (21). A spill valve (5) in the concertina bag allows excess gas to escape from the patient circuit during the expiratory phase.

When the patient makes an inspiratory effort negative pressure is transmitted from

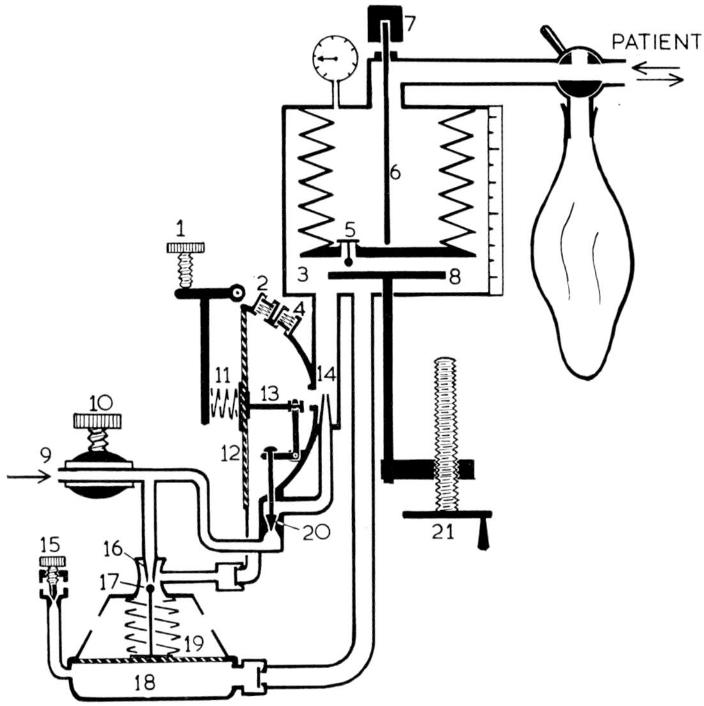

Fig. 49.2. Diagram of the Emerson 'Controller-Assistor'.

1. Patient-triggering sensitivity control
2. Air-inlet valve
3. Pressure chamber
4. Exhaust valve
5. Spill valve
6. Sliding rod
7. Adjustable weight
8. Volume-control platform
9. Driving-gas inlet
10. Pressure-reducing valve
11. Compression spring
12. Diaphragm
13. Assistor control-valve chamber
14. Injector
15. Needle valve
16. Injector
17. Ball valve
18. Timing-control chamber
19. Diaphragm
20. Valve
21. Volume-limit control

the patient circuit through the concertina reservoir bag to the chamber (13) behind the diaphragm (12). The diaphragm moves to the right and, through the link mechanism, opens the valve (20), thus allowing the driving gas to flow through the injector (14) initiating an inspiratory phase which continues until it ends as described above. The ventilator then remains in the expiratory phase either until the patient makes another inspiratory effort, or until the timing mechanism operates and initiates an inspiratory phase automatically.

If the leak-off (15) is closed, the timing mechanism is put out of action, and an inspiratory phase can only be initiated by an inspiratory effort of the patient. The sensitivity of the diaphragm (12) to an inspiratory effort, i.e. the triggering pressure, is controlled by the screw (1) which alters the force exerted by the spring (11) on the diaphragm (12).

FUNCTIONAL ANALYSIS

Inspiratory phase

The mode of operation during this phase depends upon the characteristics of the injector (14) (fig. 49.2) but is probably that of a high-constant-pressure generator, with substantial series resistance. The fresh-gas supply to the patient circuit acts as a small-constant-flow generator, supplementing the action of the main pressure generator.

Change-over from inspiratory phase to expiratory phase

This change-over is either pressure-cycled or volume-cycled, whichever limit is reached first. The system is fundamentally pressure-cycled as in the Emerson 'Assistor' but, if the concertina bag is emptied before the cycling pressure is reached in the pressure chamber, cycling follows immediately, owing to the rapid build-up of pressure to the cycling value. The system therefore becomes effectively volume-cycled. In pressure-cycled operation, if there is a weight on the concertina bag, the pressure in the pressure chamber which produces cycling is a fixed amount greater than that applied to the patient. If the supply pressure is increased by adjusting the regulator (10) this increases not only the generated pressure during the inspiratory phase but also the cycling pressure at the end of the phase. No matter whether volume-cycling or pressure-cycling occurs, since the escape of excess gas, through the spill valve, is restricted to the expiratory phase, the tidal volume of the patient is greater than that of the concertina bag, by an amount equal to the volume of fresh gas supplied during the inspiratory phase.

Expiratory phase

With no weights on the concertina bag the ventilator operates in this phase as a constant, atmospheric, pressure generator: the patient's expired gas effectively has free passage to the atmosphere at the exhaust valve (4).

With weights on the concertina bag the ventilator operates first as a constant, negative, pressure generator, owing to the weights, and later, when the bag reaches the stop, as a constant, atmospheric, pressure generator owing to the opening of the spill valve (5).

Change-over from expiratory phase to inspiratory phase

This change-over is time-cycled or patient-cycled, whichever comes first. Cycling occurs when the pressure on the right of the diaphragm (12) becomes sufficiently negative for valve (20) to open, either due to the injector (16) coming into operation at a preset time after the end of the previous inspiratory phase, or to the pressure in the pressure chamber falling as a result of an inspiratory effort from the patient. Note that, if the cycling pressure at the end of the inspiratory phase is raised, the amount of air that has to leak out of the chamber (18) before the injector (16) comes into operation is increased: the time limit to the duration of the expiratory phase is therefore increased.

CHAPTER 50

The Emerson 'Post-operative' Ventilator (electrically-operated)

DESCRIPTION

This electrically-driven ventilator (fig. 50.2) is intended for ward use. It delivers atmospheric air, with or without added oxygen, to the patient.

An a.c. mains electric motor (15) (fig. 50.1) drives a large wheel to which is attached a crank lever (23). This lever is connected to the pivoted lever (22) which carries the slide (21).

In this way the rotary motion of the large wheel is converted to an up-and-down motion of the slider (21) and this in turn is converted through the lever (20) to a reciprocating motion of the piston (11).

When the piston moves down, the one-way outlet valve (4) closes, and the one-way inlet valve (3) opens. Air is drawn into the cylinder through the filter (1) and the reservoir tube (10). The expiratory valve (7) also opens and expired gas from the patient passes freely to atmosphere through the port (8). When the piston (11) moves up, the gas contained in the cylinder is forced, past the one-way valve (4) and a hot-water humidifier (5), to the patient, the diaphragm expiratory valve (7) being held closed by the higher pressure in the cylinder. The pressure in the breathing circuit is indicated by the manometer (18).

A cam (13) on the large wheel is so shaped that it closes the microswitch (12) when the piston moves up during the inspiratory phase, and allows it to open when the piston moves down during the expiratory phase. When this switch is closed, the speed of the motor (15) depends on the setting of the 'adjust time—inhale' control (19, I) and when it is open, the speed depends on the setting of the 'adjust time—exhale' control (19, E). In this way the durations of the inspiratory and expiratory phases can be varied independently. The frequency depends on the combined settings of these two controls.

The tidal volume depends on the stroke of the piston (11) and may be varied between 80 and 1500 ml. Adjustment of the control (25) alters the position of the slider (21) on the lever (22). The nearer the slider is to the fulcrum of the lever (22), the less the reciprocating motion imparted to the piston (11) through the rod (20) and the less the tidal volume. The tidal volume set is indicated on the scale (26).

A 'sigh' mechanism (17) is connected to the breathing circuit through a one-way valve (6). This mechanism consists of an electrically-driven blower and an electric

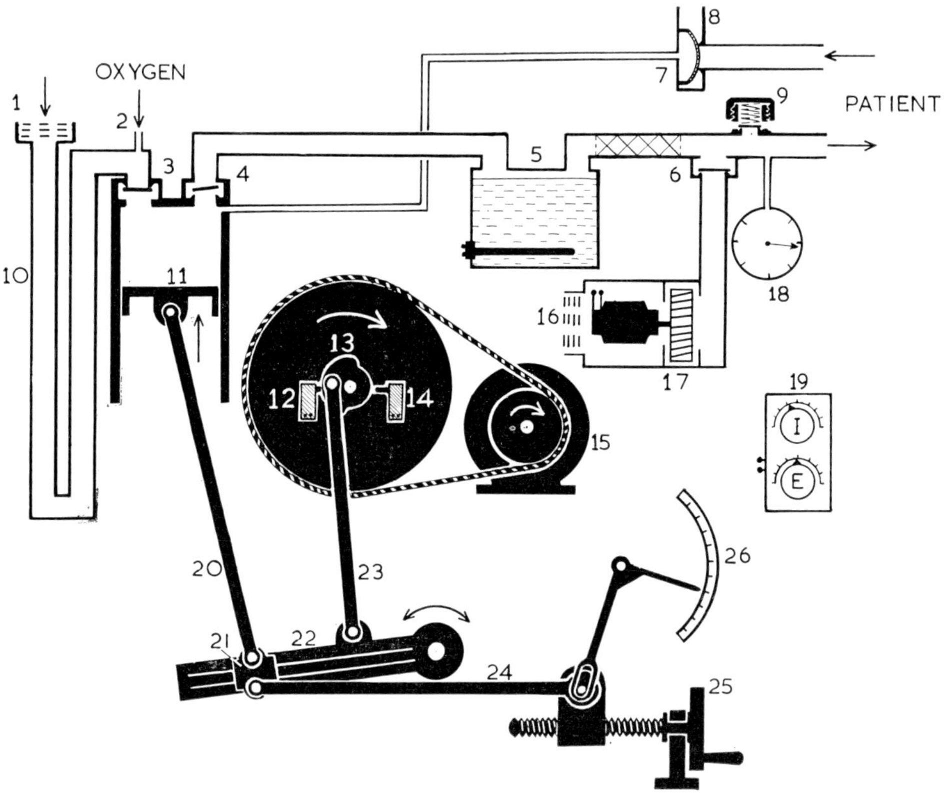

Fig. 50.1. Diagram of the Emerson 'Post-operative' ventilator (electrically-operated).

1. Filter
2. Oxygen inlet
3. One-way valve
4. One-way valve
5. Heated humidifier
6. One-way valve
7. Expiratory valve
8. Expiratory port
9. Positive-pressure safety-valve
10. Reservoir tube
11. Piston
12. Microswitch
13. Cam
14. Microswitch
15. Electric motor
16. Filter
17. Air blower
18. Manometer

19, I. 'Adjust time—inhale' control
19, E. 'Adjust time—exhale' control
20. Connecting rod
21. Slider
22. Pivoted lever
23. Crank lever
24. Connecting rod
25. Volume control
26. Volume indicator

timing circuit which automatically switches the blower on at preset intervals of between 5 and 7 minutes. The microswitch (14), operated by the cam (13), ensures that the blower can operate only during the inspiratory phase. The air drawn in through the filter (16) by the blower is therefore added to the tidal volume delivered by the piston. A positive-pressure safety-valve (9) can be set so that the blower cannot produce an excessive pressure in the patient circuit.

The humidifier (5) is heated electrically and the temperature controlled by a thermostat. Copper gauze in the tube leading to the outlet to the patient prevents water droplets entering the breathing tube.

The capacity of the reservoir tube (10) is the same as that of the cylinder (11). Therefore 100% oxygen is delivered to the patient when the flow of oxygen into the ventilator at the inlet (2) is equal to the total minute-volume ventilation. Any lower oxygen concentration can also be accurately delivered.

If desired, a volume meter can be connected to the expiratory port (8). Fig. 50.1 illustrates a special volume meter with a large scale which is available from the manufacturers.

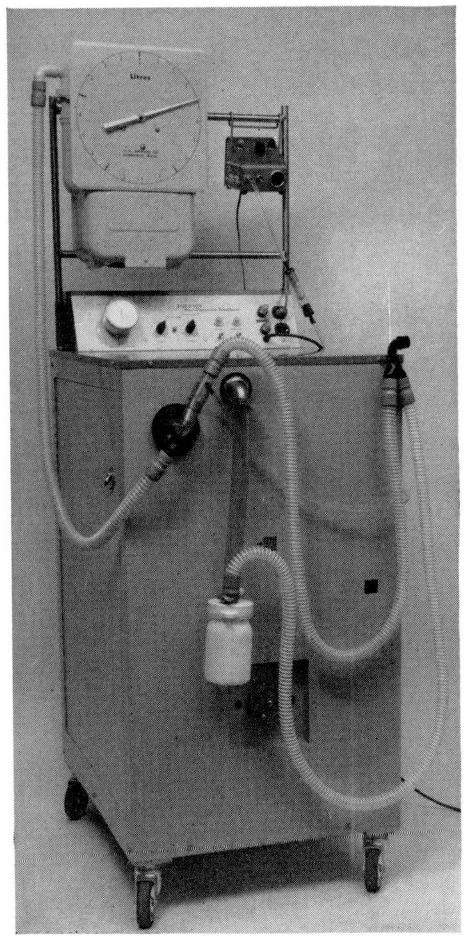

Fig. 50.2. The Emerson 'Post-operative' ventilator (electrically-operated).
Courtesy of J.H.Emerson Co.

FUNCTIONAL ANALYSIS

Inspiratory phase

In this phase, assuming that, as seems likely, the speed of the motor is constant during the phase, the ventilator operates as a non-constant-flow generator; the pattern of flow is approximately that of a half cycle of a sine wave owing to the nature of the linkages (20–23).

Change-over from inspiratory phase to expiratory phase

This change-over is both volume-cycled and time-cycled: it occurs when a preset volume has been expelled by the piston (11) in a preset time determined by the speed of the motor (15) which is controlled by the 'adjust time—inhale' control (19, I).

Expiratory phase

In this phase the ventilator operates as a constant, atmospheric, pressure generator: the patient's expired gas passes to atmosphere through the expiratory port (8).

Change-over from expiratory phase to inspiratory phase

This change-over is time-cycled: it occurs when the piston (11) has completed its return stroke in a preset time determined by the speed of the motor (15) which is controlled by the 'adjust time—exhale' control (19, E).

CHAPTER 51

The Emerson 'Post-operative' Ventilator (gas-operated)

DESCRIPTION

This ventilator (fig. 51.2) is designed for ward use. Air is drawn into the cylinder (5) (fig. 51.1) and forced to the patient by the piston (6) for which the motive power is provided by a supply of compressed gas.

The driving gas is supplied, at a pressure of 50 lb/in^2, to the pressure regulator (30), from which it flows at the operating pressure, indicated on the gauge (29), through the filter (28), to the relay valve (25, 26, 27).

During the inspiratory phase the relay valve is in its 'down' position, as shown, and driving gas flows, through the valve (26), to the lower part (23) of the high-pressure cylinder. The upper part (17) of the high-pressure cylinder is connected, through the relay valve (26), to atmosphere. The piston (18) is forced upwards and the larger piston (6) drives the gas stored in the cylinder (5), past the one-way valve (8), through the water trap (21) and the inspiratory tube (13), to the patient. The expiratory valve (9) is meanwhile held closed by the higher pressure behind its diaphragm. The pressure in the inspiratory tube (13) is indicated by the manometer (12) and can be limited by the safety-valve (10). When the piston (6) reaches the top of its stroke, the poppet valve (7) is opened, and the upper end (25) of the valve assembly is connected through it to atmosphere.

The connecting pathway between the high-pressure supply line and the upper end (25) of the relay-valve assembly offers a resistance to the driving-gas flow which is high in comparison to the resistance of the pathway between the upper end (25) of the assembly and atmosphere through the valve (7). Consequently, the pressure exerted on the upper end of the relay valve (26) now falls below the pressure exerted on its lower end, and the valve (26) is therefore moved up rapidly into its expiratory position. Driving gas now flows, through the relay valve (26), to the upper part (17) of the high-pressure cylinder, the lower part (23) being connected to atmosphere through the relay valve (26). The piston (18) is driven down, drawing down the larger piston (6). Pressure in the cylinder (5) falls immediately and the expiratory valve (9) opens. Expired gas flows along the expiratory tube (11) and through the valve (9) to atmosphere. The downward movement of the piston (6) frees the poppet valve (7), which is at once closed by its spring, blocking

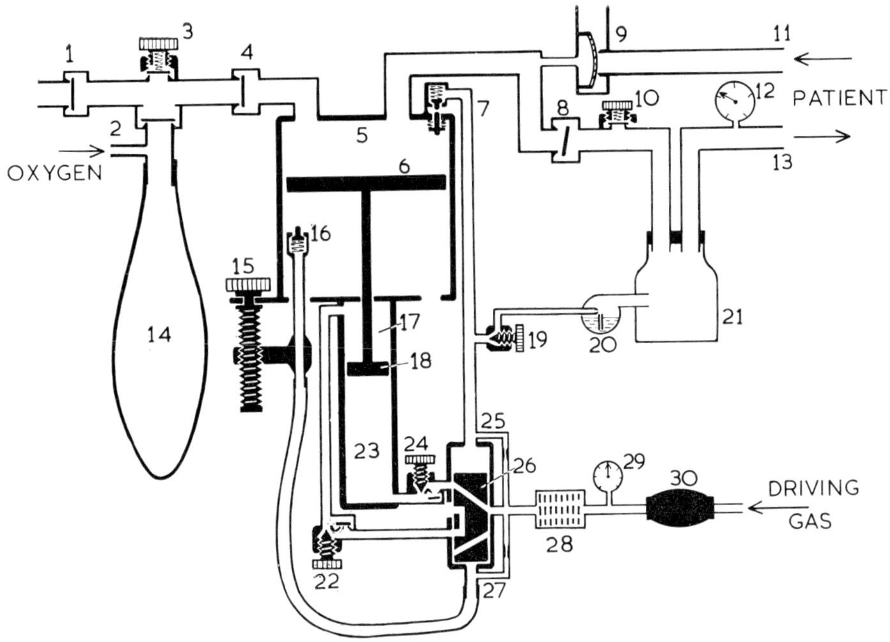

Fig. 51.1. Diagram of the Emerson 'Post-operative' ventilator (gas-operated).

1. One-way air-inlet valve
2. Oxygen inlet
3. Escape valve
4. One-way valve
5. Cylinder
6. Piston
7. Poppet valve
8. One-way valve
9. Expiratory valve
10. Safety-valve
11. Expiratory tube
12. Manometer
13. Inspiratory tube
14. Storage bag
15. 'Tidal volume' control
16. Poppet valve
17. Upper end of high-pressure cylinder
18. Piston
19. Nebulizer control
20. Nebulizer
21. Water trap
22. 'Time of cycle—inhalation' control
23. Lower end of high-pressure cylinder
24. 'Time of cycle—exhalation' control
25. Upper end of relay-valve assembly
26. Relay valve
27. Lower end of relay-valve assembly
28. Filter
29. Pressure gauge
30. Pressure regulator

the connexion between the upper part (25) of the valve assembly and atmosphere, and allowing the pressure there to rise again. At the same time the cylinder (5) refills with air through the valve (1) together with oxygen from the bag (14) if any is being added at the inlet (2). The downward movement of the pistons (6, 18) continues until the piston (6) opens the poppet valve (16). The pathway connecting the high-pressure supply line and the lower end (27) of the relay-valve assembly offers a resistance to the driving-gas flow which is high in comparison to the resistance of the pathway now connecting the lower end (27) of the relay-valve assembly to atmosphere through the poppet valve (16). There is therefore a higher pressure exerted on the upper end of the relay valve (26) which is rapidly moved down into its inspiratory position. The next inspiratory phase begins.

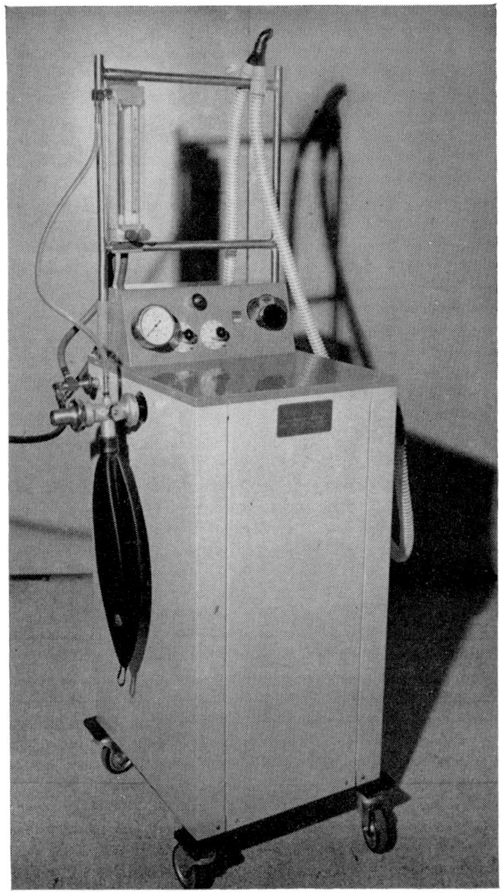

Fig. 51.2. The Emerson 'Post-operative' ventilator (gas-operated).
Courtesy of J.H.Emerson Co.

The stroke volume of the piston (6) is determined by the 'tidal volume' control (15), which sets the position of the poppet valve (16), and hence the lower limit of the excursion of the piston (6). The tidal volume of the patient exceeds the stroke volume of the piston to the extent of any driving gas flowing through the nebulizer (20) during the inspiratory phase.

For a given stroke volume the inspiratory and expiratory times depend on the speed with which the pistons are driven up and down respectively. During the inspiratory phase driving gas flows freely through the one-way by-pass valve of the control (24) to the lower end (23) of the high-pressure cylinder; but gas from the upper end (17) can escape only through the needle valve (22) and the relay valve (26). Consequently this needle valve (22) controls the speed at which the pistons are driven up and hence the inspiratory time; it is labelled 'time of cycle—inhalation'. During the expiratory phase driving gas flows freely, through the one-way by-pass of the control (22), to the upper end (17) of the high-pressure cylinder; but gas from the lower end (23) can escape only through the needle valve (24) and the relay valve (26). Accordingly this needle valve (24) governs the speed at which the pistons are driven down and hence the expiratory time. It is labelled 'time of cycle—exhalation'.

The breathing circuit is the same as that in the Emerson electrical 'Post-operative' ventilator except that the hot-water humidifier of the electrical ventilator is here replaced by the nebulizer (20) supplied through a needle valve (19) from the driving-gas line. There is no sigh attachment.

Normally the inflating gas is air, which is drawn in through the one-way valves (1, 4). Oxygen may be added at the inlet (2) and is stored in the bag (14), from which any excess can escape through the valve (3).

FUNCTIONAL ANALYSIS

Inspiratory phase

In this phase the patient is connected to a pressure transformer (see p. 89) comprising the piston (6) and cylinder (5) on the low-pressure side and the piston (18) and cylinder (17, 23) on the high-pressure side. The driving-gas pressure is very high and there is an adjustable resistance to the escape of gas from the non-driven end of the high-pressure cylinder—at the needle valve (22) during the inspiratory phase. The system can therefore be expected to act as a constant-pressure generator delivering a fairly-high pressure but with an effective series resistance which is adjusted by the 'time of cycle—inhalation' control (22). With fairly-normal lung characteristics, therefore, it probably makes a fair approximation to a constant-flow generator. Any flow from the nebulizer (20) will constitute a small-constant-flow generator in parallel with the main mechanism.

Change-over from inspiratory phase to expiratory phase

This change-over is volume-cycled: it occurs when the poppet valve (7) is opened by the piston (6) completing its preset stroke. The tidal volume of the patient exceeds the stroke volume of the piston to the extent of any volume of driving gas delivered through the nebulizer during the inspiratory phase.

Expiratory phase

During this phase the ventilator operates as a constant, atmospheric, pressure generator: the patient's expired gas passes to atmosphere through the expiratory valve (9).

Change-over from expiratory phase to inspiratory phase

This change-over is time-cycled: it occurs when the poppet valve (16) is opened by the piston (6) completing its preset return stroke at a speed which is preset by the 'time of cycle—exhalation' control (24).

CHAPTER 52

The Engström Ventilators[1, 2]

DESCRIPTION OF THE ENGSTRÖM 'UNIVERSAL RESPIRATOR' MODEL 150

This ventilator (figs. 52.1 and 52.2) provides a non-rebreathing circuit only. It can be used in the ward or operating theatre. The 'Narcosis Respirator' Model 200 (see p. 555) is substantially the same, except that the breathing circuit is modified so that it can be used either as a non-rebreathing or as a closed circuit.

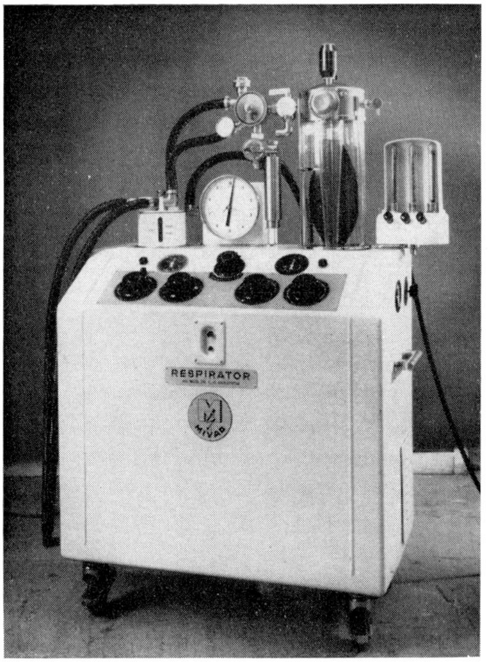

Fig. 52.1.

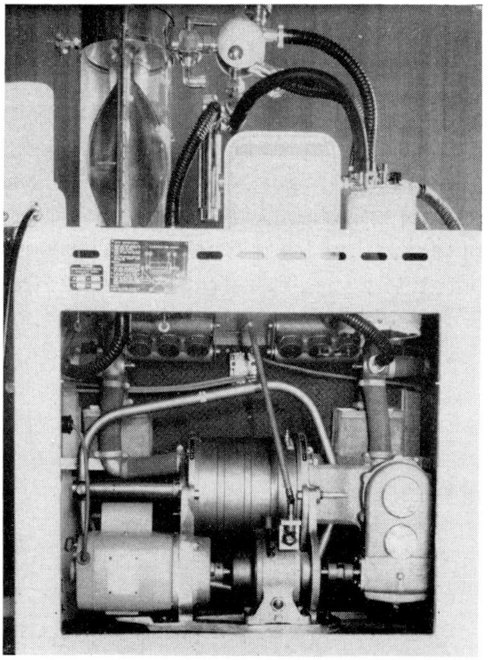

Fig. 52.2.

Fig. 52.1. The Engström 'Universal Respirator' Model 150.
Courtesy of Department of Medical Illustration, Cardiff Royal Infirmary.

Fig. 52.2. Mechanism of the Engström 'Universal Respirator' Model 150.
Courtesy of Department of Medical Illustration, Cardiff Royal Infirmary.

A piston (44) (fig. 52.3) is driven by a constant-speed a.c. mains electric motor (38) through a variable-speed gear-box (40). The 'frequency of respirations per minute' control (39) allows the frequency to be adjusted between 10 and 30 per minute. During the inspiratory phase, the piston (44) is driven to the right of the large-capacity cylinder (46), air being sucked in behind the piston through the one-way valve in the 'cuirasse/venturi selector' (31) which is set to 'venturi'. Some of the air from the right-hand side of the cylinder (46) is forced into the rigid plastic pressure chamber (24), but most of it flows, through the 'inspiration flow rate' throttle (35) and the compensating throttle (34), to atmosphere. As the pressure in the chamber (24) rises, the reservoir bag (22) is compressed and the gas contained in the bag is forced, through the one-way valve (6), the electrically-heated humidifier (3), and the inspiratory tube (1), to the patient, the expiratory valve (7) being held closed by the pressure of gas behind it. The positive pressure produced in the chamber (24) during the inspiratory phase, set by the 'inspiration flow rate' throttle (35), is shown on the manometer (37).

The positive pressure in the patient circuit is indicated by the water manometer (20), which also acts as a safety-valve. This manometer (20) consists of a conical glass container and a flexible bag. The bag rests between a fixed plate and a moveable platform, the height of which can be adjusted by the 'level water trap' control (21). By this means the volume of the bag is altered, thus varying the level of water in the conical container, and hence the pressure which must be reached before gas can ecape through it. The pressure in the patient circuit is freely transmitted to the manometer (20) through the one-way valve (11). However, a preset needle valve (10) restricts the leak of gas back from the manometer (20) during the expiratory phase. Therefore undue fluctuation between

Table 52.1. Phasing and timing of actions of the Engström ventilator.

Action	% duration of forward or reverse stroke of piston (44).	Angular rotation of output shaft of gear-box (40).
Piston starts	—	at 0°
Compression starts	after 4% of forward	at 7°
Compression stops and passive expiration starts	after 72% of forward	at 130°
Piston reverses	after 100% of forward	at 180°
Injector starts	after 13% of reverse	at 204°
Suction (refilling of bag) starts	after 28% of reverse	at 230°
Injector stops	after 87% of reverse	at 336°
Suction stops	after 96% of reverse	at 353°

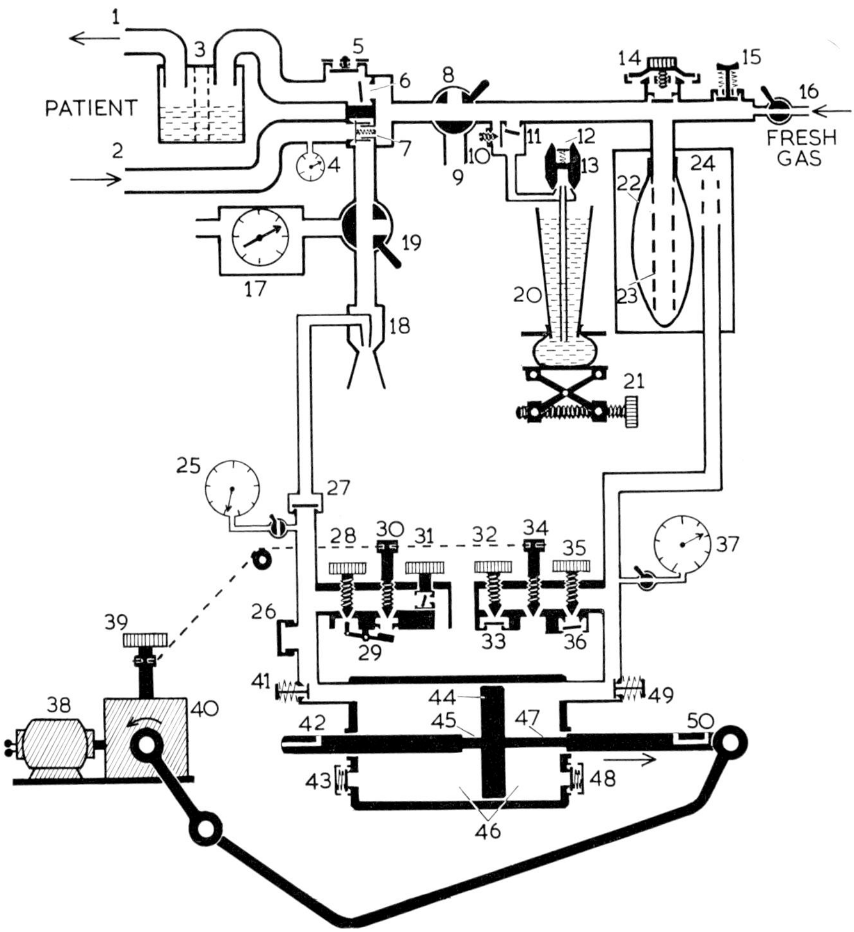

Fig. 52.3. Diagram of the Engström 'Universal Respirator' Model 150.

1. Inspiratory tube
2. Expiratory tube
3. Humidifier
4. Manometer
5. One-way air-inlet valve
6. One-way valve
7. Expiratory valve
8. 'Manual/automatic' tap
9. Port for manual reservoir bag
10. Preset needle valve
11. One-way valve
12. Spring-loaded valve
13. Reversible 'water-trap off' blocker
14. 'Dosing valve'
15. Plunger valve
16. Fresh-gas inlet
17. Spirometer
18. Injector
19. Spirometer tap
20. Water manometer
21. 'Level water-trap' control
22. Reservoir bag
23. Perforated tube
24. Rigid plastic pressure chamber
25. Cuirasse manometer
26. Connexion for cuirasse
27. One-way valve
28. 'Pressure regulator' throttle
29. Rocker valve
30. Compensating throttle
31. 'Cuirasse/venturi' control
32. 'Dosing valve calibration' throttle
33. One-way valve
34. Compensating throttle
35. 'Inspiration flow rate' throttle
36. One-way valve
37. Manometer
38. a.c. mains electric motor
39. 'Frequency of respirations per minute' control
40. Gear-box
41. Safety-valve
42. Leak channel
43. Safety-valve
44. Piston
45. Leak channel
46. Large-capacity cylinder
47. Leak channel
48. Safety-valve
49. Safety-valve
50. Leak channel

each inflation is prevented and the water manometer continuously indicates the approximate peak inspiratory pressure. In normal use the maximum pressure to which this safety-valve can be set is 35 cmH_2O. However, inflating pressures up to about 70 cmH_2O may be attained by reversing the 'water-trap off' blocker (13) from the position shown in fig. 52.3. This blocker, whose construction is more complex than can be shown in fig. 52.3, has the effect of introducing a spring-loaded valve, set to a pressure of about 35 cmH_2O, in series with the water manometer. The aneroid manometer (4) indicates the pressure at the mouth.

When 72% of the time of the forward stroke of the piston (44) has elapsed, a leak channel (47) in the piston shaft connects the pressure chamber (24) to atmosphere. Consequently, while the piston completes its forward stroke, the pressure which has been built up around the reservoir bag (22) falls rapidly to atmospheric, and inflation ceases. The one-way valve (6) closes and the pressure of the expired gas overcomes the very light spring-loading of the expiratory valve (7). Expired gas flows freely, along the expiratory tube (2), through the valve (7), the tap (19), and the diffusing tube of the injector (18), to atmosphere. The inspiratory phase therefore lasts for about two-thirds of the time of the forward stroke of the piston, i.e. for one-third of the respiratory cycle, and the inspiratory-expiratory ratio is nominally fixed at 1 : 2.

For the first one-quarter of the expiratory phase the piston is completing the last 28% of the time of its forward stroke and expiration is passive. This passive expiration is prolonged for the first 31% of the time of the return of the piston as a leak channel (42) in the piston rod allows the air in the left-hand side of the cylinder (46), which was drawn in during the previous inspiratory phase, to escape to atmosphere. Altogether passive expiration lasts for the first 31% of the expiratory phase. When the first 13% of the time of the return stroke of the piston (44) has elapsed, the leak channel (42) ceases to connect the left-hand side of the cylinder (46) to atmosphere. Air on the left of the piston (44) is now forced, through the one-way valve (27), to the injector (18), and, through the 'pressure regulator' throttle (28) and the compensating throttle (30), to atmosphere. The proportion of this air discharged through each of these pathways depends on the setting of the throttle (28). When there is a flow of air through the injector (18), it creates a negative pressure in the expiratory pathway. This effect lasts until 87% of the time of the return stroke of the piston (44) has elapsed, whereupon the leak channel (45) allows the remaining air in the left-hand side of the cylinder (46) to escape to atmosphere. Negative pressure, therefore, can be applied for 56% of the total expiratory time.

When 28% of the time of the return stroke of the piston has elapsed, the leak channel (47) ceases to connect the pressure chamber (24) to atmosphere. The pressure within the right-hand side of the cylinder (46), and hence in the chamber (24), now falls below atmospheric, the negative pressure produced being regulated by the 'dosing valve calibration' throttle (32) and the compensating throttle (34). The reservoir bag (22) now fills with a mixture of fresh gas and/or air. The flow of fresh gas is controlled by flowmeters connected to the inlet (16); the flow of air depends on the setting of the 'dosing valve' (14), which acts as an air-inlet control. The 'dosing valve' (14) is calibrated in litres per minute; this calibration is correct when the peak negative pressure, regulated by the control (32), is sufficient to move the pointer of the manometer (37) to the red mark on the dial. This corresponds to a negative pressure of about -30 cmH_2O.

Since the stroke of the piston (44) is fixed, any change made in the frequency alters the rate at which air is drawn into, or forced out of, either side of the cylinder (46). During the inspiratory and expiratory phases this would alter the positive and negative pressures produced in the chamber (24) for any particular settings of the throttles (35, 32) respectively. The throttle (34), connected to the frequency control (39), partly compensates for these effects, and therefore reduces the adjustment which must be made to the throttles (35, 32). Similarly, the throttle (30), also connected to the frequency control, reduces the adjustment which must be made to the throttle (28) in order to maintain the desired expiratory pressure when the frequency is altered. When the throttle (28) is fully closed, a rocker valve (29) blocks the inlet of the compensating throttle (30) and so ensures that maximum negative pressure is produced irrespective of the frequency. The throttle (28) can only be set in this way by pressing a button to release a limit stop, and then turning the control (28) to the upper part of its 'high' range.

In using this ventilator, the patient's ventilation requirement is estimated. The flow of fresh gas from the anaesthetic machine, together with any flow of air indicated by the calibrated 'dosing valve' (14), is made equal to the desired total minute-volume ventilation. The frequency of ventilation, and hence the tidal volume, and the maximum positive and negative pressures are set separately. In order to ensure a constant tidal volume the bag (22) must be collapsed at the end of each inflation, and for this reason the positive pressure in the driving circuit, indicated by the manometer (37), should be set, by the control (35), to at least 40 cmH_2O.

An occluder, on top of the one-way inlet valve (5), can be opened so that, should the patient attempt to breathe spontaneously, air can enter the inspiratory tube. The occluder must be closed if negative pressure is used, in which case the patient can draw gas only from the reservoir bag and that only during the very short time (about 5% of the expiratory cycle) between the cessation of negative pressure *in the pressure chamber* (24) and the start of active inflation.

Positive-pressure safety-valves (43, 48) and negative-pressure safety-valves (41, 49) set overall limits to the pressures produced in the cylinder (46), and eliminate any possibility of overloading the motor (38).

When it is wished to check the total minute-volume ventilation, the three-way tap (19) is turned temporarily to 'rebreathing position–spirometer' so as to direct the expired gas through the spirometer (17) instead of the injector (18). This does not alter the ventilation, provided the reservoir bag (22) is still completely emptied during each inspiratory phase. In the third, 'danger', position of this tap (19) the expiratory pathway is partly or wholly blocked to prevent the complete loss of positive pressure by the end of the expiratory phase.

If it is desired to empty the bag (22), or to allow it to fill quickly with air, the plunger valve (15) must be depressed during the inspiratory or expiratory phase respectively. A trap for condensed moisture is provided in the expiratory tubing. If manual ventilation is desired, a reservoir bag, connected to the port (9), may be brought into use by turning the tap (8). An electric elapsed-time indicator, mounted in the ventilator, shows the accumulated hours of use.

The ventilator may be used to drive a cuirasse which is connected to the port (26), here shown capped. The 'cuirasse/venturi' control (31) must be turned through 180° to the 'cuirasse' position, thereby reversing the action of the one-way valve within it and ensuring that the forward stroke of the piston (44) is effective in producing negative pressure in the cuirasse. The negative pressure in the cuirasse is set by the control (28) and indicated on the manometer (25) which is used only in this circumstance. On the return stroke of the piston, the reversed valve (31) allows a free escape of air from the left-hand side of the cylinder (46) to atmosphere.

In an earlier model the pressure produced by the movement of the piston to the left was used to inflate an 'expiration belt' which was placed around the lower thorax of the patient, so producing a mechanical compression of the chest during the expiratory phase.

DESCRIPTION OF THE ENGSTROM 'NARCOSIS RESPIRATOR' MODEL 200

The driving mechanism of this ventilator (fig. 52.4), which is intended for anaesthetic use, is the same as that described for the Engström 'Universal Respirator', the only differences being in the arrangement of the breathing circuits.

During the inspiratory phase, the reservoir bag (30) (fig. 52.5) is compressed, and the gas within it is forced, through the one-way valve (7) and the inspiratory tube (1), to the patient, the expiratory valve (8) being held closed by the pressure of the gas behind it. The 'to absorber/to shunt' tap (4) allows the inflating gas to be diverted through the soda-lime canister (3).

During the expiratory phase, the one-way valve (7) is closed, and expired gas flows, through the expiratory tube (2) and the expiratory valve (8), to the three-position tap (23).

When the tap (23) is set to the position marked 'venturi', the expired gas flows, through the diffuser tube of the injector (24), to atmosphere. The circuit is now a non-rebreathing one similar to that of the 'Universal Respirator', Model 150. There are two ways of setting the total minute-volume ventilation. If the 'dosing valve' (18) is closed the total fresh-gas flow, made up of oxygen and/or anaesthetic gases, supplied at the inlet (22) from flowmeters, must be set to equal the desired total minute-volume ventilation. Alternatively, part or all of the gas required for inflation consists of air, admitted through the port (19) and the 'dosing valve' (18), if the control (20) is in the 'non-rebreathing' position.

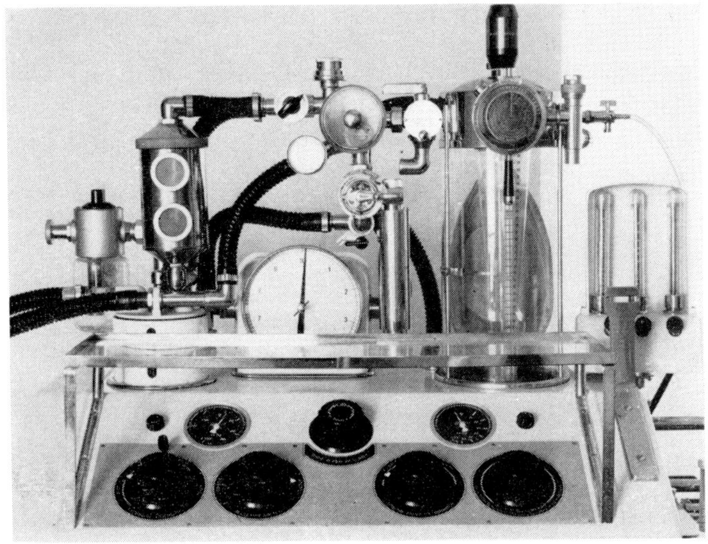

Fig. 52.4. The Engström 'Narcosis Respirator' Model 200.
Courtesy of Department of Medical Photography, Sully Hospital.

When the tap (23) is set to the position marked 'rebreathing position—spirometer', the expired gas flows through it to the spirometer control (25), by means of which it may be directed through or around the spirometer (26), and thence through the spring-loaded one-way valve (12). During the first, passive, part of the expiratory phase, the expired gas is stored in the bag (28). The subsequent course of the expired gas depends on the settings of the 'dosing valve' (18), the circuit control (20), and the spill valve (13).

The 'dosing valve' (18) is calibrated in 'litres/min', this figure indicating the volume of gas drawn into the bag (30) per minute, either from the storage bag (28) or from atmosphere depending on the setting of the control (20).

The control (20) has three settings; 'filling', 'rebreathing', and 'non-rebreathing'. The 'filling' position is intended only for use during the setting-up of the ventilator with either the non-rebreathing or the closed circuit. In this position, the 'dosing valve' (18) is rendered inoperative whatever it may be set to, since the air inlet (19) and the pathway from the storage bag (28) are both closed. The fresh-gas flow must now be set to equal the desired total minute-volume ventilation, and the spill valve (13) must be opened. Having established the desired respiratory pattern, the change to the closed circuit is made as follows. The calibrated 'dosing valve' (18) is set to the volume/min of expired gas which it is desired to draw into the reservoir bag (30) from the storage bag (28). The fresh-gas flow is then reduced to a level equal to the difference between the desired total minute-volume ventilation and the setting of the 'dosing valve' (18). As soon as this has been done, the control (20) is turned to the 'rebreathing' position (shown in fig. 52.5). During each expiratory phase a volume of expired gas, equal to the volume set on the 'dosing

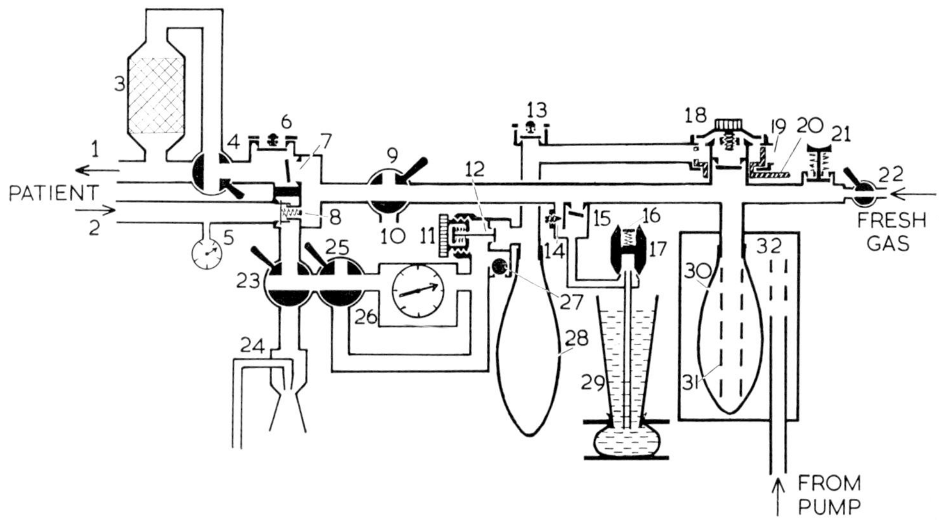

Fig. 52.5. Diagram of the breathing circuit of the Engström 'Narcosis Respirator' Model 200.

1. Inspiratory tube
2. Expiratory tube
3. Soda-lime canister
4. 'To absorber/to shunt' tap
5. Manometer
6. Air-inlet valve
7. One-way valve
8. Expiratory valve
9. 'For manual operation' tap
10. Port for connexion of manual bag
11. 'Expiratory resistance' control
12. Spring-loaded one-way valve
13. Spill valve
14. Preset needle valve
15. One-way valve
16. Spring-loaded valve
17. Reversible 'water-trap off' blocker
18. 'Dosing valve'
19. Air-inlet port
20. 'Rebreathing/filling/non-rebreathing' control
21. Spring-loaded valve
22. Fresh-gas inlet
23. 'Spirometer/venturi/danger' tap
24. Injector
25. Spirometer by-pass tap
26. Spirometer
27. Air-inlet safety-valve
28. Storage bag
29. Water manometer
30. Reservoir bag
31. Perforated tube
32. Rigid plastic pressure chamber

valve' (18) divided by the respiratory frequency, is now drawn into the reservoir bag (30) from the storage bag (28).

When a completely-closed circuit is to be used, the initial procedure is the same, but the setting of the 'dosing valve' (18) is now increased to equal the desired total minute-volume ventilation, and the fresh-gas flow is reduced to a basal-metabolic flow of oxygen. The soda-lime canister must be brought into the circuit and the spill valve (13) must be closed. When this has been done the control (20) is turned to the 'rebreathing' position.

For ward use, the ventilator may be used in exactly the same way except that oxygen and/or compressed air is substituted for anaesthetic gases. If room air is to be used, however, the control (20) is set to the 'non-rebreathing' position, in which the pathway between the bags (28) and (30) is closed and the air-inlet port (19) is open. All expired gas is now discharged through the valve (13) when the tap (23) is set to 'spirometer', or through the injector (24) when it is set to 'venturi', in which case negative pressure can be applied during the expiratory phase. The bag (30) is refilled with a mixture of air and fresh gas, the composition of which depends on the settings of the 'dosing valve' (18) and the fresh-gas flow.

It is essential that the storage bag (28) should neither overfill nor completely empty. If the bag (28) is emptied by the filling of the bag (30) air is drawn into the circuit through the ball valve (27), until such time as the fresh-gas flow is suitably increased. This prevents the transfer of the negative pressure within the bag (30) to the patient, but, of course, dilutes the anaesthetic mixture with air.

The 'end-expiratory pressure' valve (12) may be adjusted by the control (11) so as to maintain, if desired, a positive pressure in the expiratory pathway throughout the expiratory phase. It is calibrated in cmH_2O.

When the tap (23) is set to its 'danger' position, the expiratory pathway is partly or wholly blocked and there is a progressive rise in the end-expiratory pressure and in the functional residual capacity of the lungs.

An electrically-heated humidifier, identical with that in the 'Universal Respirator', Model 150, is available for connexion into the inspiratory pathway between the soda-lime canister (3) and the patient. An ether/halothane vaporizer is also available for connexion between the humidifier and the patient. The manufacturers state that flammable agents should not be allowed to enter the reservoir bag (30) at any time, and therefore such agents should be used only with the non-rebreathing circuit.

FUNCTIONAL ANALYSIS

This functional analysis and the 'Controls' section which follows, together with all the recordings of figs. 52.6, 52.7 and 52.8, refer to a 'Universal Respirator' Model 150 (non-rebreathing) ventilator. Some notes are added at the end of each section on the 'Narcosis Respirator' Model 200 which permits closed-circuit operation. The notes on the 'Narcosis Respirator' are based on published material and not on any physical tests or recordings.

Inspiratory phase

During this phase the piston (44) is driven to the right by the constant-speed motor (38) according to a preset pattern of movement so that it generates part of a virtually-perfect sine wave of flow. However, the volume of gas displaced, before the leak channel (47) opens to discharge the remainder of the stroke to atmosphere, is about 5 litres. Therefore the great majority of the flow generated by the piston must normally be blown to waste past the resistance of the throttles (34, 35) and the pattern of flow past this resistance is not greatly altered, even by large changes of tidal volume, and is hardly affected at all by moderate changes of lung characteristics. Therefore the pattern of pressure-drop across the resistance of the throttles is determined by the ventilator, and is little influenced by lung characteristics, i.e. the ventilator operates as a pressure generator during the inspiratory phase.

The pattern of generated pressure is not constant, nor is it the same as the pattern of flow through the throttles: this pattern of flow combines with the compliance of the large pressure chamber (24) (about 9 ml/cmH_2O), with the diminishing compliance of the cylinder volume to the right of the piston (44), and with the turbulent nature of the flow through the throttles (34, 35), to generate a pattern of pressure in the pressure chamber which, after a short delay, rises fairly steadily to some level at which it may remain for a further short time before the end of the phase. The rate of rise of pressure, the maximum pressure attained, and the period during which the maximum is maintained, all vary with the settings of the controls. They are also a little influenced by lung characteristics, but only when the changes of lung characteristics are sufficient to be accompanied by large changes in the waveform of flow into the patient. These statements are based on recordings (not reproduced here) of flow into the lungs, and of the pressure in the pressure chamber, made under a wide variety of extreme circumstances. They are supported by the recordings reproduced by Engström.[3] The statements confirm the deduction of the previous paragraph that the ventilator operates as a pressure generator during the inspiratory phase. However, there is a volume limit, set by the volume of gas in the reservoir bag at the start of the phase, and this limit is normally reached in each inspiratory phase. There are also pressure limits set by the blow-off valves (20, 48) but these do not normally operate. In addition, any fresh-gas flow entering the ventilator at (16) constitutes a small-constant-flow generator in parallel with the main pressure generator. Until the volume limit is reached, the flow-generating action is largely overridden by the action of the main pressure generator but, once the reservoir bag is fully collapsed, the ventilator operates as a pure flow generator. With this background information it is now possible to consider the effects of the changes of compliance and resistance shown in figs. 52.6 and 52.7.

In fig. 52.6 there was no fresh-gas flow, air being drawn in through the 'dosing valve' (14), and no negative pressure was applied during expiration. The gradually increasing pressure generated in the pressure chamber then leads to a gradually increasing pressure in the alveoli and at the mouth, while the flow also increases, at first rapidly then more slowly. These patterns are to be expected from the theory of the application of a steadily increasing pressure to a compliance and resistance in series. If continued long enough the flow would eventually reach a steady limit equal to the product of the rate of increase of generated pressure and the compliance, but here the volume limit, set by the reservoir bag, comes into play well before this limiting flow is achieved. The operation of the volume limit is clearly shown in fig. 52.6 by the cessation of flow, and by the equalization of mouth and alveolar pressures, in the last part of the inspiratory phase. The slight oscillation of flow about zero in this period is associated with 'bounce' of the wall of the reservoir bag when it is collapsed. The gradual decline in flow from the peak, particularly

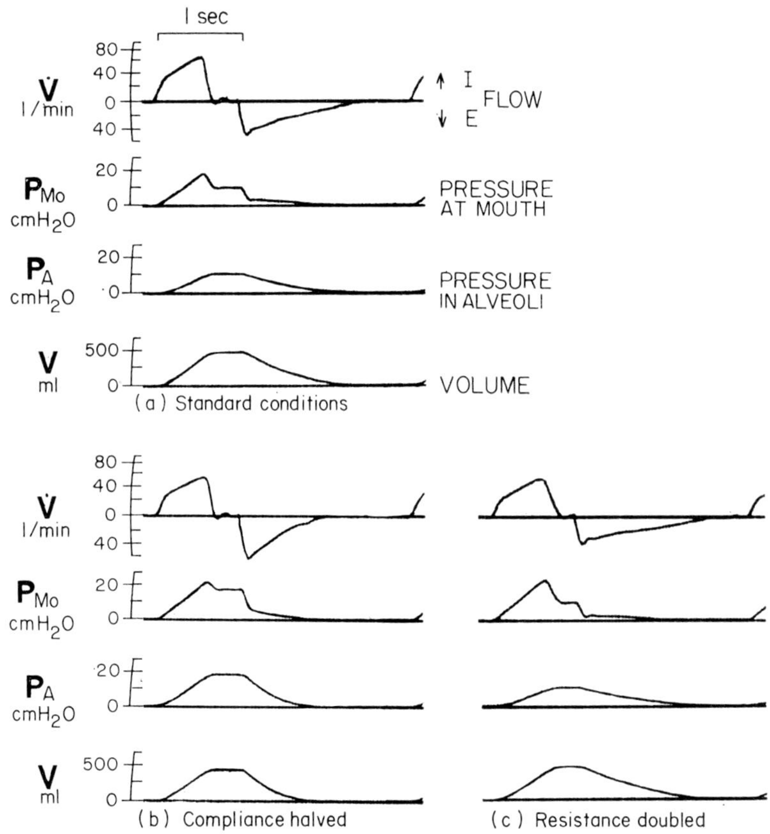

Fig. 52.6. Engström 'Universal Respirator' Model 150. Recordings, with the 'dosing valve' open but with no fresh-gas flow and with no negative pressure, showing the effects of changes of lung characteristics.

Standard conditions: 'selector switch' ((31) fig. 52.3) and three-way tap (19), set to 'venturi'; 'pressure regulator' (28), set to minimum; respiratory frequency, 20/min; fresh-gas flow, zero; 'dosing valve' (14), set to produce a tidal volume of 500 ml; 'emptying pressure' (35), set to give a peak reading of 55 cmH_2O on the dial manometer (37); 'dosing valve' calibration (32), set so that the needle of the dial manometer (37) just reached the red mark during the expiratory phase.

when the resistance is doubled, indicates that the volume limit is not abrupt: quite a large pressure difference, of the order of 50 cmH_2O, is required across the wall of the bag in order to mould the bag to the shape of the perforated tube (23) and expel the last 50 or 100 ml from the bag. Since the pressure chamber, in which the driving pressure is generated, is separated from the mouth by some resistance (equal to about half the 'standard' airway resistance) halving the compliance or doubling the airway resistance leads to some increase in the pressure recorded at the mouth (fig. 52.6b and c). However there is a reduction in peak flow under these conditions and close inspection will reveal that, when the resistance is doubled, the peak flow occurs later in the phase.

In fig. 52.7 the waveforms are made more complicated by the development of negative pressure in the expiratory phase and by a fresh-gas flow which supplies the whole of the patient's total minute-volume ventilation. When, towards the end of the return stroke of the piston, the negative pressure in the pressure chamber falls to a lesser magnitude than the negative pressure in the alveoli, gas begins to flow from the reservoir bag into the lungs giving an initial pulse of flow in what would otherwise have been part of the expiratory phase. Towards the end of the inspiratory phase, when the volume limit of the reservoir bag has been reached, the flow falls, not to zero, but to a value equal to the fresh-gas flow which is, of course, unaffected by changes of lung characteristics. On the other hand the mouth pressure at this time is considerably different in the three sets of tracings in fig. 52.7. During the central part of the phase the basic, increasing-pressure-generating mechanism is operative. The peak flow is less than in fig. 52.6 because it occurs earlier in the phase (when the generated pressure is less), but it is still somewhat reduced by a decrease in compliance or increase in resistance and again it occurs a little later when the resistance is increased.

In summary, therefore, the Engström ventilator operates, during the inspiratory phase, as an increasing-pressure generator with a volume limit which is normally reached during each phase. Once the volume limit is reached any fresh-gas flow acts as a small constant-flow generator.

Change-over from inspiratory phase to expiratory phase

This is time-cycled. It occurs when the piston has moved far enough to the right, in a time determined by the constant-speed motor (38) and the variator (40), for the leak channel (47) to open and release the pressure from the pressure chamber, so that the expiratory valve (7) opens. However, it is the time interval from the end of the previous *inspiratory* phase which is fully controlled by the ventilator: the time from the end of the previous expiratory phase may vary a little (see below).

Expiratory phase

With the 'pressure regulator' set to minimum, that is with the throttle (28) wide open, and therefore with no drive to the injector (18) (as in fig. 52.6), or with the three-way tap (19) set to 'spirometer', the ventilator operates as a constant, atmospheric, pressure generator, with the patient expiring freely to atmosphere at the injector (18) or at the outlet of the spirometer (17). There is some resistance between either of these points and the mouth so that the pressure at the mouth in fig. 52.6 does not fall to atmospheric immediately at the beginning of the phase. However, the characteristic changes of flow pattern, with changes of lung characteristics, show clearly in fig. 52.6: the peak flow is greater and the decay is more rapid when the compliance is halved (b) and the reverse is true when the resistance is doubled (c).

When the three-way tap (19) is set to 'Danger' the resistance to expiration is greatly increased, so that flow decays only very slowly (fig. 52.8f); but the action is still that of an atmospheric-pressure generator.

When the three-way tap is set to 'Venturi', and the 'pressure regulator' is set above

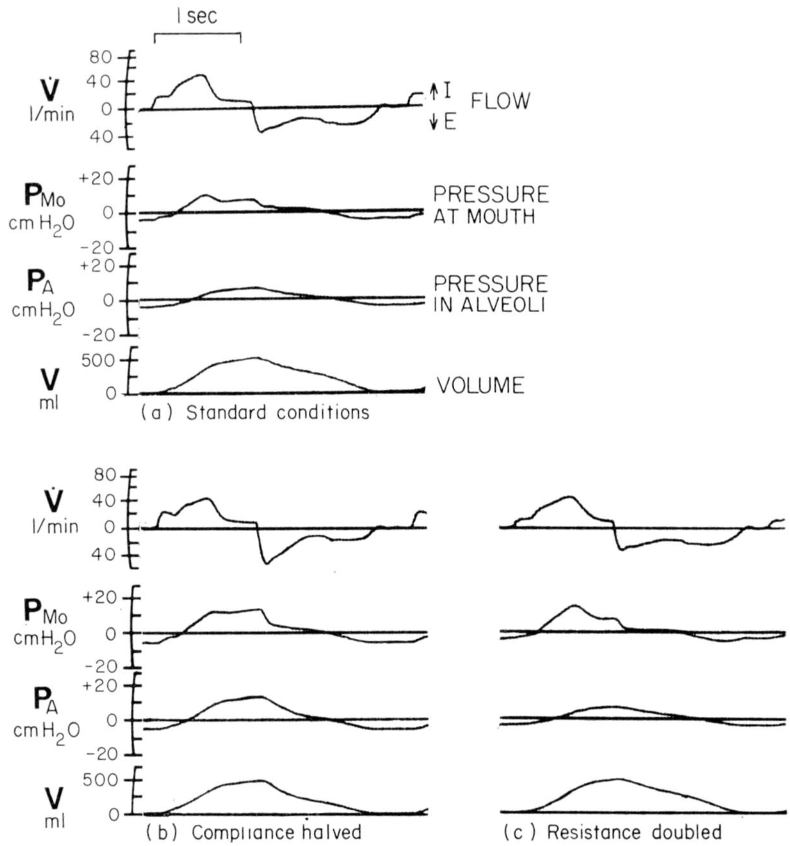

Fig. 52.7. Engström 'Universal Respirator' Model 150. Recordings, with the 'dosing valve' closed, with a continuous fresh-gas flow, and with negative pressure in the expiratory phase, showing the effects of changes of lung characteristics.

Standard conditions: 'selector switch' ((31) fig. 52.3) and three-way tap (19), set to 'venturi'; 'dosing valve' (14), closed; respiratory frequency, 20/min; fresh-gas flow, set to produce a tidal volume of 500 ml; 'emptying pressure' (35), set to give a peak reading of 55 cmH_2O on the dial manometer (37); 'dosing valve calibration' (32), set so that the needle of the dial manometer (37) just reached the red mark during the expiratory phase (since the 'dosing valve' was closed this was not strictly necessary but it was desirable because, with negative pressure in the lungs during the expiratory phase, the pattern of negative pressure in the pressure chamber could influence the time of onset of inspiratory flow—see the functional analysis); 'pressure regulator' (28), set to produce an end-expiratory alveolar pressure of -3 cmH_2O.

minimum, the injector (18) is activated by a near-sine wave of flow during most of the return stroke of the piston, that is during most of the last three-quarters of the expiratory phase. The characteristics of the injector are such that it then generates a half cycle of a near-sine wave of negative pressure. The pressure at the mouth in fig. 52.7 varies a little with lung characteristics because of the resistance between the mouth and the injector. In addition, when the generated pressure falls to a value which is less negative than the pressure which has then been developed in the alveoli, the expiratory valve (7) closes and the system behaves as a zero-flow generator for the remainder of the phase: there is no flow into or out of the lungs because both the inspiratory (6) and the expiratory (7) valves are held closed by pressure differences. In fig. 52.7 it can be seen that, for all values of lung characteristics used, there is a period at the end of the expiratory phase in which there is no flow and in which the mouth pressure is equal to the alveolar pressure, and steady at some negative value.

Change-over from expiratory phase to inspiratory phase

Superficially this change-over would appear to be time-cycled, occurring as soon as the piston has moved far enough to the right to prevent escape of gas from the cylinder through the leak channel (50) and start building up pressure in the pressure chamber. However, if the resistance to expiration is very high, due either to a very high airway resistance or (fig. 52.8f) to the three-way tap (19) being set to 'Danger', the alveolar pressure at the end of the expiratory phase is positive and inspiratory flow cannot start (i.e. the change-over does not occur) until some later time at which the pressure in the pressure chamber exceeds the pressure in the alveoli. Similarly, if a negative pressure is developed in the alveoli during the expiratory phase, inspiratory flow will start at some earlier moment, in what would otherwise be the expiratory phase. This moment is when the negative pressure in the pressure chamber has fallen to a value which is slightly less negative than the pressure in the alveoli. Thus in fig. 52.7, for which negative pressure was used, the expiratory phase is appreciably shorter than in fig. 52.6, for which no negative pressure was used. Even when the alveolar pressure is atmospheric at the end of the expiratory phase, it is still true to say that inspiratory flow does not commence until the pressure in the pressure chamber exceeds the pressure in the alveoli. Therefore the most general statement that can be made about this change-over is that it is pressure-cycled: it occurs when the pressure in the pressure chamber becomes positive with respect to the alveolar pressure. It is legitimate to make this statement because, although the pattern of pressure in the pressure chamber is almost entirely determined by the ventilator and is practically uninfluenced by lung characteristics, the alveolar pressure at the end of the expiratory phase, and therefore the moment at which the pressure difference becomes such as to initiate inspiratory flow, does indeed depend upon lung characteristics.

However, the rise of pressure in the pressure chamber, after the leak channel (50) has become inoperative, is fairly rapid in relation to the highest positive pressure likely to be encountered in the lungs at the end of the expiratory phase. Therefore, the change-over will never be much delayed beyond the closing of the leak channel (50). Similarly, with negative pressure in the alveoli at the end of the expiratory phase, the change-over will never occur much before the opening of the leak channel (50). Therefore the maximum variation in the time of change-over is from a little before the leak channel (50) opens on the reverse stroke of the piston to a little after it closes on the forward stroke — a little more than 7% of a respiratory cycle. Furthermore, a change from one extreme to the other would rarely occur in response to a change in lung characteristics. Therefore, for practical purposes, the change-over can be regarded as time-cycled, but the timing is earlier when negative pressure is developed in the alveoli. The inspiratory-expiratory ratio is then changed from 1 : 2 (fig. 52.6) to 1 : 1·5 (fig. 52.7).

'Narcosis Respirator' Model 200

When the closed circuit is used on this model, negative pressure cannot be applied and the ventilator operates as a constant-pressure generator throughout the expiratory phase. The generated pressure can be made positive by adjustment of the valve (11, 12) (fig. 52.5). Since negative pressure cannot be developed in the alveoli the change-over from the expiratory phase to the inspiratory phase is almost perfectly time-cycled.

CONTROLS

Total ventilation

This can be directly controlled and is nominally equal to the sum of the fresh-gas flow and of the ventilation set on the calibrated 'dosing valve' (14). However, this is only so provided that the 'emptying pressure' control is set high enough (throttle (35) is sufficiently closed) for the reservoir bag (22) to be emptied in each inspiratory phase. In addition, the calibration marks on the 'dosing valve' (14) are accurate only if, during the expiratory phase, the needle of the manometer (37) just reaches the red mark, indicating a peak negative pressure in the pressure chamber (24) of about -30 cmH_2O. This must be regulated by means of the 'dosing valve calibration' control (32). Therefore, unless the 'dosing valve' (14) is set to zero, any change in the setting of the respiratory-frequency control (39) must be followed by an adjustment of the 'dosing valve calibration' control (32) in order to ensure that the reservoir bag is refilled with the correct volume during each expiratory phase and so prevent a change of ventilation. In addition, whether the 'dosing valve' is in use or not, a change in the settings of some of the other controls may need to be followed by an increase in the 'emptying pressure' (a screwing down of the throttle (35)). This is in order to ensure that, whatever volume is drawn into the reservoir bag during the expiratory phase, it is all delivered to the patient during the inspiratory phase; otherwise the total ventilation would fall. Since the 'standard conditions' of fig. 52.8 were with the 'dosing valve' closed and with the 'emptying pressure' set high enough to ensure emptying of the reservoir bag early in the inspiratory phase, the changes of control settings tried were not sufficient to alter the total ventilation accidentally.

Reminders are engraved at the side of the 'dosing valve calibration' (32) and 'emptying pressure' (35) controls, of the need to keep them adjusted in the manner described, in order to maintain the ventilation set by the fresh-gas flow and 'dosing valve' (14). Even when these reminders are acted upon, the ventilation received by the patient is always a little less than the sum of the fresh-gas flow and the ventilation set on the 'dosing valve'. This is because an appreciable fraction of the volume discharged from the reservoir bag in each inspiratory phase is absorbed in the compliance of the humidifier (3) and breathing tubes (about 5 ml/cmH_2O with adult breathing tubes). Allowances are made for this in the 'Ventilation Nomogram' supplied with the machine, but it should be noted that the allowance to be made varies with changes of lung characteristics. Of the changes tried here the one which had the biggest effect was when the compliance was halved in the absence of negative pressure (compare (b) with (a) in (fig. 52.6)). This increased the end-inspiratory pressure at the mouth (and hence in the humidifier) by 10 cmH_2O so that a further 50 ml was absorbed in the humidifier compliance and the tidal volume was reduced from 500 ml to 450 ml and hence the total ventilation was reduced from 10 to 9 litres/min. Apart from this effect, of the compliance of the humidifier and breathing tubes, a large drop in the patient's compliance or a large rise in resistance could lead to a failure of the reservoir bag to empty and hence to a fall in ventilation, unless the 'emptying pressure' were increased.

When the total ventilation is deliberately changed by means of the fresh-gas flow or 'dosing valve' setting it is the tidal volume which is changed while the respiratory frequency is unaltered (fig. 52.8b). When the increase is achieved by means of an adjustment to the 'dosing valve' it is necessary also to adjust the 'dosing valve calibration' control (32) to maintain the validity of the calibration on the 'dosing valve'.

Tidal volume

This cannot be directly controlled but is equal to the total ventilation, set in the manner and subject to the variations described above, divided by the respiratory frequency.

Respiratory frequency

This is directly and exclusively controlled by the respiratory-frequency control (39). It is quite uninfluenced by other controls or by lung characteristics. When the respiratory frequency is changed the total ventilation is unaltered (subject to the provisos discussed above) and therefore the tidal volume is changed in inverse proportion (fig. 52.8c).

Inspiratory-expiratory ratio

This cannot be directly controlled but is subject to some incidental variation. The start of the expiratory phase coincides with the opening of the leak channel (47) to atmosphere, about two-thirds of the way through the forward stroke of the piston. However the start of the inspiratory phase is not rigidly related to any moment in the forward or reverse strokes of the piston; instead it occurs when the pressure in the pressure chamber first exceeds the pressure in the alveoli. As explained in the functional analysis above, this results in an inspiratory-expiratory ratio of about 1 : 2 if the end-expiratory alveolar

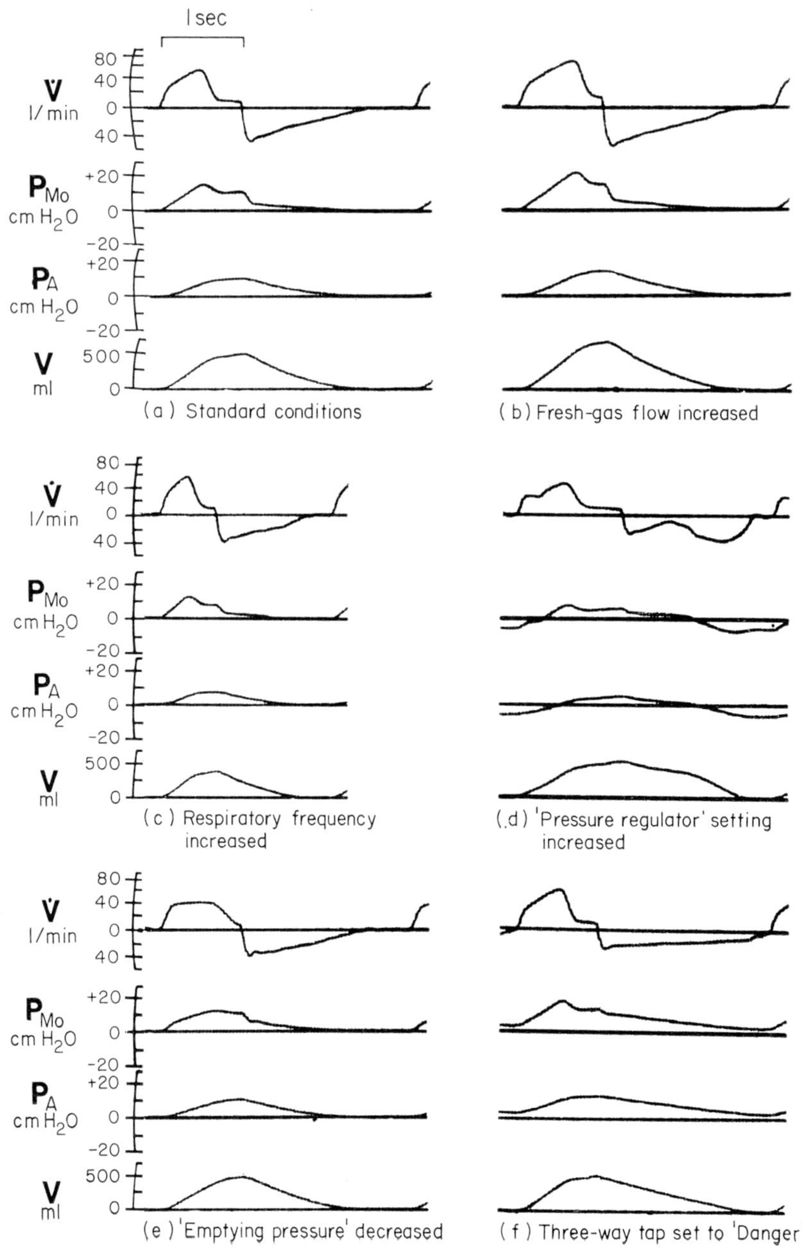

pressure is atmospheric or above (fig. 52.8 except d) but of about 1 : 1·5 if it is negative (fig. 52.8d). Thus the change from one value to the other is occasioned mainly by the introduction or removal of the injector action but, if negative pressure is being applied during the expiratory phase, the change of inspiratory-expiratory ratio may occur as a result of changes of lung characteristics if these change the end-expiratory alveolar pressure from negative to positive or vice versa. The precise value of the ratio in either condition depends to a very small extent upon the settings of other controls and on lung characteristics.

Inspiratory waveforms

During the inspiratory phase this ventilator operates as an increasing-pressure generator with a volume limit, and the effect of this on the lungs determines the flow waveforms. The flow increases, rapidly at first, and then more slowly to a maximum; it then declines, usually reaching a value equal to the fresh-gas flow before the end of the phase. The waveform of inspiratory flow can be altered by changing the rate of increase of pressure (the setting of the 'emptying pressure' control (35)) although the flow waveform also depends upon lung characteristics. If the rate of increase of pressure is high in relation to the tidal volume, the peak flow occurs early in the phase and the lungs are held inflated for the later part of the phase (fig. 52.6a). On the other hand, if the rate of increase of pressure is low, the peak flow occurs later in the phase and the inspiratory flow falls off only at the very end of the phase, so that the delivery of the tidal volume is spread more evenly over the duration of the phase (fig. 52.8e). However, if the fresh-gas flow supplies all the total ventilation then, even with a high rate of increase of generated pressure, a moderate rate of inflation is maintained to the very end of the phase (fig. 52.7 and fig. 52.8 except (e)).

When the tidal volume is increased by increasing the fresh-gas flow (fig. 52.8b) or the setting of the 'dosing valve' (14), it takes longer to empty the reservoir bag so that flow goes on increasing for a greater fraction of the inspiratory phase: the peak flow is higher and occurs later in the phase.

When the respiratory frequency was increased from 20/min to 30/min under other-

---

Fig. 52.8. Engström 'Universal Respirator' Model 150. Recordings, with the 'dosing valve' closed, with a continuous flow of fresh gas, but with no negative pressure during the expiratory phase, showing the effects of changes in the settings of the controls.

(a) Standard conditions as in fig. 52.7 except that the 'pressure regulator' (28) was set to minimum.

(b) Fresh-gas flow increased 50%.

(c) Respiratory frequency increased to 30/min.

(d) 'Pressure regulator' (28) setting increased to the maximum of the 'medium' range.

(e) 'Emptying pressure' (35) decreased to minimum giving a peak reading on the dial manometer of about 20 cmH_2O.

(f) Three-way tap (19) turned in the direction of 'Danger' as far as '2 o'clock', that is, not so far as to bring the pointer to the '0' of the 0–5 scale.

wise 'standard conditions' (compare (c) with (a) in fig. 52.8) the flow waveform was 'compressed' in the time dimension but not much altered otherwise.

Expiratory waveforms

This ventilator operates as a pressure generator for all or most of the expiratory phase so that the expiratory flow waveform is determined by the effect of the generated pressure on the lungs and varies with lung characteristics (figs. 52.6 and 52.7). However, the pattern of generated pressure and hence the resultant pattern of flow can be altered. When the injector (18) is not in use during the expiratory phase the ventilator operates as a constant, atmospheric, pressure generator (fig. 52.6 and 52.8 except (d)) giving the characteristic flow pattern of an initial peak followed by a gradual decay. The initial peak can be reduced and the decay made slower by increasing the resistance in series with the pressure generator, by means of turning the three-way tap (19) to 'Danger'. However, even before the pointer reaches the '0' of the 0–5 scale of 'Danger', the resistance is high enough for the alveolar pressure not to fall to atmospheric during the expiratory phase under otherwise 'standard' conditions (fig. 52.8f).

When the injector is brought into use by setting the three-way tap (19) to 'Venturi' and the 'pressure regulator' control (28) above minimum, a half cycle of a near-sine wave of negative pressure is developed in about the last three-quarters of the expiratory phase giving a surge of flow at that time (fig. 52.8d). In addition the initial peak of flow, during the atmospheric-pressure-generating part of the phase, is reduced because of the lower end-expiratory, and hence end-inspiratory, alveolar pressures. Another corollary of using the injector is that, as discussed in the functional analysis, when the generated pressure becomes less negative than the pressure developed in the alveoli, the ventilator operates as a zero-flow generator for the remainder of the expiratory phase, with both inspiratory (6) and expiratory (7) valves held closed by pressure differences.

Pressure limits

When the injector is not in use the alveolar pressure during the expiratory phase approaches the atmospheric pressure which is generated throughout the phase. In most of the recordings of figs. 52.6 and 52.8 it does so very closely; but the approach is not close when resistance to expiration is high as a result, either of setting the three-way tap (19) to 'Danger' (fig. 52.8f), or of a high respiratory resistance (higher than that of fig. 52.6c).

When the injector is in use the alveolar pressure will normally fall to a negative value, but not necessarily so if the respiratory resistance is very high. The end-expiratory alveolar pressure which is in fact developed depends on the interaction of the generated pressure and the lung characteristics and probably also, to some extent, on the total ventilation and respiratory frequency.

The peak alveolar pressure at the end of the inspiratory phase cannot be directly controlled; whatever the minimum alveolar pressure at the end of the expiratory phase happens to be, the peak alveolar pressure exceeds it by an amount equal to the tidal volume divided by the compliance.

'Narcosis Respirator' Model 200

When the closed circuit is used on this model negative pressure cannot be applied and the consequent variation in inspiratory-expiratory ratio is absent. Also, the lower limit of alveolar pressure, at the end of the expiratory phase, cannot be negative, but the constant generated pressure, to which the alveolar pressure approaches during the phase, can be made positive by means of the 'end-expiratory pressure' valve (11) (fig. 52.5). In all other respects the actions of the controls appear to be similar to those in the 'Universal Respirator' Model 150.

REFERENCES

1 ENGSTRÖM C.G. (1954) Treatment of severe cases of respiratory paralysis by the Engström Universal Respirator. *Br. med. J.* **2**, 666.

2 BJÖRK V.O., ENGSTRÖM C.G., FRIBERG O., FEYCHTING H. and SWENSSON A. (1956) Ventilatory problems in thoracic anaesthesia; a volume-cycling device for controlled respiration. *J. thorac. Surg.* **31**, 117.

3 ENGSTRÖM C.G. (1963) The clinical application of prolonged controlled ventilation. *Acta anaesth. Scand.* Supp. **13**, 25.

CHAPTER 53

The 'Fazakerley' Ventilator[1]

DESCRIPTION

This ventilator (fig. 53.2) is driven by a supply of compressed gas from a cylinder or from a compressor. In the case of the former, an injector fitted close to the cylinder to entrain air considerably economizes in the use of the compressed gas. The pressure at the apparatus should be in the range of 2–7 lb/in^2.

Fig. 53.1 shows the ventilator during the expiratory phase. Driving gas enters the ventilator at (6) and flows through the jet of an injector (8) which is raised or lowered by the control (7). With the control (7) screwed down as far as it will go, the maximum negative pressure is created, sucking gas out of the pressure chamber (2) which contains the reservoir bag (3). When the control (7) is unscrewed, the injector nozzle (8) is withdrawn leaving a space between it and the main housing of the valve; the entrainment action is now lost because driving gas entering at (6) escapes around the injector (8).

The small concertina bag (14), which was distended during the inspiratory phase, slowly collapses as its contents leak out through the constriction (9) which controls the duration of the expiratory phase. When the volume within the bag (14) falls to a certain level, the 1-inch diameter steel ball (11) rolls onto and closes the exhaust valve (12). The inspiratory phase begins.

During the inspiratory phase the valve (12) is shut and the bag (14) begins to fill through the Kendrick one-way valve (15). Gas enters the pressure chamber (2) compressing the reservoir bag (3) and forcing the gas within it, through the breathing tube (1), to the patient. The pressure in the patient circuit is shown on the water manometer (5) which also acts as a safety-valve. However, at the end of the expiratory phase, any excess gas within the patient circuit can spill out through the valve (4) which can be set to some maximum positive pressure. As the reservoir bag (3) is compressed the bag (14) gradually expands until, at some preset pressure determined by the control (10), which alters the tension of the spring (13), the steel ball (11) rolls down and snaps open the exhaust valve (12), initiating the next expiratory phase. The pressure in the chamber (2) is freely transmitted to the bag (14) through the Kendrick valve (15). During the expiratory phase, gas can only escape from the bag (14) through the control (9).

The frequency of ventilation is varied by adjustment of the duration of the expiratory

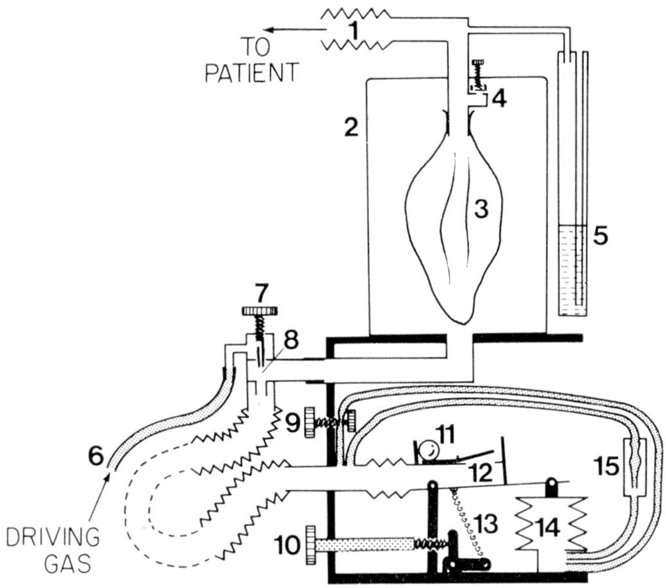

Fig. 53.1. Diagram of the 'Fazakerley' ventilator.

1. Breathing tube
2. Rigid plastic pressure chamber
3. Reservoir bag
4. Spill valve
5. Water manometer and safety-valve
6. Driving-gas inlet
7. Negative-pressure control
8. Injector
9. Expiratory-time control
10. Cycling-pressure control
11. Steel ball
12. Exhaust valve
13. Spring
14. Concertina bag
15. Kendrick one-way valve

phase by the control (9) but also depends on the cycling pressure set by the control (10).

Fig. 53.3 shows the 'Fazakerley' ventilator with a compressor in a single unit.[2]

FUNCTIONAL ANALYSIS

Inspiratory phase

When driven by a positive-displacement-pump type of compressor, the ventilator operates as a constant-flow generator owing to the characteristics of the pump (see p. 85).

When driven by a compressed-gas cylinder via an injector, the mode of operation depends upon the injector characteristics but is probably that of a high-constant-pressure generator with substantial series resistance.

In either case the fresh-gas supply to the patient circuit acts as a small-constant-flow generator, supplementing the action of the main flow or pressure generator.

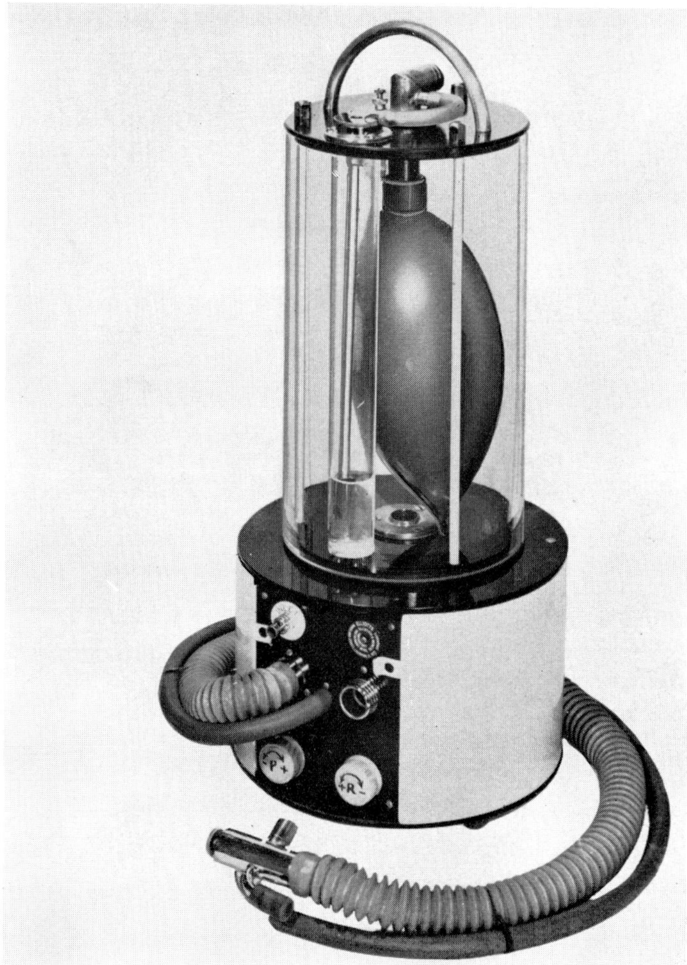

Fig. 53.2. The 'Fazakerley' ventilator.

Courtesy of Elliotts (Liverpool) Ltd.

Change-over from inspiratory phase to expiratory phase

This change-over is pressure-cycled: the pressure in the control concertina bag (14) which produces cycling is that applied to the patient via the reservoir bag.

Expiratory phase

In this phase the ventilator operates as a constant, negative, pressure generator with substantial series resistance, owing to the characteristics of the injector (8). The fresh-gas flow now slightly impedes the main pressure-generating action.

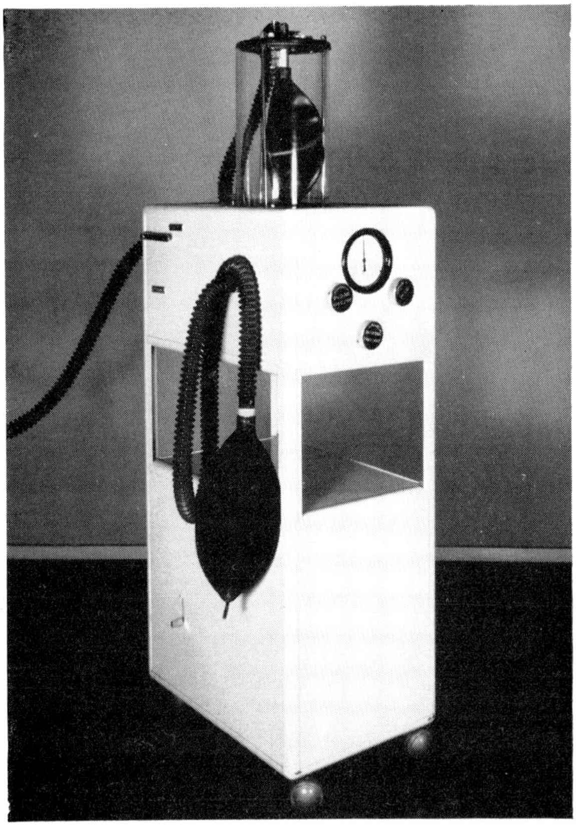

Fig. 53.3. The Hillard self-contained 'Fazakerley' ventilator.

Courtesy of *Anaesthesia*.[2]

Change-over from expiratory phase to inspiratory phase

This change-over is time-cycled: the expiratory time is equal to the time in which enough air leaks out of the control concertina bag (14) for cycling to occur. This time is uninfluenced by the patient; but it depends on the force of the spring (13) as well as on the setting of the control (9). Therefore raising the cycling pressure at the end of the inspiratory phase, by means of extending this spring further, shortens the expiratory phase.

REFERENCES

1 Esplen J.R. (1956) The Fazakerley respirator. *Br. J. Anaesth.* **28**, 176.
2 Hillard E.K. (1958) A self-contained respirator. *Anaesthesia*, **13**, 347.

CHAPTER 54

The Frumin Ventilator[1]

DESCRIPTION

This ventilator (fig. 54.1) is intended primarily for anaesthetic use but may also be used in the ward. It may be used with a non-rebreathing or a closed circuit. It is shown in fig. 54.1 combined with flowmeters and a halothane vaporizer for anaesthetic use.

Driving gas at a pressure of 25–60 lb/in^2 is supplied at the inlet (26) (fig. 54.2), and flows through the filter (25), the pressure regulator (22), and the 'on/off' tap (15). It flows

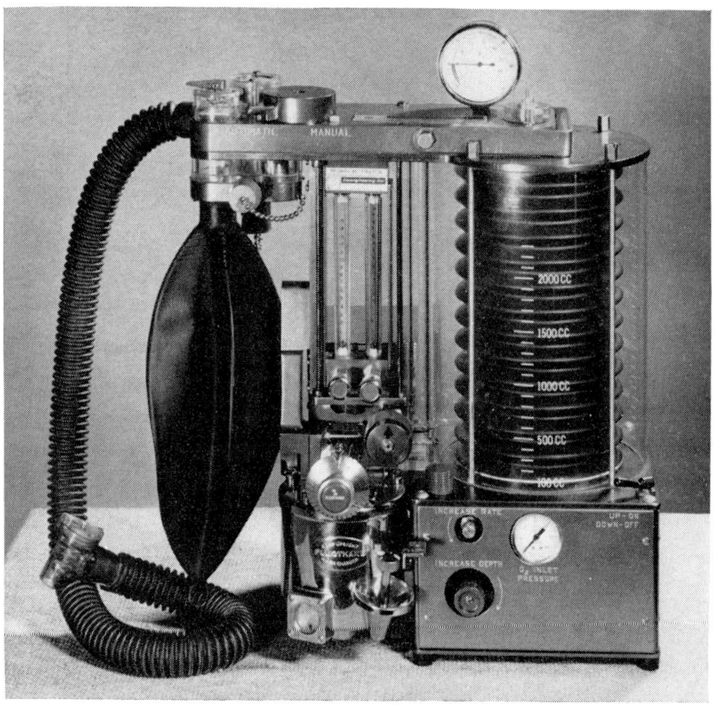

Fig. 54.1. The Frumin ventilator.

Courtesy of Invengineering Inc.

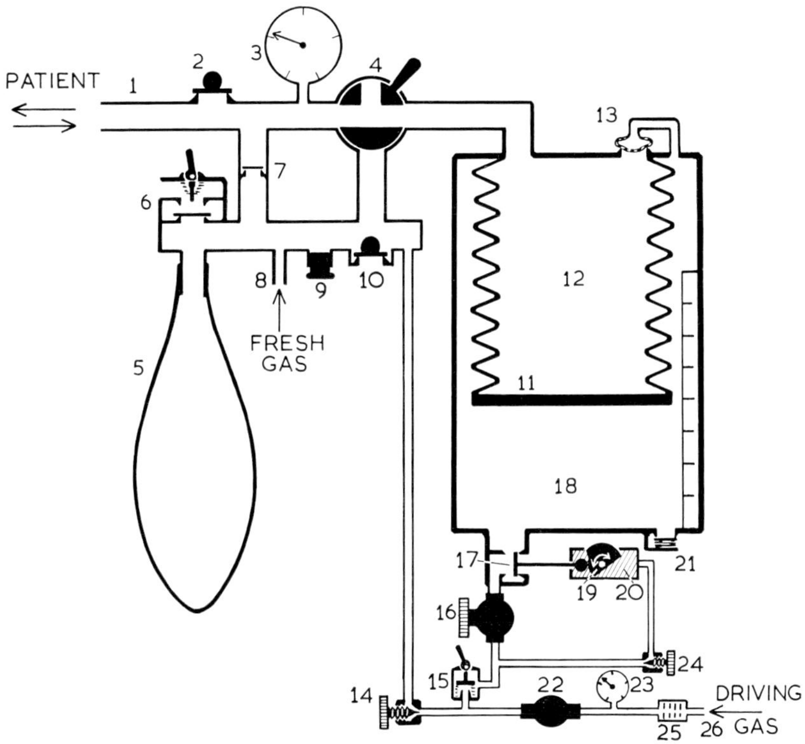

Fig. 54.2. Diagram of the Frumin ventilator.

1. Breathing tube
2. Safety-valve
3. Manometer
4. 'Manual/automatic' tap
5. Reservoir bag
6. Steen 'pressure-equalizing' valve
7. One-way valve
8. Fresh-gas inlet
9. Stopper
10. Emergency air inlet
11. Weight
12. Concertina reservoir bag
13. Inflatable mushroom valve
14. Oxygen supply valve
15. On/off tap
16. 'Increase depth' control
17. Valve
18. Rigid plastic pressure chamber
19. Oscillating cam
20. Compressed-air motor
21. Safety-valve
22. Pressure regulator
23. Pressure gauge
24. 'Increase rate' control
25. Filter
26. Driving-gas inlet

continuously, past the 'rate' control (24), to the compressed-air motor (20), which oscillates the cam (19), alternately opening and closing the valve (17). During the inspiratory phase, the outlet port of the valve (17) is closed, and driving gas flows, through the 'depth' control (16) and the valve (17), to the rigid plastic pressure chamber (18). The concertina reservoir bag (12) is compressed and, since the mushroom valve (13) is distended, the gas within the bag is forced past the 'automatic/manual' tap (4) to the patient. The inspiratory pressure is limited to about 35 cmH_2O by the safety-valve (2). The maximum pressure may be increased to about 50 cmH_2O by adding weights to this

CHAPTER 55

The Greer and Donald Ventilator[1]

DESCRIPTION

Driving gas at a pressure of 10 lb/in^2 enters at (21) (fig. 55.2) passing, through a needle valve (20) and a solenoid-operated inlet valve (18), to the rigid plastic pressure chamber (11). Pressure builds up in this chamber (11) and compresses the concertina reservoir bag (1), forcing the gas within it to the patient. When bag (1) reaches the top of its stroke

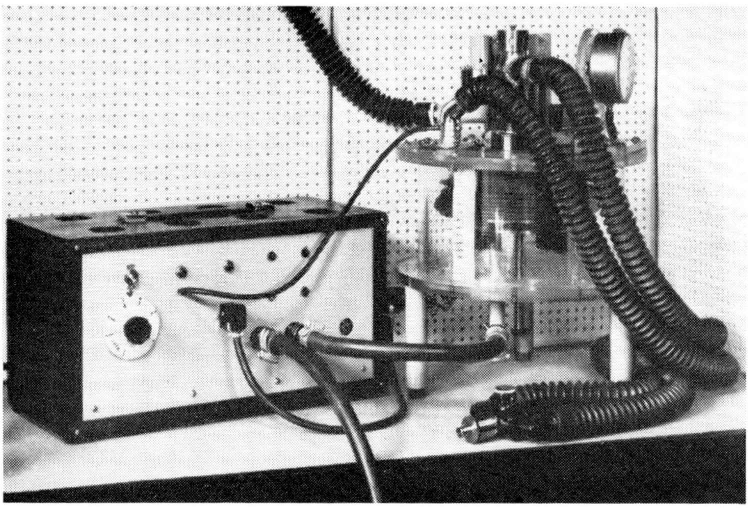

Fig. 55.1. The Greer and Donald ventilator.

Courtesy of *British Journal of Anaesthesia*.[1]

it presses a microswitch (4). This switch completes the circuit of one of the operating coils of the relay (14), the action of which is reversed. The electrical circuit to the solenoid valve (18) is completed and the circuit to the solenoid valve (17) is interrupted. The driving-gas supply to the chamber (11) is now cut off, and the contents of the chamber are vented to atmosphere through the exhaust valve (17) and the port (16).

The reservoir bag expands under the influence of a weight in its base and expired

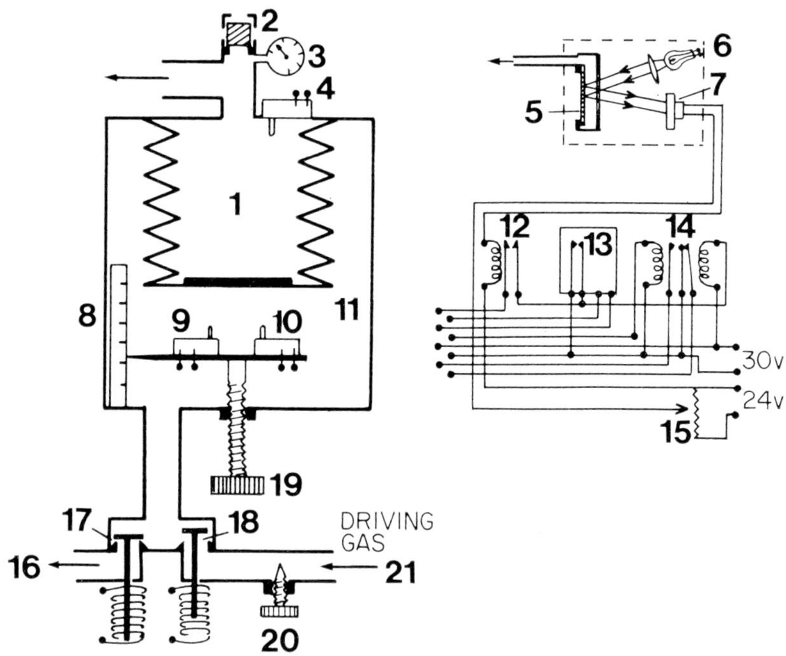

Fig. 55.2. Diagram of the Greer and Donald ventilator.

1. Concertina reservoir bag with weighted base
2. Safety-valve
3. Manometer
4. Microswitch
5. Aluminized Terylene flap
6. Light source
7. Phototransistor
8. Volume scale
9. Microswitch
10. Microswitch
11. Rigid plastic pressure chamber
12. Relay
13. Electronic timer
14. Double relay
15. Patient-triggering-sensitivity control
16. Driving-gas exhaust outlet
17. Solenoid-operated exhaust valve
18. Solenoid-operated inlet valve
19. Tidal-volume control
20. Needle valve
21. Driving-gas inlet

gas flows into it. When the bag has descended sufficiently, its bottom plate makes contact with the microswitches (9, 10). The switch (10) starts the timer (13) which, after a preset delay, energizes the second coil of the relay (14), the action of which is again reversed. The electrical circuit to the solenoid-operated valve (17) is completed, and the circuit to the solenoid valve (18) is interrupted. The valve (17) closes, the valve (18) opens, pressure builds up in the chamber (11), and the next inspiratory phase begins.

The speed of inflation is governed by the needle valve (20) which controls the rate of delivery of driving gas to the chamber (11). The duration of the expiratory phase is determined by the electronic timer (13). The tidal volume delivered from the bag (1) is adjusted by the screw (19) which alters the height of the plate carrying the switches

(9, 10). This volume is indicated on the scale (8). The safety-valve (2) consists of a weight lifted by any escaping gas. It limits the positive pressure attainable to 25 cmH_2O. The manometer (3) indicates the pressure in the patient circuit.

If the patient takes a breath while the apparatus is in the expiratory phase and the bag (1) has closed the microswitch (9), the slight negative pressure produced by the patient is transmitted through a narrow-bore tube running from the inspiratory tube to a small chamber containing a light aluminized Terylene flap (5). When the flap is in its resting position the light from the lamp (6) is focused and reflected on to a phototransistor (7), which passes enough current to hold the relay (12) open. When the flap is lifted by the negative pressure, the light no longer falls on the phototransistor (7) and the relay (12) closes. The circuit of the relay coil (14) is completed and an inspiratory phase commences. The speed of operation of this trigger is only 0·1 second. The phototransistor (7) and the relay (12) are so connected with the microswitch (9) that they can only operate when the switch (9) is closed. The current from the phototransistor is controlled by the resistance (15). This resistance therefore determines the degree of negative pressure needed to initiate an inspiratory phase, i.e. the sensitivity of the patient-triggering mechanism.

This apparatus is primarily intended as an assister of respiration. Should spontaneous breathing fail, automatic ventilation commences. The delay timer (13) incorporates a relay whose contacts close at any preset interval up to 5 seconds after the switch (10) has been closed by the downward movement of the bag (1). Thus, if the patient fails to take a breath during this preset period, an inspiratory phase commences automatically.

Two methods of connecting this ventilator to the patient have been described. In one (fig. 55.3) the ventilator forms part of a closed circuit with carbon-dioxide absorption. In this method it is recommended that the expiratory valve on the Y-piece at the patient be left slightly open to act as a blow-off valve for the venting of excess gas. In the other (fig. 55.4) all rebreathing is eliminated, all the expired gas being vented to atmosphere. In this arrangement the rate of the fresh-gas flow limits the minute-volume ventilation.

FUNCTIONAL ANALYSIS

Closed circuit (fig. 55.3)

Inspiratory phase

In this phase the ventilator operates as a constant-flow generator, owing to the constant high pressure of the driving gas applied to the resistance of the needle valve (20) (fig. 55.2). A pressure limit due to the blow-off valve on the Y-piece comes into operation shortly before the end of the phase.

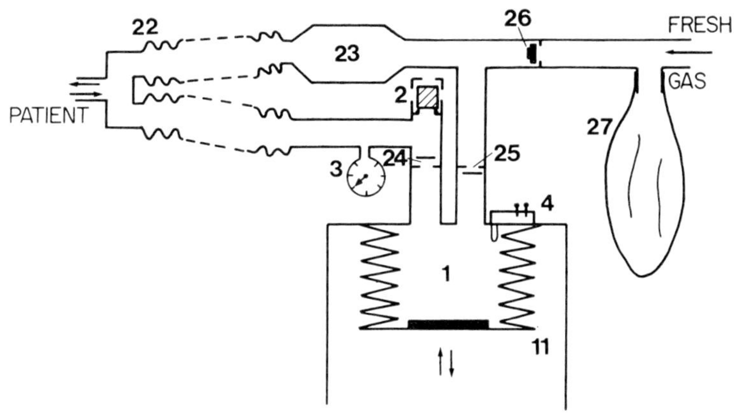

Fig. 55.3. Diagram of the Greer and Donald ventilator connected to a carbon-dioxide absorption circuit.

1. Concertina reservoir bag
2. Safety-valve
3. Manometer
4. Microswitch
11. Rigid plastic pressure chamber
22. Y-piece for connexion to patient
23. Soda-lime canister
24. One-way inspiratory valve
25. One-way expiratory valve
26. Weighted one-way valve. This opens during the expiratory phase to admit fresh gas
27. Storage bag for fresh gas

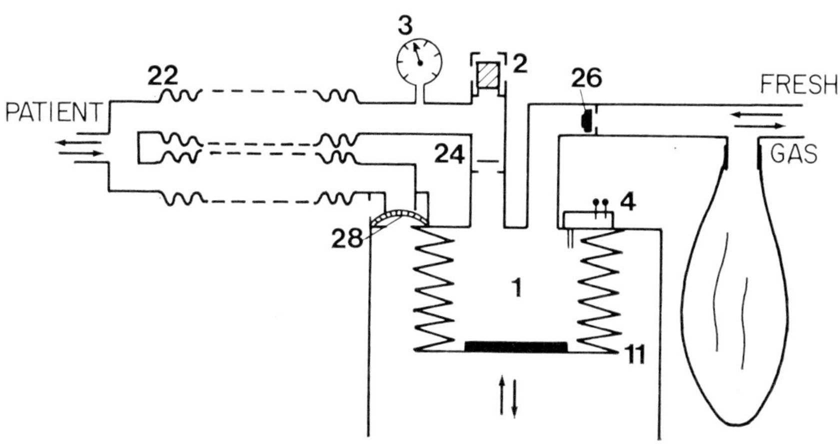

Fig. 55.4. Diagram of the Greer and Donald ventilator connected to a non-rebreathing ('total loss') circuit.

1. Concertina reservoir bag
2. Safety-valve
3. Manometer
4. Microswitch
11. Rigid plastic pressure chamber
22. Y-piece for connexion to patient
24. One-way inspiratory valve
26. Weighted one-way valve. This opens during the expiratory phase to admit fresh gas
28. Diaphragm. This is distended by pressure in (11) and occludes the expiratory outlet during the inspiratory phase

Change-over from inspiratory phase to expiratory phase
This change-over is volume-cycled: the phase ends when the base of the concertina bag has travelled from the lower microswitches to the upper one, and a preset volume has been expelled. The volume entering the lungs is less than this by the amount lost through the blow-off valve at the end of the inspiratory phase, which must equal the volume of fresh gas drawn in during the expiratory phase.

Expiratory phase, Part I. (Expansion of the concertina bag)
In this part of the phase the ventilator operates as a constant, negative, pressure generator, owing to the weight in the bag.

Change-over from Part I of expiratory phase to Part II
This change-over is volume-cycled: Part I of the expiratory phase ends when the base of the concertina bag has travelled from the upper microswitch to the lower ones and a preset volume has been drawn in. The volume leaving the patient's lungs will be less than this by the amount of fresh gas which enters the storage bag over the time of one respiratory cycle.

Expiratory phase, Part II. (Concertina bag at rest in the expanded position)
In this part of the phase the ventilator operates as a zero-flow generator: the bag and lungs form a closed system with no movement of gas.

Change-over from expiratory phase to inspiratory phase
This change-over is time-cycled or patient-cycled, whichever comes first. Cycling occurs when the relay (14) is reversed: either by a signal from the delay timer (13), at a preset time after the end of Part I of the expiratory phase; or by a signal from the patient-triggering circuit, when the patient makes an inspiratory effort.

Non-rebreathing circuit (fig. 55.4)

Inspiratory phase
In this phase the ventilator operates as a constant-flow generator, as with the closed circuit.

Change-over from inspiratory phase to expiratory phase
This change-over is volume-cycled, as with the closed circuit, except that the whole of the contents of the concertina bag enters the lungs.

Expiratory phase, Part I. (Expansion of the concertina bag)
In this part of the phase the ventilator operates as a constant, atmospheric, pressure

generator: the patient's expired gas passes freely to atmosphere at the expiratory valve (28).

Change-over from Part I of expiratory phase to Part II
This change-over is time-cycled: it occurs when the concertina bag has refilled at a rate, and therefore in a time, which is determined by characteristics of the ventilator, including the fresh-gas flow rate, and is uninfluenced by the patient.

Expiratory phase, Part II. (Concertina bag at rest in the expanded position)
In this part of the phase the ventilator continues to operate as a constant, atmospheric, pressure generator.

Change-over from expiratory phase to inspiratory phase
This change-over is time-cycled or patient-cycled, whichever comes first—as with the closed circuit.

REFERENCE

1 Greer J.R. and Donald I. (1958) A volume controlled patient-cycled respirator for adults. *Br. J. Anaesth.* **30**, 32.

CHAPTER 56

The Gullberg 'Positive-Pressure Attachment'[1]

DESCRIPTION

This is a positive-pressure attachment for simultaneous use with the Kifa Freiberger Cuirasse (fig. 56.1). The electric motor (19) (fig. 56.2) not only drives the concertina

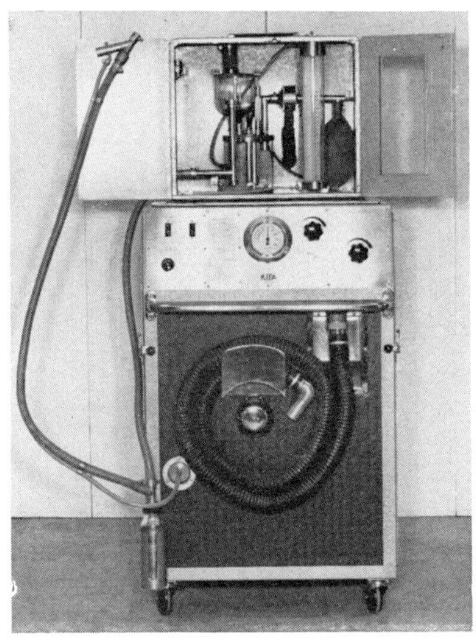

Fig. 56.1. The Kifa 'Freiberger Gullberg Universal' ventilator.
Courtesy of Kifa, Sweden.

reservoir bag (15) but also, through a gear-box (17), the large bellows for the cuirasse. An eccentric drive (18) on the output shaft of this gear-box operates a link rod (16) which alternately compresses and expands the positive-pressure concertina bag (15).

On the compression stroke the one-way valve (10) closes and the one-way valve (9) opens, allowing the contents of the bag to be forced, through an electrically-heated thermostatically-controlled humidifier (7) and a condensation trap (14), to a Y-piece (1) which is connected to an endotracheal tube. At the same time pressure is transmitted

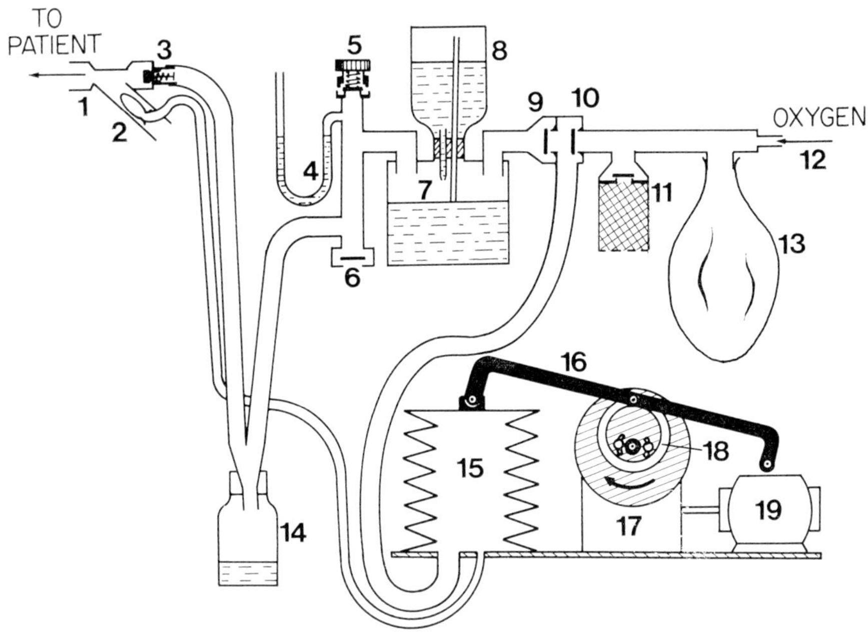

Fig. 56.2. Diagram of the Gullberg 'Positive-Pressure Attachment'.

1. Y-piece for connexion to patient
2. Balloon
3. Non-return valve
4. Manometer
5. Blow-off valve
6. Air-inlet valve
7. Humidifier
8. Water reservoir
9. One-way valve
10. One-way valve
11. Air inlet and filter
12. Oxygen inlet
13. Oxygen storage bag
14. Condensation trap
15. Concertina reservoir bag
16. Connecting rod
17. Gear-box
18. Eccentric drive on output shaft of gear-box
19. Electric motor

directly from the bag (15) to the small balloon (2) in the expiratory outlet of the Y-piece. The balloon is inflated and blocks the expiratory outlet.

At the end of the compression stroke the balloon (2) collapses and expired gas passes freely to atmosphere through the expiratory outlet. The spring-loaded one-way valve (3) prevents any expired gas passing back into the apparatus. The expansion of the bag (15) closes the valve (9) and opens the valve (10).

Oxygen may be supplied through the inlet (12) and, during the inspiratory phase, collects in the storage bag (13). If the supply of oxygen is sufficient, pure oxygen will be drawn into the bag (15). Lower flows of oxygen result in the patient receiving a mixture of air drawn in through the filter and valvc (11) and oxygen drawn from the bag (13).

A water manometer (4) indicates the pressure. A blow-off valve (5) limits the positive pressure developed and is adjusted to control the tidal volume, since the stroke of the concertina bag (15) is fixed. The one-way valve (6) allows air to be drawn in, preventing any negative pressure being developed. This is necessary because the eccentric drive (18) can be adjusted so that the positive-pressure attachment is slightly out of phase with the cuirasse.

A water container (8) maintains the level of water in the humidifier (7) at a constant level.

FUNCTIONAL ANALYSIS

Inspiratory phase

In this phase the ventilator operates fundamentally as a near-sine-wave-flow generator, owing to the nature of the driving mechanism and the constant speed of the motor. A pressure limit, due to the blow-off valve (5), comes into operation before the end of the phase whenever the patient's tidal volume is required to be less than the fixed stroke volume of the concertina bag.

Change-over from inspiratory phase to expiratory phase

This change-over is time-cycled: the constant-speed electric motor expels a fixed volume of gas from the concertina bag (15) in a preset time, but the volume entering the patient's lungs is normally less than this and is governed by the setting of the blow-off valve (5).

Expiratory phase

In this phase the ventilator operates as a constant, atmospheric, pressure generator: the expired gas passes freely to atmosphere at the expiratory outlet.

Change-over from expiratory phase to inspiratory phase

This change-over is time-cycled: the expiratory phase ends and the inspiratory phase begins after the driving motor has expanded the bag in a preset time.

REFERENCE

1 Lassen H.C.A. (1956) *Management of life-threatening poliomyelitis*, p. 67. Edinburgh: Livingstone.

CHAPTER 57

The Howells Ventilator[1]

DESCRIPTION

This ventilator (figs. 57.1 and 57.2) is intended for ward or anaesthetic use. It is of such size that it will stand on the commonly-used British anaesthetic trolley. It is operated by the anaesthetic gas mixture, or the compressed air or oxygen, with which the patient's lungs are to be inflated. The ventilator operates as a non-rebreathing circuit.

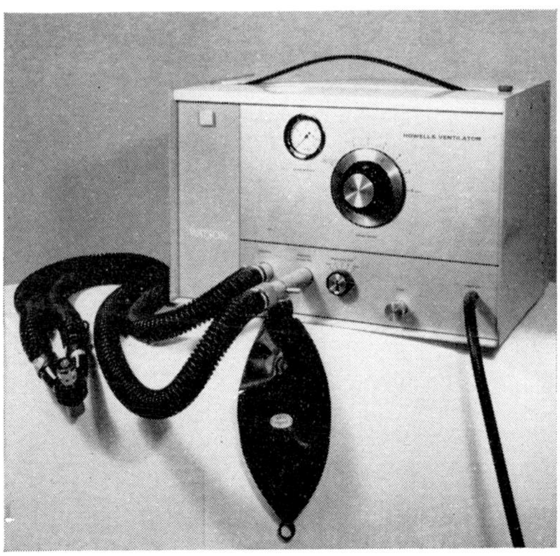

Fig. 57.1.

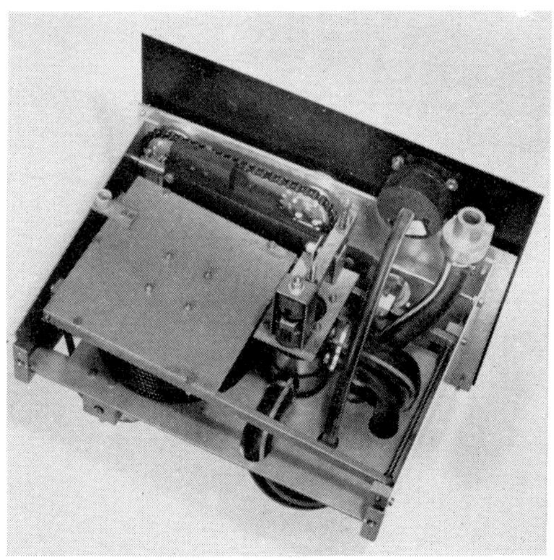

Fig. 57.2.

Fig. 57.1. The Howells ventilator.
Courtesy of Department of Medical Illustration, Cardiff Royal Infirmary.

Fig. 57.2. The mechanism of the Howells ventilator.
Courtesy of Department of Medical Illustration, Cardiff Royal Infirmary.

All the gas supplied to the ventilator, provided that the flow is not excessive, is delivered to the patient. This gas should be derived from a source of at least 5 lb/in^2, e.g. the regulators on the anaesthetic apparatus. The flow must be regulated by a suitable needle valve. It is desirable also that the flow be monitored by a flowmeter. During anaesthesia, the controls and flowmeters of the anaesthetic machine are used.

During the expiratory phase, inflating gas enters at the inlet (11) and fills the concertina reservoir bag (12) expanding it against the pull of the twin coil springs (10), the inspiratory valve (18) being closed. When the bag has expanded sufficiently for the stop

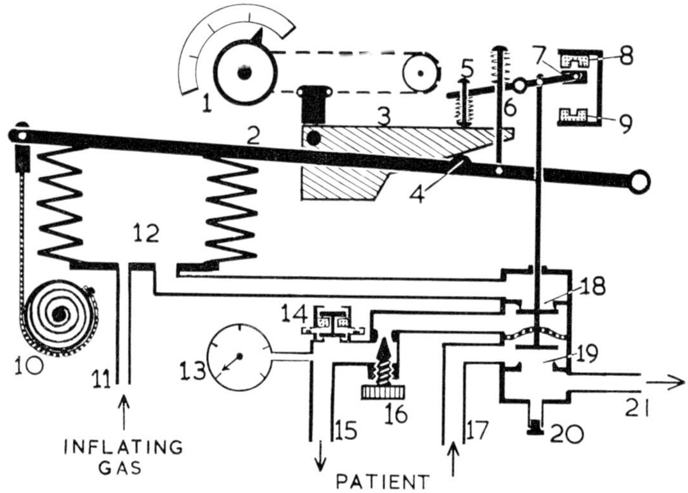

Fig. 57.3. Diagram of the Howells ventilator.

1. 'Volume selector'
2. Top-plate
3. Wedge
4. Stop
5. Pin
6. Pin
7. Soft-iron block
8. Magnet
9. Magnet
10. Coil springs
11. Inflating-gas inlet
12. Concertina reservoir bag
13. Manometer
14. Magnetic safety-valve
15. Inspiratory tube
16. 'Inspiratory time' control
17. Expiratory tube
18. Inspiratory valve
19. Expiratory valve
20. Drain plug
21. Expiratory port

(4) on the top-plate (2) to strike the pivoted wedge (3), further movement of the top-plate (2) raises the narrower end of the wedge and pushes up the pin (5), compressing the spring on it. When the force exerted by this spring is sufficient to overcome the pull of the magnet (8) on the soft-iron block (7), the lever flicks over and the block (7) is held by the magnet (9). The inspiratory valve (18) is opened and the expiratory valve (19) is closed. The gas stored in the reservoir bag (12), together with fresh gas entering the bag, flows, at a pressure determined by the coil spring (10), past the inspiratory valve (18) and the 'inspiratory time' control (16), to the patient.

As the reservoir bag (12) empties and the top-plate (2) moves down, the pin (6), attached to the top-plate, compresses the spring around it until, when the bag (12) is collapsed, the force exerted by the spring overcomes the pull of the magnet (9). The lever flicks over, and the inspiratory valve (18) is closed and the expiratory valve (19) is opened.

Expired gas now passes freely, through the expiratory tube (17), the expiratory valve (19), and the port (21), to atmosphere. At the same time the reservoir bag (12) is refilling.

All gas supplied at the inlet (11) is delivered to the patient. The tidal volume is made up of the volume stored in the reservoir bag (12) at the start of the inspiratory phase and the inflating-gas flow during the phase. The volume stored in the bag depends on the setting of the control (1), which determines the lateral position of the pivoted wedge, and hence the thickness of that part of the wedge which lies between the stop (4) and the lower end of the pin (5), i.e. the distance which the top-plate (2) has to rise before the cycling mechanism is switched to the inspiratory position. The duration of the expiratory phase is the time required for the inflating-gas flow to deliver this volume to the bag (12).

The duration of the inspiratory phase is the time taken for the pressure in the bag (12) to deliver the tidal volume. It depends on the total airway resistance and the patient's compliance. The 'inspiratory time' control (16) allows the airway resistance to be increased if it is desired to prolong the inspiratory phase. The manometer (13) indicates pressure in the inspiratory tube which is limited to 50 cmH_2O by the magnetic safety-valve (14). This valve is so designed that, if the pressure exceeds 50 cmH_2O, a free pathway to atmosphere is established and is maintained until the pressure in the tube has fallen nearly to atmospheric. This will occur only when the bag (12) has emptied sufficiently to reverse the valves to the expiratory position. Any gas still in the patient's lungs can now empty through the expiratory port (21).

If manual ventilation is desired a separate reservoir bag, which is supplied, is incorporated in the respiratory pathway, between the port (15) and the patient. An expiratory valve forms part of the Y-piece connecting the two breathing tubes near the patient. The 'volume selector' (1) must be set to the 'manual' position, in which the thickest part of the wedge (3) lies between the stop (4) and the pin (5), thus holding the cycling mechanism with the inspiratory valve open and the expiratory valve closed. The concertina reservoir bag (12) is now held in its collapsed position by the coil spring (10). The inflating gas flows continuously to the inspiratory tube (15).

The drain (20) allows the expiratory-valve chamber to be emptied of condensed water. A Wright respirometer may be attached to the expiratory port (21).

FUNCTIONAL ANALYSIS

Inspiratory phase

Fundamentally this ventilator is a pressure generator due to the force exerted by the coil springs (10) on the concertina reservoir bag (12). The pressure decreases as the bag empties (fig. 57.4) due, no doubt, partly to the characteristics of the springs and partly to the elasticity of the wall of the bag. However, the generated pressure is always high (mostly between 80 and 120 cmH_2O) and a high series resistance is normally maintained in the inspiratory pathway by means of the 'inspiratory time' control (16) so that the ventilator

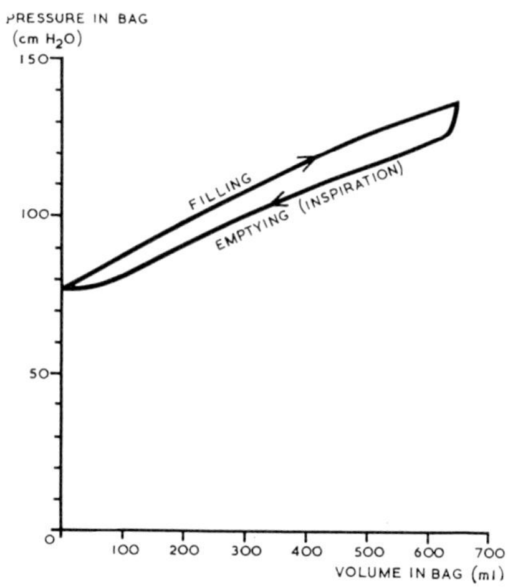

Fig. 57.4. Howells ventilator. Pressure-volume characteristics of the concertina reservoir bag. Volume is expressed in terms of the volume which the contents of the bag would occupy when expanded to atmospheric pressure without change of temperature.

approximates well to a decreasing-flow generator. This is confirmed by fig. 57.5 in which comparison of (b) and (c) with (a) shows that halving the compliance or doubling the airway resistance has very little effect on the flow waveform but substantially alters the pressure waveforms.

Change-over from inspiratory phase to expiratory phase

This is volume-cycled. It occurs when the concertina bag has emptied from a preset volume. The tidal volume exceeds this volume by the amount of inflating gas which enters the ventilator during the phase. Since the ventilator approximates to a flow generator during the inspiratory phase the inspiratory flow is little affected by changes in lung characteristics. Therefore the time taken for the positive-pressure concertina bag to empty, the inspiratory time, is also little affected by such changes; hence the change-over from the inspiratory phase to the expiratory phase can be considered to be time-cycled as well as volume-cycled. A very low compliance or a very high resistance could reduce the inspiratory flow a little and so increase the inspiratory time and hence, because of the continuous entry of inflating gas, increase the tidal volume; but in fig. 57.5 the changes of compliance and resistance are not big enough to show this effect.

Expiratory phase

Here the ventilator is a constant, atmospheric, pressure generator with the patient expiring freely to the atmosphere at the port (21).

All the figures show the pressure at the mouth falling very rapidly almost to zero at the start of the phase. The flow and alveolar-pressure tracings show the typical decline to

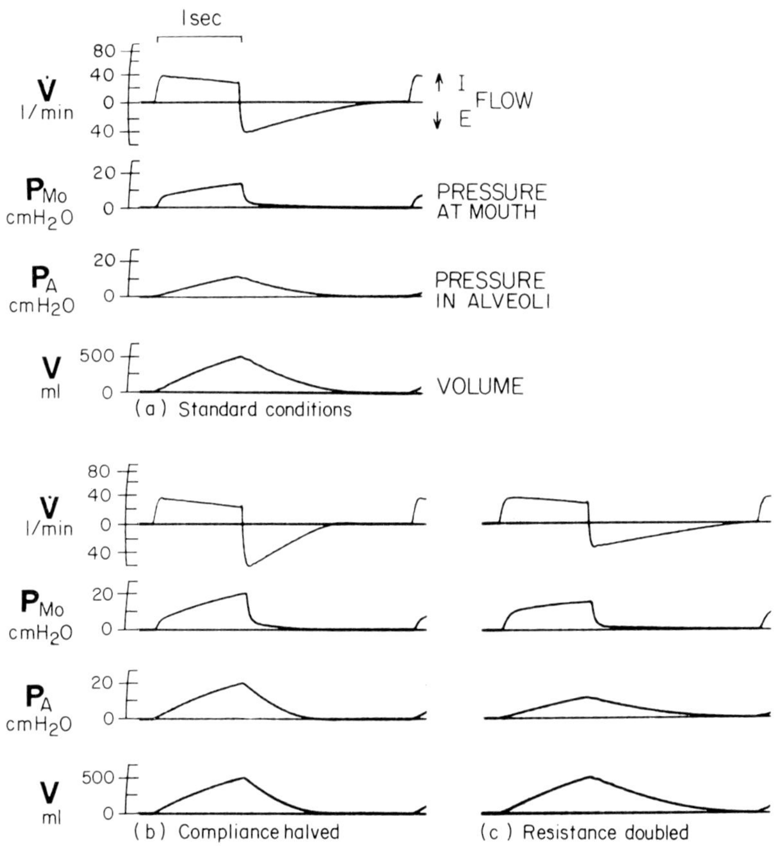

Fig. 57.5. Howells ventilator. Recordings showing the effects of changes of lung characteristics.

Standard conditions: inflating-gas, from a 60 lb/in^2 pipe-line and needle valve, set to give a total ventilation of 10 litres/min (Rotameter reading when corrected to atmospheric pressure was nearly 11 litres/min); 'volume selector' and 'inspiratory time', set for a tidal volume of 500 ml and an inspiratory-expiratory ratio of 1 : 2.

zero with the time constant of the decline depending on the product of compliance and resistance.

Change-over from expiratory phase to inspiratory phase

This occurs when the preset inflating-gas flow has expanded the concertina bag by a preset volume. It is therefore time-cycled, as is evident from the tracings.

CONTROLS

Total ventilation

Since this ventilator is a minute-volume divider (see p. 140) the total ventilation is directly controlled by, and is nominally equal to, the inflating-gas flow. The only source of loss, apart from leaks, is the compliance of the breathing tubes. With those tubes supplied with the ventilator this loss approached 10% of the inflating-gas flow under the 'standard' conditions.

Increasing the total ventilation, by increasing the inflating-gas flow, increases both the tidal volume and the respiratory frequency (fig. 57.6b); it also increases inspiratory time and decreases expiratory time thereby changing the inspiratory-expiratory ratio. This is because the higher inflating-gas flow refills the concertina bag more rapidly (shorter expiratory time) and adds a greater volume to the volume excursion of the bag to make up the increased tidal volume. This bigger tidal volume takes longer to deliver at the fixed inspiratory flow.

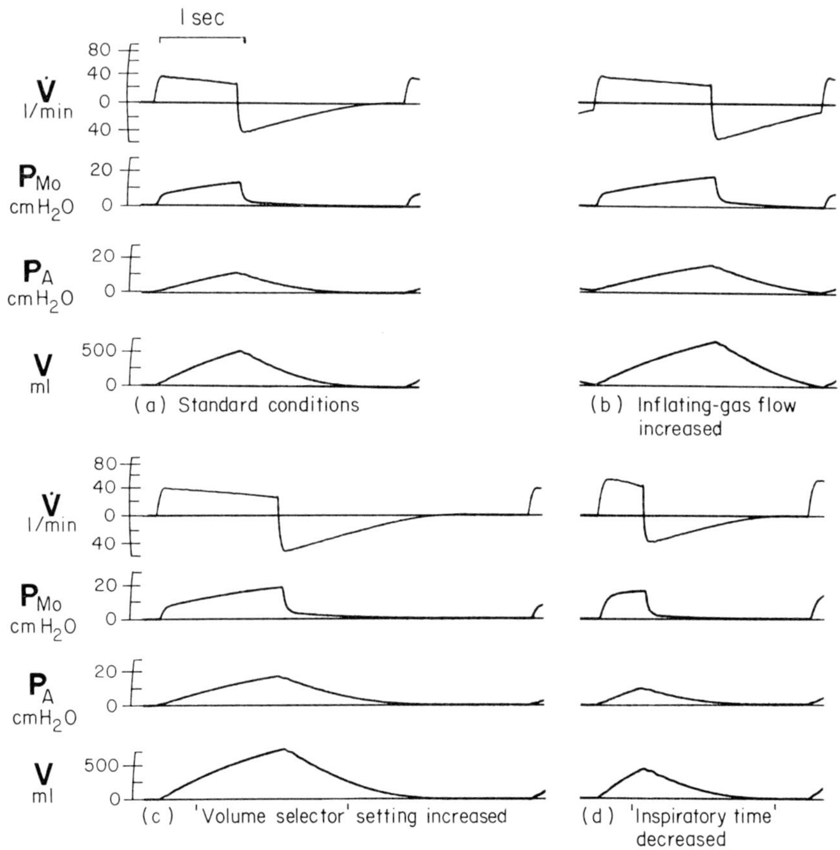

Fig. 57.6. Howells ventilator. Recordings showing the effects of changes in the settings of the controls.

(a) Standard conditions as in fig. 57.5.

(b) Inflating-gas flow increased to 16·5 litres/min (corrected to atmospheric pressure).

(c) 'Volume selector' setting increased (from '3·25' to '4·5') to give a tidal volume of 750 ml.

(d) 'Inspiratory time' decreased from '4·3' to '3'.

Tidal volume

This is directly controlled by adjustment of the excursion of the concertina bag by means of the 'volume selector' (1), (fig. 57.6c) but it is also influenced by any factor which alters the volume of inflating gas entering during the inspiratory phase. It is increased by increasing the inflating-gas flow (fig. 57.6b) or slightly decreased by decreasing the resistance to inspiration by means of the 'inspiratory time' control (16) (fig. 57.6d). Changes in compliance and airway resistance should have little influence on tidal volume because the ventilator approximates well to a time-cycled flow generator; certainly the effect of the changes tried in fig. 57.5b and c is negligible.

Increasing the tidal volume, by increasing the excursion of the concertina bag (fig. 57.6c), necessarily reduces the frequency because the total ventilation is fixed. The expiratory time is necessarily increased in the same proportion as the bag excursion, because the rate of refilling of the bag is constant. On the other hand, the degree of prolongation of the inspiratory phase needed to deliver the increased tidal volume depends on a number of factors and, unlike the prolongation of the expiratory phase, it is not, in general, in the same proportion as the increase in bag excursion. Therefore the inspiratory-expiratory ratio is usually altered. In fig. 57.6c the inspiratory phase occupies a shorter fraction of the respiratory cycle than in the standard conditions of fig. 57.6a.

Respiratory frequency

This is not directly controlled but is mathematically equal to the inflating-gas flow divided by the tidal volume delivered from the machine. Decreasing the setting of the 'inspiratory time' control (16) increases the frequency: the effect may be regarded as a direct one, or as one which is mediated by the associated reduction in tidal volume (see below). The respiratory frequency is hardly affected by the changes in lung characteristics tried here.

Inspiratory-expiratory ratio

The main means of controlling this parameter is the 'inspiratory time' control (16), that is, the resistance to inspiration (fig. 57.6d); but this also affects the tidal volume. If the tidal volume is then reset by adjusting the excursion of the concertina bag this, in turn, usually affects the inspiratory-expiratory ratio to some extent (see above). Therefore, if precise values of tidal volume and inspiratory-expiratory ratio are required, a second, or third, adjustment to each control may be necessary. If the total ventilation should then be altered by adjusting the inflating-gas flow this will upset the inspiratory-expiratory ratio (fig. 57.6b, see above) and necessitate further adjustment of the other controls.

Since the ventilator is time-cycled at the end of the expiratory phase, and effectively so at the end of the inspiratory phase, the inspiratory-expiratory ratio is virtually uninfluenced by changes in lung characteristics.

Inspiratory waveforms

In the inspiratory phase the flow waveform is set by the ventilator and the pressure waveforms result from the interaction of this flow waveform with the lung characteristics. Although the flow can be varied, by adjusting the 'inspiratory time' control (16), its level will normally have been determined on the basis of the required tidal volume and required inspiratory time. The way in which flow falls off slightly during the phase cannot be deliberately varied and is only slightly altered by the changes in lung characteristics tried here.

Expiratory waveforms

Throughout the expiratory phase atmospheric pressure is applied, via the expiratory pathway, to the patient's lungs. It cannot be varied in any way. The expiratory flow which results depends on the effect of this pressure on the lungs.

Pressure limits

The range of pressure in the alveoli is determined by the tidal volume divided by the compliance. Since atmospheric pressure is applied to the lungs throughout the expiratory phase the pressure in the alveoli will normally fall very nearly to atmospheric pressure by the end of the phase. Only an expiratory resistance higher than any in the tracings, or an expiratory time shorter than any in the tracings, will keep the minimum alveolar pressure appreciably above atmospheric. The maximum alveolar pressure is the minimum pressure plus the pressure range.

REFERENCE

1 Howells T.H. (1960) A new mechanical ventilator. *Br. J. Anaesth.*, **32**, 438.

CHAPTER 58

The James Ventilator[1,2]

DESCRIPTION

In this ventilator a concertina reservoir bag (1) (fig. 58.2) is compressed and expanded twenty times a minute by a sparkless constant-speed electric motor (3), through a link (4) and sliding pivot (5) mechanism similar to the valve-gear link motion used on some locomotives. This link system (4, 5) permits changes in the stroke volume to be made easily by the crank and worm (2) without stopping the electric motor (3).

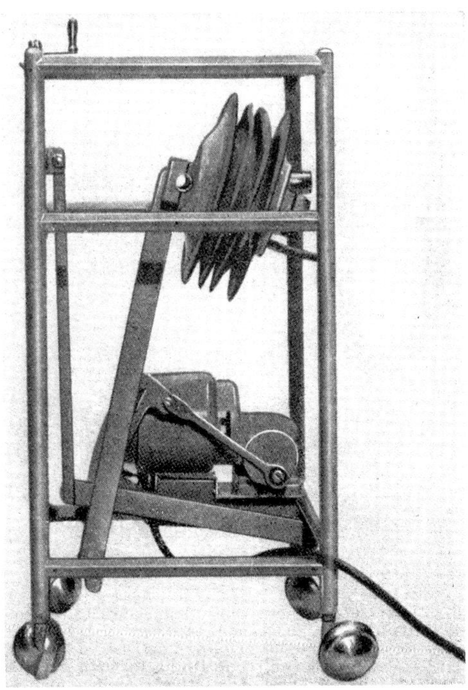

Fig. 58.1. The James ventilator.

Courtesy of *Medical Journal of Australia*.[1]

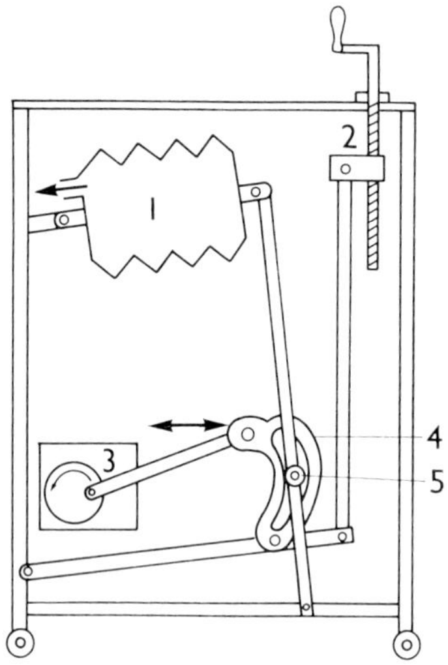

Fig. 58.2.

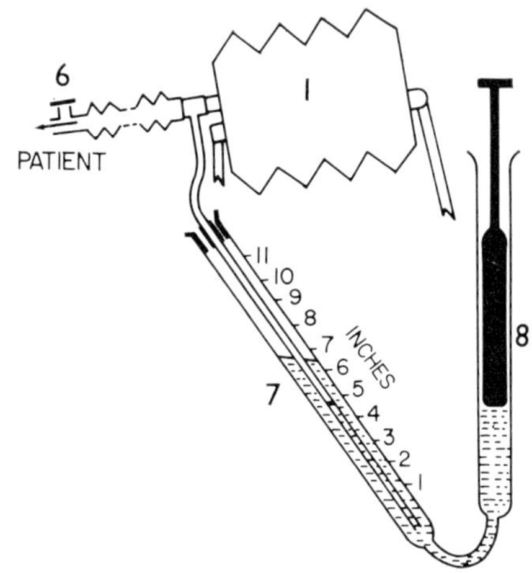

Fig. 58.3.

Fig. 58.2. Diagram of the James ventilator.

Courtesy of *British Journal of Anaesthesia.*[2]

Fig. 58.3. Diagram of the manometer of the James ventilator.

1. Concertina reservoir bag
2. Crank and worm
3. Electric motor
4. Link
5. Sliding pivot
6. Blow-off valve
7. Water manometer and safety-valve
8. Adjustable plunger

Courtesy of *British Journal of Anaesthesia.*[2]

A water manometer (7) (fig. 58.3) indicates the pressures produced and also acts as a safety-valve. The peak pressure is set by adjusting the water level in the manometer. To permit the escape of surplus gas when using nitrous oxide and oxygen mixtures, a spring-loaded blow-off valve (6) is provided and is set to blow off just before the manometer (7) reaches peak pressure. By pushing the adjustable displacement plunger (8) down, the safety pressure can be increased and is indicated by the water level on the scale. If this pressure is exceeded, gas will bubble audibly and visibly through the water and escape through openings at the top. The manometer (7) is set to a suitable pressure, say 20–30 cmH_2O. Further adjustments may be made as the anaesthetic proceeds. Obstruction of the airway or forcible compression of the lungs will be shown at once by the escape of gas, either through the blow-off valve (6) or through both it and the water manometer.

The inspiratory-expiratory ratio is fixed at 1 : 1.

FUNCTIONAL ANALYSIS

Inspiratory phase

In this phase the ventilator operates as a near-sine-wave-flow generator owing to the nature of the driving mechanism and the constant speed of the motor. A pressure limit, due to the blow-off valve, comes into operation during the phase. Until then, the fresh-gas supply to the patient circuit acts as a small-constant-flow generator, supplementing the main flow generator.

Change-over from inspiratory phase to expiratory phase

This change-over is both volume-cycled and time-cycled: the constant-speed electric motor expels a preset volume of gas from the concertina bag in a fixed time. Since the supply of anaesthetic gas is continuous, while its escape, through the blow-off valve, is restricted to the inspiratory phase, the patient's tidal volume is less than the stroke volume of the bag, by an amount equal to the volume of fresh gas supplied during the expiratory phase (see p. 146).

Expiratory phase

In this phase the ventilator again operates as a near-sine-wave-flow generator, except that the fresh-gas flow is now subtracted from, instead of added to, the main flow pattern.

Change-over from expiratory phase to inspiratory phase

This change-over is volume-cycled and time-cycled: the motor draws a preset volume of gas into the bag in a fixed time. The volume leaving the patient's lungs is slightly less than this—by an amount equal to the volume of fresh gas which enters the patient circuit during the expiratory phase.

REFERENCES

1 James N.R. (1950) Automatic machine for controlled respiration. *Med. J. Aust.* **1**, 325.
2 Mushin W.W. and Rendell-Baker L. (1954) Modern automatic respirators. *Br. J. Anaesth.* **26**, 131.

CHAPTER 59

The Jefferson Ventilator

DESCRIPTION

In its first version (1955) (fig. 59.1) the superficial similarity between the Jefferson and the Allbritten ventilator from which it evolved was close. However, by changing the driving mechanism from a windscreen wiper to a pressure-actuated piston controlled by a pneumatic timer, the functional character was changed. The Allbritten ventilator is fundamentally volume-cycled, while the Jefferson is time-cycled.

In later versions (fig. 59.2) the reservoir bag is of concertina pattern and the timing-control mechanism has been further refined.

Driving gas at 16 lb/in^2 is delivered to the timing-control unit at (22) (fig. 59.3). If the pressure of the driving gas is higher than 16 lb/in^2 it must be reduced by a regulator or needle valve until a pressure of 16 lb/in^2 is shown on the pressure gauge (23). The compressed air is held in the chamber (21) by a spring-loaded ball valve (20). It can, however, pass the constriction (19). Pressure builds up quickly above the diaphragm (18) moving it down and forcing the ball valve (20) off its seating. Driving gas can now flow from the chamber (21), through the delivery tube (15), to the bottom of the cylinder (14), forcing the piston upwards. This upward movement of the piston compresses the concertina bag (8). The pressure thus built up in the pressure chamber (9) compresses the concertina bag (4), inflating the lungs.

In the control unit, pressure is meanwhile building up slowly in the chamber (17), at a rate controlled by the needle valve (16). The diaphragm (10) is double, the upper leaf having a smaller diameter than the lower one. Thus a pressure balance between the two sides of the diaphragm (10) will be reached before the pressure in (17) reaches that in (13). At a slightly higher pressure in (17) the diaphragm (10) is forced up and the ball valve (12) lifted from its seat. This opens the chamber (13) to atmosphere and there is a drop in pressure above the constriction (19). The diaphragm (18) moves up to its normal position and the ball valve (20) shuts. Pressure in the cylinder (14) falls since its contained gas can escape to atmosphere through the space between the two leaves of the diaphragm (18) and the orifice in the centre of the lower leaf. The piston now falls. Pressure in the chamber (17) falls as air escapes, past the needle valve (16), through the chamber (13), and past the ball valve (12), to atmosphere. The diaphragm (10) returns to its resting

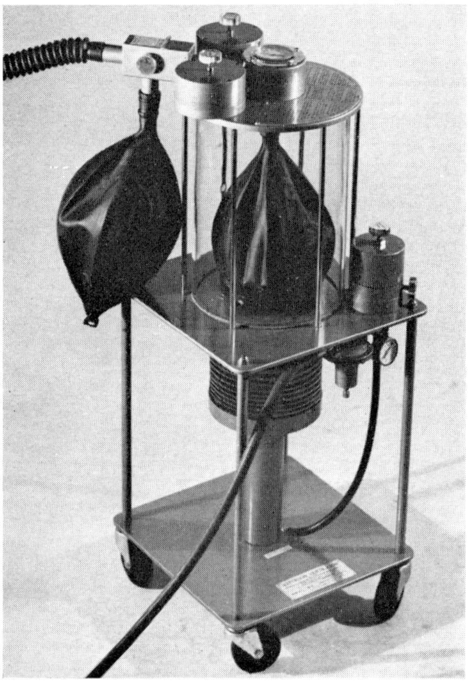

Fig. 59.1.

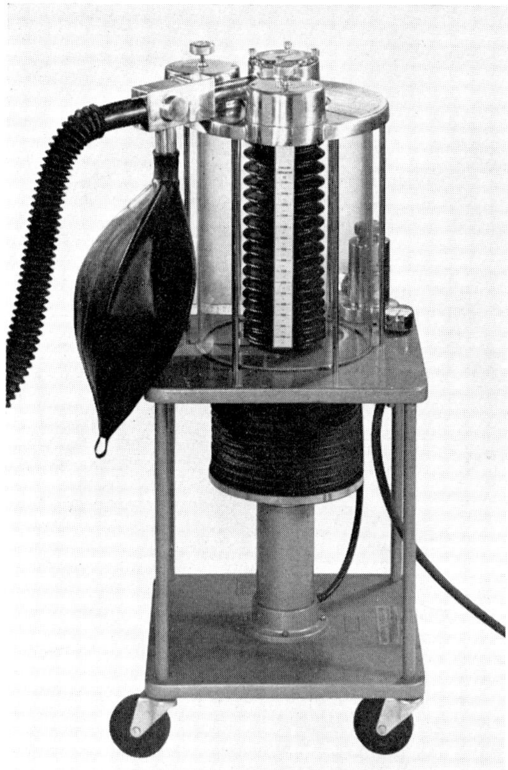

Fig. 59.2.

Fig. 59.1. The Jefferson ventilator—early model.

Courtesy of Air-Shields Inc.

Fig. 59.2. The Jefferson ventilator.

Courtesy of Air-Shields Inc.

position allowing the ball valve (12) to reseat. Pressure now builds up again and another inspiratory phase commences.

During the expiratory phase the concertina bag (8) descends under the influence of a weight in its base. The amount of negative pressure this transfers to the patient circuit can be varied by the negative-pressure-limiting valve (1). The maximum negative pressure is -15 cmH_2O. An adjustable blow-off valve (2) limits the positive pressure during the inspiratory phase, the maximum being 40 cmH_2O.

The frequency of cycling is controlled by the needle valve (16). The control (11) is known as the 'Phase control'. The tension of the phase-control spring alters the relative durations of the inspiratory and expiratory phases. When there is little tension on the spring the inspiratory phase comes to an end soon after the gas enters the chamber (17) pushing up the diaphragm (10). There is thus a shorter inspiratory phase and a longer

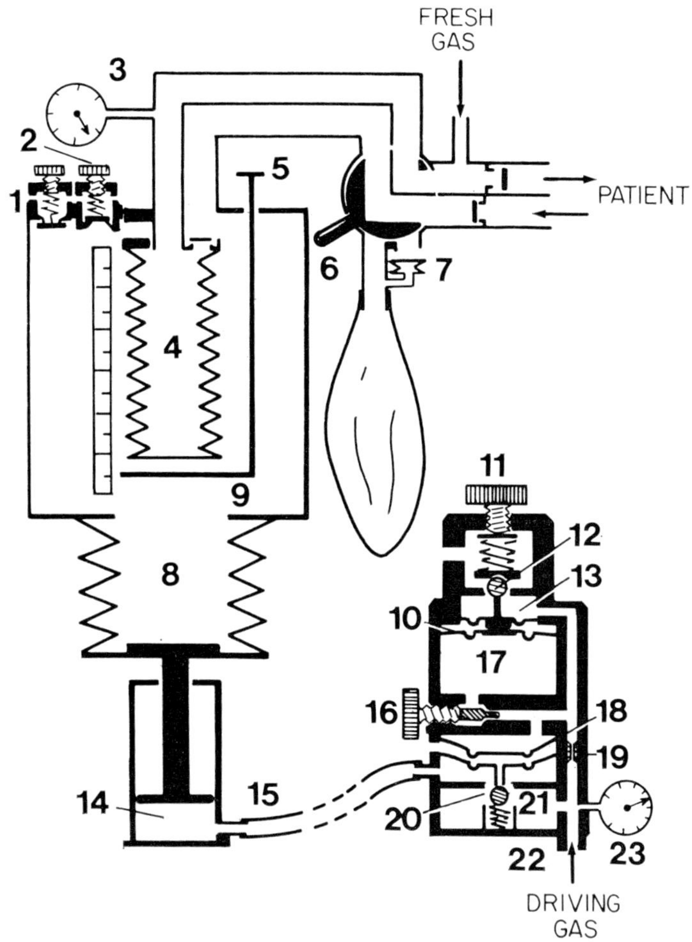

Fig. 59.3. Diagram of the Jefferson ventilator with 'NRB head'.

1. Negative-pressure-limiting valve
2. Positive-pressure-limiting valve
3. Manometer
4. Concertina reservoir bag
5. Control for adjusting height of volume-limiting plate
6. 'Manual/Auto' control
7. Valve
8. Driving concertina bag
9. Pressure chamber
10. Double diaphragm
11. 'Phase control' for adjusting the inspiratory-expiratory ratio
12. Ball valve
13. Chamber
14. Cylinder
15. Connecting tube
16. Needle valve controlling frequency of cycling
17. Chamber
18. Double diaphragm
19. Constriction
20. Ball valve
21. Chamber
22. Driving-gas inlet
23. Pressure gauge

expiratory one. When the tension of the phase-control spring is high the diaphragm (10) moves more slowly and the ball valve (12) is not opened until later. The expiratory phase is thus correspondingly shorter. The phase control (11) is normally set by the manufacturers so that the inspiratory-expiratory ratio is 1:1·5.

Movement of the rod (5) limits the volume of the bag (4) during the expiratory phase. This attachment is used when the tidal volume is to be limited to a particular figure. In this circumstance the blow-off valve (2) is set at a high pressure, ensuring that the whole of the contents of bag (4) is delivered to the patient. Although the tidal volume can thus be limited to a given figure, cycling does not occur until the lapse of a preset time interval.

In another mode of operation, the reservoir bag (4) can expand to its fullest (1,500 ml). The volume delivered to the patient is then governed by the setting of the positive-pressure-limiting valve (2). The pressure within the lungs remains at this level until the expiratory phase begins.

In use the pressure and respiratory frequency desired are selected with the apparatus functioning but with the tap (6) set to 'Manual'. The tap (6) is then turned to 'Auto'.

The concertina reservoir bag (4) may take the place of the reservoir bag of a carbon-dioxide absorption circuit. A single breathing tube (fig. 59.2) then connects the ventilator and absorber. Excess anaesthetic gas is vented into the pressure chamber at the end of the expiratory phase through a spill valve in the head of the concertina bag (4). The diagram (fig. 59.3) shows the 'Non-rebreathing attachment' which can be fitted to the standard ventilator. The lungs are inflated by the compression of the bag (4) but the expired gas and any excess fresh gas pass along a second breathing tube into the outer chamber (9).

The manometer (3) indicates the pressure in the patient circuit. A bag for manual control of respiration can be brought into action by the tap (6). When this bag is squeezed the lungs are inflated because the expiratory outlet is occluded by the valve (7). The expired gas passes freely to atmosphere.

A modified 'closed-circuit' head, which incorporated a patient-triggering mechanism, was available for use with this ventilator.

Further modifications were also made to the timing mechanism. These had the effects of almost fixing the inspiratory time at about 1 second and of providing a single control which regulated the expiratory time and hence the respiratory frequency.

FUNCTIONAL ANALYSIS

This ventilator contains a pressure transformer (see p. 89) with a constant driving pressure and some resistance on the input side. It therefore operates fundamentally as a pressure generator with some series resistance. The volume displacement of the driving concertina bag (8) (fig. 59.3) is much greater than the tidal volume normally required from the reservoir bag (4), so that there is a large volume difference which passes in and out through the pressure-limiting valves.

Inspiratory phase

In this phase the ventilator operates as a constant-pressure generator with some series resistance, owing to the pressure-transformer characteristics. The valve (2) on the pressure chamber introduces a pressure limit, and there is a volume limit equal to the volume of gas in the reservoir bag at the start of the phase. One of these limits will normally be reached during the phase. The steady flow of fresh anaesthetic gas acts as a small-constant-flow generator, supplementing the action of the main pressure generator, except for any part of the phase in which the pressure limit is operative but the volume limit is not. The volume of gas which enters the lungs exceeds the volume expelled from the reservoir bag by an amount equal to the volume of fresh gas entering the patient circuit during the inspiratory phase at a rate at least equal to the patient's total ventilation.

Change-over from inspiratory phase to expiratory phase

This change-over is time-cycled: the duration of the inspiratory phase is determined by the pneumatic timing mechanism.

Expiratory phase

In this phase the ventilator operates as a constant, negative, pressure generator with some series resistance, owing to the pressure-transformer characteristics. The valve (1) introduces a negative-pressure limit. Until this limit is reached the fresh-gas supply acts as a small-constant-flow generator, slightly impeding the main pressure-generator action, because it helps to expand the reservoir bag within the pressure chamber and so absorb some of the energy of the driving bag.

Change-over from expiratory phase to inspiratory phase

This change-over is time-cycled: the duration of the expiratory phase is determined by the pneumatic timing mechanism.

CHAPTER 60

The Lundia 'Special' Ventilator Model B

DESCRIPTION

This ventilator (figs. 60.1 and 60.2) is intended for ward use.

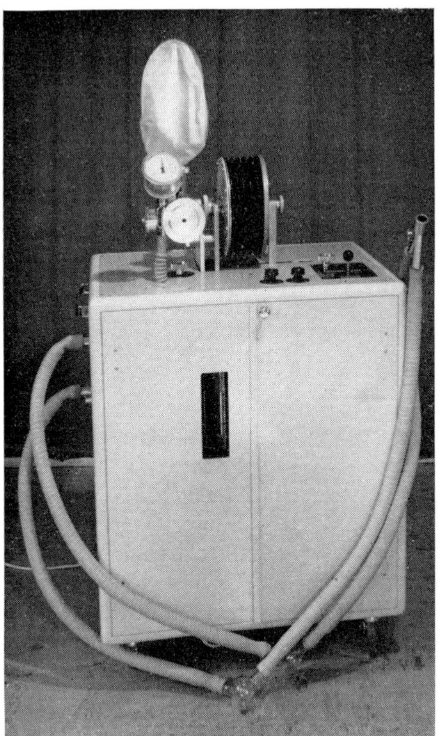

Fig. 60.1.

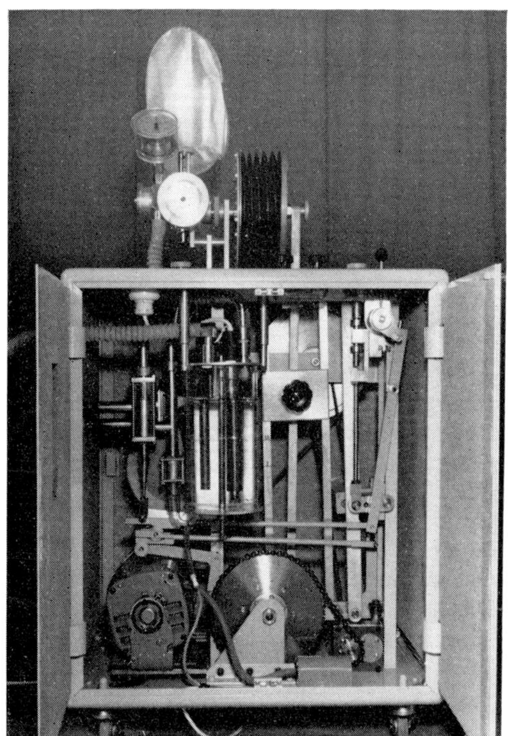

Fig.60.2.

Fig. 60.1. The Lundia 'Special' ventilator Model B.
Courtesy of Department of Medical Illustration, Cardiff Royal Infirmary

Fig. 60.2. Mechanism of the Lundia 'Special' ventilator Model B.
Courtesy of Department of Medical Illustration, Cardiff Royal Infirmary.

A constant-speed a.c. mains electric motor (32) (fig. 60.3) is connected to a gear-box (31) by a series of belt drives. The output shaft of the gear-box is connected by a chain drive to a large sprocket wheel (28). This wheel has an eccentric groove cut in its face which imparts motion to the three rods (23, 24, and 27) as the wheel turns.

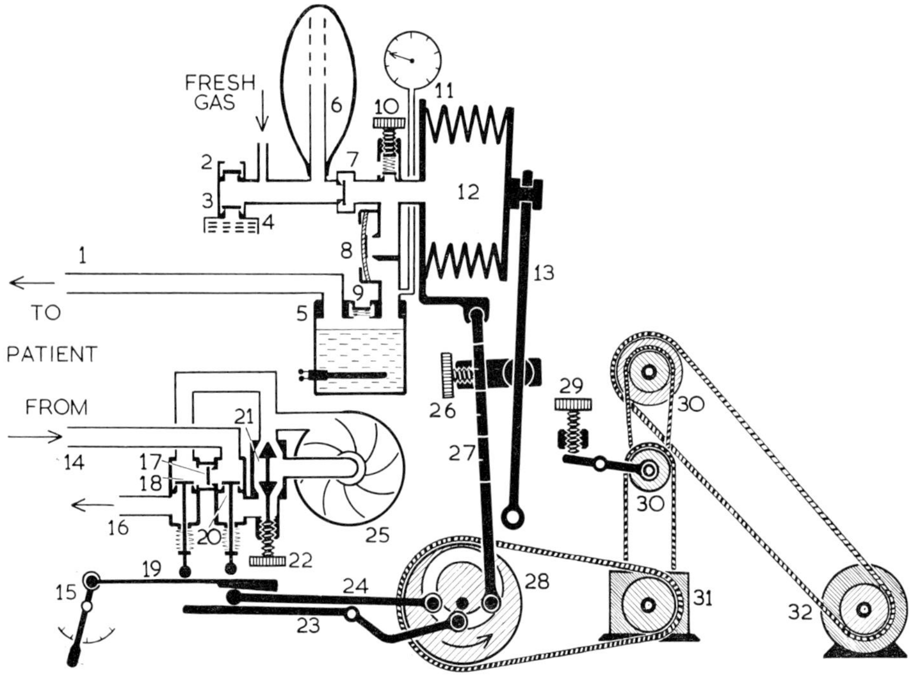

Fig. 60.3. Diagram of the Lundia 'Special' ventilator Model B.

1. Inspiratory tube
2. One-way spill valve
3. One-way inlet valve
4. Filter
5. Heated humidifier
6. Storage bag
7. One-way valve
8. Diaphragm valve
9. Air-inlet valve
10. Safety-valve
11. Manometer
12. Concertina reservoir bag
13. Connecting rod
14. Expiratory tube
15. Negative-pressure-timing control
16. Exhaust port
17. One-way valve
18. Poppet valve (open for expiration)
19. Rod
20. Poppet valve (open for negative pressure)
21. Double valve
22. Negative-pressure-magnitude control
23. Pivoted rod
24. Sliding rod
25. Blower
26. 'Stroke volume' control
27. Crank rod
28. Sprocket wheel
29. Frequency control
30. Expanding pulleys
31. Gear-box
32. Electric motor

The rod (27) is pivoted at its upper end and is connected, by an adjustable pivot (26), to another rod (13). One end of the rod (13) is fixed to the concertina reservoir bag (12) while the other end is pivoted. Movement of the rod (27), therefore, alternately compresses and expands the bag (12).

As soon as the bag (12) begins its expansion stroke the diaphragm valve (8) closes, so preventing expired gas being drawn into the bag. At the same time air is drawn into the bag (12) through the filter (4) and the one-way valves (3) and (7). If required, oxygen is added through the fresh-gas inlet. During the inspiratory phase this oxygen is stored in the bag (6) ready to be drawn into the concertina reservoir bag (12) during the next expiratory phase. If the flow of oxygen is excessive a one-way outlet valve (2) allows it to escape to atmosphere when the storage bag (6) is filled.

During the compression stroke of the bag (12) the one-way valve (7) is held closed and the gas stored within the bag is forced, past the diaphragm valve (8), through the hot-water humidifier (5), to the patient. A safety-valve (10) can be set to limit the maximum pressure during the inspiratory phase to any level up to 60 cmH_2O. The manometer (11) indicates the inflating pressure.

When compression of the bag (12) is almost complete the lever (23) lifts the two rods (24) and (19) and opens the expiratory valve (18) which is normally held closed by its spring. The inspiratory phase ends, and expired gas flows, through the one-way valve (17) and the valve (18), to atmosphere.

A blower (25) runs continuously and either recirculates air through its connecting tubes or produces a negative pressure below the valve (20) depending on the position of the double valve (21). This position, and hence the magnitude of the negative pressure, can be adjusted by means of the negative-pressure-magnitude control (22). Any negative pressure produced in this way is applied to the expiratory pathway only when the valve (20) is opened.

Whether the valve (20) is opened at all, and if so at what interval after the start of the expiratory phase, depends on the setting of the control (15) which alters the position of the wedge-shaped end of the pivoted rod (19). The wedge-shaped end of the rod (19) is lifted by the traverse of the sliding rod (24) and the upward movement of the pivoted rod (23). When the control (15) is in the 'positive pressure' position, the rod (19) is over to the right and its wedge-shaped end never makes contact with the stem of the valve (20) which remains closed. The further the control (15) is set towards the 'negative pressure' position, the further the rod (19) is moved to the left, and the earlier the valve (20) is opened.

When expansion of the bag (12) is almost complete the lever (23) moves down away from the stems of the valves (18) and (20). The valves close and the expiratory phase ends.

The valve (9) allows the patient to draw in air if he should make an inspiratory effort. The stroke volume of the concertina reservoir bag (12) is set by adjusting the position of the sliding coupler (26) from 0–2000 ml. The maximum negative pressure obtainable is -12 cmH_2O. The speed of the final drive can be varied by setting the control (29). This allows the respiratory frequency to be set between 12 and 46 per minute.

The inspiratory-expiratory ratio is nominally fixed at 1 : 1·7.

A simplified version of this ventilator, the Lundia 'Heim' Model, is available. It has no provision for negative pressure during the expiratory phase, and the frequency is not continuously variable, there being a choice of five preset frequencies (16, 18, 20, 22 and 24 per minute).

FUNCTIONAL ANALYSIS

Inspiratory phase

Fundamentally the Lundia is a non-constant flow generator in the inspiratory phase because the concertina reservoir bag (12) is compressed according to a preset pattern of movement by the constant-speed electric motor (32). The waveform is determined by the eccentric groove in the sprocket wheel (28) and the linkage (13, 26, 27) and is approximately sinusoidal, but with the peak flow occurring late in the phase.

However, the high compliance of the concertina bag (about 10 ml/cmH_2O) and the operation of the diaphragm valve (8) serve to modify this fundamental action somewhat. Thus, when the compliance of the lung model is halved or its resistance is doubled (fig. 60.5) the increased pressure at the mouth (and hence in the concertina bag) in the later part of the phase leads to some of the generated flow being absorbed in the compliance of the bag. Therefore the flow at the mouth in the last two-thirds of the phase is slightly diminished. The flow pattern in the first one-third of the phase is influenced by the valve (8). With negative pressure in the lungs at the end of the expiratory phase, this valve does not open until a positive pressure has been built up in the concertina bag. Therefore, when it does open, there is a rapid rush of gas as the compliance of the concertina bag 'discharges' into the compliance of the lungs (see p. 98). This is particularly marked when the lung compliance is halved because of the more-negative alveolar pressure at the end of the expiratory phase. In extreme circumstances the valve (8) may even close again momentarily before reopening finally for the main part of the inspiratory phase (fig. 60.6f).

Change-over from inspiratory phase to expiratory phase

This is both volume-cycled and time-cycled. It occurs when the moving plate of the concertina reservoir bag (12) has been swept through a preset volume in a preset time by the drive from the constant-speed motor. In practice (fig. 60.5) the tidal volume is very slightly influenced by lung characteristics, because of the compliance of the concertina bag (12). The inspiratory time is also slightly influenced by lung characteristics because of resultant variation in the delay in the opening of valve (8).

Expiratory phase

At the start of this phase the ventilator operates as a constant, atmospheric, pressure generator with the patient expiring freely to atmosphere past the one-way valve (17). Fig. 60.5 shows that the pressure at the mouth, which is separated from the generated pressure by some resistance, always declines fairly rapidly to atmospheric at the beginning of the phase, despite changes of lung characteristics; on the other hand the flow pattern alters considerably with lung characteristics.

Later in the phase, at a time determined by the setting of the negative-pressure timing lever (15), the negative-pressure mechanism is brought into play. In fig. 60.5 it can be seen that, towards the end of the expiratory phase, when the flow has fallen to zero, or very nearly so, and the mouth and alveolar pressures have fallen to atmospheric, there is a period in which the flow suddenly increases again and the mouth pressure suddenly becomes negative. The mode of operation in this period depends on the setting of the negative-pressure-magnitude control (22). When this is set to maximum (curve (a) in fig. 60.4) the mechanism forms a good approximation to a constant-pressure generator;

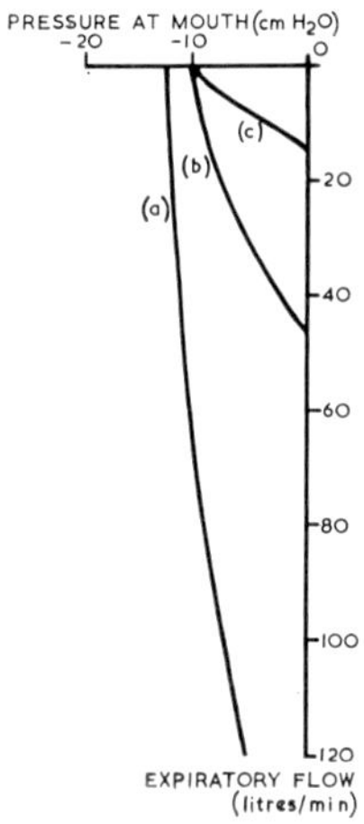

Fig. 60.4. Lundia 'Special' ventilator Model B. Flow-pressure characteristics of the negative-pressure mechanism. Negative-pressure-magnitude control knob (22) set to (a) 10 (i.e. maximum) (b) $3\frac{1}{2}$ (c) $2\frac{1}{4}$ turns above minimum setting. These measurements were made with the belt drive disconnected from the main ventilator mechanism, which was stopped in the expiratory position, so that continuous negative pressure was available at the 'expiration' port (14).

large flows do not diminish the pressure very much. At lower settings (curves (b) and (c) in fig. 60.4) the pressure at the mouth falls off much more rapidly as the flow increases, and the mechanism is best regarded as a constant-pressure generator with substantial series resistance, the resistance arising primarily at the valve (21). (The mechanism does not approximate to a flow generator because the generated pressure is not much larger than that which may be required in the alveoli.) It can be seen in fig. 60.5 (for which the setting of the negative-pressure-magnitude control knob (22) was as for curve (b) in fig. 60.4) that decreasing the compliance or increasing the airway resistance decreases the flow in the negative-pressure part of the phase, but also allows the mouth pressure to approach the generated pressure (about -10 cmH_2O) more closely, because of the reduced pressure drop across the resistance in series with the generated pressure.

Finally, there is usually a short period of zero-flow generation at the end of the expiratory phase, after the expiratory valve (18) has closed, and before the pressure in the concertina bag (12) has built up sufficiently to open the inspiratory valve (8). In fig. 60.5 the flow is always zero during this part of the phase whereas the pressure at the mouth is different for different lung characteristics.

Change-over from expiratory phase to inspiratory phase

Primarily this is time-cycled in that, because of the constant speed of the electric motor,

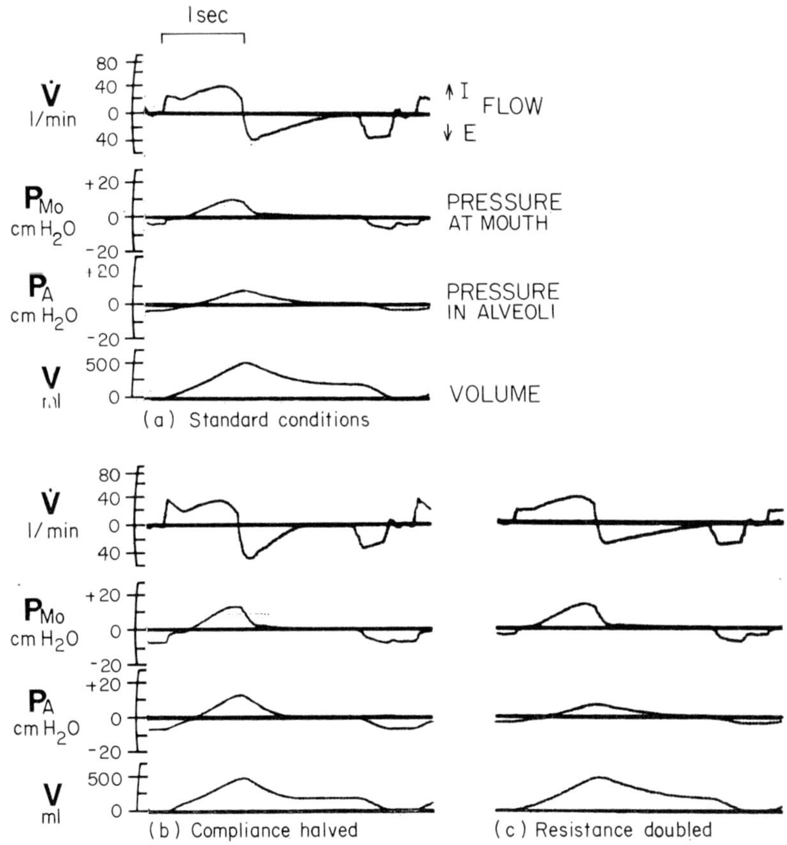

Fig. 60.5. Lundia 'Special' ventilator Model B. Recordings showing the effects of changes of lung characteristics.

Standard conditions: positive-pressure safety-valve, set to maximum; air-inlet valve (9), closed; fresh-gas flow, 16 litres/min oxygen; tidal-volume control, set to produce a tidal volume of 500 ml; respiratory-frequency control, set to 20/min; negative-pressure timing lever, set one-quarter of the way from minimum towards maximum; negative-pressure-magnitude control knob, set to produce a minimum alveolar pressure of -3 cmH_2O ($3\frac{1}{2}$ turns, out of 10 turns, from minimum to maximum).

the expiratory valve (18) closes at a preset time after it opens. However, there is a small delay between the closing of the expiratory valve and the opening of the inspiratory valve (8), due mainly to the need to build up some pressure in the concertina reservoir bag (12) first. Variations in this delay are small, so the resultant percentage variations in expiratory time are very small indeed. Fig. 60.5 shows that the expiratory time is negligibly affected by changes of lung characteristics, whereas the pressure at the mouth at the end of the phase varies substantially, and the phase does not end immediately some critical volume has come out of the lungs.

CONTROLS

Total ventilation

This is not directly controlled but is equal to the product of the separately-controlled tidal volume and respiratory frequency.

Tidal volume

This is directly controlled (fig. 60.6b) by the stroke-volume control (26) which alters the swept volume of the moving plate of the concertina reservoir bag (12). The only way in which the tidal volume can differ markedly from this is if some gas escapes through the adjustable safety-valve (10). Otherwise, the tidal volume is little affected by changes of lung characteristics or by changes in the settings of other controls. However, since the concertina bag has a high compliance (about 10 ml/cmH_2O) large changes in the pressure at the mouth, and hence the pressure in the concertina bag, at the end of the inspiratory phase, can produce some change in the tidal volume delivered to the patient. The biggest change in our recordings occurred when negative pressure was applied for the whole of the expiratory phase (fig. 60.6f). This led to a very low mouth pressure at the end of the expiratory phase, and hence also at the end of the inspiratory phase, with the result that the tidal volume was 10% greater than under the standard conditions (fig. 60.6a).

Respiratory frequency

This is directly controlled by the respiratory-frequency control (29) and is quite uninfluenced by changes of lung characteristics (fig. 60.5) or by changes in the settings of the other controls (fig. 60.6).

Inspiratory-expiratory ratio

The expiratory valve is closed for about two-fifths of each respiratory cycle so that potentially the inspiratory-expiratory ratio is about 2 : 3 or 1 : 1·5.

However, since the inspiratory valve does not open until pressure has been built up in the concertina reservoir bag some time after the expiratory valve has closed, the inspiratory-expiratory ratio is in fact less than 1 : 2. It cannot be deliberately altered in any way although it does vary slightly with lung characteristics and the settings of some of the controls.

Inspiratory waveforms

Since this ventilator operates mainly as a flow generator in this phase, it is primarily the flow waveform which is determined by the ventilator while the pressure waveforms depend on the interaction of this flow waveform with the lung characteristics. The nature of the basic flow waveform is determined by the eccentric groove (28) and therefore cannot be altered. However, because of the large compliance of the concertina reservoir bag and the action of the inspiratory valve the actual flow waveform is slightly modified by changes of lung characteristics (fig. 60.5). For the same reason it is also modified when, because of negative pressure being applied throughout the expiratory phase (fig. 60.6f), the mouth pressure at the end of the phase is very low.

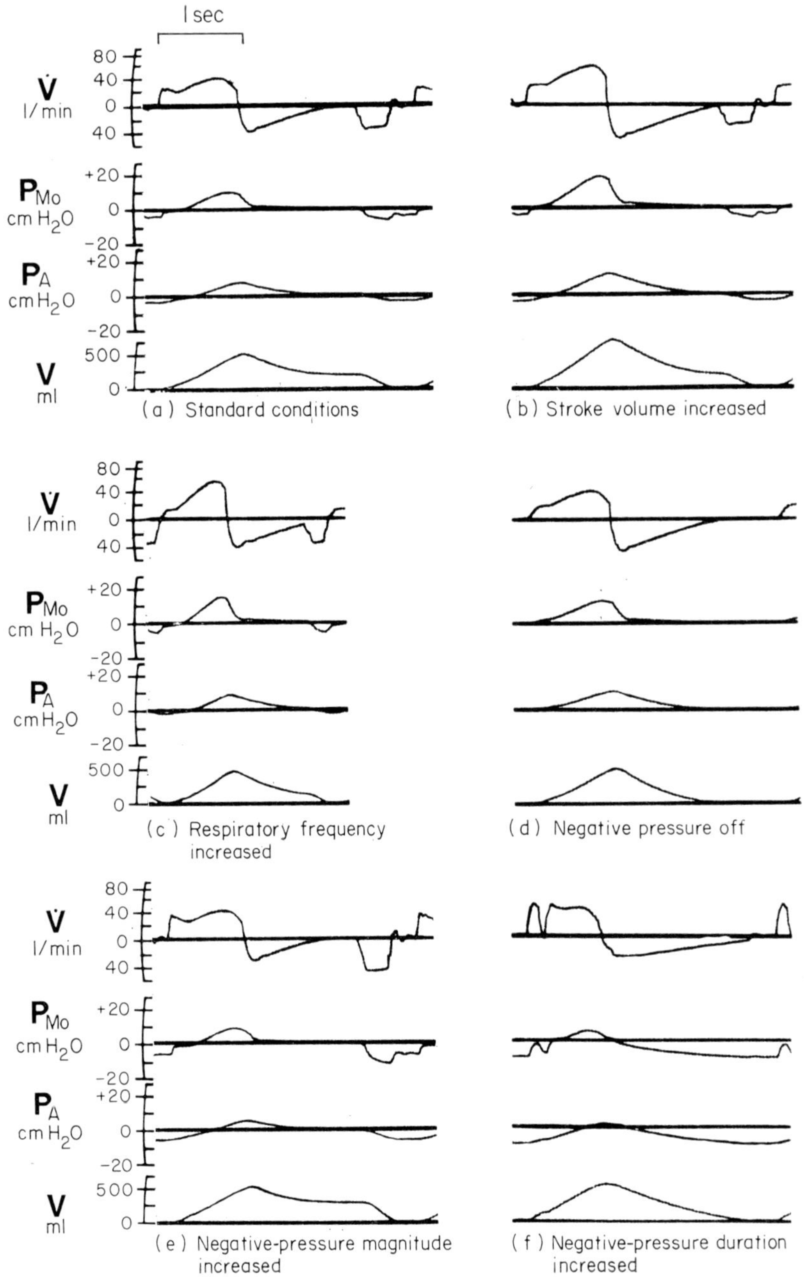

The amplitude of the flow waveform is increased when the tidal volume or respiratory frequency is increased (fig. 60.6b and c).

Expiratory waveforms

In the expiratory phase it is the applied pressure which is determined by the ventilator, apart from the short period of zero-flow generation at the end of the phase. The generated pressure is first atmospheric and then negative. The magnitude and duration of the negative pressure can be independently varied by the controls (22) and (15) (fig. 60.6e and f) respectively. Therefore it is possible, for instance by increasing the magnitude but decreasing the duration of negative pressure, to make a real change in the expiratory waveforms without changing the pressure at the end of the phase or, indeed, any other parameter of ventilation.

Pressure limits

If either of the negative-pressure controls (15) (22) is set to minimum, constant, atmospheric, pressure generation continues throughout the phase and the alveolar pressure always falls to atmospheric, unless the airway resistance is very high or the expiratory time very short (i.e. respiratory frequency very high). The minimum alveolar pressure may be made negative, and the degree of negativity controlled, by adjusting the negative-pressure-timing lever (15) or the negative-pressure-magnitude control (22). However, only if negative pressure is applied for most of the phase (timing lever (15) at or near maximum as in fig. 60.6f) will there be time for the alveolar pressure to approach the generated pressure closely. With negative pressure applied for only a short time the minimum alveolar pressure varies with changes of lung characteristics (fig. 60.5) and with the setting of the respiratory-frequency control (29) (fig. 60.6c).

The peak alveolar pressure at the end of the inspiratory phase cannot be directly controlled; whatever the minimum alveolar pressure at the end of the expiratory phase happens to be, the peak alveolar pressure exceeds it by an amount equal to the tidal volume divided by the compliance.

Fig. 60.6. Lundia 'Special' ventilator Model B. Recordings showing the effects of changes in the settings of the controls.

(a) Standard conditions as in fig. 60.5.
(b) Stroke-volume-control setting increased to produce a tidal volume of 750 ml.
(c) Respiratory frequency increased to 30/min.
(d) Negative-pressure-magnitude control knob set to minimum.
(e) Negative-pressure-magnitude control knob set to maximum.
(f) Negative-pressure-timing lever set to maximum.

CHAPTER 61

The Manley Ventilator[1]

DESCRIPTION

This ventilator (figs. 61.1 and 61.2) is intended for ward or anaesthetic use, and is available with or without a negative-pressure phase. It is of such size that it will stand on

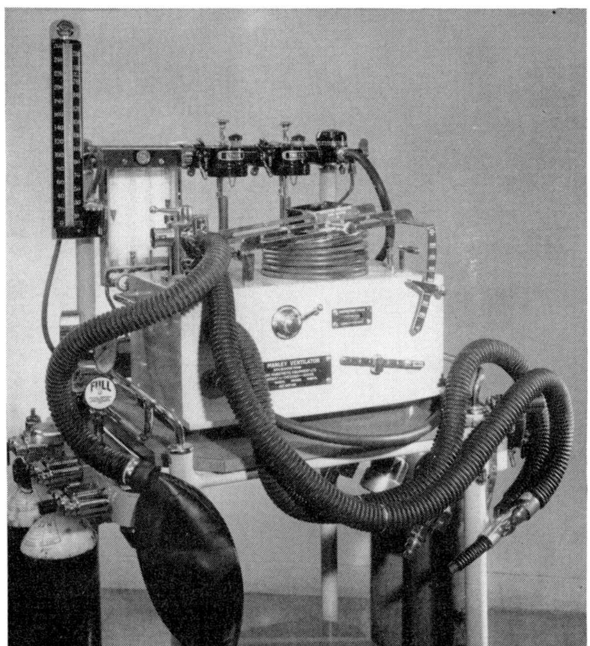

Fig. 61.1. The Manley ventilator.
Courtesy of Department of Medical Illustration, Cardiff Royal Infirmary.

the commonly-used British anaesthetic trolley. It is operated by the anaesthetic gas mixture or by the compressed air or oxygen with which the patient's lungs are to be inflated. The ventilator operates as a non-rebreathing circuit.

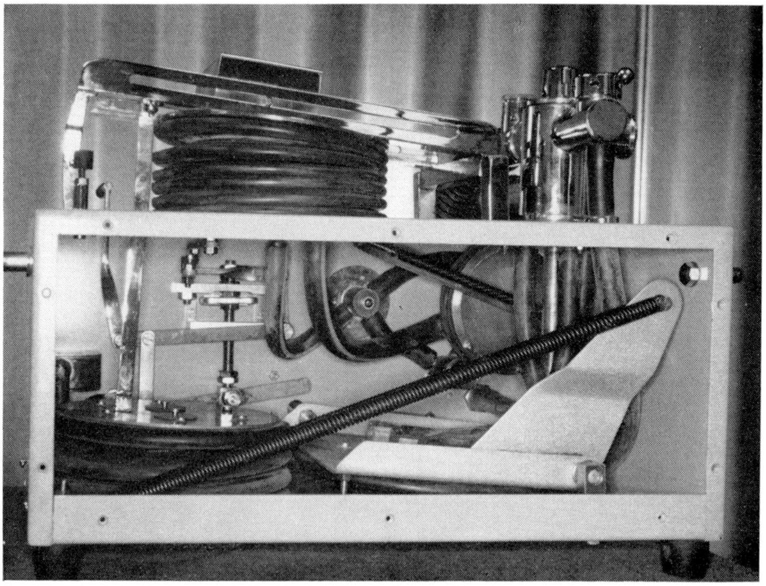

Fig. 61.2. Mechanism of the Manley ventilator.
Courtesy of Department of Medical Illustration, Cardiff Royal Infirmary.

All the gas supplied to the ventilator, provided that the flow is not excessive, is delivered to the patient. The driving gas should be derived from a source of at least 5 lb/in^2 (e.g. the regulators on the anaesthetic apparatus). The flow must be regulated by a suitable needle valve. It is desirable also that the flow be monitored by a flowmeter. During anaesthesia, the controls and flowmeters of the anaesthetic machine are used.

The gas is delivered through the inlet (26) (fig. 61.3) to the small concertina bag (25) which is compressed by the spring (27). This bag acts as a small reservoir in which the pressure is maintained by the spring (27) between 110 and 150 cmH_2O. If at any time the concertina bag (25) becomes nearly empty, any further outflow of gas from the bag is prevented by the closure of the valve inside the bag. This ensures that, however low the flow of fresh gas into the bag (25), the pressure within the bag cannot fall below that determined by the spring (27). Undue fluctuation of the flowmeter readings which would otherwise result is thus prevented.

During the expiratory phase the valve (6), which is operated by the click mechanism (5), is open, and gas flows, from the small concertina bag (25), into the main reservoir bag (8). This concertina bag (8) expands, lifting the top-plate with its moveable weight (7), and with it the arm (2), until the adjustable stop (4) strikes the arm (3), reversing the click mechanism (5); this allows the valve (6) to be closed by its spring. Now that the flow of gas from the concertina bag (25) to the bag (8) is stopped, the pressure in the

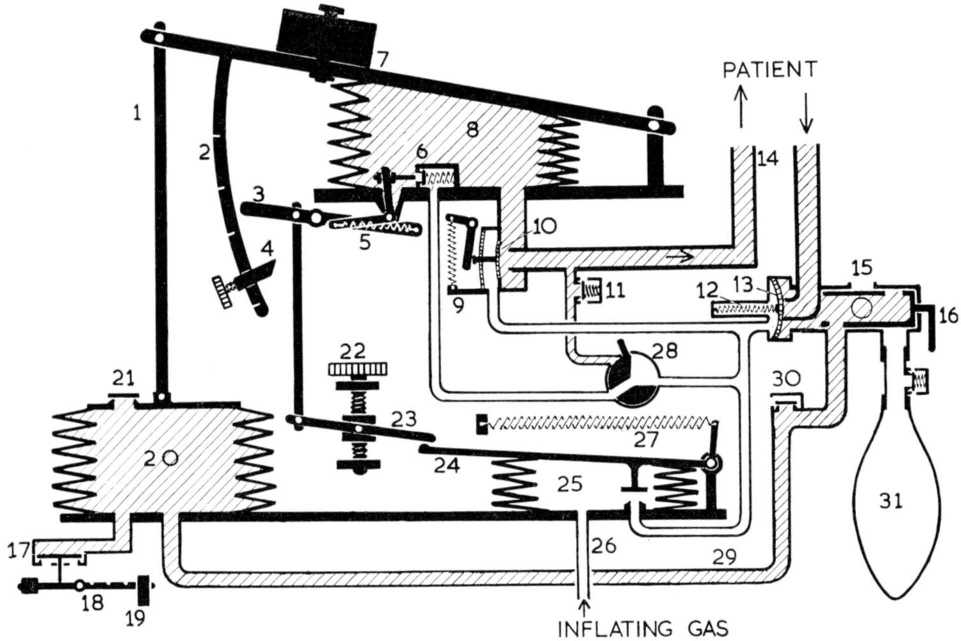

Fig. 61.3. Diagram of the Manley ventilator.

1. Connecting rod
2. Arm
3. Lever of click mechanism
4. Adjustable stop, limiting tidal volume
5. Click mechanism
6. Inlet valve of main concertina bag
7. Top-plate of main concertina bag with moveable weight
8. Main concertina reservoir bag
9. Expansion spring of inspiratory valve
10. Inspiratory valve
11. Safety-valve
12. Expansion spring of expiratory valve
13. Diaphragm of expiratory valve
14. Inspiratory tube
15. Port
16. 3-position tap
17. Inlet valve
18. Arm
19. Counterweight
20. Negative-pressure concertina bag
21. One-way valve
22. 'Inspiratory phase' control
23. Lever of click mechanism
24. Top-plate of small concertina bag
25. Small concertina bag
26. Inflating-gas inlet
27. Expansion spring
28. 'Manual/automatic' control
29. Connecting tube
30. One-way valve
31. Reservoir bag for manual inflation

circuit between them rises towards that in the bag (25). This pressure rise also occurs behind the diaphragm (13) of the expiratory valve and between the diaphragms of the inspiratory valve (10). When this pressure has risen sufficiently, the pull of the spring (12) on the diaphragm (13) is overcome; the diaphragm (13) moves over and closes the expiratory valve. As the pressure continues to rise the force on the larger diaphragm of the inspiratory valve (10) becomes sufficient to overcome both the force on the smaller diaphragm and the pull of the spring (9), thus opening the inspiratory valve, and allowing the weight (7) to force the contents of the bag (8), through the inspiratory tube (14), to the patient. The safety-valve (11) limits the positive pressure in the inspiratory tube to 35 cmH_2O. It will only come into operation if the weight (7) is near its maximum setting and some partial or total obstruction causes the pressure in the delivery tube (14) to approach that in the concertina bag (8).

During the inspiratory phase fresh gas continues to enter the concertina bag (25) which expands until the top-plate (24) hits the lever (23), reversing the click mechanism (5) and reopening the valve (6). The pressure in the tube connecting the bags (25) and (8) falls. The gas stored under pressure in the small bag (25) is now rapidly discharged into the main reservoir bag (8). When the pressure in the connecting tube has fallen sufficiently the inspiratory valve (10) closes. As the pressure continues to fall, the expiratory valve (13) opens and the expiratory phase commences.

Provided the inspiratory phase is long enough, and the pressure generated by the weight (7) is high enough, the main reservoir bag (8) is completely emptied. The volume delivered to the patient therefore depends on the volume in the concertina bag (8) at the beginning of the inspiratory phase. This is determined by the position of the stop (4) on the arm (2). Further, insomuch as all fresh gas entering the ventilator is finally delivered to the patient, the fresh-gas flow and the minute-volume ventilation are equal. The time taken for one complete respiratory cycle is then the time taken for one tidal volume of fresh gas to enter the ventilator. Of this time, the duration of the inspiratory phase is the time taken for the fresh-gas flow to fill the small bag (25) sufficiently for the plate (24) to strike the lever (23) and reverse the click mechanism (5). The small bag (25) is, in fact, always collapsed at the end of the expiratory phase, and hence the time taken for it to fill is dependent, not only on the inflating-gas flow, but also on the height of the lever (23), set by the 'inspiratory phase' control (22). Once the inflating-gas flow and the control (22) have been set, a change in the setting of the tidal volume on the arm (2) will alter the duration of a complete respiratory cycle, but not of the inspiratory phase. There is no independent control for the duration of the expiratory phase, which is the difference between the duration of the complete respiratory cycle and the duration of the inspiratory phase. The expiratory phase is in fact the time needed for the main concertina bag (8) to expand sufficiently for the stop (4) to reverse the click mechanism, i.e. for a tidal volume to enter the bag. However, it should be noted that part of this tidal volume accumulates in the small bag (25) during the inspiratory phase, at the end of which it is discharged rapidly into the main bag (8). The rest of the tidal volume is the gas which enters steadily throughout the expiratory phase. The duration of the expiratory phase therefore, for any set tidal volume and inflating-gas flow, depends on the amount which was stored in the small bag (25), i.e. on the duration of the inspiratory phase.

When the inflating-gas flow and the tidal volume are set, and hence the duration of each respiratory cycle is fixed, the inspiratory-expiratory ratio depends on the setting of the control (22). If the inflating-gas flow is altered, but the tidal volume unchanged, then the duration of one respiratory cycle is altered, but, unless the control (22) is also adjusted, the inspiratory-expiratory ratio remains the same. Conversely, if the tidal volume is altered, but the inflating-gas flow is unchanged, then the duration of one respiratory cycle is altered, the duration of the inspiratory phase remains the same, and the inspiratory-expiratory ratio is therefore altered.

The time taken for the tidal volume to enter the lungs depends on two factors. The first is the pressure generated in the main bag (8) by the weight (7). The second is a combination of the patient's compliance and the total resistance of the gas pathway from the bag (8) to the alveoli. This time is not necessarily as long as the duration of the inspiratory phase. For example, if the gas can flow rapidly enough into the lungs, the main bag (8) will reach the bottom of its stroke before the end of the inspiratory phase. This occurs if the pressure in the main bag (8) is set high enough by the weight (7), if the patient's compliance is high enough, if there is a leak in the gas pathway, or if the tidal volume is set low enough. On the other hand, if the flow of gas into the lungs is slow, the main bag (8) may not reach the bottom of its stroke before the end of the inspiratory phase. This may arise because the inflating pressure is set too low, the patient's compliance is low, the resistance of the gas pathways is high, or too large a tidal volume is set.

A convenient method of setting the controls in practice is as follows. The weight (7) is moved to the position for maximum pressure. The inflating-gas flow (i.e. the minute-volume ventilation), the tidal volume, and the inspiratory-expiratory ratio are then set in that order. Finally the position of the weight (7) is adjusted so that the emptying of the main bag (8) occupies the desired fraction of the inspiratory phase.

The expiratory tube from the patient leads to a tap (16) which, in the positive-pressure version of the ventilator, has only two positions: one in which the expired gas flows freely to atmosphere through the port (15), and one in which the expiratory tube is connected to a reservoir bag (31), with an adjustable blow-off valve, for manual inflation. In the positive-negative version (illustrated in fig. 61.3) the tap (16) has a third position which allows negative pressure to be applied during the expiratory phase.

The top of the negative-pressure concertina bag (20) is connected by the rod (1) to the top-plate of the main concertina bag (8). During the expiratory phase the main bag (8) is filling, and its upward movement expands the negative-pressure bag (20). An adjustable air-inlet valve (17) at the base of the bag (20) sets a limit to the negative pressure. This limit is determined by the position of the counterweight (19) on the arm (18). During the inspiratory phase the negative-pressure bag (20) is compressed and, since the expiratory valve (13) is closed, the contents of the bag (20) are voided to atmosphere through the one-way valve (21). A one-way outlet valve (30) near the 3-position tap (16) allows expired gas to spill to atmosphere if it flows from the patient faster than the bag (20) is expanded.

For manual inflation the taps (16) and (28) are turned to the 'manual' position bringing the reservoir bag (31) into use. Tap (28) by-passes the main concertina bag (8) and directs the fresh gas to the inspiratory tube (14). The safety-valve (11) limits the pressure within this circuit to 35 cmH_2O which is insufficient to reverse the valves (10) and (13). These valves are therefore held closed and open respectively, by the force of their springs.

FUNCTIONAL ANALYSIS

Inspiratory phase

Since the mechanism for inflation in this ventilator is a weighted concertina bag (8), it might be expected to operate as a constant-pressure generator. However, a number of factors serve to modify or obscure this fundamental mode of operation.

Firstly, the volume limit, set by the volume of gas contained within the bag, is commonly reached before the end of the phase; this occurs in all instances in fig. 61.5 and in most instances in fig. 61.6. Once this limit is reached the ventilator operates as a zero-flow generator for the remainder of the phase. Secondly, the elasticity of the wall of the bag causes an appreciable fall of pressure in the bag as it empties (fig. 61.4), so that the

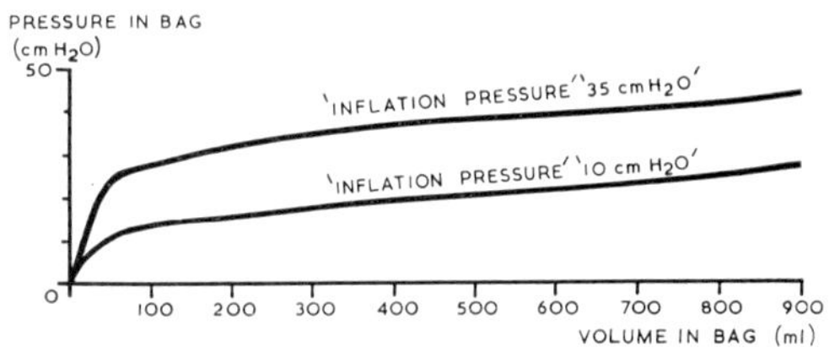

Fig. 61.4. The Manley ventilator. Pressure-volume characteristics of the main, positive-pressure, concertina reservoir bag.

mechanism is better regarded as a discharging compliance (see p. 98). Thirdly, the build-up of pressure at the mouth at the start of the phase is gradual rather than abrupt; this can probably be accounted for by a gradual opening of the inspiratory valve (10). Finally, the inertia of the weight (7) imposes some oscillations on the pressure in the bag.

The result of these various factors is that the waveforms in fig. 61.5 differ substantially from those for an ideal constant-pressure generator (fig. 3.4, p. 75) or even those for a discharging compliance. However, in the brief period between the attainment of peak flow and the operation of the volume limit, the flow waveform can be seen to change with lung characteristics in the expected manner: halving the compliance, and so reducing the time constant of the system, produces a more rapid decline of flow; doubling the airway resistance produces a slower decline of flow. In all instances the expected long tail of the decline is cut off by the attainment of the volume limit. At the start of the ensuing, zero-flow-generating part of the phase, the pressure at the mouth falls abruptly to that which has previously been built up in the alveoli.

Change-over from inspiratory phase to expiratory phase

This change-over is time-cycled: it occurs when a preset volume of gas (preset by the 'inspiratory phase' control (22)) has been delivered to the small concertina bag (25) by the preset inflating-gas flow. It can be seen in fig. 61.5 that the inspiratory time is the same in all three conditions whereas the pressure at the mouth at the end of the phase is greatly altered by halving the compliance. The tidal volume is the same in all conditions but this is due to the attainment of the volume limit and not to any volume-cycling mechanism: it can be seen that each volume trace has a long 'flat' at its maximum, indicating that the inspiratory phase does not end until some considerable time after the volume limit has been reached. In some conditions, not shown in figs. 61.5 or 61.6, time-cycling will occur before the volume limit is reached.

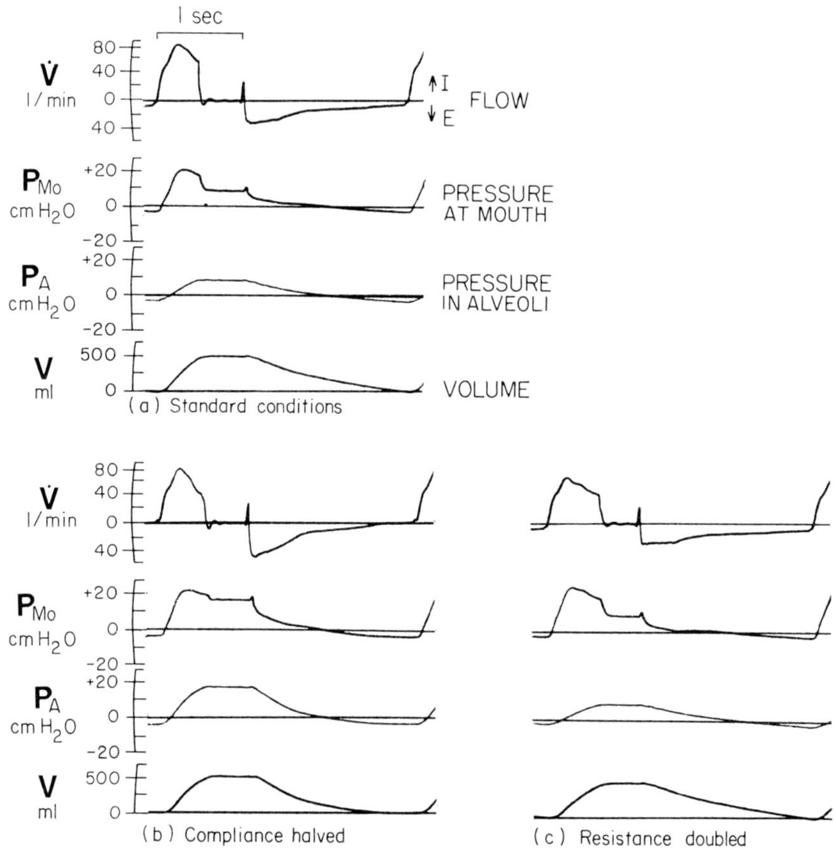

Fig. 61.5. The Manley ventilator. Recordings showing the effects of changes of lung characteristics.

Standard conditions: inflating gas, oxygen from a 60 lb/in^2 pipe-line and needle valve, set to give a total ventilation of 10 litres/min (Rotameter reading when corrected to atmospheric pressure was 11 litres/min); 'inflation pressure', '35 cmH_2O'; 'negative phase', '3 cmH_2O'; 'tidal volume', set for a tidal volume of 500 ml; 'inspiratory phase', set for an inspiratory-expiratory ratio of 1 : 2.

Expiratory phase

When the negative-pressure circuit is not in use (fig. 61.6f) the patient is simply connected to atmosphere at the expiratory port (15) during the expiratory phase and therefore the ventilator acts as a constant, atmospheric, pressure generator. In fig. 61.6f the slow fall to atmospheric of the mouth pressure can probably be mainly attributed to gradual opening of the valve (13).

When the negative-pressure circuit is in use (fig. 61.5 and fig. 61.6a–e) it is necessary to distinguish three parts of the phase. Throughout the phase expired gas can enter the negative-pressure concertina bag only at a rate equal to the rate at which the bag is expanding. If, as is usually the case, the initial flow rate of expired gas exceeds this, the excess spills to atmosphere through the one-way valve (30) and the ventilator operates as a constant, atmospheric, pressure generator during this first part of the phase.

In the second part of the phase, when the expiratory flow has fallen to equal the flow into the negative-pressure concertina bag (20), there is no excess expired gas to escape and the ventilator operates as a flow generator. This is due to the negative-pressure concertina bag being expanded by its mechanical linkage to the positive-pressure concertina bag (8) which, in turn, is expanded by the entry of inflating gas. Since the pressure in the small, internal, positive-pressure concertina bag (25) is about 110 cmH_2O at this time, and the pressure in the main positive-pressure reservoir bag (8) increases by about 10 cmH_2O in the course of filling (fig. 61.4), the flow of gas into the main positive-pressure reservoir bag declines slightly during the phase. Therefore the rate of expansion of both the positive-pressure and the negative-pressure bags, and the flow generated by the negative-pressure bag, all decline slightly during the phase.

Finally, if the pressure in the negative-pressure concertina bag falls to the negative-pressure limit set by the mechanism (17–19), there will be a third part of the phase in which the ventilator operates as a constant, negative, pressure generator.

In relating this theoretical analysis to the experimental curves in fig. 61.5 it must be remembered that there is resistance (and therefore flow-dependent pressure difference) between the mouth, where pressure is recorded, and the valve (30) at which atmospheric pressure is generated, or the valve (17) at which negative pressure is generated. Thus the evidence of the initial, atmospheric-pressure-generating part of the phase is the variation in the flow waveform in the different conditions, rather than any constancy in the pressure waveform at the mouth. The middle, flow-generating, part of the phase can be seen fairly clearly, allowing for the decline in flow mentioned above. This flow-generating section is very short when the compliance is halved, because the given generated flow then drops the pressure more rapidly to the point at which the negative-pressure limit (17–19) comes into play. The final, negative-pressure-generating part of the phase is also characterized by variability of flow rather than by constancy of pressure at the mouth. However in fig. 61.5b it can be seen that with the compliance halved (and therefore a short time constant) the flow has fallen to zero before the end of the phase and the mouth and alveolar pressures are both equal to the generated pressure and steady.

In certain circumstances some of the three modes of functioning in the expiratory phase may be missing. For instance, if the airway resistance or the compliance is very high (beyond the range used in fig. 61.5) the conditions may be such that free expiration to atmosphere would result in a lower initial flow than that generated by the negative-pressure concertina bag. In this case there will be no initial period of constant, atmospheric, pressure generation. In extreme cases, the negative-pressure-limit valve may open at the very start of the phase so that the ventilator then operates as a constant, negative, pressure generator throughout the phase.

Change-over from expiratory phase to inspiratory phase

This change-over occurs when the main positive-pressure concertina bag (8) has refilled with inflating gas. The volume required to refill the bag is equal to the tidal volume which left it in the previous inspiratory phase. The fresh gas which supplies this volume enters the ventilator at a constant flow throughout the respiratory cycle. (The fraction that enters during the inspiratory phase is stored temporarily in the small, internal, positive-pressure concertina bag (25)). Therefore the change-over occurs at a time, after the end of the previous *expiratory* phase, equal to the tidal volume divided by the inflating-gas flow.

If the volume limit is always reached in the inspiratory phase the tidal volume is constant and therefore so is the duration of the respiratory cycle. Since the change-over from the inspiratory phase to the expiratory phase is also time-cycled (it occurs at a preset time after the end of the expiratory phase) the change-over from the expiratory phase to the inspiratory phase can be said to be time-cycled in the conventional sense: it occurs at a preset time after the end of the inspiratory phase irrespective of changes of lung characteristics.

If the volume limit is not reached during the inspiratory phase then the tidal volume, and hence the volume required to refill the positive-pressure concertina bag, varies with the patient's lung characteristics and therefore so also does the duration of the expiratory phase and of the whole respiratory cycle. In these circumstances all that can be said is that the change-over from the expiratory phase to the inspiratory phase occurs at a time, after the end of the previous expiratory phase, equal to the previous tidal volume divided by the inflating-gas flow. Although the inflating-gas flow is determined by the ventilator (regarding the flowmeter controls as forming part of the ventilator) the tidal volume in these circumstances will vary with lung characteristics.

In both cases, whether the volume limit is reached or not during the inspiratory phase, the duration of the expiratory phase, and of the whole respiratory cycle, is in fact somewhat longer than the above argument indicates because, in the three models of this ventilator tested, some of the gas stored in the small, internal, positive-pressure concertina bag (25), instead of being simply transferred to the main positive-pressure bag (8), escaped past the inspiratory valve (10) and expiratory valve (13) just as the change-over was occurring. This was because the expiratory valve started to open before the inspiratory valve was completely shut. However in the model used to make the recordings in figs. 61.5 and 61.6, the volume lost in this way had been reduced to about 25 ml in each cycle. This escape of gas from the small, internal, concertina bag explains the 'spike' of inspiratory flow which can be seen in all tracings at the very end of the inspiratory phase: the sudden brief rush of gas through the inspiratory and expiratory tubes raises the mouth pressure sufficiently (see the small 'pip' on the mouth-pressure tracings) to drive a little more gas into the patient—although the amount is barely detectable on the volume tracing.

In fig. 61.5 the volume limit is reached during the inspiratory phase in all three cases and it can be seen that the expiratory time is uninfluenced by changes in compliance or resistance. On the other hand the pressure at the mouth at the end of the expiratory phase varies a little and, when the compliance is halved, the full volume has come out of the lungs some time before the change-over occurs.

CONTROLS

Total ventilation

Since this ventilator is a minute-volume divider (see p. 140) the total ventilation is directly controlled by the inflating-gas flow. Ideally the total ventilation is equal to the inflating-gas flow but in practice is always a little less. This is partly because of the compliance of the breathing tubes (about 25 ml of the stroke volume of the bag is lost in this way under the 'standard conditions') and partly because, in the three models tested, at the very end of the inspiratory phase some of the gas in the small, internal, concertina bag (25) escapes to atmosphere via the main positive-pressure reservoir bag (8) and the inspiratory and expiratory valves. In the model used to make the recordings of figs. 61.5 and 61.6 the volume lost in this second way in each respiratory cycle was only about 25 ml. Under the 'standard' conditions the total loss from both causes made the total ventilation fall short of the inflating-gas flow by 10%.

When the inflating-gas flow is increased the inspiratory time, the time required to fill the small, internal, concertina bag (25), is always decreased; the effect on other parameters depends on whether or not the volume limit is still reached (whether or not the main positive-pressure reservoir bag (8) still empties) within this shortened inspiratory phase.

If the volume limit is still reached during the inspiratory phase (fig. 61.6b) the tidal volume is unaltered and the increased ventilation is produced by a proportionate increase in respiratory frequency. Since the rate of filling of the small concertina bag (25), which controls the inspiratory time, and the rate of filling of the main concertina bag (8), which controls the expiratory time, are increased to the same extent by the increase in inflating-gas flow, the inspiratory-expiratory ratio is unaltered. The shortening of the expiratory time prevents the mouth and alveolar pressures from approaching the negative generated pressure so closely at the end of the expiratory phase. Therefore pressures are higher throughout the whole respiratory cycle and the mean pressure is raised.

If the volume limit is not reached during the inspiratory phase when the inflating-gas flow is increased (not illustrated in fig. 61.6) the tidal volume is decreased and the respiratory frequency must increase more than in proportion to the inflating-gas flow. In addition a smaller volume of gas is required to refill the main positive-pressure bag (8) so

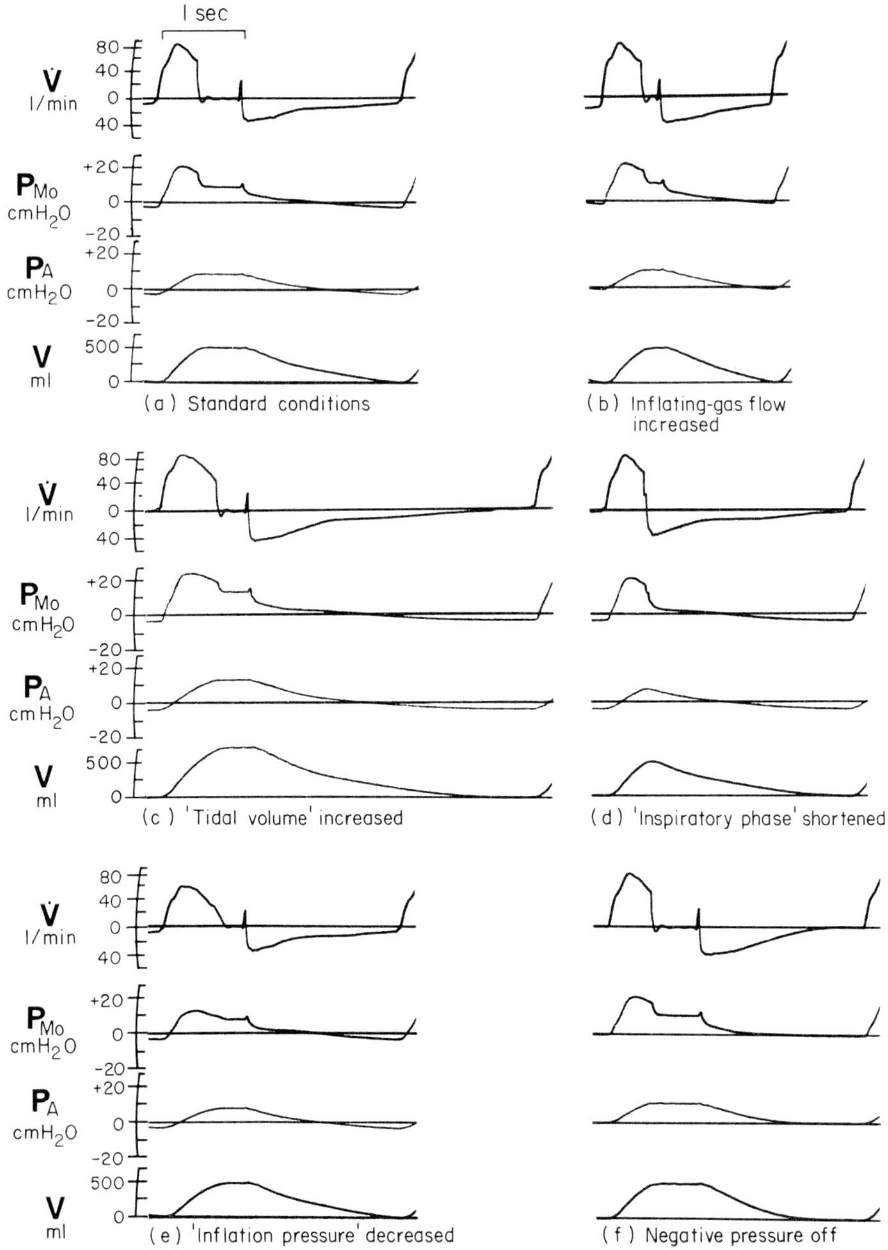

that, with the increased inflating-gas flow, the rate of refilling of the main bag (controlling the expiratory time) is increased relatively more than the rate of refilling of the small, internal, bag (controlling the inspiratory time) and so the inspiratory-expiratory ratio is altered.

Tidal volume

This can be directly controlled by adjusting the excursion of the main positive-pressure concertina bag (8) provided that it always empties during the inspiratory phase. Since the total ventilation is unaltered by this procedure, increasing the tidal volume (fig. 61.6c), must decrease the respiratory frequency. However, the inspiratory time, the time to fill the small, internal, concertina bag (25), is unaltered; the increase in the respiratory period all arises from the increased time taken for the inflating-gas flow to deliver the increased volume to the main positive-pressure bag during the expiratory phase. The inspiratory-expiratory ratio is therefore altered. Also the inspiratory waveforms are modified in that flow continues for a longer part of the inspiratory phase.

If the conditions are such that the volume limit is not reached, i.e. that the main positive-pressure bag does not empty, during the inspiratory phase (not illustrated in fig. 61.6), then the tidal volume can be deliberately increased by either (a) increasing the generated pressure by adjusting the weight (7) on the main positive-pressure bag, or (b) increasing the inspiratory time by the 'inspiratory phase' control (22), or (c) increasing the negative pressure in expiration by adjusting the control (19). Under these conditions, of incomplete emptying of the main positive-pressure bag, the tidal volume also increases with any increase in compliance or decrease in airway resistance.

As already mentioned, increasing the total ventilation may lead to a decrease in tidal volume in certain circumstances.

Respiratory frequency

This cannot be directly controlled but is mathematically determined by the total ventilation, which ideally is equal to the inflating-gas flow, divided by the tidal volume, which is usually the volume excursion set for the main positive-pressure concertina bag.

Inspiratory-expiratory ratio

This is primarily controlled by the 'inspiratory phase' control (22). Adjusting this control (fig. 61.6d) alters the volume excursion of the small, internal, concertina bag and hence changes the inspiratory time. So long as the volume limit is still reached within the

---

Fig. 61.6. The Manley ventilator. Recordings showing the effects of changes in the settings of the controls.

(a) Standard conditions as in fig. 61.5.
(b) Inflating-gas flow increased to 16·5 litres/min (corrected to atmospheric pressure).
(c) 'Tidal volume' increased for a tidal volume of 750 ml.
(d) 'Inspiratory phase' control moved several turns to the right.
(e) 'Inflation pressure' reduced to '15 cmH_2O'.
(f) 'Selector valve' (16) switched to 'negative off'.

new inspiratory time, the duration of the respiratory period, which is the time taken for one tidal volume of fresh gas to enter the machine, is unaltered and the expiratory time is therefore increased by the amount by which the inspiratory time is decreased. In fig. 61.6d the inspiratory time has been reduced to a point at which the volume limit is just reached within the inspiratory phase. Further reduction would have decreased the tidal volume and increased the frequency.

The inspiratory-expiratory ratio is also changed by any change, deliberate or accidental, in tidal volume because this results in a change in expiratory time without any change in inspiratory time (see above).

Inspiratory waveforms

The inspiratory waveforms can be deliberately modified by adjusting the generated pressure by means of the weight (7) on the main, positive-pressure, concertina bag. Reducing the nominal generated pressure (the 'inflation pressure') from 35 cmH_2O (fig. 61.6a) to 15 cmH_2O (fig. 61.6e) results in a reduction in mouth pressure. Consequently the peak flow is reduced and flow continues for a longer fraction of the inspiratory phase before the volume limit is reached.

Expiratory waveforms

The expiratory waveforms are somewhat dependent upon the setting of the negative-pressure control (19) but this setting will normally be determined by the amount of negative pressure required.

Pressure limits

The mouth and alveolar pressures at the end of the expiratory phase can be adjusted by altering the setting of the negative-pressure limit (19) or by switching out negative pressure altogether (fig. 61.6f). However, when the negative-pressure circuit is in use, the closeness with which the mouth and alveolar pressures approach the generated pressure depends to some extent on the patient's compliance and resistance (fig. 61.5) and on the duration of the expiratory phase (fig. 61.6b, c).

The peak mouth pressure in the inspiratory phase approaches the generated pressure but the peak alveolar pressure is determined indirectly. It exceeds the alveolar pressure at the end of the expiratory phase by an amount equal to the tidal volume divided by the compliance and so is changed by changes in these parameters (figs. 61.6 and 61.5b). For any given tidal volume and compliance, any change in the alveolar pressure at the end of the expiratory phase is accompanied by an equal change in the alveolar pressure at the end of the inspiratory phase and, indeed, at almost every point throughout the respiratory cycle. The mean alveolar pressure is therefore also changed by the same amount.

REFERENCE

1 Manley R.W. (1961) A new mechanical ventilator. *Anaesthesia*, **16**, 317.

CHAPTER 62

The Mautz Ventilator[1, 2, 3, 4]

DESCRIPTION

A continuous flow of driving gas enters at the inlet (7) (fig. 62.2) and flows to the plastic pressure chamber (1) surrounding the reservoir 'breathing' bag (2) connected to the patient. A windscreen-wiper motor (5) intermittently opens a disc exhaust valve (4) so

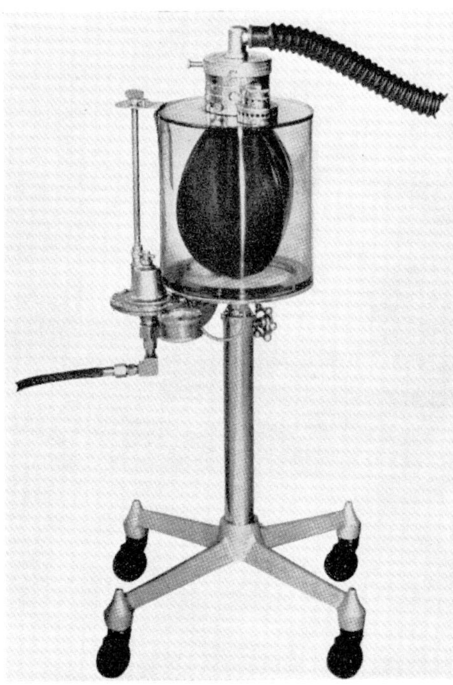

Fig. 62.1. The Mautz ventilator.

Courtesy of Ohio Chemical & Surgical Equipment Co.

that the pressure within the pressure chamber (1) alternates between atmospheric and a maximum determined by the setting of a separate spring-loaded blow-off valve (3). The

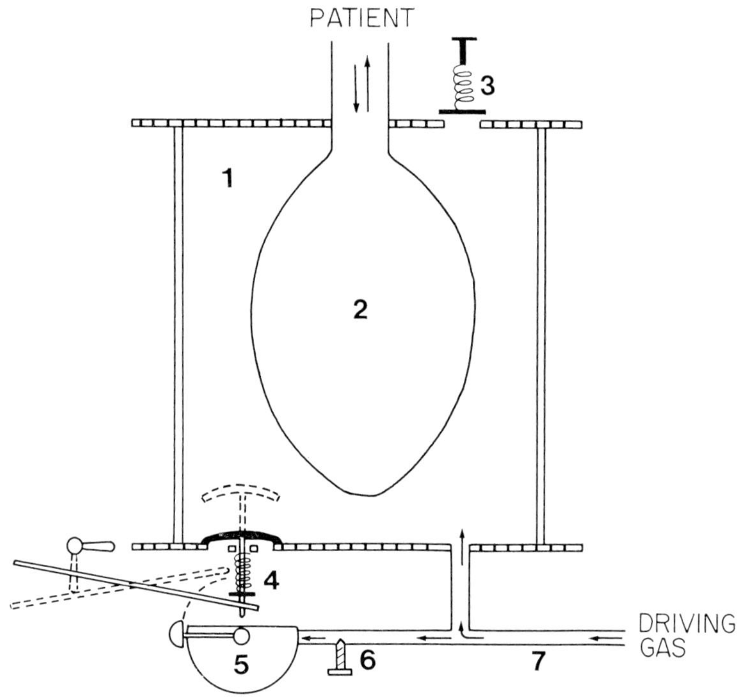

Fig. 62.2. Diagram of the Mautz ventilator.

1. Plastic pressure chamber
2. Reservoir bag
3. Pressure-limiting valve
4. Exhaust valve
5. Windscreen-wiper motor
6. Needle valve
7. Driving-gas inlet

Courtesy of the Scandinavian Society of Anaesthesiologists.[4]

incorporation of either a blow-off valve, spill valve, or a constant leak in the patient circuit allows excess inflating gas to escape.

The frequency of ventilation is controlled by a needle valve (6) in the driving-gas supply to the windscreen wiper (5).

FUNCTIONAL ANALYSIS

In this analysis it is assumed that a spill valve is the means used to vent excess gas from the patient circuit.

Inspiratory phase

In this phase the ventilator operates as a constant-flow generator owing to the constant pressure of the supply (which must be high in order to drive the wiper motor) applied to the resistance (not shown in fig. 62.2) which must separate it from the pressure chamber in order to limit the flow. The pressure-limiting valve (3) on the pressure chamber introduces a pressure limit which governs the patient's tidal volume. Until it comes into operation the fresh-gas supply to the patient circuit acts as a small-constant-flow generator, supplementing the main flow generator.

Change-over from inspiratory phase to expiratory phase

This change-over is time-cycled: the duration of the phase is determined by the wiper motor.

Expiratory phase

In this phase the ventilator operates as a constant, atmospheric, pressure generator: the patient's expired gas effectively has free passage to atmosphere, at the exhaust valve (4).

Change-over from expiratory phase to inspiratory phase

This change-over also is time-cycled: the duration of the expiratory phase is determined by the wiper motor.

REFERENCES

1 MAUTZ F.R. (1939) Mechanical respirator as an adjunct to closed system anesthesia. *Proc. Soc. exp. Biol. (N.Y.)* **42**, 190.
2 MAUTZ F.R. (1941) Mechanism for artificial pulmonary ventilation in the operating room. *J. thorac. Surg.* **10**, 544.
3 MAUTZ F.R., BECK C.S. and CHASE H.F. (1948) Augmented and controlled breathing in transpleural operations. *J. thorac. Surg.* **17**, 283.
4 MÖRCH E.T. and BENSON D.W. (1955) *Proceedings of the Third Congress of the Scandinavian Society of Anaesthesiologists, Copenhagen*, 1954, p. 30.

CHAPTER 63

The 'Minivent'[1]

DESCRIPTION

This tiny ventilator (figs. 63.1 and 63.2) is little bigger than an expiratory-valve assembly. It is designed for anaesthetic use, fitting into a non-rebreathing circuit on the patient side of the standard reservoir bag. It is operated by the pressure built up in the reservoir bag by the steady inflow of gas from the anaesthetic apparatus. This gas flow must be set to equal the desired total minute-volume ventilation.

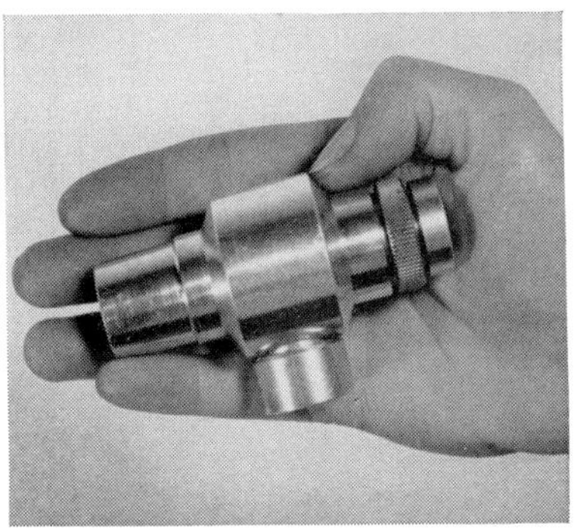

Fig. 63.1.

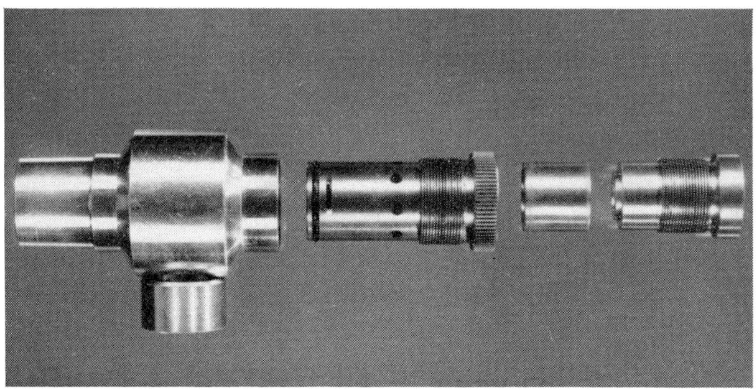

Fig. 63.2.

Fig. 63.1. The 'Minivent'.
Courtesy of Department of Medical Illustration, Cardiff Royal Infirmary.

Fig. 63.2. The components of the 'Minivent'.
Courtesy of Department of Medical Illustration, Cardiff Royal Infirmary.

At rest, the bobbin (5) is held in the position shown in fig. 63.3 by the magnet (2), and there is a free communication, through the port (6), the ports (8, 8) in the bobbin carrier (9), and the expiratory port (7), between the patient and atmosphere. The steady flow of anaesthetic gas into the reservoir bag, to which the 'Minivent' is connected by way of the port (1), distends the bag, causing a rise of pressure within it. This pressure is exerted on the face of the bobbin (5) and when it has increased sufficiently it overcomes the pull of

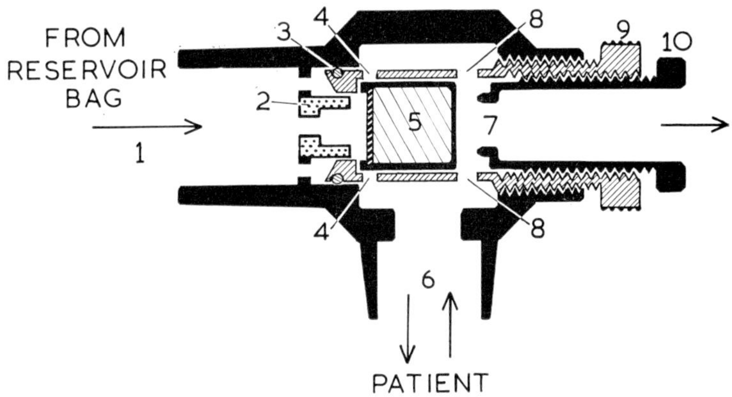

Fig. 63.3. Diagram of the 'Minivent'.

1. Port
2. Magnet
3. Rubber O-ring
4. Slotted ports
5. Bobbin
6. Port
7. End stop and expiratory port
8. Ports
9. Brass 'knurled control knob' of bobbin carrier
10. Aluminium 'smooth control knob' of end stop

the magnet (2) on the bobbin (5). The bobbin (5) is now forced away from the magnet (2), closing the ports (8, 8) and seating on the end stop (7), thereby closing the expiratory port (7). Gas now flows from the reservoir bag, past the magnet (2), through the slotted ports (4, 4) in the bobbin carrier, and the port (6), to the patient, and the inspiratory phase begins. As inflation continues, the pressure within the distended reservoir bag falls until it reaches a level at which the force exerted on the bobbin (5) is overcome by the attraction of the magnet (2), and the bobbin returns to its resting position. The flow of gas from the reservoir bag to the patient is cut off, and the expiratory phase begins. This mode of cycling is discussed in fuller detail in the functional analysis.

The distance between the magnet (2) and the bobbin (5) when the latter is in its resting (expiratory) position is determined by the position of the bobbin carrier (9) which is adjusted by the brass 'knurled control knob' (9). The setting of this control, therefore, determines the pressure required in the reservoir bag to move the bobbin to its inspiratory position. The distance between the magnet (2) and the bobbin (5) when the latter is in its inspiratory position is determined by the position of the end stop (7) which is adjusted by the aluminium 'smooth control knob' (10). The setting of this control, therefore, determines the level to which the pressure within the reservoir bag must fall before the bobbin can be drawn back by the magnet (2) to its resting (expiratory) position. The combined settings of these two controls, therefore, determine the working-pressure range within the reservoir bag, and hence, for any given inflating-gas flow and any particular patient, the durations of the inspiratory and expiratory phases and the tidal volume. The total minute-volume ventilation depends solely on the inflating-gas flow.

FUNCTIONAL ANALYSIS

Inspiratory phase

During this phase the 'Minivent' is best regarded as a discharging compliance (see p. 98). During the previous expiratory phase the compliance of the reservoir bag (fig. 63.4) has

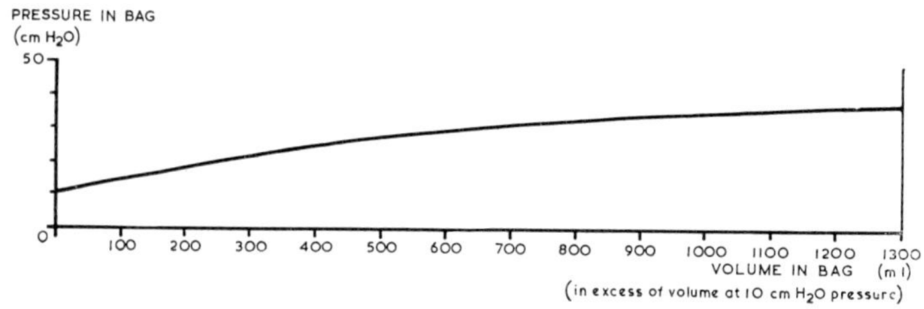

Fig. 63.4. 'Minivent'. Pressure-volume characteristic of the new, two-litre reservoir bag used in conjunction with the 'Minivent' to obtain the recordings shown in figs. 63.5 and 63.6. The characteristic plotted is the mean of those determined immediately before and after the bag had been used for making all the recordings. The absolute volume required to produce a given pressure was a little higher after use but, in terms of volume in excess of that at 10 cmH_2O pressure, there was no appreciable difference. The very first inflation of the new bag gave an appreciably more rapid rise of pressure with volume to a higher maximum.

been charged to a high pressure by the inflating-gas flow, and the compliance of the patient's lungs has discharged to atmospheric pressure through the expiratory port (7 in fig. 63.3). During the inspiratory phase the bag compliance discharges into the patient's compliance: the bag pressure falls, the alveolar pressure rises, and the flow, after rising very rapidly to a high initial level, falls. All three variables change in a manner (discussed on p. 99) which is dependent upon the bag's compliance, the patient's compliance, the total resistance between the bag and the alveoli, and the inflating-gas flow. Thus changes in the patient's lung characteristics produce changes in both the flow and the bag-pressure waveforms. This is shown directly in fig. 63.5, since this includes a tracing of bag pressure in place of the tracing of mouth pressure shown with all other ventilators.

There is another characteristic of the discharging compliance with a continuous inflow of inflating gas which is of importance in the functioning of this ventilator. If, for any reason, the inspiratory phase becomes very prolonged, the bag pressure does not fall indefinitely but reaches a minimum and then rises again (see p. 101 and fig. 3.14).

Change-over from inspiratory phase to expiratory phase

This change-over occurs when the bobbin (5) moves to its leftward position in fig. 63.3. To a first approximation this occurs when the pressure in the bag has fallen far enough for the force it exerts on the piston to be overcome by the attraction of the magnet. If this were exactly true, since the change-over from the expiratory phase to the inspiratory phase occurs at another (higher) bag pressure, the inspiratory phase would end when a given change in bag pressure had occurred, in other words when a given volume had come out of the bag. Thus the ventilator could be considered to be volume-cycled, although the tidal volume would exceed the volume discharged from the bag by the amount of inflating gas which entered during the inspiratory phase.

However, it can be seen from fig. 63.5 that, when the patient's compliance is halved, the tidal volume is decreased and the bag pressure at the end of the inspiratory phase is increased. This is because the exact mode of cycling is more complex than the approximation given above. Firstly, the pressure on the left face of the bobbin is not the same as the

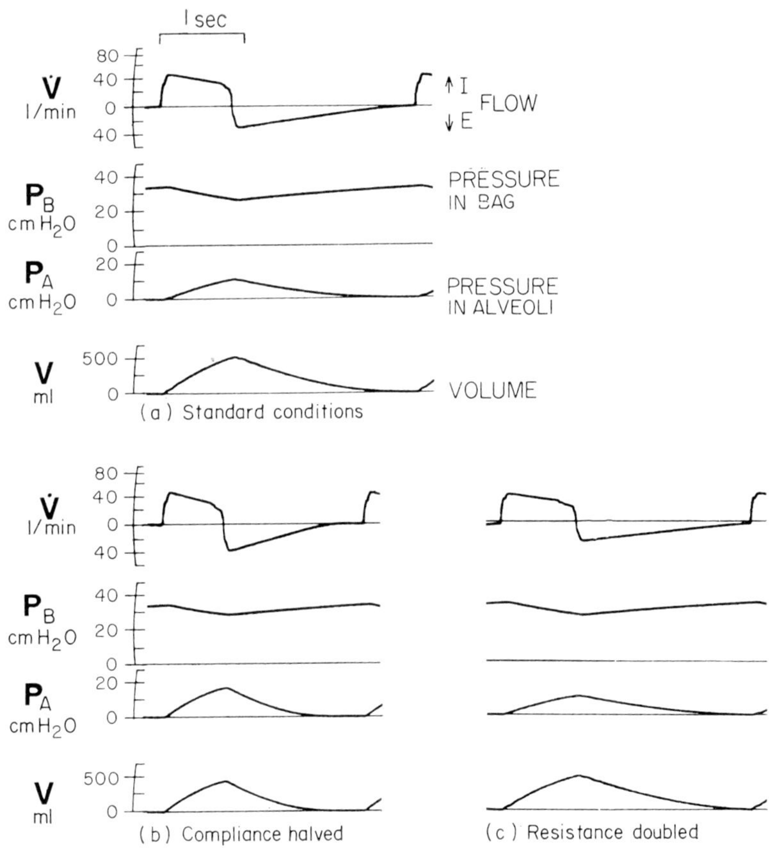

Fig. 63.5. 'Minivent'. Recordings showing the effects of changes of lung characteristics. Note that the second tracing in each set is of bag pressure and not of mouth pressure as with the other ventilators.

Standard conditions: inflating gas, oxygen from a 60 lb/in² pipe-line and needle valve set to give a Rotameter reading of 10 litres/min; aluminium 'smooth control knob' (10 in fig. 63.3) fully screwed in; brass 'knurled control knob' (9) unscrewed $2\frac{1}{8}$ turns to give a tidal volume of 500 ml.

bag pressure: it is intermediate between the pressure in the bag and the pressure at the mouth of the patient. These two pressures are substantially different because the resistance to flow through and around the magnet (2) is about three-quarters of the 'standard' airway resistance of the model lung, while the resistance of the ports (4) is one-and-a-half to two times the standard airway resistance. Secondly, when the bobbin (5) is against the expiratory port (7), only the small central portion of the right face is exposed to atmospheric pressure; the outer, annular, portion is subjected to the pressure at the patient's mouth via the ports (8). (If the aluminium 'smooth control knob' (10) is so far unscrewed that the ports (8) are occluded with the bobbin to the right, the outer annulus of the right face of the piston will be subjected to a pressure which is somewhere between that at the patient port and atmospheric.) Therefore the pressure difference between the left face of the bobbin and the outer annulus of the right face is the pressure drop across the ports (4) and hence is dependent on flow. On the other hand, the pressure difference between the left face and the central portion of the right face is simply the pressure on the left face of the piston, which pressure, it has just been shown, is intermediate between bag pressure and mouth pressure. Since the inspiratory phase ends when the sum of the rightward forces, due to the two pressure differences, falls to a critical level, equal to the force of magnetic attraction, the change-over mechanism is a mixture of flow-cycling and pressure-cycling.

Thus, when the compliance is halved, the flow declines more rapidly and the bag pressure falls less rapidly during the inspiratory phase so that the critical force for the change-over is reached at a higher bag pressure and a lower flow. This can be seen by comparing (b) with (a) in fig. 63.5, although the difference in flow at the end of the phase is somewhat obscured by the rounding of the flow waveform at the end of the phase. This arises from the fact that the start of the leftward movement of the bobbin is often somewhat sluggish because, as it begins to move, the pressure on the outer annulus of the right face begins to fall to atmospheric thereby increasing the rightward force on the piston and impeding its leftward movement.

The effect of doubling the airway resistance (fig. 63.5c) is very small because, in view of the high resistance around the magnet (2) and through the ports (4), the resultant percentage change in total resistance is quite small.

In the 'Controls' section which follows the change-over from the inspiratory phase to the expiratory phase is occasionally spoken of as though it depended only on the bag pressure. This is done in the interests of brevity but it should always be borne in mind that flow as well as pressure influence the moment of change-over.

Expiratory phase

During this phase the ventilator operates as a constant, atmospheric, pressure generator: expiration to atmosphere occurs through the ports (8) and the expiratory port (7). The resistance of this pathway varies with the setting of the aluminium 'smooth control knob' (10) but is comparable to the standard airway resistance of the model lung so that the mouth pressure is always about half the alveolar pressure during the phase. This is not recorded in fig. 63.5, but the characteristic changes of flow pattern, which occur with a constant pressure generator when the lung characteristics are altered, especially when the compliance is halved, can be clearly seen.

Change-over from expiratory phase to inspiratory phase

This change-over occurs when the pressure in the reservoir bag has risen to a point at which the force it exerts on the bobbin is sufficient to overcome the attraction of the magnet. In this sense the change-over is pressure-cycled but the pressure concerned is quite unrelated to any pressure in the patient. A more useful way of specifying this change-over can be deduced as follows. When the bag pressure has reached the critical level the bag volume must also have reached a precisely-defined level—the same volume in each respiratory cycle. This occurs when whatever tidal volume entered the patient in the previous inspiratory phase has been replaced by the inflating-gas flow. This is achieved in a time, from the start of the previous *inspiratory* phase, equal to the previous tidal volume divided by the inflating-gas flow. However, although the inflating-gas flow is determined by the ventilator, the tidal volume is dependent upon lung characteristics because of the nature of the change-over mechanism at the end of the inspiratory phase. Therefore the time of change-over at the end of the expiratory phase also depends on lung characteristics.

CONTROLS

Total ventilation

This is directly controlled by and, provided there are no leaks, is exactly equal to the inflating-gas flow. In fact, there is inevitably some leakage each time the bobbin (5) changes position but, from the measurements made, it appears that this is always negligible at the end of the expiratory phase and is usually very small at the end of the inspiratory phase.

When the inflating-gas flow is increased the initial inspiratory flow rate is unaltered but a smaller fraction of it comes from the bag so that the bag pressure falls less rapidly, the inspiratory time is increased and the tidal volume is also increased (fig. 63.6b). In the expiratory phase the bag is refilled more rapidly so that the expiratory time is decreased —to such an extent in fig. 63.6b that the alveolar pressure does not fall to atmospheric. Thus the increase in total ventilation is brought about partly by an increase in tidal volume but mostly by an increase in respiratory frequency; it is accompanied by a large change in inspiratory-expiratory ratio and perhaps a rise in the lower limit of alveolar pressure. If the inflating-gas flow is increased too far the bag pressure may never fall far enough for the bobbin to return to its expiratory position so that the ventilator becomes arrested in the inspiratory phase. Then the alveolar pressure and bag pressure rise together towards the maximum bag pressure (fig. 3.14). Under the conditions used for the recordings of fig. 63.6 this occurred at an inflating-gas flow of 18 litres/min. Even if the inflating-gas flow is increased to a level which is somewhat less than that necessary to

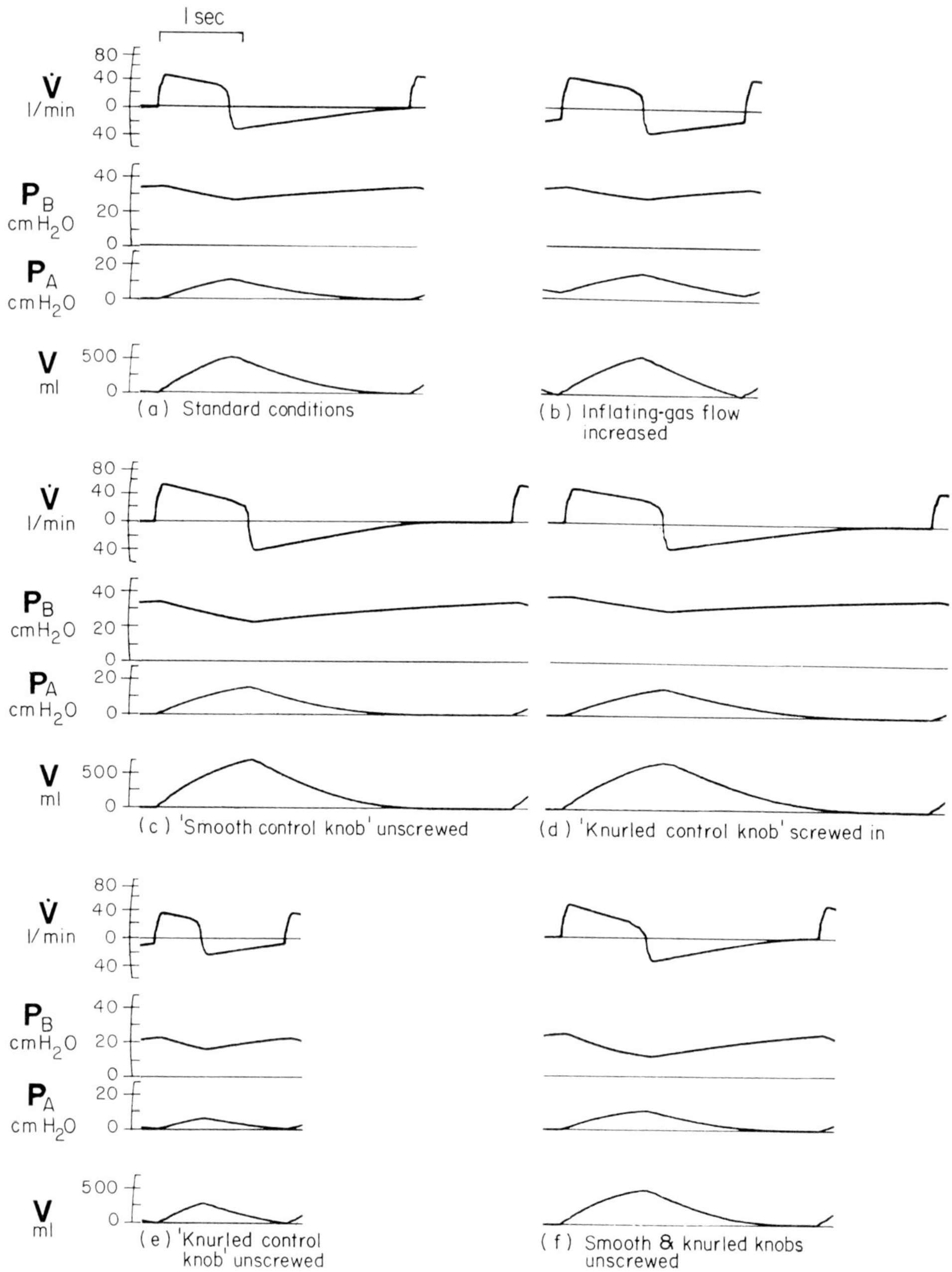

cause arrest of the ventilator in the inspiratory phase, a subsequent drop in the patient's compliance may result in such an arrest. This is because the resultant, more-rapid rise of alveolar pressure prevents the bag pressure falling as far as before, perhaps to the extent that the bag pressure starts to rise again before falling far enough to cause the piston to change to the expiratory position. The same effect could arise from a large increase in resistance.

Tidal volume

This depends on the range of pressures between which the bag is constrained to operate and on the compliance of the bag. It is increased by increasing the inflating-gas flow (see above), and decreased somewhat by a decrease in the compliance of the patient (fig. 63.5b). It is little influenced by changes of airway resistance (fig. 63.5c) because of the high resistance within the 'Minivent'.

If the aluminium 'smooth control knob' (10) is unscrewed the bag pressure for the start of the inspiratory phase is unaltered, but the pressure for the ending of the phase is decreased. Therefore the tidal volume is increased (fig. 63.6c) and, in consequence, the respiratory frequency is decreased. The inspiratory-expiratory ratio, however, is little altered. If the aluminium 'smooth control knob' (10) is unscrewed too far the bag pressure required for ending the inspiratory phase becomes less than the minimum to which the bag pressure falls and the ventilator is arrested in the inspiratory phase. In the circumstances of the present tests, unscrewing the 'smooth control knob' (10) from its fully 'in' position by $1\frac{1}{8}$ turns was sufficient to arrest the ventilator. Even at a lesser degree of unscrewing, a drop in the patient's compliance or a large increase in resistance may bring about arrest by raising the minimum bag pressure: in the conditions used for fig. 63.6c, halving the patient's compliance was just sufficient to cause arrest.

If instead of unscrewing the aluminium 'smooth control knob' (10) the brass 'knurled control knob' and bobbin carrier (9) is screwed in, the bag pressures at which the inspiratory phase starts and ends are both increased. The difference between the pressures is slightly increased but, at the generally higher pressure level in the bag, the compliance of the bag is increased, as can be seen from the gentler slope of the pressure-volume curve

---

Fig. 63.6. 'Minivent'. Recordings showing the effects of changes in the settings of the controls. Note that the second tracing in each set is of bag pressure and not of mouth pressure.

(a) Standard conditions as in fig. 63.5.

(b) Inflating-gas flow increased to give a Rotameter reading of 15 litres/min.

(c) Aluminium 'smooth control knob' (10 in fig. 63.3) unscrewed $\frac{3}{4}$ of a turn to give a tidal volume of 750 ml.

(d) Brass 'knurled control knob' (9) screwed in by $\frac{3}{8}$ of a turn to give a tidal volume of 750 ml.

(e) Brass 'knurled control knob' unscrewed by $\frac{5}{8}$ of a turn to give a tidal volume of 250 ml.

(f) Aluminium 'smooth control knob' unscrewed by one turn and brass 'knurled control knob' unscrewed by $\frac{1}{4}$ turn to give a tidal volume of 500 ml.

(fig. 63.4) at higher pressures. Therefore, screwing in the brass 'knurled control knob' (9) increases the tidal volume and hence decreases the respiratory frequency (fig. 63.6d). In the circumstances of fig. 63.6, there is little effect on the inspiratory-expiratory ratio (compare (d) with (a)). However, when the brass 'knurled control knob' (9) is turned in the reverse direction and unscrewed far enough to reduce the tidal volume markedly (fig. 63.6e) there is a much bigger effect on the inspiratory-expiratory ratio. The total ventilation is fixed (by the inflating-gas flow) but the reduced bag pressure results in a reduced mean inspiratory flow; therefore the inspiratory time occupies a larger fraction of the respiratory cycle. Thus, comparing (e) with (a) in fig. 63.6, unscrewing the 'knurled control knob' (9) sufficiently to reduce the tidal volume from 500 ml to 250 ml has changed the inspiratory-expiratory ratio from 1 : 2·6 to 1 : 1·8.

If the 'knurled control knob' (9) is screwed in too far the ventilator becomes arrested in the expiratory phase because the pressure required to move the bobbin to the inspiratory position is greater than the maximum bag pressure.

Respiratory frequency

This is not directly controlled but, because of the preset total ventilation, varies inversely with tidal volume. Thus it may be deliberately increased by screwing in the aluminium 'smooth control knob' (10) or by unscrewing the brass 'knurled control knob' (9). It is also increased by any fall in compliance or large rise in resistance. If the total ventilation is increased by increasing the inflating-gas flow this results in an increase in respiratory frequency.

Inspiratory-expiratory ratio

This is influenced by many factors. The inspiratory phase occupies a larger fraction of the respiratory cycle when the inflating-gas flow (and hence the total ventilation) is increased, when the tidal volume is decreased, and, to a small extent, when the patient's compliance is decreased or the respiratory resistance increased. However, for given values of all these parameters there is little possibility for deliberately altering the inspiratory-expiratory ratio. Thus the 'standard' conditions of fig. 63.6a were obtained with the 'smooth control knob' (10) fully screwed in and the 'knurled control knob' (9) $2\frac{1}{8}$ turns unscrewed, resulting in an inspiratory-expiratory ratio of 1 : 2·6. The tracings in fig. 63.6f were obtained by unscrewing both the knurled knob ($\frac{1}{4}$ turn) and the smooth knob (1 turn) so that the same tidal volume was delivered at the same respiratory frequency. This was achieved with a lower mean bag pressure, and hence a lower mean inspiratory flow rate, operating for an inspiratory time which occupied a larger fraction of the respiratory cycle. However, the result of this manipulation was to change the inspiratory-expiratory ratio only from 1 : 2·6 to 1 : 2 and, after the change, a halving of the patient's compliance was sufficient to arrest the ventilator in the inspiratory phase. A somewhat wider range of variation would be possible with a bag with higher maximum pressure.

Inspiratory waveforms

Since the ventilator operates as a discharging compliance in the inspiratory phase both the flow and the driving pressure decline during the phase in a manner which varies with changes of lung characteristics. The only possibility for deliberately altering the inspiratory waveform lies in altering the compliance of the bag. This can be achieved to some extent by altering the range of pressure over which a given bag works in the course of each respiratory cycle. Thus, in fig. 63.6f unscrewing both control knobs (9 and 10) has caused the bag to work at generally-lower pressures than in fig. 63.6a so that the bag's compliance is less (fig. 63.4), the time constant of the system is less, and flow declines more rapidly during the phase (fig. 63.6f). However, the setting of the knurled and smooth control knobs for a given total ventilation and tidal volume may already have been decided in order to achieve a particular inspiratory-expiratory ratio. In that case, the only possibility of altering the inspiratory waveform would be to use a special bag of very low compliance but capable of developing very high pressures—a small, thick-walled bag. Then the bag pressure, and hence the inspiratory flow, would start at higher initial values and decline much more rapidly during the phase, while still delivering the same tidal volume in the same inspiratory time.

Expiratory waveforms

During the expiratory phase atmospheric pressure is applied, via the expiratory port (7), to the lungs. It cannot be varied in any way. The expiratory flow which results depends on the effect of this pressure on the lungs.

Pressure limits

During the expiratory phase the alveolar pressure approaches the generated, atmospheric, pressure. In many cases it reaches this limit by the end of the phase but, because of the resistance to expiration through the 'Minivent' (about the same as the 'standard' airway resistance of the model lung) the short expiratory times which occur in some circumstances (fig. 63.6b) stop the phase while the alveolar pressure is still positive.

The peak alveolar pressure in the inspiratory phase depends in a complex way on the setting of the controls and on the lung characteristics. Since changes of lung characteristics have less effect on the tidal volume than on the peak alveolar pressure itself, it is probably most useful to consider that the peak alveolar pressure in the inspiratory phase exceeds the minimum alveolar pressure in the expiratory phase by an amount which is equal to the tidal volume divided by the patient's compliance. But then it must be remembered that the tidal volume is reduced by any decrease in the patient's compliance or large increase in resistance.

REFERENCE

1 COHEN A.D. (1966) The Minivent respirator. *Anaesthesia*, **21**, 563.

CHAPTER 64

The Mörch I Ventilator[1, 2]

DESCRIPTION

An electrically-driven air compressor both supplies compressed air to a 'compressed air' storage tank and produces a negative pressure in a 'suction' tank (fig. 64.2).

The 'mercury pressure switch' contains two pairs of contacts. One pair is closed during the inspiratory phase completing the circuit for the solenoid-operated inspiratory valve, and holding it open. Compressed air flows from the storage tank to the plastic pressure chamber containing the reservoir bag. As the pressure in the pressure chamber increases, the contents of the bag are forced to the patient.

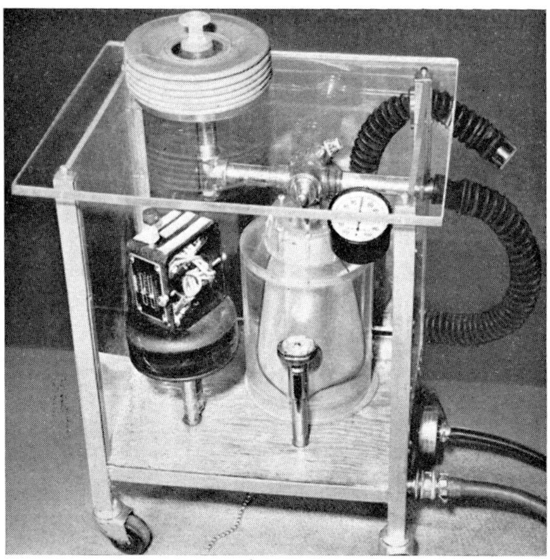

Fig. 64.1. The Mörch I ventilator.

Courtesy of the Scandinavian Society of Anaesthesiologists.[1]

At the same time the compressed air expands a small concertina bag connected to the pressure chamber. When this bag has been expanded sufficiently, it tips the mercury switch over. The circuit for the inspiratory valve is broken and that for the expiratory valve is closed. The compressed air in the pressure chamber is now drawn into the

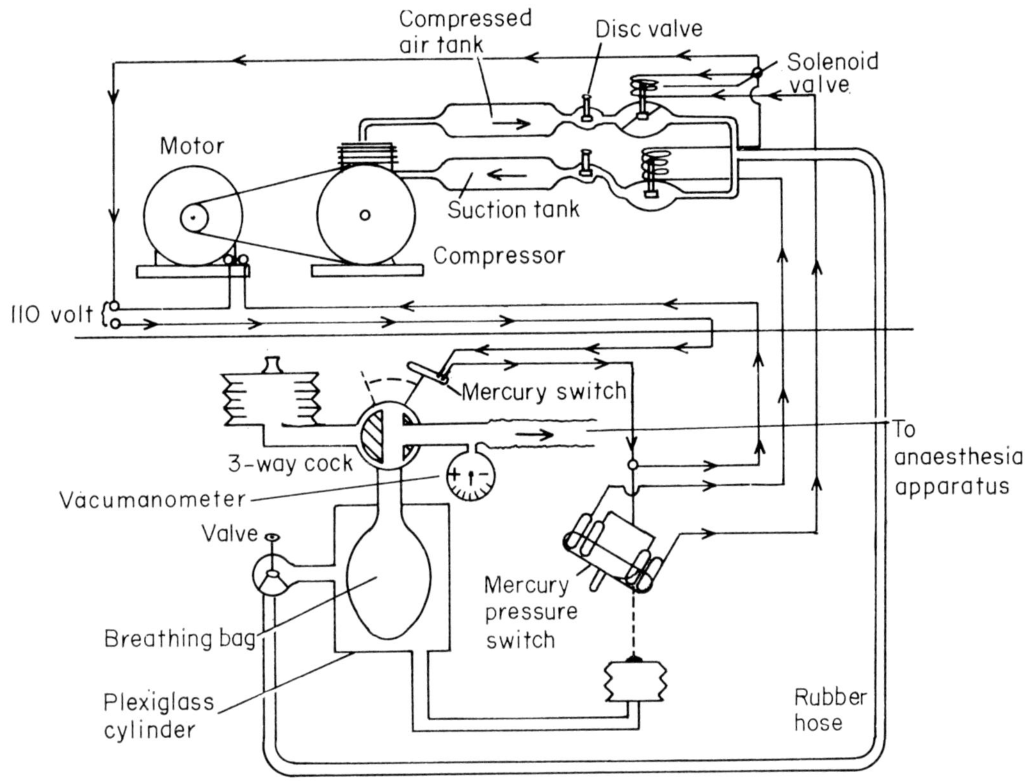

Fig. 64.2. Diagram of the Mörch I ventilator.[2]

suction tank and the reservoir bag fills with expired gas. When the small control concertina bag has collapsed sufficiently, the mercury switch tips back and the next inspiratory phase begins.

A three-way tap in the patient circuit allows inflation to be performed manually. When the machine is set to 'Manual control' the electrical supply to the ventilator is cut off by a second mercury switch connected to the three-way tap.

A manometer indicates the pressure in the patient circuit. The diagram in fig. 64.2 does not show a spill valve for excess gas in the patient circuit. The expiratory valve in the anaesthetic circuit must be used for this purpose.

FUNCTIONAL ANALYSIS

In this analysis it is assumed that the pressures in the compressed-air and suction tanks are regulated at a few pounds per square inch, positive and negative respectively.

Inspiratory phase

In this phase the ventilator operates as a constant-flow generator owing to the constant high pressure in the tank applied to the resistance of the disc valve. A pressure limit, due to the blow-off valve which must be incorporated in the patient circuit to vent excess gas, comes into operation during the phase. Until then, the fresh-gas supply to the patient circuit acts as a small-constant-flow generator, supplementing the main flow generator.

Change-over from inspiratory phase to expiratory phase

Superficially this change-over appears to be pressure-cycled: the pressure in the small control concertina bag which is sufficient to tilt the mercury switch and produce cycling is that applied to the patient via the reservoir bag. However, the blow-off valve in the patient circuit must open at less than the cycling pressure in order to vent excess gas. Therefore the pressure in the patient circuit can never rise to the cycling pressure. However, the pressure in the pressure chamber rises to the cycling pressure, and therefore produces the change-over, very shortly after the reservoir bag has been emptied. From this it might appear that the change-over is volume-cycled, but even this is not true in the conventional sense of the term. A precisely similar situation arises in the 'Cyclator CAV'; in the functional analysis of that ventilator it is shown that the change-over can best be described in the following way.

If the fresh-gas flow to the patient circuit is large, the only way of describing the change-over is to say that it is volume-cycled but that the volume involved (that in the reservoir bag at the beginning of the inspiratory phase) includes the tidal volume which happened to be expired by the patient in the previous respiratory cycle and which is dependent upon lung characteristics. If the fresh-gas flow is small, the above statement is still true, but there is now so little excess gas to be vented through the blow-off valve that the change-over occurs almost immediately the blow-off valve opens. Therefore the change-over is effectively pressure-cycled at the opening pressure of the blow-off valve.

Expiratory phase

In this phase also the ventilator operates as a constant-flow generator owing to the constant large negative pressure applied to the resistance of the disc valve. The fresh-gas flow is now subtracted from, instead of added to, the main flow.

Change-over from expiratory phase to inspiratory phase

This change-over is pressure-cycled: the pressure in the small concertina bag which produces cycling is that applied to the patient via the reservoir bag.

REFERENCES

1 MÖRCH E.T. and BENSON D.W. (1955) *Proceedings of the Third Congress of the Scandinavian Society of Anaesthesiologists, Copenhagen*, 1954, p. 30.

2 MUSHIN W.W. and RENDELL-BAKER L. (1953) *Principles of Thoracic Anaesthesia*, p. 100. Oxford: Blackwell.

CHAPTER 65

The Mörch II 'Surgical' Ventilator

DESCRIPTION

Driving gas at a pressure of 50 lb/in^2 enters the ventilator through the filter (27) (fig. 65.2) and the reducing valve (16) which is set to 10–14 lb/in^2. It passes through the pneumatic relay (15) and acts upon the diaphragm in the three-way valve (11). The diaphragm is forced over to the right, compressing the spring and pushing the valve on to its exhaust seating, thereby closing the exhaust port. Driving gas can now flow from the T-junction (18) through the control (24) which regulates its flow. The gas passes through the three-way valve (11) into the cylindrical pressure chamber (6), compressing the concertina reservoir bag (5) and forcing the gas within it through the breathing tube (1) to the patient.

As the pressure rises in the pressure chamber (6), the 6-inch diameter soft diaphragm (9) is distended and the rod (10) descends, pushing down the free end of the pivoted lever (22). The circular coil-spring (20), held captive to the lever (22), is forced down over the pear-shaped cam (17).

When the spring (20) passes the thickest portion of the cam (17), the cam snaps upwards, lifting the valve and thus sealing the supply port and opening the exhaust port. The driving-gas pressure behind the diaphragm in the three-way valve (11) can now escape through the relay. The spring in the three-way valve (11) forces the valve back onto its inlet seating, and opens the exhaust port, thus allowing the air within the pressure chamber (6) to escape to atmosphere through the control (14) and the silencer (26). The control (14) varies the resistance to expiration. As the pressure in the pressure chamber (6) falls, the concertina reservoir bag (5) expands, assisted in its descent by the heavy weight (7) in its base. A negative pressure is thereby produced overcoming the resistance of the control (14). The plate (8) can be raised or lowered by the rack-and-pinion mechanism (25) to limit the tidal volume, which is read off from the scale.

During the expiratory phase the pressure in the pressure chamber falls until the diaphragm (9) is pushed up by the action of spring (19) on the lever (22) and on the rod (10). As the lever (22) is raised, the captive circular spring (20) again passes over the widest part of the cam (17) and snaps the cam and valve down, thus initiating the next inspiratory phase.

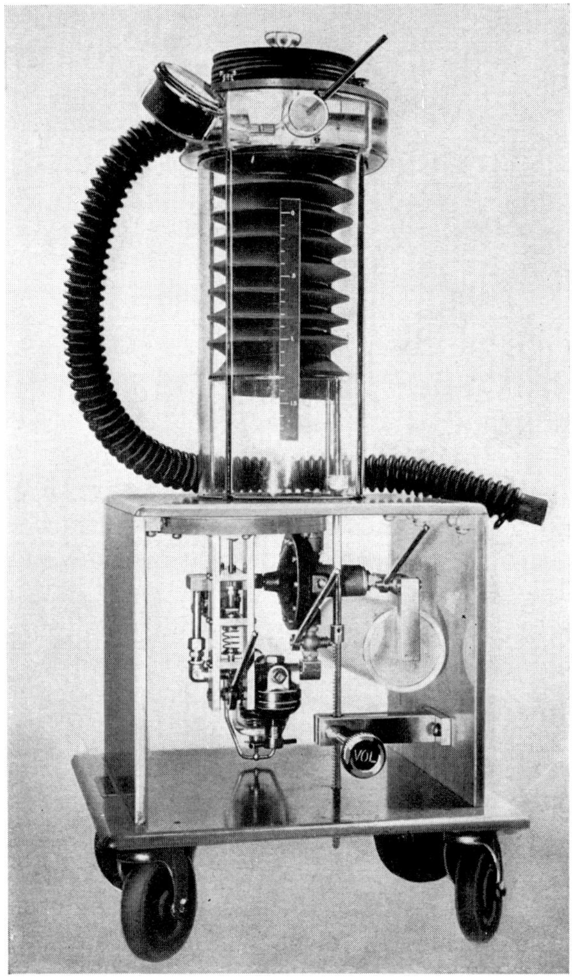

Fig. 65.1. The Mörch II 'Surgical' ventilator.

Courtesy of Dr. E.T. Mörch.

The cycling pressure is determined by the force of the spring (21) which opposes the descent of the diaphragm (9) and the rod (10). The compression of the spring (21) may be varied by the lever (23) and its eccentric cam. The safety-valve (12) limits the maximum pressure in the pressure chamber (6).

Negative pressure in the patient circuit is produced by the weight (7) in the bottom of the reservoir bag (5). The maximum negative pressure will not be developed if there is appreciable resistance to the outflow of gas from the chamber (6) through the control (14) and the silencer (26). Some of the force exerted by the weight (7) is dissipated in overcoming this resistance.

The one-way valve (13) makes it possible for the patient to inspire spontaneously

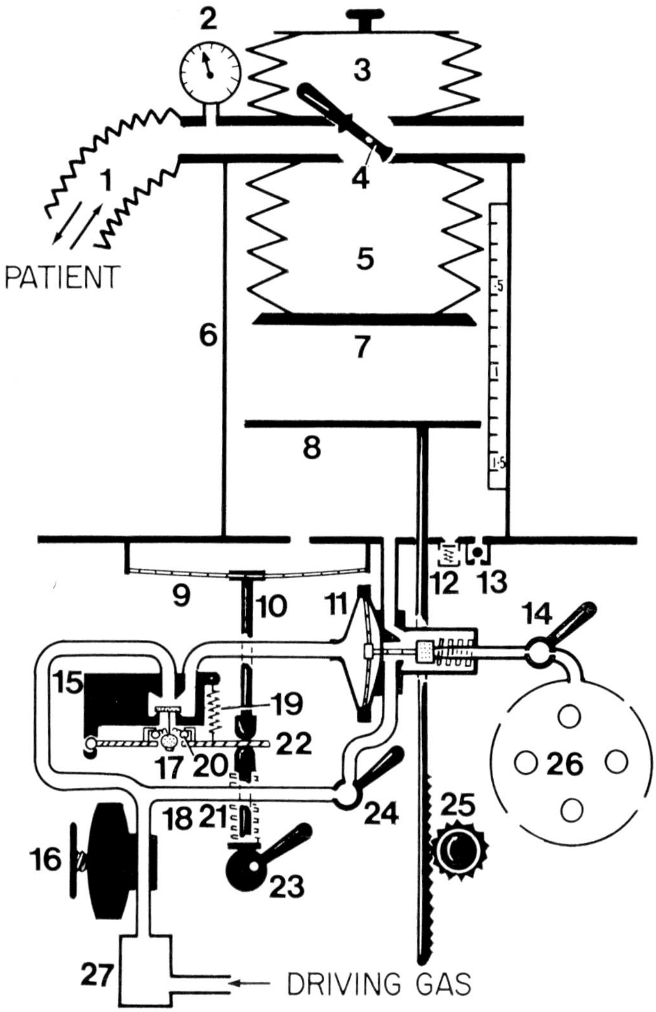

Fig. 65.2. Diagram of the Mörch II 'Surgical' ventilator.

1. Breathing tube
2. Manometer
3. Concertina bag for manual ventilation
4. 'Manual/Auto' control
5. Concertina reservoir bag
6. Rigid plastic pressure chamber
7. Weight
8. Adjustable plate
9. Diaphragm
10. Connecting rod
11. Three-way valve
12. Safety-valve
13. One-way valve
14. Adjustable resistance to expiration
15. Pneumatic relay
16. Pressure-reducing valve
17. Pear-shaped cam
18. T-junction
19. Expansion spring
20. Circular coil-spring
21. Compression spring
22. Pivoted lever
23. Cycling-pressure control
24. Driving-gas flow-rate control
25. Rack-and-pinion mechanism
26. Silencer
27. Driving-gas filter

while the ventilator is in operation. In this circumstance air can enter the plastic chamber (6) through this valve.

The frequency of respiration is adjusted primarily by varying the duration of the expiratory phase. The inspiratory phase is normally kept short by adjustment of the flow control (24). The duration of the expiratory phase is adjusted by the control (14) which imposes a resistance to the escape of gas from the chamber (6) and therefore effectively puts this resistance in the path of the expired gas.

Manual control of ventilation may be assumed at any time by reversing the position of the tap (4) which connects either of the two bags (3 or 5) to the patient.

The two valves (15, 11) were commercially-available; one, the relay (15), being used in the control of air conditioning, and the other, the three-way valve (11), in plumbing!

An expiratory valve in the anaesthetic circuit is used as a blow-off valve to vent excess gas.

FUNCTIONAL ANALYSIS

Inspiratory phase

In this phase the ventilator operates as a constant-flow generator owing to the constant high pressure from the reducing valve, applied to the resistance of the control (24) (fig. 65.2). There is a pressure limit, due to the blow-off valve which must be incorporated in the patient circuit to vent excess gas,* which comes into operation during the phase. Until then, the fresh-gas supply to the patient circuit acts as a small-constant-flow generator, supplementing the main flow generator.

Change-over from inspiratory phase to expiratory phase

This change-over is fundamentally pressure-cycled: the pressure at the cycling mechanism is the same as that in the pressure chamber surrounding the concertina bag. However, the pressure in the patient circuit differs from this on two counts. Firstly, the pressure inside the bag is less than that outside because of the weight in it. Secondly, to vent excess anaesthetic gas, the blow-off valve in the patient circuit must be set to open at a pressure less than the cycling pressure by an amount greater than the pressure difference due to the weight. Thus cycling does not occur until immediately after the concertina bag has completely emptied, allowing the surrounding pressure to build up rapidly to the cycling value. In this way, the system becomes volume-cycled. However, if in the previous expiratory phase the reservoir bag did not expand as far as the adjustable plate (8), the volume at which cycling occurs is not controlled by the ventilator but depends upon the lung characteristics in the manner which is explained fully in the account of the 'Cyclator CAV'.

Since the fresh-gas supply is continuous but its escape, through the blow-off valve, is

* An 'automatic spill-valve' was incorporated in a later model. This account refers to the earlier model.

restricted to the inspiratory phase, the patient's tidal volume is less than the stroke volume of the concertina bag by an amount equal to the volume of fresh gas supplied during the expiratory phase (see p. 146).

Expiratory phase

In this phase the ventilator operates as a constant, negative, pressure generator, owing to the weight in the concertina bag, with substantial series resistance, due to control (14). The fresh-gas flow now slightly impedes the main pressure-generator action.

Change-over from expiratory phase to inspiratory phase

This change-over is pressure-cycled or volume-cycled, whichever limit is reached first. The system is fundamentally pressure-cycled as at the end of the inspiratory phase. If the expansion of the bag is not limited by the adjustable plate (8), the pressure in the bag at cycling will be less than the cycling pressure by a fixed amount, owing to the weight in the bag. Thus, although the cycling pressure in the chamber is positive, that in the bag is doubtless negative. If the expansion of the bag is stopped by the limiting plate, before the pressure has fallen that far, the pressure in the chamber will then fall rapidly, producing immediate cycling, so that the system becomes volume-cycled. No matter whether volume-cycling or pressure-cycling occurs, the volume leaving the patient is less than that entering the bag by an amount equal to the volume of fresh gas which enters the patient circuit during the expiratory phase.

CHAPTER 66

The Mörch III 'Piston' Ventilator[1, 2]

DESCRIPTION

This simple pump-type apparatus (fig. 66.1) was designed for prolonged use in cases of poliomyelitis. The electric motor (1) (fig. 66.2) drives a piston (7) through a mechanical

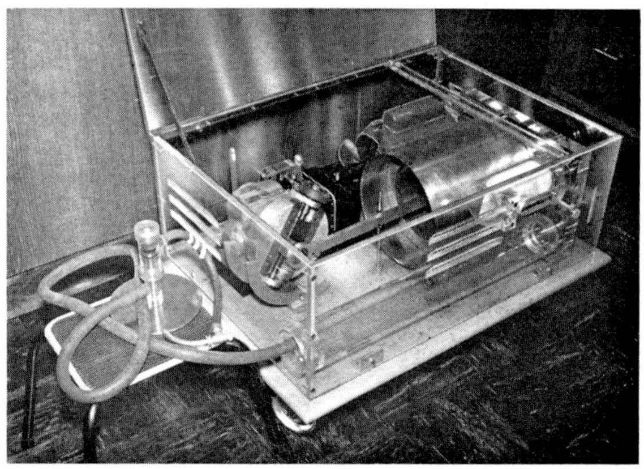

Fig. 66.1. The Mörch III 'Piston' ventilator.

Courtesy of *Journal of Thoracic Surgery*.[2]

stepless variable-speed gear (2). The crank which connects the speed gear (2) and the piston (7) can be adjusted by the control (4) to produce a variable stroke. This permits the volume of air delivered to the patient to be controlled. On its outward stroke the piston (7) draws in air from the atmosphere through the filter (5), together with any oxygen which may be added. On its compression, or inward, stroke the contents of the cylinder (8) are driven through the humidifier (10) to the inspiratory-expiratory valve (9). The force of the air-flow lifts the light metal weight within this valve (9) to the upper part of its chamber, allowing the gas to flow to the patient. The one-way valve (6) prevents leakage of gas to the atmosphere during the inspiratory phase. At the end of inflation, the weight in the valve (9) falls to the lower part of its chamber and expired gas flows freely through the valve orifice to atmosphere.

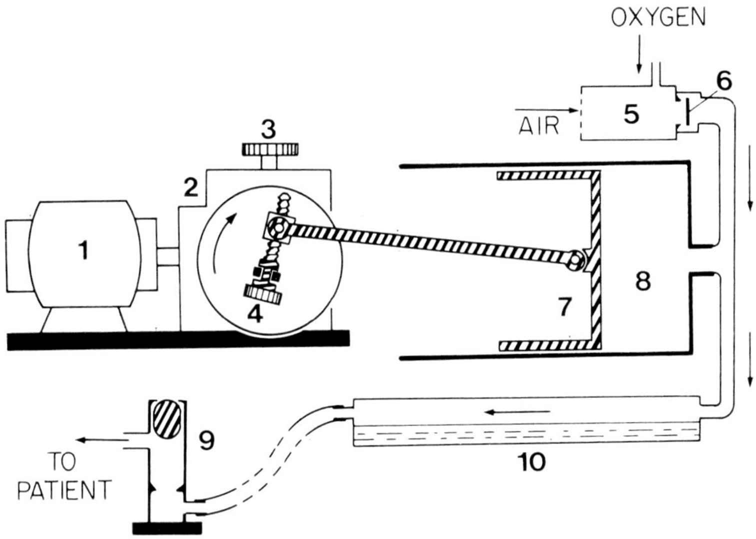

Fig. 66.2. Diagram of the Mörch III 'Piston' ventilator.

1. Electric motor
2. Gear-box
3. Frequency control
4. Stroke-volume control
5. Filter
6. One-way valve
7. Piston
8. Cylinder
9. Inspiratory-expiratory valve
10. Humidifier

The valve (9) has an additional function; during the outward stroke of the piston (7) the one-way character of this valve prevents any expired gas being drawn into the cylinder (8).

The inspiratory-expiratory ratio is fixed by the nature of the mechanism at 1 : 1.

No safety-valve is provided and reliance is placed on leakage round an endotracheal tube to avoid excessive pressure in the respiratory tract.

FUNCTIONAL ANALYSIS

Inspiratory phase

During this phase the ventilator operates fundamentally as a near-sine-wave-flow generator, owing to the nature of the driving mechanism and assuming the speed of the electric motor to be constant. This behaviour is modified by the leakage which it is recommended should be allowed around the endotracheal tube, there being no safety-valve.

Change-over from inspiratory phase to expiratory phase

This change-over is both volume-cycled and time-cycled: the constant-speed motor expels a preset volume of gas from the cylinder in a preset time. The volume entering the lungs is less than this, due to the recommended leakage around the endotracheal tube.

Expiratory phase
In this phase the ventilator operates as a constant, atmospheric, pressure generator: expired gas passes freely to atmosphere at the expiratory outlet.

Change-over from expiratory phase to inspiratory phase
This change-over is time-cycled: it occurs after the motor has driven the piston through its return stroke in a preset time.

REFERENCES

1 Mörch E.T. and Benson D.W. (1955) *Proceedings of the Third Congress of the Scandinavian Society of Anaesthesiologists, Copenhagen*, 1954, p. 30.
2 Avery E.E., Mörch E.T. and Benson D.W. (1956) Critically crushed chests; a new method of treatment with continuous mechanical hyperventilation to produce alkalotic apnea and internal pneumatic stabilization. *J. thorac. Surg.* **32**, 291.

CHAPTER 67

The Mortimer Ventilator[1]

DESCRIPTION

This ventilator (fig. 67.1) is made from a 'Tex' suction-operated car windscreen-wiper motor and the concertina bag from a Coxeter-Mushin absorber.[2] Normally a hospital

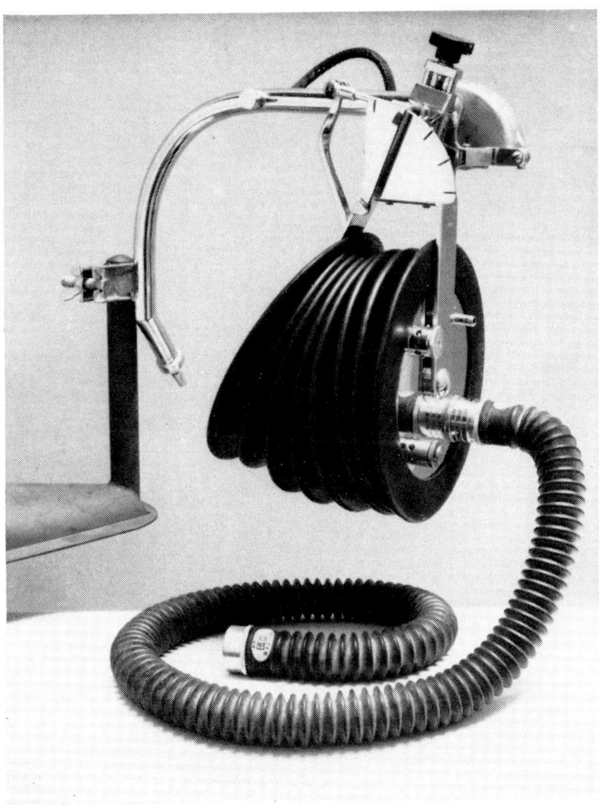

Fig. 67.1. The Mortimer ventilator.

Courtesy of Coventry & Jeffs Ltd

suction line is used to drive the motor, but any efficient portable sucker is suitable, provided it develops the necessary 15–20 inHg vacuum. The movement of the paddle within the windscreen-wiper motor is transferred through a system of levers which alternately compresses and expands the concertina bag. Since there is active expansion of the bag by the wiper motor, negative pressure can be produced during the expiratory phase. The levers are so arranged that a rotation of the main spindle of the motor through 90° expels 2 litres of air from the concertina bag.

Two modifications have been made to the windscreen-wiper motor. The first allows the arc of throw of the paddle to be altered, thus varying the amplitude of the bag movement and hence the tidal volume.

The second allows adjustment independently of the speeds of inflation and expiration. This in fact permits adjustment of the inspiratory-expiratory ratio. By means of these modifications and by adjusting the pinch-cock on the vacuum supply tube, the functioning of the ventilator can be varied within wide limits. The positive pressure produced during compression of the concertina bag depends upon a number of factors such as the stroke volume and the compliance of the patient's chest. An expiratory valve is provided to blow off excess gas. A similar apparatus was described two years later.[3]

FUNCTIONAL ANALYSIS

This ventilator contains a pressure transformer (see p. 89) with adjustable resistances and a constant driving pressure on the input side. It therefore acts as a high-constant-pressure generator with a substantial series resistance between it and the patient.

Inspiratory phase

In this phase the ventilator operates as a high-constant-pressure generator with substantial series resistance, owing to the pressure-transformer characteristics. A pressure limit, due to the blow-off valve, comes into operation during the phase. Until then, the fresh-gas supply to the patient circuit acts as a small-constant-flow generator, supplementing the action of the main pressure generator.

Change-over from inspiratory phase to expiratory phase

This change-over is volume-cycled: the phase ends when the driving mechanism reaches the end of its stroke and a preset volume has been expelled from the concertina bag. Since the supply of anaesthetic gas is continuous, but its escape through the blow-off valve is restricted to the inspiratory phase, the patient's tidal volume is less than the stroke volume of the bag, by an amount equal to the volume of fresh gas supplied during the expiratory phase (see p. 146).

Expiratory phase

In this phase the ventilator operates as a constant, negative, pressure generator with substantial series resistance, owing to the pressure-transformer characteristics. The fresh-gas flow now slightly impedes the main pressure-generating action.

Change-over from expiratory phase to inspiratory phase

This change-over also is volume-cycled: it occurs when the driving mechanism reaches the beginning of its stroke and a preset volume has been drawn into the concertina bag. The volume leaving the patient's lungs is less than this, by an amount equal to the volume of fresh gas which enters the patient circuit during the expiratory phase.

REFERENCES

1 MORTIMER P.L.F. (1954) A simple respirator. *Anaesthesia*, **9**, 312.
2 MUSHIN W.W. (1943) A new circle type carbon dioxide absorber. *Br. J. Anaesth.* **18**, 97.
3 KEATING V. (1956) Simple respiration pump. *Curr. Res. Anesth. Analg.* **35**, 538.

CHAPTER 68

The Naess Ventilator[1]

DESCRIPTION

This is an automatic ventilator designed for laboratory experimental animals but has been used clinically.[2] The plate (5), with a slot, is oscillated by a windscreen-wiper

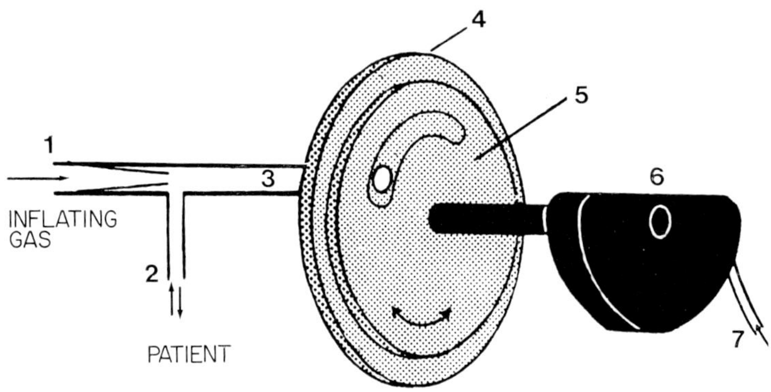

Fig. 68.1. Diagram of the Naess ventilator.

1. Inflating-gas entry and injector
2. Connexion to patient
3. Expiratory outlet
4. Fixed plate
5. Slotted plate oscillated by windscreen-wiper motor
6. Windscreen-wiper motor
7. Vacuum supply

motor (6) to-and-fro over the fixed plate (4) containing the outlet of the gas delivery tube (3). Fresh anaesthetic or other inflating gas is led into the apparatus at (1) through an injector. During the inspiratory phase the opening of the tube (3) is occluded by the moveable plate (5). The gas enters the endotracheal tube (2) to inflate the animal's lungs. During the expiratory phase the inflating gas and the expired gas pass to the atmosphere through the wide-bore tube (3) and the holes in the two plates (4, 5). Emptying of the lungs is assisted by the negative pressure created as the anaesthetic gas passes through the injector. The frequency of ventilation can be varied between 20 and 90 per minute by adjusting the degree of vacuum driving the motor (6).

The durations of the inspiratory and expiratory phases can be varied by adjusting the position of the slot in the plate (5) relative to the fixed plate (4). By this means the inspiratory-expiratory ratio may be varied from 1:0·75 to 1:3. The settings of these two controls in combination with the fresh-gas flow determine the tidal volume.

FUNCTIONAL ANALYSIS

Inspiratory phase
In this phase, assuming that the inlet (1) (fig. 68.1) is connected direct to flowmeters, the ventilator operates as a constant-flow generator.

Change-over from inspiratory phase to expiratory phase
This change-over is time-cycled: the duration of the phase is determined by the wiper motor and the slotted plate.

Expiratory phase
In this phase the ventilator operates as a constant, negative, pressure generator with substantial series resistance owing to the injector characteristics.

Change-over from expiratory phase to inspiratory phase
This change-over also is time-cycled: the duration of the expiratory phase is determined by the wiper motor and the slotted plate.

REFERENCES

1 Naess K. (1951) A simple apparatus for artificial respiration, built of a vacuum window wiper. *Acta physiol. scand.* **22**, 376.

2 Mörch E.T. and Benson D.W. (1955) *Proceedings of the Third Congress of the Scandinavian Society of Anaesthesiologists, Copenhagen*, 1954, p. 30.

CHAPTER 69

The 'Newcastle I' Ventilator*[1, 2]

DESCRIPTION

This ventilator is a modification of the Bang ventilator. It consists of a cylinder of compressed air (1) fitted with a reducing valve set to 5–7 lb/in², a reservoir bag (6) which

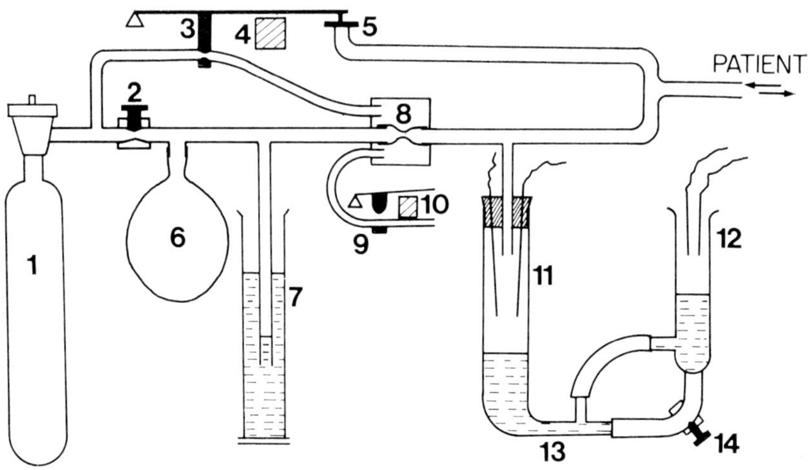

Fig. 69.1. Diagram of the 'Newcastle I' ventilator.

1. Compressed-air cylinder and reducing valve
2. Flow control
3. Pinch-cock
4. Electrical relay
5. Relay-actuated expiratory valve
6. Reservoir bag
7. Water-seal safety-valve
8. Gas-actuated inspiratory valve
9. Pinch-cock
10. Electrical relay
11. Electrodes
12. Electrodes
13. Manometer containing electrolyte solution
14. Screw clip

Courtesy of *British Journal of Anaesthesia*.[2]

* A series of ventilators are labelled 'Newcastle' and we have attached roman numerals in chronological order. Most of these ventilators are characterized by the cheapness, the ease, and the speed with which they may be constructed, for they were in the main intended to satisfy needs, such as arise during an epidemic of poliomyelitis, when these factors are important.

provides a supply of air at low pressure, a water-seal safety-valve (7), a relay-actuated expiratory valve (5), a gas-actuated inspiratory valve (8), and a manometer (13), filled with a solution of sodium sulphate, containing the two sets of electrodes (11, 12). The two electrical relays (4, 10) control the pinch-cocks (3, 9) on the entry and exit tubes from the inspiratory-valve chamber. By opening one pinch-cock and closing the other, the thin-rubber tube of the inspiratory valve is either collapsed or patent.

The height of the electrodes (12) is adjusted to give the desired cycling pressure. The flow of air from the cylinder (1) is set by the flow control (2) to the desired minute-volume ventilation, and the depth of the tube in the water-seal safety-valve (7) adjusted to about 50 cmH_2O so that ample working pressure is available. Air flows at a steady rate from the cylinder (1) and fills the reservoir bag (6).

During the inspiratory phase air passes through the inspiratory valve (8) to the patient. The relay (4) is held closed, both occluding the expiratory valve (5) and closing the pinch-cock (3). As the pressure in the lungs rises, the electrolyte level in the right-hand limb of the manometer (13) rises until it reaches the contacts (12). When the circuit at (12) is closed, the actions of the two relays are reversed; (10) closes the pinch-cock (9), and (4) opens the expiratory valve (5) and the pinch-cock (3). Air from the reducing valve then flows into the outer chamber of the inspiratory valve (8) causing the thin-rubber tubing to collapse. Expired gas flows out of the open expiratory valve (5).

During this expiratory phase the pressure in the lungs falls rapidly, and the electrolyte in the right-hand limb of the manometer falls until, at a certain level, the contacts (11) are closed, energizing the relay (4) and closing the expiratory valve (5). The next inspiratory phase begins.

The rate of fall of the electrolyte, and with it the duration of the expiratory phase, is controlled by the screw clip (14). The siting of the upper rubber tube permits rapid response to the increase of pressure during the inspiratory phase, coupled with an adjustable delay in the fall in liquid level during the expiratory phase.

The source of electricity is a series of car batteries, though the apparatus has been adapted for a.c. mains by means of suitable relays and a transformer.[2]

FUNCTIONAL ANALYSIS

Inspiratory phase

As in the Clevedon ventilator, the mode of operation during this phase depends on the average degree of inflation of the reservoir bag (6). If it is inflated to the 50 cmH_2O mentioned in the 'Description' above, the bag will probably be on the 'plateau' of its pressure-volume characteristic (see fig. 3.12 and p. 96). The ventilator will then operate as a constant-pressure generator during the phase. If it is inflated only to somewhat lower pressures it will be on the steep part of its pressure-volume characteristic. Then it will operate as a discharging compliance (see p. 98).

Change-over from inspiratory phase to expiratory phase

This change-over is pressure-cycled: the pressure in the manometer at which cycling occurs is that applied to the patient.

Expiratory phase

In this phase the ventilator operates as a constant, atmospheric, pressure generator: expired gas passes freely to atmosphere through the expiratory valve.

Change-over from expiratory phase to inspiratory phase

This change-over is time-cycled: the time taken for the electrolyte level in the left-hand limb of the manometer (13) to rise to the contacts (11) is uninfluenced by the patient.

REFERENCES

1 PASK E.A. (1953) A simple respirator. *Lancet*, **2**, 141.

2 MUSHIN W.W. and RENDELL-BAKER L. (1954) Modern automatic respirators. *Br. J. Anaesth.* **26**, 131.

CHAPTER 70

The 'Newcastle II' Ventilator[1]

DESCRIPTION

This ventilator (fig. 70.1) needs a supply of air at a pressure of about 35 cmH_2O. The air may come from a cylinder, from a compressor, or from a vacuum cleaner adapted for 'blowing'. In the case of the first two sources, to maintain a driving pressure as low as 35 cmH_2O, a 'self-regulating reservoir bag' (fig. 70.2) acts as a second-stage reducing valve. A 4-litre bag, arranged as shown, is filled with gas. A wooden flap, to which the supply tube is fixed, is raised. When the bag is inflated to a certain extent and the pressure

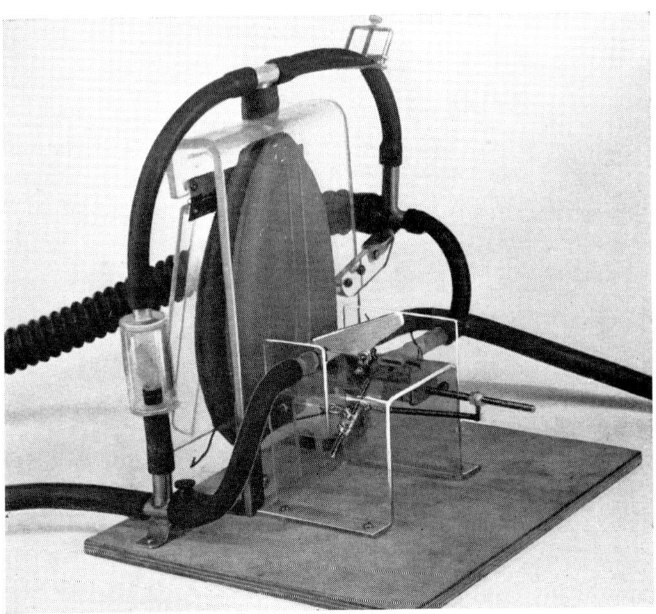

Fig. 70.1. The 'Newcastle II' ventilator.

Courtesy of Prof. E.A. Pask.

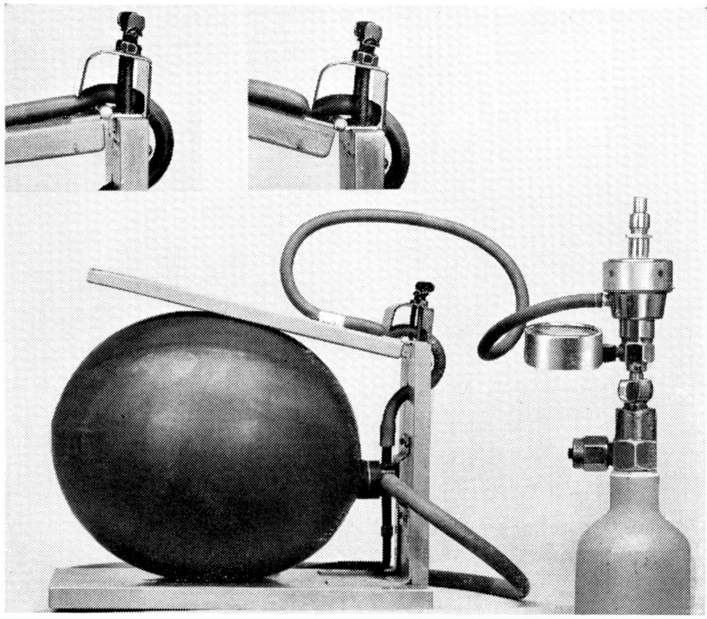

Fig. 70.2. The second-stage pressure-reducing unit of the 'Newcastle II' ventilator.
Courtesy of *The Lancet*.[1]

within it is about 35 cmH_2O, the supply tube is nipped between the flap and a metal edge attached to the wooden framework.

During the inspiratory phase (fig. 70.3) air enters through the tube (8) and flows, through the valve (5) and along the tube (9), to the patient. The metal paddle (6), which is attached to a toggle mechanism taken from a common electric-light switch, keeps the expiratory valve (7) closed. At the same time some of the air flows through the one-way valve (10) into the control bag (4). As this bag is distended it raises the hinged flap (11) and so pulls on the cord (12). The rod (13) is gradually pulled over against the tension of the spring (14) until, when it reaches its critical position, the switch mechanism flicks over and the paddle (6) alters position to close the inspiratory valve (5) and allow the expiratory valve (7) to open. The supply of inflating gas is now cut off.

The expiratory phase now begins, and expired gas flows along the corrugated tube (1) and escapes to the atmosphere through the expiratory valve (7). The tension of the spring (14) maintains a pull on the rod (13) and therefore on the hinged flap (11), maintaining a positive pressure in the bag (4). The bag (4) empties through the tube (2), the rate of emptying being controlled by a screw clip (3). When the bag (4) has emptied sufficiently the rod is again back at its critical point, the paddle (6) is flicked over, and the next inspiratory phase begins. The pressure in the bag (4), which is the same as that in the patient circuit during the inspiratory phase, at which inflation is cut off may be

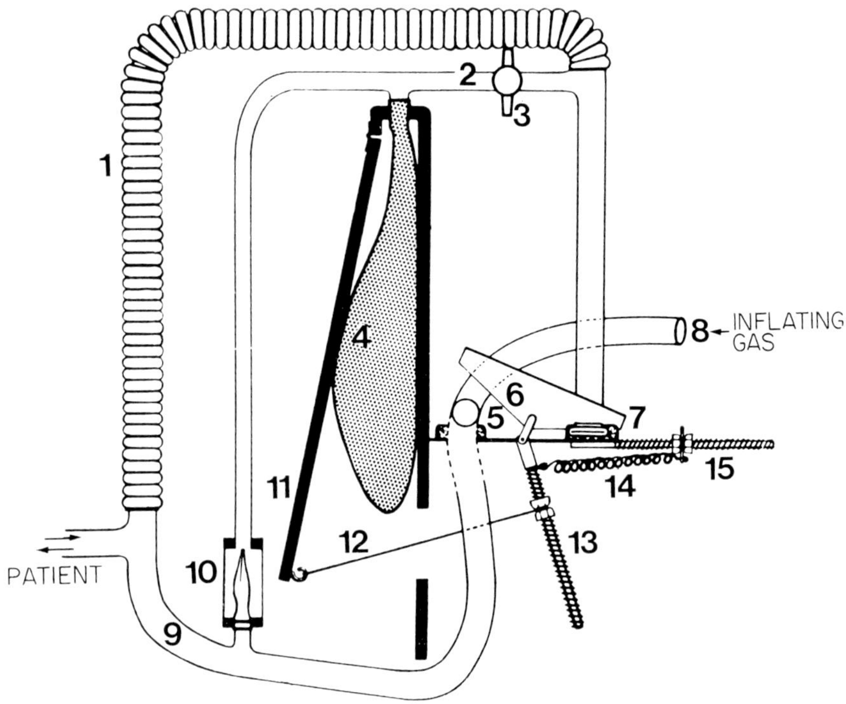

Fig. 70.3. Diagram of the 'Newcastle II' ventilator.

1. Corrugated tube
2. Outlet tube
3. Screw clip
4. Control bag
5. Inspiratory valve
6. Metal paddle
7. Expiratory valve
8. Inflating-gas supply tube
9. Supply tube to patient
10. One-way valve
11. Hinged flap
12. Cord
13. Threaded rod
14. Spring
15. Threaded rod

Courtesy of *The Lancet*.[1]

varied by adjustment of the attachment of the cord (12) to the rod (13); the nearer this is to the toggle mechanism the less is the leverage exerted on the rod (13) and the greater is the pressure attained in the bag (4). If a still-higher pressure is desired, the attachment of the spring (14) on the rod (15) can also be moved. The rate of inflow of air during inflation may be reduced by placing a screw clip on the tube (9). The duration of the expiratory phase depends on the rate of escape of air from the bag (4) through the screw clip (3). If the patient has an irremediable respiratory obstruction a premature cutting-off of inflation, due to a rapid build-up of pressure within the bag (4), may be prevented by placing a screw clip above the one-way valve (10), thereby slowing the rate of filling of the bag (4).

The valves (5) and (7) consist of short lengths of latex Penrose drainage tube, lying on cushions of orthopaedic sponge rubber.

FUNCTIONAL ANALYSIS

Inspiratory phase

In this phase the ventilator operates as a constant-pressure generator when used with a second-stage reducing valve.

Change-over from inspiratory phase to expiratory phase

This change-over is pressure-cycled: the pressure in the control bag (4) (fig. 70.3) which produces cycling is that applied to the patient.

Expiratory phase

In this phase the ventilator operates as a constant, atmospheric, pressure generator: the patient's expired gas passes freely to atmosphere at the expiratory valve (7).

Change-over from expiratory phase to inspiratory phase

This change-over is time-cycled: the duration of the expiratory phase is equal to the time in which enough air leaks out of the control bag (4) for cycling to occur. This time is uninfluenced by the patient but depends on the force of the spring (14) and the point of attachment of cord (12) on the rod (13), as well as on the setting of screw clip (3). Therefore, raising the cycling pressure at the end of the inspiratory phase, by means of extending spring (14) or adjusting the point of attachment of cord (12), shortens the expiratory phase.

REFERENCE

1 Pask E.A. (1954) Emergency intermittent positive-pressure respirator. *Lancet*, **2**, 217.

CHAPTER 71

The 'Newcastle III' Ventilator[1]

DESCRIPTION

Air or a mixture of anaesthetic gases at a pressure of about 40–90 cmH_2O is supplied at (19) (fig. 71.2). A flow of at least 60 litres/min is desirable. If this is not available, a

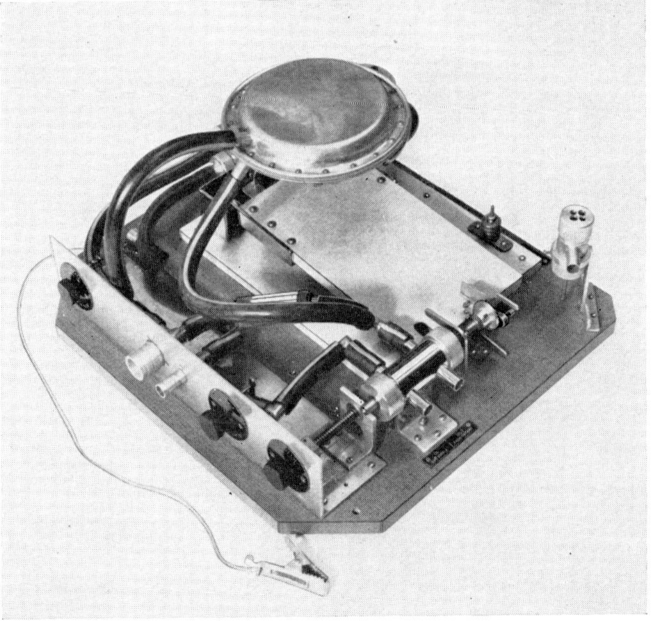

Fig. 71.1. The 'Newcastle III' ventilator.
Courtesy of British Oxygen Company Ltd.

two-gallon storage bag in a restraining net (20) is added. A water-seal (18) acts as a safety-valve. During the inspiratory phase gas flows freely through one channel of the rotary valve (10) and past an adjustable clip (17) to the patient. It also flows from the rotary valve through the tube (16) and the one-way valve (3), filling the control bag (6).

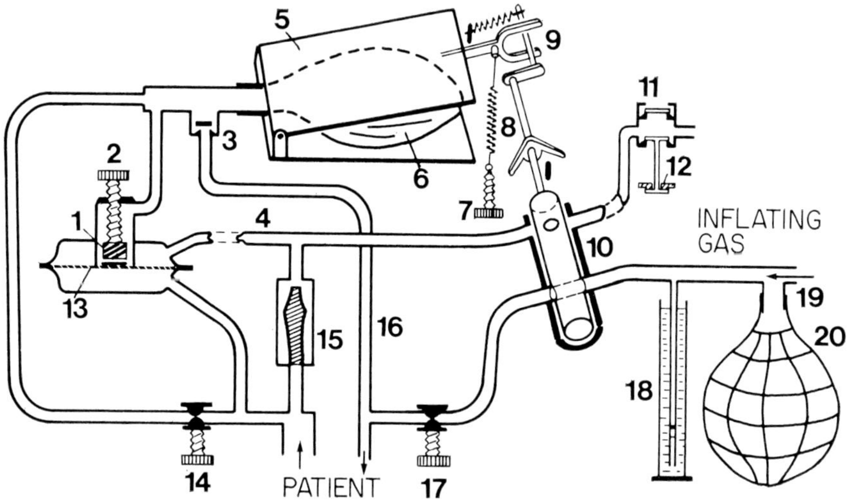

Fig. 71.2. Diagram of the 'Newcastle III' ventilator.

1. Magnet
2. Patient-triggering sensitivity control
3. One-way valve
4. Connecting tube
5. Hinged flap
6. Control bag
7. Cycling-pressure control
8. Spring
9. Fork
10. Rotary inspiratory-expiratory valve
11. One-way expiratory valve
12. Air-inlet valve with adjustable weight
13. Diaphragm
14. Screw clip
15. One-way valve
16. Connecting tube
17. Screw clip
18. Water-seal safety-valve
19. Inflating-gas inlet
20. Storage bag with restraining net

This lifts the hinged plate (5) against the pull of the spring (8) until the flick mechanism (9) operates and rotates the valve (10) through 90°, cutting off the supply of inflating gas.

During the expiratory phase the expired gas escapes through the one-way valve (15) and the expiratory channel in the valve (10). If negative pressure is required during the expiratory phase, suction may be applied to the expiratory outlet of the rotary valve (10). In this case the weighted air-inlet safety-valve (12) limits the negative pressure produced in the respiratory tract. This limit may be varied by altering the weights on the valve (12).

Meanwhile, the gas contained in the bag (6) escapes past the screw clip (14). When the bag has emptied sufficiently the plate (5) again operates the flick mechanism (9), reversing the rotary valve (10) and starting the next inspiratory phase. The clip (17) controls the speed of inflation and the clip (14) the duration of the expiratory phase. The screw (7), by altering the tension of the spring (8), determines the pressure which must be reached in the circuit before inflation is cut off.

If the patient attempts to take a breath during the expiratory phase a negative pressure is produced in the chamber below the diaphragm (13). The diaphragm is drawn downwards and the gas stored in the bag (6) can now escape rapidly through the diaphragm chamber and along the tube (4). In this way the expiratory phase is cut short and inflation commences immediately. The diaphragm (13) is normally kept in place by the pull of the magnet (1). The negative pressure required to overcome this pull and so initiate inflation may be varied by the control (2) which alters the position of the magnet.

FUNCTIONAL ANALYSIS

Inspiratory phase

The mode of operation in this phase depends on the source of the inflating gas. If the source is a second-stage pressure regulator the ventilator will operate as a constant-pressure generator. If a storage bag in a restraining net is used, as in fig. 71.2, the ventilator will operate as a discharging compliance (see p. 98).

Change-over from inspiratory phase to expiratory phase

This change-over is pressure-cycled: the pressure in the control bag (6) which produces cycling is that applied to the patient.

Expiratory phase

With no suction applied, the ventilator operates during this phase as a constant, atmospheric, pressure generator: the expired gas passes freely to atmosphere at the one-way valve (11) or directly at the expiratory outlet of the rotary valve (10).

With suction applied, the ventilator operates as a constant, negative, pressure generator owing to the negative-pressure-limiting valve (12).

Change-over from expiratory phase to inspiratory phase

This change-over is either time-cycled or patient-cycled, whichever comes first: it occurs when sufficient gas has escaped from the control bag (6). This may occur either gradually, past the screw clip (14) in a preset time; or suddenly, through the patient-cycling valve (1), when the patient makes an inspiratory effort. Note that the time limit set by the gradual escape of gas is shortened when the cycling pressure at the end of the inspiratory phase is raised—as in the 'Newcastle II'.

REFERENCE

1 HORTON J.A.G., INKSTER J.S. and PASK E.A. (1956) Two more respirators. *Br. J. Anaesth.* **28**, 169.

CHAPTER 72

The 'Newcastle IV' Ventilator[1]

DESCRIPTION

This ventilator, like the 'Newcastle III', is driven either by anaesthetic gases or by compressed air at low pressure. The gas enters at (20) (fig. 72.1) and during the inspiratory phase passes, through the inspiratory valve (19) and the delivery tube (16), to the patient. It also flows, through the expiratory tube (10) and the side tubes (3, 5), into the concertina bag (1). There is a non-return valve (2) at the top of the tube (3). The concertina bag (1) rises, taking with it the rod (8). The sprung collar (9) now makes contact with the stirrup (12), and the spring (11) is compressed until the force it exerts on the rod (14) overcomes the attraction of the magnet (18) for the plate (17). The rod (14) snaps up and the valve (19) is shut, cutting off the supply of inflating gas.

The expiratory valve (13) is opened, and expired gas escapes to atmosphere through the port (15). At the same time the contents of the bag (1) flow, through the constricted tube (5), into the expiratory tube (10) and the bag collapses. When the bag has dropped far enough for the cut-away section of the rod (8) to come in line with the port (6), emptying of the bag (1) is rapidly completed. The sprung collar (9) no longer holds up the rod (14) and the pull of magnet (18) on the plate (17) now snaps it down. The expiratory valve (13) is closed and the inspiratory valve (19) is opened, allowing the next inspiratory phase to begin.

The cycling pressure is set by weights on top of the bag (1). The duration of the expiratory phase depends on the constriction in tube (5) which may be varied by the control (4). A patient-triggering device, similar to that of the 'Newcastle III', can be connected at (7).

FUNCTIONAL ANALYSIS

Inspiratory phase

The mode of operation in this phase depends on the supply source used—as in the 'Newcastle III'.

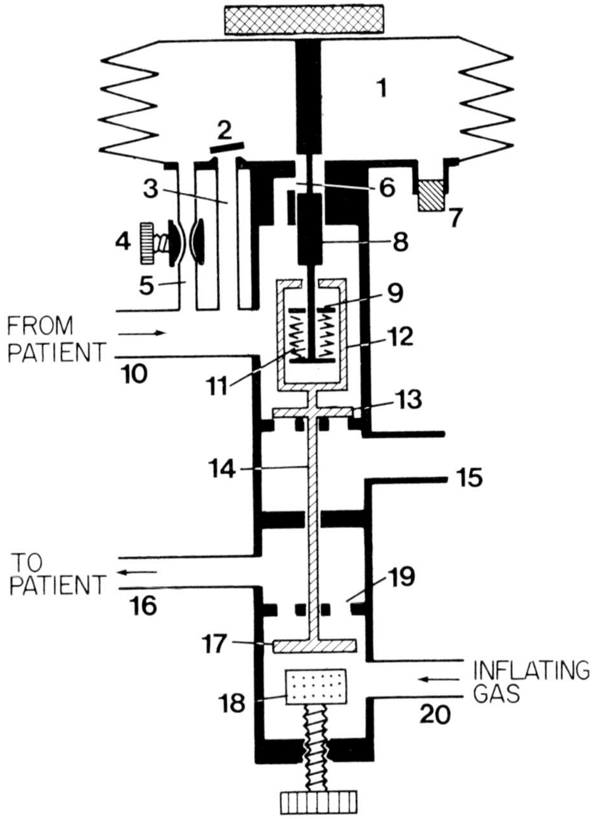

Fig. 72.1. Diagram of the 'Newcastle IV' ventilator.

1. Control concertina bag, with adjustable weight
2. One-way valve
3. Connecting tube
4. Screw clip
5. Connecting tube
6. Port
7. Plugged hole for connexion to patient-triggering unit
8. Rod
9. Sprung collar
10. Expiratory tube
11. Spring
12. Stirrup
13. Expiratory valve
14. Valve rod
15. Expiratory outlet
16. Inspiratory tube
17. Soft-iron plate
18. Magnet
19. Inspiratory valve
20. Inflating-gas inlet

Change-over from inspiratory phase to expiratory phase

This change-over is pressure-cycled: the pressure in the control concertina bag (1) (fig. 72.1) which produces cycling is that applied to the patient.

Expiratory phase

In this phase the ventilator operates as a constant, atmospheric, pressure generator: the expired gas passes freely to atmosphere at the expiratory outlet (15).

Change-over from expiratory phase to inspiratory phase

This change-over is time-cycled: the duration of the expiratory phase is governed by the escape of gas from the control concertina bag past the screw clip (4) and is shortened when the cycling pressure at the end of the inspiratory phase is raised—as in the 'Newcastle II'.

REFERENCE

1 Horton J.A.G., Inkster J.S. and Pask E.A. (1956) Two more respirators. *Br. J. Anaesth.* **28**, 169.

CHAPTER 73

The 'Newcastle V' Ventilator[1]

DESCRIPTION

This is a very simply-constructed device (fig.73.1) made from materials readily available

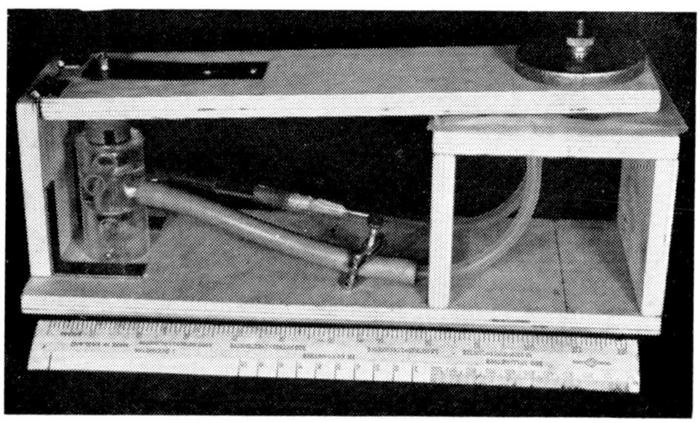

Fig. 73.1. The 'Newcastle V' ventilator.

Courtesy of *The Lancet*.[1]

in a small workshop. During the inspiratory phase (fig. 73.2) a supply of inflating gas at a pressure of 70–140 cmH_2O enters at the inlet (1) and flows freely, through the valve-box (5) and the port (2), to the patient. It also passes through the one-way valve (6), filling the control bag (9). As this bag expands it lifts the hinged flap (8) against the downward force of the weight (10). The upward movement of the flap (8) carries the magnet (4), suspended by a springy strip, away from the soft-iron disc (3) on the valve spindle. When the attraction of the magnet for the disc becomes too weak to hold the valve open, the valve drops suddenly under the influence of its own weight and the gas pressure above it.

The supply of inflating gas is now cut off (fig. 73.3) and the expired gas escapes freely, through the lower opening of the valve-box (5), to atmosphere. The opening of the valve also allows the gas in the control bag (9) to escape past the screw clip (7). As soon as the bag has emptied enough for the magnet (4) to exert its attraction on the iron

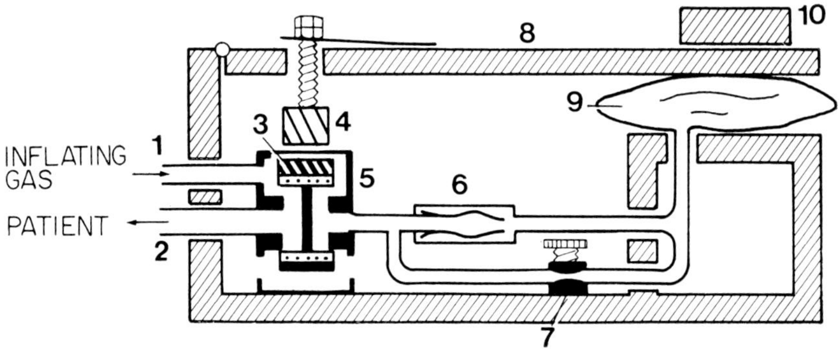

Fig. 73.2. Diagram of the 'Newcastle V' ventilator—beginning of inspiratory phase.

1. Inflating-gas inlet
2. Port
3. Soft-iron disc
4. Magnet
5. Valve-box
6. One-way valve
7. Screw clip
8. Hinged flap
9. Control bag
10. Adjustable weight

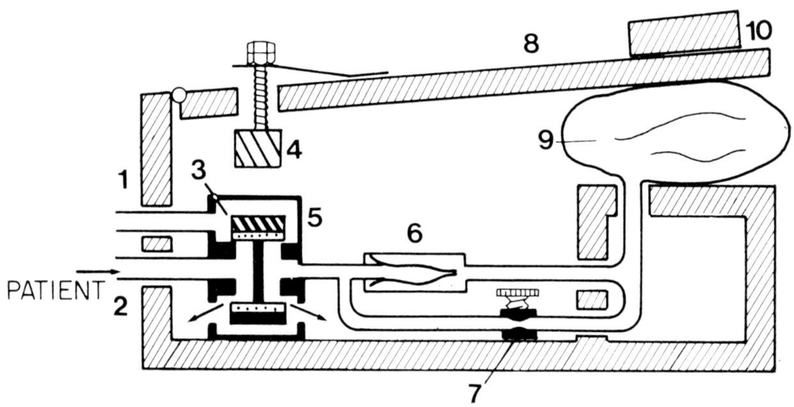

Fig. 73.3. Diagram of the 'Newcastle V' ventilator—beginning of expiratory phase.

disc (3) again, the valve is lifted sharply and the next inspiratory phase begins. The cycling pressure depends on the weight (10) and the duration of the expiratory phase on the setting of the screw clip (7) which delays the emptying of the control bag (9).

FUNCTIONAL ANALYSIS

Inspiratory phase

The mode of operation in this phase depends on the supply source used—as in the 'Newcastle III'.

Change-over from inspiratory phase to expiratory phase

This change-over is pressure-cycled: the pressure in the control bag (9) (fig. 73.2) which produces cycling is that applied to the patient.

Expiratory phase

In this phase the ventilator operates as a constant, atmospheric, pressure generator: the expired gas passes freely to the atmosphere at the expiratory outlet.

Change-over from expiratory phase to inspiratory phase

This change-over is time-cycled: the duration of the expiratory phase is governed by the escape of gas from the control bag, and is shortened when the cycling pressure at the end of the inspiratory phase is raised—as in the 'Newcastle II'.

REFERENCE

1 PASK E.A. (1953) A simple respirator. *Lancet*, **2**, 141.

CHAPTER 74

The Ohio (Monaghan) Model 120 L 'IPPB Unit'

DESCRIPTION

This ventilator (fig. 74.1) is intended for ward or domestic use. The basic control mechanism is similar to that in the Ohio (Monaghan) Model 300/DO 'Anesthesia Ventilator', but the driving gas is now supplied to the patient instead of compressing a bag-in-bottle.

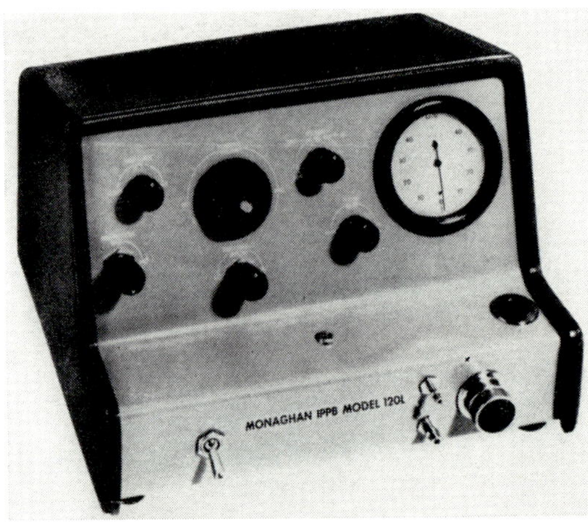

Fig. 74.1. The Ohio (Monaghan) Model 120 L 'IPPB Unit'.
Courtesy of the Monaghan Co., Denver.

Driving gas supplied at the inlet (1) (fig. 74.2) at a pressure of 45–50 lb/in^2 flows, through the on/off tap (2) and the sliding valve (14), to the injector (5) where it entrains air through the filter (7) before passing the 'flow control' (4) and entering the main chamber (15). The proportion of air entrained in the mixture entering the main chamber depends on the proportion of the driving-gas flow which is delivered through the side port of the injector by adjustment of the 'oxygen concentration control' (8). If the driving gas is oxygen the proportion of oxygen in the gas mixture delivered to the patient depends on the setting of this control; the control is calibrated between 40 and 100% oxygen in the inflating-gas mixture.

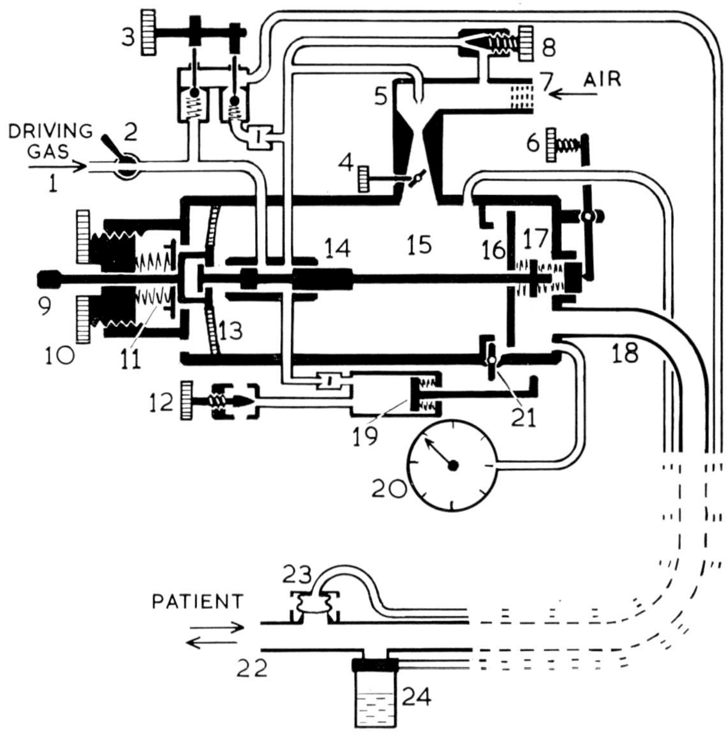

Fig. 74.2. Diagram of the Ohio (Monaghan) Model 120 L 'IPPB Unit'.

1. Gas inlet
2. On-off tap
3. Nebulizer control
4. 'Flow rate' control
5. Injector
6. 'Triggering effort' control
7. Filter
8. 'Oxygen %' control
9. Manual control button
10. 'Positive pressure' control
11. Spring
12. 'Respiration rate' control
13. Diaphragm
14. Sliding valve
15. Main chamber
16. 'Actuator disc'
17. Springs
18. Delivery tube
19. Piston
20. Manometer
21. Lever
22. Patient outlet
23. Inflatable capsule
24. Nebulizer

During the inspiratory phase the 'actuator disc' (16) is off its seating and the gas mixture flows, through the delivery tube (18) and the breathing tube (22), to the patient, the expiratory port of the inflating valve being held closed by the inflated capsule (23). As pressure rises in the main chamber (15), the diaphragm (13) is quickly moved to the left until it is stopped by the spring (11). Pressure in the chamber continues to rise and, when it becomes high enough to overcome the force exerted by the spring (11), outward movement of the diaphragm (13) recommences. The diaphragm now takes the shaft of the sliding valve (14) with it. This closes the sliding valve (14), and the flow of driving gas to the injector is cut off. The 'actuator disc' (16), which has been held off its seating by the pressure difference across it overcoming the light resistance of the spring (17), now comes to rest on its seating, lying against the small lever (21). The gas in the main chamber rapidly escapes to atmosphere through the air-entrainment port (7) of the injector; the pressure falls; and the diaphragm (13) is returned to its resting position by the spring (11) and its own elasticity. At the same time the capsule (23) deflates and expired gas flows past it to atmosphere.

The expiratory phase is terminated either when the patient makes an inspiratory effort, or after a time set by the expiratory-time control (12). In the patient-triggered mode the negative pressure produced by the patient's inspiratory effort produces a pressure difference across the 'actuator disc' (16), lifting it off its seating and moving over the sliding valve (14). The sensitivity of this patient-triggering mechanism is determined by the setting of the 'triggering effort' control (6). In the time-cycled mode the expiratory phase ends when the pivoted arm (21) moves the 'actuator disc' (16) which takes with it the sliding valve (14). During the previous inspiratory phase driving gas flowed from the sliding valve into the chamber behind the piston (19) which was driven over against the force of its spring. The time taken during the expiratory phase for the piston to be returned to its resting position depends on the rate at which the gas stored in the chamber can escape to atmosphere. This is determined by the setting of the 'respiration rate' control (12).

The pressure in the delivery tube is shown on the manometer (20). The 'nebulizer cont/off/int' control (3) allows humidification throughout the respiratory cycle, not at all, or during the inspiratory phase only. The control acts by supplying driving gas to the nebulizer (24).

The 'flow rate' control (4) may be adjusted so as to deliver flows between 25 and 100 litres/min. Positive pressure is in the range 0–40 cmH_2O. The maximum frequency is 45/min. The ventilator may be cycled at any time by pushing or releasing the button (9), which, in this model, is spring-loaded.

In the 1741 Model, intended for domestic use, the controls are reduced to three—positive pressure, flow through the nebulizer (which is continuous), and the manual push-button.

FUNCTIONAL ANALYSIS

Inspiratory phase

Assuming that the characteristics of the injector are similar to those of the injectors in the Ohio (Monaghan) Model 300/DO 'Anesthesia Ventilator' this ventilator will approximate to a constant-flow generator at the start of this phase. Any flow to the nebulizer will supplement this generated flow. Later, when the slide valve (14) begins to cut off the supply of driving gas to the injector, the operation can be expected to approach that of a pressure generator as in the pressure-cycled mode of the 300/DO.

Change-over from inspiratory phase to expiratory phase
This change-over is pressure-cycled: it occurs when the pressure in chamber (15) has risen sufficiently to overcome the force of the spring (11) and shut off the supply of driving gas to the injector by means of the slide valve (14).

Expiratory phase
In this phase the ventilator operates as a constant, atmospheric, pressure generator: the patient's expired gas passes freely to atmosphere through the valve (23).

Change-over from expiratory phase to inspiratory phase
This change-over is either time-cycled or patient-cycled whichever mechanism operates first. At a preset time after the end of the inspiratory phase the pressure in the cylinder (19) has decayed sufficiently past the needle valve (12) of the 'respiration rate' control for the striking arm to operate the lever (21) and move the 'actuator disc' (16) to the right, thereby opening the slide valve (14). If the patient makes an inspiratory effort before this, the pressure difference produced across the actuator disc (16) will move it to the right and open the slide valve (14).

CONTROLS

This 'Controls' section, unlike all but one of the others (Dräger 'Pulmomat'), has been deduced purely theoretically from data supplied by the manufacturer and from our laboratory tests on the Ohio (Monaghan) Model 300/DO 'Anesthesia Ventilator'.

Total ventilation
This cannot be directly controlled but is equal to the product of tidal volume and respiratory frequency.

Tidal volume
This can be indirectly controlled by changing the cycling pressure by means of the 'positive pressure' control (10). It also depends on the patient's compliance and resistance, particular the former.

Increasing the tidal volume by means of the cycling pressure will result in some increase in the inspiratory time and hence in a decrease in respiratory frequency and a change in inspiratory-expiratory ratio.

Respiratory frequency and inspiratory-expiratory ratio
Neither of these factors can be directly controlled but both are determined by the separately-variable inspiratory and expiratory times.

The inspiratory time is not directly controlled; it is simply the time taken to deliver the tidal volume. It therefore varies with any change, deliberate or otherwise, in tidal volume. However, for a given tidal volume, the inspiratory time can be altered by adjusting the generated inspiratory flow by means of the throttle (4) of the 'flow' control. The total generated flow, and therefore the inspiratory time, is also affected by the setting of the nebulizer control (3).

When the patient makes no inspiratory effort the ending of the expiratory phase is directly controlled by the pneumatic timer (19). The expiratory time can therefore be adjusted by means of the needle valve (12) of the 'rate' control but is uninfluenced by lung characteristics or by other controls except possibly in the manner mentioned for the pressure-cycled mode of operation of the 300/DO.

Therefore the respiratory frequency is primarily controlled by the 'rate' control (12). However it is also influenced by the setting of the 'flow' (4) and 'nebulizer' (3) controls and by any changes in tidal volume due to changes in the cycling pressure ('positive pressure') control (10) or to changes in lung characteristics. When the respiratory frequency is changed by adjusting the 'rate' control (12) the inspiratory-expiratory ratio is altered.

The inspiratory-expiratory ratio can be adjusted by means of the 'flow' control (4) but it is also influenced by the setting of the 'nebulizer' (3) and 'rate' (12) controls and by changes in tidal volume.

When the ventilator is being patient-cycled from the expiratory phase to the inspiratory phase the respiratory frequency is, of course, controlled by the patient except that the timing mechanism sets a lower limit to the frequency.

Inspiratory waveforms

At the start of the phase the flow waveform is determined by the flow-generating characteristics of the injector and the nebulizer supply and the magnitude of the flow can be adjusted by means of the 'flow' (4) and 'nebulizer' (3) controls. However, the nebulizer control will normally be set in accordance with nebulization requirements and the setting of the flow control may already have been decided in order to achieve a particular inspiratory-expiratory ratio at a particular frequency. The pressure waveforms then depend on the interaction of this flow waveform with the lung characteristics.

Later in the phase, when the slide valve (14) begins to cut off the supply of driving gas to the injector, the ventilator can be expected, as in the 300/DO in the pressure-cycled mode, to generate a pressure in the chamber (15) which is close to the cycling pressure.

Expiratory waveforms

Throughout the expiratory phase atmospheric pressure is applied to the lungs at the valve (23). It cannot be varied in any way. The expiratory flow which results depends on the effect of this pressure on the lungs.

Pressure limits

The peak inspiratory pressure at the mouth is equal to the cycling pressure. If there is indeed a period at the end of the inspiratory phase in which the ventilator generates a pressure nearly equal to the cycling pressure the peak alveolar pressure may be nearly as high as the cycling pressure. During the expiratory phase the alveolar pressure must fall to atmospheric unless the airway resistance is very high or the expiratory time very short.

CHAPTER 75

The Ohio (Monaghan) Model 300/DO 'Anesthesia Ventilator'

DESCRIPTION

This ventilator (fig. 75.1), which may be clamped to the side of an anaesthetic trolley, is designed for use during closed-circuit anaesthesia. It has three modes of operation (a) automatic ('controller'), (b) patient-triggered ('assistor'), and (c) patient-triggered with automatic override ('assistor-controller'). In all of these modes some negative pressure is applied during the expiratory phase. The ventilator is powered by compressed gas.

The driving gas is supplied to the control unit through an on/off tap (2) (fig. 75.2); ideally the supply pressure should be 50 lb/in^2, since this is the pressure for which the 'inspiratory flow rate' control is calibrated by the manufacturers. However, any pressure between 45 and 75 lb/in^2 will operate the ventilator. During the inspiratory phase the sliding valve (7) is open, as shown, and the driving gas flows to a bank of injectors (3), and also past a non-return valve (15) to the timing cylinder (16). There are five injectors in the bank (3), each having different characteristics. Four of them have spring-loaded inlet valves and one-way outlet valves. The inlet valves can be held open by the cams of the 'inspiratory flow rate' control (1), which are so arranged that any combination of these four injectors can be brought into use, thus giving a choice of as many as 15 different flow rates. In earlier models of the ventilator this choice was limited to 11. The fifth injector (4) has no inlet or outlet valve and is therefore always in operation during the inspiratory phase. Its characteristics are such that the flow from it is relatively small compared to the flow from any of the other injectors. The function of this injector will be discussed later.

The mixture, of driving gas and entrained air from those injectors in use, flows into the main chamber (8) of the control unit. The capsule (29) is inflated, blocking the outlet from the rigid plastic pressure chamber (38). The 'actuator disc' (9) is off its seating and gas flows to the manifold containing the linked valves (21) and (27). The sharp rise in pressure above the valve (27) is sufficient to overcome the effect of the counterweight (19), and the valve (27) opens. The gas mixture now flows into the pressure chamber (38). The valve (21) is held closed by the combined effect of the pressure within the manifold and the pressure difference across the valve (27). At the same time, the pressure difference across the 'actuator disc' (9) is sufficient to overcome the force of the light springs (10) and so hold the 'actuator disc' in the open position. As the pressure in the pressure chamber (38) rises, the concertina reservoir bag (36) is compressed and its contents are delivered to the patient. The spill valve (31) is held closed by the pressure difference between the outside and the inside of the reservoir bag.

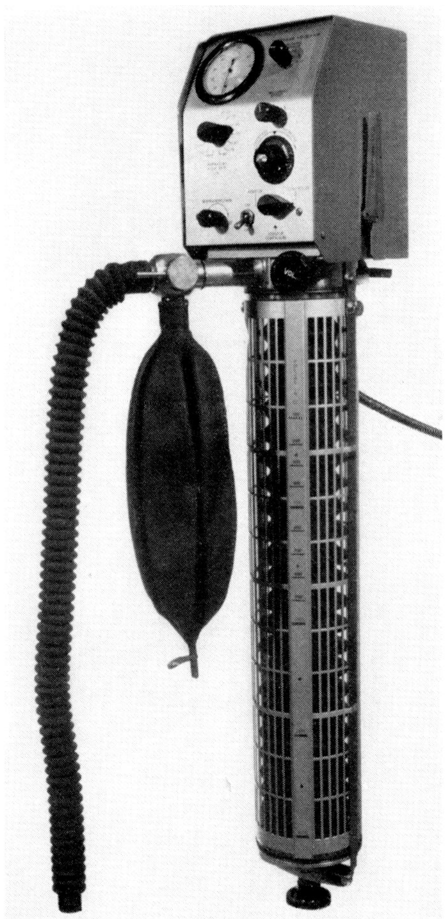

Fig. 75.1. The Ohio (Monaghan) Model 300/DO 'Anesthesia Ventilator'.
Courtesy of Department of Medical Illustration, Cardiff Royal Infirmary.

As the pressure rises within the main chamber (8) of the control unit, the diaphragm (13) is quickly pushed outwards until it is stopped by the spring (12). Pressure in the chamber (8) continues to rise and, when it becomes high enough to overcome the force exerted by the spring (12), outward movement of the diaphragm (13) recommences. The diaphragm now takes the shaft of the sliding valve (7) with it. This closes the sliding valve (7), and the flow of driving gas to the injectors (3) is cut off. The 'actuator disc' (9) comes to rest on its seating, and so lies against the small lever (18). The gas within the chamber (8) rapidly escapes to atmosphere through the valveless injector (4), the pressure falls, and the diaphragm (13) is returned to its resting position by the spring (12) and its own elasticity. At the same time the capsule (29) deflates, the gas within the chamber (38) escapes to atmosphere past the throttle valve (28), and expiration into the reservoir bag (36) commences.

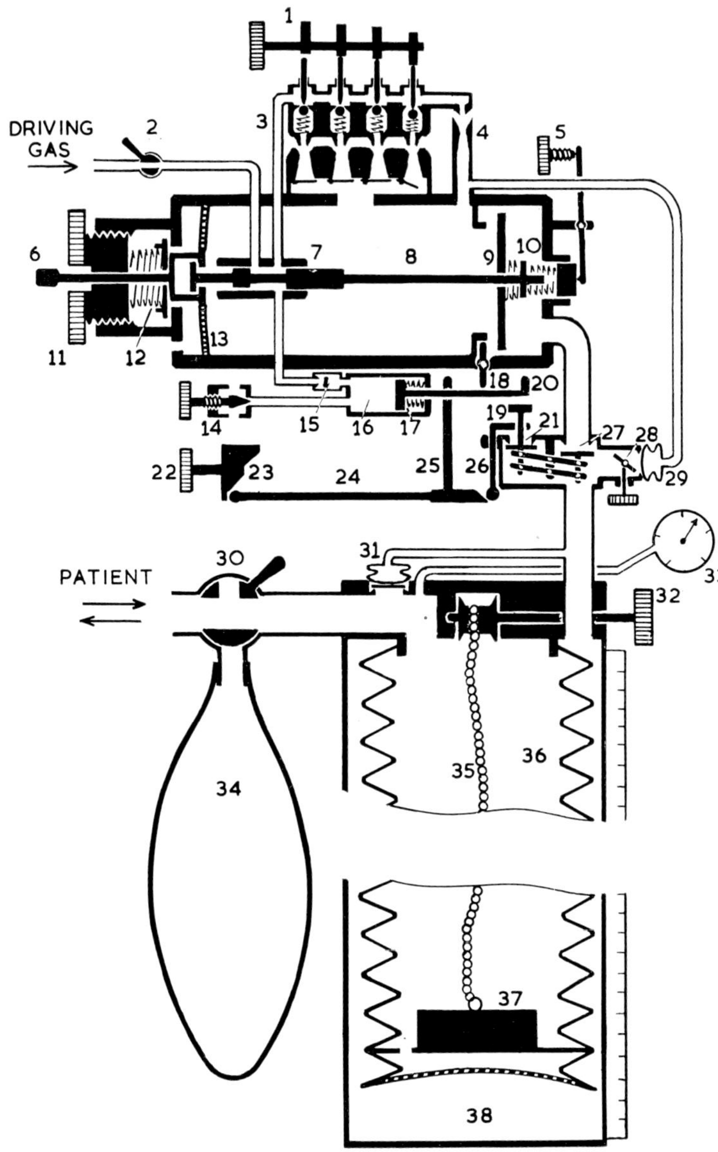

Until the escape of gas past the capsule (29) is virtually complete, the valve (21) is held in the closed position by the pressure within the manifold. When the sliding valve (7) is closed, gas escaping from the cylinder (16) through the needle valve (14) is not replaced. The piston (17) is gradually pushed by its spring until the striking arm (20) moves over the lever (18), thereby pushing the 'actuator disc' (9) to the right and re-opening the slide valve (7). The next inspiratory phase commences.

The expansion of the reservoir bag (36) during the expiratory phase is assisted by a weight (37) in the base of the bag and impeded by the resistance of the throttle (28). The flow of gas from the lungs into the reservoir bag must displace an equal flow from the pressure chamber (38) past the throttle (28). If the pressure drop across the throttle (28) is less than the pressure difference produced by the weight (37), then the pressure in the bag will be negative. If, on the other hand, the pressure drop across (28) is more than the pressure difference produced by the weight, then the pressure in the bag will be positive. By varying the resistance of the throttle by the 'negative pressure' control (28), the pressure in the reservoir bag (36) during the expiratory phase can be varied.

The control (22) turns a cam (23) which sets the sliding rod (24) in one of three positions.

In the first, 'controller', position, as shown in fig. 75.2, the push-rod (26) is not engaged and the linked valves (21, 27) move in the manner already described until, during the expiratory phase, the expansion of the concertina bag (36) is complete and the pressure in the manifold has fallen to atmospheric. The force exerted by the weight (19) now opens the valve (21), maintaining a free pathway between the pressure chamber (38) and atmosphere, and closes the valve (27). The linked-valve mechanism (21, 27) is, in

---

Fig. 75.2. Diagram of the Ohio (Monaghan) Model 300/DO 'Anesthesia Ventilator'.

1. 'Inspiratory flow rate' control
2. On/off tap
3. Bank of four injectors
4. Valveless injector
5. 'Triggering effort' control
6. Knob for manual cycling
7. Sliding valve
8. Main chamber of control unit
9. 'Actuator disc'
10. Springs
11. 'Positive pressure' control
12. Spring
13. Diaphragm
14. 'Respirations/min' control
15. One-way valve
16. Cylinder of expiratory timer
17. Piston
18. Lever
19. Weight
20. Striking arm
21. Linked valve
22. Mode selector
23. Cam
24. Sliding rod
25. Locking arm
26. Push rod
27. Linked valve
28. Throttle valve ('Negative pressure' control)
29. Check valve
30. Manual/automatic tap
31. Spill valve
32. 'Volume' control
33. Manometer
34. Reservoir bag for manual inflation
35. Bead chain
36. Concertina reservoir bag
37. Weight
38. Rigid plastic pressure chamber

fact, incorporated only to ensure that, in this 'controller' mode of operation, no inspiratory effort by the patient can affect the triggering mechanism. During the inspiratory phase the flow of gas from the main chamber (8) easily overcomes the force of the weight (19), opening the valve (27) and closing the valve (21).

In the second, 'assistor-controller', position of the cam (23), the rod (24) is moved over sufficiently to lift the push-rod (26) far enough to hold up the weight (19) and so lock the linked valves (21) and (27) in the closed and open positions respectively. The part of the concertina bag (36) below the weight (37) is particularly flexible. Therefore, once the weight is supported by the chain (35), the slightest inspiratory effort by the patient creates a negative pressure in the chamber (38). As the 'actuator disc' (9) has a large area, only a small fall in pressure on the patient's side of it is needed to move the disc over, against the force exerted by the light springs (10), and thus initiate an inspiratory phase. The force exerted by the light springs (10), and hence the negative pressure required to trigger the ventilator, can be adjusted by the 'triggering effort' control (5). If the patient fails to make an inspiratory effort, the expiratory timing mechanism (16, 17, 18, 20) operates in the normal way.

In the third, 'assistor', position of the control (22) the rod (24) is moved further over, and the linked valves (21, 27) remain locked, as in the second, 'assistor-controller', position of the control (22). However, the locking arm (25) now holds the lever (18) away from the 'actuator disc' (9), with the result that automatic cycling can no longer occur. Ventilation is now exclusively patient-triggered.

The ventilator may be cycled, from either phase to the other, by pushing or pulling the knob (6).

A bead chain (35) connected to the weight in the reservoir bag (36) allows the stroke volume to be preset by the 'volume' control (32). A scale on the chamber (38) indicates the volume delivered from the reservoir bag. The maximum inflating pressure can be varied between 5 and 40 cmH_2O by adjusting the compression of the spring (12) by the 'positive pressure' control (11). The pressure in the patient circuit is indicated on the manometer (33).

The needle valve (14) of the 'respirations/min' control regulates the leak of gas from the cylinder (16), and hence the expiratory time.

By turning the tap (30) the patient can be connected to the reservoir bag (34) for manual inflation.

Excess gas in the patient circuit can escape through the spill valve (31) during the expiratory phase. During the inspiratory phase the pressure of the driving gas distends the capsule of this valve sufficiently to hold it closed.

A lever marked 'Release' allows the section of the ventilator containing the respiratory pathways to be removed for cleaning and sterilization.

The 'Anesthesia Ventilator' Model 300/SO (Standard) is similar to the Model 300/DO (Deluxe) described above. It differs in that only a single inspiratory flow rate, nominally 60 litres/min, is provided.

FUNCTIONAL ANALYSIS

This ventilator has two modes of operation for the change-over from the inspiratory phase to the expiratory phase: volume-cycled and pressure-cycled. The tracings of figs. 75.4 and 75.5 are confined to the volume-cycled mode and were obtained from a 300/DO (Deluxe) model.

Inspiratory phase

Fundamentally the ventilator approximates to a constant-flow generator in this phase because the characteristics of the injectors (fig. 75.3) are such that the flow does not fall

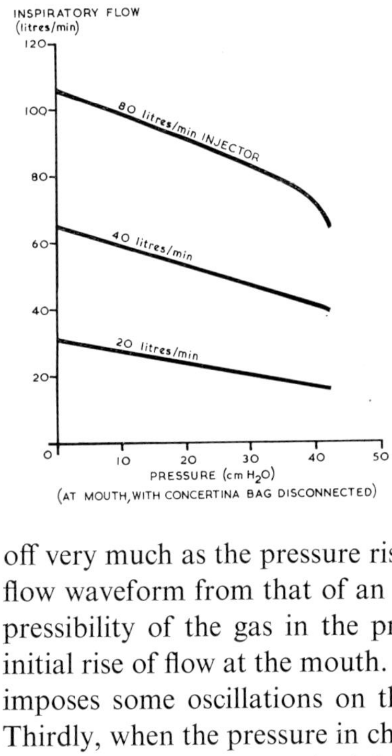

Fig. 75.3. Ohio (Monaghan) Model 300/DO. Flow-pressure characteristics of injectors. For this test the driving gas was oxygen at 50 lb/in^2, the 'positive pressure' (cycling pressure) control was set to maximum, the spill valve (31, fig. 75.2) was blocked by a rubber bung, and the concertina reservoir bag was disconnected from its mount so that the gas from the injectors flowed directly to the 'patient'. Since, in normal operation, there is a pressure drop of about 10 cmH_2O across the bag wall, the true flow at any given mouth pressure will be that indicated by the above graph for a mouth pressure about 10 cmH_2O greater than the given pressure.

off very much as the pressure rises. However, a number of factors operate to distort the flow waveform from that of an ideal flow generator shown in fig. 3.6. Firstly, the compressibility of the gas in the pressure chamber (38, fig. 75.2) results in a rather slow initial rise of flow at the mouth. Secondly, the inertia of the weight in the concertina bag imposes some oscillations on the flow waveform, especially at the start of the phase. Thirdly, when the pressure in chamber (8) has risen sufficiently for the valve (7) to begin to cut off the supply to the injector, the reduced supply results in a reduced entrained flow and hence a slower build-up to the full pressure in chamber (8) necessary to cut off the supply of driving gas completely and thereby permit the change-over to expiration. Thus, in the later part of the phase, there is usually a gradual decline of flow, rather than a sharp cut off. This effect is less noticeable at higher inspiratory flow rates (compare (d) with (a) in fig. 75.5) and more marked with low inspiratory flow rates (not shown here). It seems to occur at all inspiratory flow rates in the pressure-cycled mode of operation. However, despite these various distortions from the 'ideal', it can clearly be seen from fig. 75.4 that, in the volume-cycled mode of operation, the flow waveform is little affected by changes of compliance or resistance whereas the mouth-pressure waveform is considerably altered. In the pressure-cycled mode of operation, on the other hand, (not shown here) the ventilator operates as a flow generator only in the early part of the phase. In the later part, while the slide valve (7) is gradually closing, the action of the ventilator seems in practice to approximate more closely to that of a constant-pressure generator.

With both modes of cycling, during that part of the phase in which the ventilator operates as a constant-flow generator, the fresh-gas flow to the patient circuit acts as a small-constant-flow generator, supplementing the main flow generator.

Change-over from inspiratory phase to expiratory phase

Fundamentally this change-over is pressure-cycled: it occurs when the pressure in chamber (8) has risen sufficiently for the valve (7) to cut off the supply of gas to the injectors. If the volume of the reservoir bag is set to a large value and the cycling pressure is not set too high, the pressure in chamber (8) will be closely related to that at the patient's mouth (after allowing for the pressure-drop due to the weight in the bag) and the change-over will indeed be pressure-cycled.

However, the change-over may alternatively be made effectively volume-cycled by setting the bag volume to about the desired tidal volume and the cycling pressure to a high value which is more than sufficient to deliver the desired tidal volume. Then the pressure in chamber (8) will not rise to the cycling pressure (and the change-over to expiration will not occur) until the bag has completely emptied—more or less irrespective of the pressure required to achieve this. Once the bag has emptied, the pressure in the pressure chamber (38) rises rapidly and therefore the pressure in the chamber (8) quickly reaches the cycling pressure. For the tracings of fig. 75.4 the 'positive pressure' control, that is the cycling pressure, was set to maximum and the bag volume was set to deliver a tidal volume of 500 ml. It can be seen that this volume was still delivered when the compliance was halved (fig. 75.4b) or the resistance was doubled (fig. 75.4c).

Since the ventilator approximates to a flow generator during the inspiratory phase it takes a nearly-fixed time to deliver a fixed volume and therefore the change-over is also effectively time-cycled: fig. 75.4 shows that the inspiratory time is barely affected by changes in lung characteristics. On the other hand the pressure at the mouth at the end of the inspiratory phase is considerably altered by the changes in lung characteristics.

Expiratory phase

At the start of this phase the ventilator operates as a constant, negative, pressure generator owing to the weight in the concertina bag. There is some delay before any negative pressure appears at the mouth because the high pressure left in the pressure chamber (38) at the end of the expiratory phase has to decay by the escape of gas through the throttle (28) and past the valve (29) which inevitably have some resistance, even with

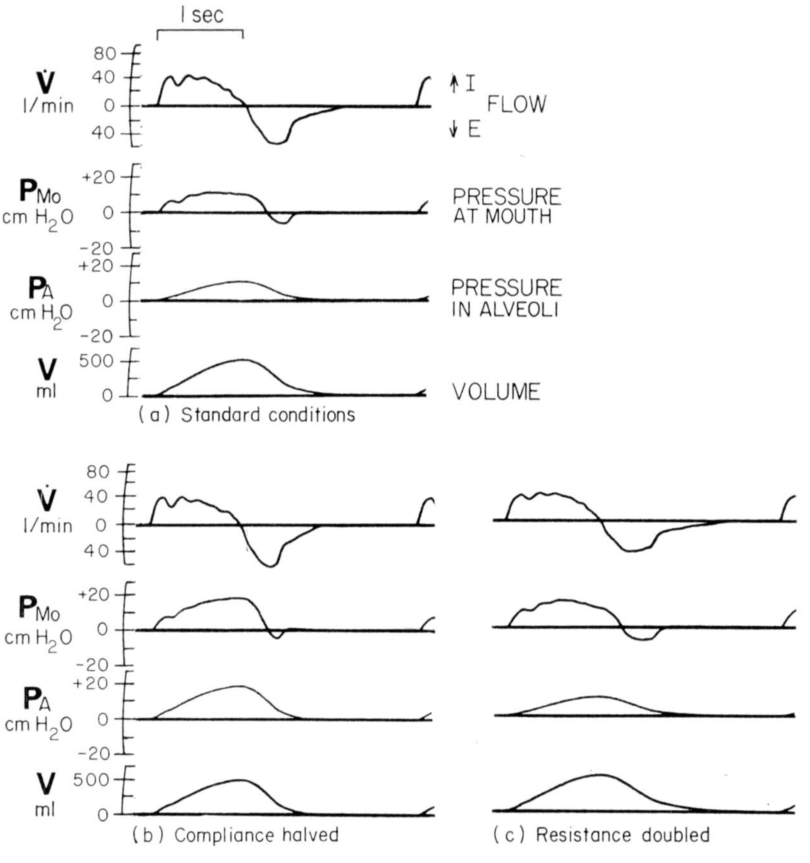

Fig. 75.4. Ohio (Monaghan) Model 300/DO in the volume-cycled mode of operation. Recordings showing the effects of changes of lung characteristics.

Standard conditions: driving gas, oxygen at 50 lb/in^2; selector switch, on 'Controller'; 'positive pressure', maximum; 'negative pressure', maximum; fresh-gas flow, 0·5 litre/min; 'volume', set for a tidal volume of 500 ml; 'inspiratory flow rate' control, set (at '40 litres/min') to give an inspiratory time of approximately 1 sec; 'respirations/min', set for a frequency of 20/min.

the 'negative pressure' control (28) set at maximum, i.e. with the resistance of the throttle set at minimum. Even when the excess pressure has been released from the pressure chamber there is still a continuing flow of gas through the resistance of throttle and valve (28, 29) owing to the re-expansion of the concertina bag by the patient's expiration. Therefore the negative pressure at the mouth is somewhat flow-dependent. However, it can be seen in fig. 75.4 that the flow pattern at the start of the expiratory phase is modified by changes of lung characteristics.

Once the concertina bag has expanded to the limit set by the volume control (32) the weight in the bag is supported by the chain (35) and therefore no longer generates negative pressure. Once this occurs the ventilator operates as a constant, atmospheric, pressure generator with expired gas escaping to atmosphere through the spill valve (31). From fig. 75.4 it can be seen that, in the later part of the expiratory phase, the pressure at the mouth is constant, and atmospheric, in all conditions, whereas the pattern of flow varies with changes in lung characteristics.

Change-over from expiratory phase to inspiratory phase

This change-over is either time-cycled or patient-cycled (patient-triggered). With the selector switch (22) set to 'Controller', as when the recordings of figs. 75.4 and 75.5 were made, the change-over is purely time-cycled. It occurs when the pressure in the cylinder (16) of the pneumatic timer has decayed sufficiently through the needle valve (14) of the 'respirations/min' control to allow the striking arm (20) to operate the lever (18) and 'actuator disc' (9) thereby opening the slide valve (7). This mechanism is quite unconnected with the patient and it can be seen from fig. 75.4 that the inspiratory phase commences at a fixed time after the start of the expiratory phase, irrespective of lung characteristics, and not when some critical volume has come out of the lungs nor immediately some critical pressure has been reached at the mouth.

With the selector switch set to 'Assistor' the change-over is purely patient-cycled; it occurs when a small inspiratory effort from the patient moves the 'actuator disc' (9) thereby opening the slide valve (7).

With the selector switch set to 'Assistor/Controller' the change-over is either time-cycled or patient-cycled; it occurs when the 'actuator disc' (9) is operated either by the decay of pressure in the pneumatic timer or by an inspiratory effort from the patient, whichever occurs first.

CONTROLS

Total ventilation

This cannot be directly controlled but is equal to the product of tidal volume and respiratory frequency.

Tidal volume

In the volume-cycled mode of operation the tidal volume is directly controlled by the setting of the volume control which limits the expansion of the concertina bag. It is therefore unaffected by changes in lung characteristics (fig. 75.4). However, the tidal volume exceeds the volume of gas leaving the concertina bag by the amount of fresh gas which enters the patient circuit during the inspiratory phase. Therefore increasing the fresh-gas flow (fig. 75.5f) increases the tidal volume. Increasing the duration of the inspiratory phase, by means of decreasing the inspiratory flow rate, will also increase the tidal volume, especially when the fresh-gas flow is high. This is because more fresh gas can then enter during the phase. (This effect is not shown in fig. 75.5). Since the ventilator operates as a flow generator during the inspiratory phase, increasing the tidal volume, by means of adjusting the volume control (fig. 75.5b), results in an increase in the inspiratory time. However, the expiratory time remains unaltered (in the 'Controller' mode of operation). Therefore the inspiratory-expiratory ratio is altered, the duration of the respiratory period is increased, and the respiratory frequency is decreased. These features can all be seen by comparing (b) with (a) in fig. 75.5.

In the pressure-cycled mode of operation the tidal volume can be varied by changing the cycling pressure but it also depends on the patient's compliance and resistance.

Respiratory frequency and inspiratory-expiratory ratio

Neither of these parameters can be directly controlled; both are influenced by many factors. However, both are determined by the separately-variable inspiratory and expiratory times.

The inspiratory time is not directly controlled; it is simply the time taken to deliver the tidal volume. It therefore varies with any change, deliberate or otherwise, in tidal volume. However for a given tidal volume, the inspiratory time can be altered by adjusting the 'inspiratory flow rate' control. Fig. 75.5d shows that increasing the inspiratory flow rate decreases the inspiratory time. Since the ventilator operates as a flow generator in the inspiratory phase the inspiratory time does not vary so long as the tidal volume is constant. Therefore, in the volume-cycled mode of operation, changes of lung characteristics do not affect the inspiratory time. However, in the pressure-cycled mode of operation, any change, at least of compliance, does alter the inspiratory time as a result of the alteration it produces in tidal volume.

In the 'Controller' mode of operation the expiratory time is directly controlled by the pneumatic timer and is uninfluenced by other controls or by lung characteristics. The only exception to this is when, as a result of a very gradual cut-off of the slide valve (7), the pressure in the cylinder (16) is below the supply pressure at the start of the expiratory phase. The expiratory time will then be shortened. However, this does not occur in the volume-cycled mode of operation.

Therefore the respiratory frequency can be controlled by the 'respirations/min' control. However, it is also influenced by the 'inspiratory flow rate' control and by changes in tidal volume, due to changes either in the settings of the ventilator controls or, in the pressure-cycled mode of operation, in the lung characteristics. Changing the respiratory frequency by means of the 'respirations/min' control also changes the inspiratory-expiratory ratio.

The inspiratory-expiratory ratio can be adjusted by means of the 'inspiratory flow rate' control but it is also influenced by the setting of the 'respirations/min' control and by changes in tidal volume. In the volume-cycled mode of operation neither the respiratory frequency nor the inspiratory-expiratory ratio is affected by changes in lung characteristics.

In the 'Assistor' mode the respiratory frequency is entirely controlled by the patient. In the 'Assistor/Controller' mode the frequency is primarily controlled by the patient but the timing mechanism sets a lower limit.

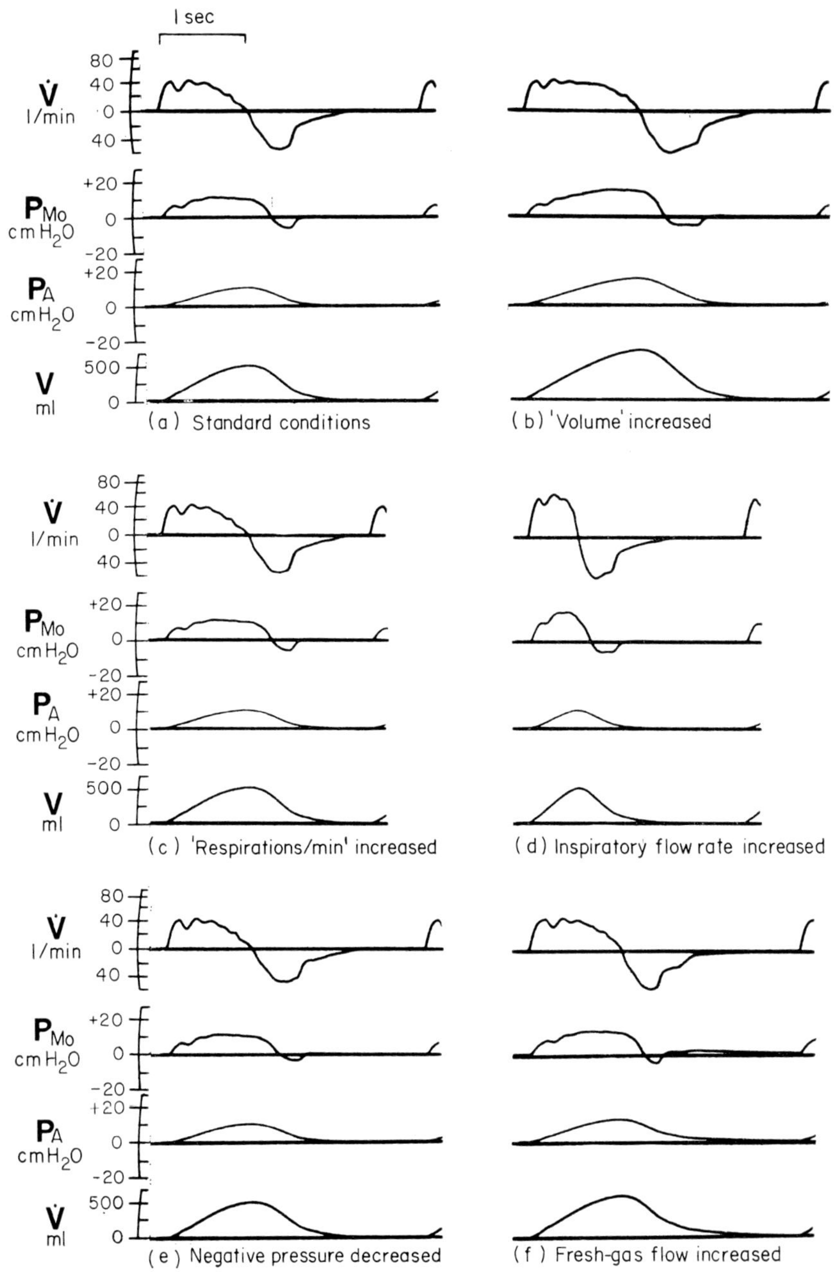

Inspiratory waveforms

In the volume-cycled mode of operation the flow waveform is controlled by the ventilator while the pressure waveforms are the result of the interaction of the flow waveform with the lung characteristics. The magnitude of the flow can be varied by adjusting the 'inspiratory flow rate' control (fig. 75.5d) but the setting of this control may already have been decided in order to achieve a particular inspiratory-expiratory ratio in combination with a particular respiratory frequency. In the pressure-cycled mode of operation the waveforms are more complex (see the functional analysis above) but the same limitations apply to deliberate control of the waveforms.

Expiratory waveforms

In the expiratory phase it is the pressure waveform which is controlled by the ventilator, initially in the form of constant, negative, pressure generation by the weight in the concertina bag and, afterwards, in the form of constant, atmospheric, pressure generation by the escape of gas through the spill valve (31). The only method of control is by altering the resistance to expiration during the negative-pressure part of the phase by means of the throttle (28). Comparison of (e) with (a) in fig. 75.5 shows the smallness of the effect of changing this resistance from minimum to maximum, that is, of altering the setting of the 'negative pressure' control (28) from maximum to minimum.

Pressure limits

If the fresh-gas flow exceeds the sum of the patient's oxygen and anaesthetic uptake, together with any leaks that may occur, then some gas must escape through the spill valve (31) at the end of the expiratory phase. Therefore, although negative pressure is developed in the concertina bag while it is falling, this can do no more than increase the expiratory flow rate in the early part of the phase; once the bag has refilled gas must spill through valve (31) and therefore the alveolar pressure cannot fall below atmospheric. This can be seen in all the tracings in figs. 75.4 and 75.5. With a high airway resistance or a short expiratory time it is possible that the alveolar pressure may not fall even as far as this, but the negative generated pressure in the early part of the phase helps to prevent this and it does not occur in any of the tracings in figs. 75.4 or 75.5. In the volume-cycled mode of operation the peak alveolar pressure will then equal the preset tidal volume divided by the compliance. In the pressure-cycled mode of operation

---

Fig. 75.5. Ohio (Monaghan) Model 300/DO in the volume-cycled mode of operation. Recordings showing the effects of changes in the settings of the controls.

(a) Standard conditions as in fig. 75.4.
(b) 'Volume' increased to deliver a tidal volume of 750 ml.
(c) 'Respirations/min' increased $\frac{3}{8}$ of a turn for a frequency of 25/min.
(d) 'Inspiratory flow rate' increased to '80 litres/min'.
(e) 'Negative pressure' set to minimum.
(f) Fresh-gas flow set to 4 litres/min.

the peak mouth pressure is determined by the cycling pressure and the pressure drop across the wall of the concertina bag. In addition, since, with pressure cycling, the flow is usually small at the end of the inspiratory phase, the peak alveolar pressure will be almost the same as the peak mouth pressure.

The only circumstance in which the ventilator can produce a negative pressure in the alveoli is when the fresh-gas flow is less than the sum of the patient's oxygen and anaesthetic uptake together with any leaks. Then the concertina bag will not fall to the limit set by the chain and negative pressure will be applied to the mouth throughout the expiratory phase, that is the ventilator will operate as a constant, negative, pressure generator throughout the phase and the alveolar pressure will approach this pressure approximately exponentially. However, in this situation, the bag will progressively empty from one respiration to the next so that, after a time, no matter whether the volume-cycled or the pressure-cycled mode of operation is employed, the bag completely empties in each inspiratory phase. The stroke of the bag, and hence the tidal volume, will then decrease further until the mean airway pressure is low enough to reduce the leak to a point at which, together with the patient's oxygen and anaesthetic uptake, it just balances the fresh-gas flow. In these circumstances, therefore, the minimum alveolar pressure, at the end of the expiratory phase, will equal, or nearly equal, the negative generated pressure, while the maximum alveolar pressure will depend in a complex way on the nature of the leak. The tidal volume will be the difference between these pressures divided by the compliance and will not be controlled by the limit set to the reservoir bag volume by the volume control (32) nor by the cycling-pressure control (11).

CHAPTER 76

The Pierce Ventilator[1]

DESCRIPTION

This apparatus was originally intended for use in the experimental laboratory. A Folberth windscreen-wiper motor (W) rhythmically interrupts a flow of compressed air into the trachea of the experimental animal. Compressed air enters the apparatus at (H).

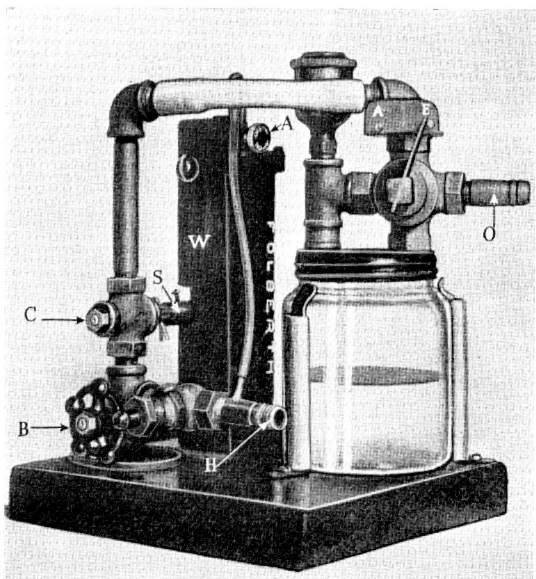

Fig. 76.1. The Pierce ventilator.

A. Needle valve controlling respiratory frequency
B. Needle valve controlling inspiratory flow
C. Motor-operated tap, rhythmically interrupting flow
H. Compressed-air inlet
O. Delivery tube for connexion to animal
S. Control for adjusting the inspiratory-expiratory ratio
W. Windscreen-wiper motor

Courtesy of *Journal of Laboratory and Clinical Medicine.*[1]

Some of the air passes through the narrow-bore tubing and the control (A) to actuate the windscreen-wiper motor. The rest passes through the needle valve (B) to the tap (C) which is opened and shut by the motor of the windscreen wiper. The flow of compressed air passing to the animal through the tube (O) is therefore interrupted in rhythmic fashion. No expiratory valve is included. The apparatus is connected to an endotracheal tube of small bore relative to the trachea, so that expiration occurs round it. There is thus inevitably considerable leakage round the tube during the inspiratory phase.

The speed of the motor, and with it the frequency of ventilation, is controlled by the needle valve (A). The flow of air passing to the animal is controlled by (B). The relative durations of the inspiratory and the expiratory phases may be varied by loosening the set screw (S) and rotating the sleeve on the motor shaft. The volume of air blown into the trachea depends on the flow (control B) and on the duration of the inspiratory phase (controls S and A). On the right-hand side is an ether bottle. By moving the lever above it either air (A) or ether and air (E) is delivered.

FUNCTIONAL ANALYSIS

Inspiratory phase

During this phase the ventilator operates fundamentally as a constant-flow generator, owing to the constant high pressure of the driving gas and the high resistance of needle valve (B) (fig. 76.1). However, because of the leak around the endotracheal tube, it behaves effectively as a constant-pressure generator with series resistance (see p. 85).

Change-over from inspiratory phase to expiratory phase

This change-over is time-cycled: the duration of the phase is determined by the wiper motor.

Expiratory phase

In this phase the ventilator operates as a constant, atmospheric, pressure generator: the expired gas passes to atmosphere around the endotracheal tube.

Change-over from expiratory phase to inspiratory phase

This change-over is time-cycled: the duration of the expiratory phase is determined by the wiper motor.

REFERENCE

1 Pierce H.F. (1923) Artificial respiration and ether apparatus for use with compressed air. *J. Lab. clin. Med.* **9**, 197.

CHAPTER 77

The Pires and Mentz Ventilator[1]

DESCRIPTION

A domestic vacuum cleaner (12) (fig. 77.2) drives air through an injector (13). The sources of positive and negative pressure thus provided are connected to the ventilator at (6) and (7) respectively.

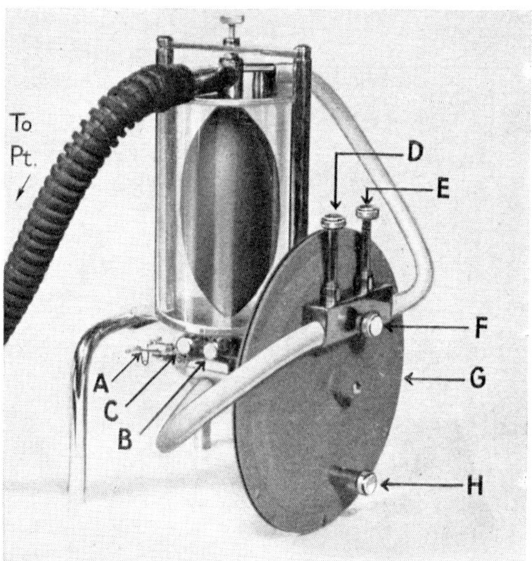

Fig. 77.1. The Pires and Mentz ventilator.
A. Spring system
B, C, D, E, F. Needle valves
G. Diaphragm
H. Tap connecting the diaphragm chamber to atmosphere
Courtesy of *Revista Brasileira de Anestesiologia.*[1]

During the inspiratory phase compressed air flows, through the control valve (6) and the piston chamber, to the glass pressure chamber (9) containing the reservoir bag (10), forcing the anaesthetic gas within the bag (10), through the breathing tube (11), to the patient.

As the pressure in the pressure chamber (9) increases, the diaphragm (4) becomes

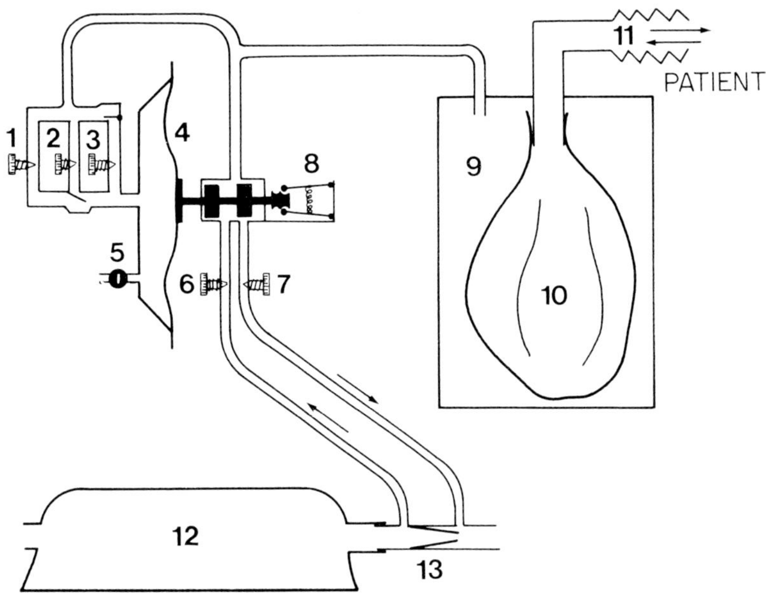

Fig. 77.2. Diagram of the Pires and Mentz ventilator.

1. Needle valve
2. Needle valve
3. Needle valve
4. Diaphragm
5. Tap
6. Needle valve
7. Needle valve
8. Spring
9. Glass pressure chamber
10. Reservoir bag
11. Breathing tube
12. Vacuum cleaner
13. Injector

distended until the tension of the spring (8) is overcome and the control piston is pushed outwards and takes up the expiratory position.

In the expiratory phase the gas under pressure in the pressure chamber (9) and behind the diaphragm (4) can flow out through the control valve (7) aided by the negative pressure exerted by the injector (13). As the pressure falls, air behind the diaphragm (4) leaks away through the needle valves (1 and 3), until once again the tension of the spring at (8) is overcome and the control piston is pulled to the left to assume the inspiratory position.

The working of this device will be understood more easily if the effects of adjustment of each of the six controls are considered.

Tap (6) controls the flow of gas during the inspiratory phase and hence the speed of inflation, and so affects the duration of this phase.

Tap (7) imposes a resistance in series with the negative pressure. It therefore affects the speed of expiration and so the duration of the phase.

Tap (2) controls the rate of build-up of pressure behind the diaphragm (4) by regulating the flow of driving gas, through the one-way valve at its exit, to the diaphragm chamber. It therefore affects the duration of the inspiratory phase.

Tap (3) has the same action as (2) during the expiratory phase.

Tap (1) provides a further path for the entry and exit of gas from the diaphragm chamber. It therefore primarily controls the frequency of respiration.

Tap (5) opens the diaphragm chamber to the atmosphere and allows the apparatus to be held in either the inspiratory or expiratory position at the anaesthetist's will.

FUNCTIONAL ANALYSIS

Inspiratory phase

The mode of operation during this phase depends upon the characteristics of the vacuum cleaner but, like other blowers (see p. 88), it probably operates as a fairly-high-constant-pressure generator with substantial series resistance. There is a pressure limit, owing to the blow-off valve in the patient circuit, which comes into operation during the phase. Until then the fresh-gas supply to the patient circuit acts as a small-constant-flow generator, supplementing the action of the main pressure generator.

Change-over from inspiratory phase to expiratory phase

This change-over is a hybrid mixture of time-cycled and pressure-cycled. Cycling occurs when the pressure around the reservoir bag (10) (fig. 77.2) has raised the pressure behind the diaphragm (4) to the cycling value. Thus the time at which cycling occurs depends partly on the pattern of pressure build-up around the bag, which is that applied to the patient until the blow-off valve opens, and partly by the setting of controls (1) and (2) between this pressure and the diaphragm.

Expiratory phase

In this phase the ventilator operates as a constant, negative, pressure generator with substantial series resistance owing to the injector characteristics and the tap (7). The fresh-gas flow now slightly impedes the main pressure-generating action.

End of expiratory phase

This change-over also is a hybrid mixture of time-cycled and pressure-cycled—as at the end of the inspiratory phase. Cycling occurs when the pressure behind the diaphragm (4) has fallen to the cycling value.

REFERENCE

1 PIRES F.K. and MENTZ E. (1953) A respiração controlada, automática, ativa em ambas as fases respiratórias, regulável em freqüência, pressões e proporções, por meio do alternator. *Rev. bras. Anestes.* **3**, 75.

CHAPTER 78

The 'Pneumotron'

DESCRIPTION

This ventilator (fig. 78.1) is a commercial development of the Donald ventilator. It can be used for either assisted or fully-controlled respiration in infants or adults.

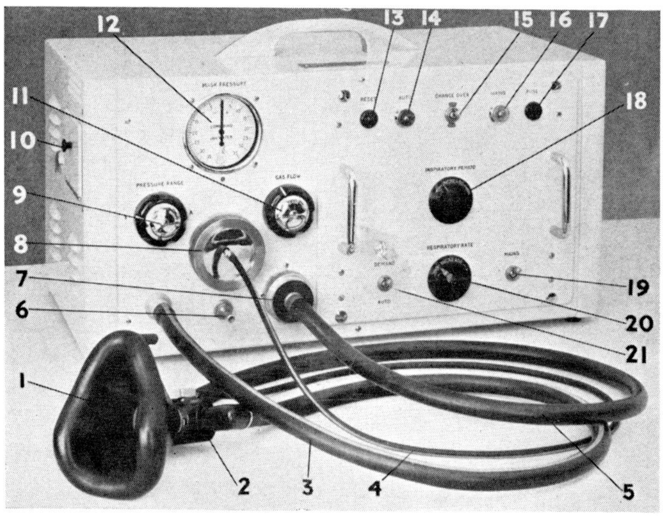

Fig. 78.1. The 'Pneumotron'.

1. Face mask
2. Swivel mount
3. Inspiratory tube
4. Tube to manometer and trigger mechanism
5. Expiratory tube
6. Connexion to injector-operated sucker
7. Expiratory valve
8. 'Germ barrier' cover
9. Pressure-limit selector
10. Inspection cover for trigger-unit lamp
11. Gas-flow control
12. Manometer
13. Reset button for restoring circuit to 'Demand'
14. 'Auto' indicator lamp
15. Change-over switch. This can be used to inactivate the automatic 'change-over' from 'Demand' to 'Auto'
16. Mains pilot light
17. Fuse
18. Control for adjusting the inspiratory-expiratory ratio
19. Mains on/off switch
20. Respiratory-frequency control
21. 'Auto/Demand' switch

Courtesy of British Oxygen Company Limited.

Connexions to the a.c. mains and to a supply of compressed gas at 60 lb/in^2 are needed. Instead of the a.c. mains a battery-supplied power pack (3) (fig. 78.2) may be used.

When the patient makes an inspiratory effort the electrical mechanism is triggered, the inspiratory valve (17) is opened and the expiratory valve (26) is closed. After a set time the mechanism reverses the valves (17, 26) and expired gas passes to atmosphere through the valve (26). The expiratory valve (26) is then held open until the patient makes another inspiratory effort and initiates a new inspiratory phase.

The slight negative pressure produced by the patient's inspiratory effort is transmitted through the tube (22) and deflects the sensitive metal diaphragm (23). A shutter fixed to the diaphragm is moved, allowing a beam of light to fall on the photo-electric cell (24). This operates a relay (25) which closes the contacts (9). The relay (14) is now energized through the contacts (4) and closes the three pairs of contacts (11, 12, 13). The closing of the contacts (13) completes the electrical circuit of the solenoid-operated inspiratory and expiratory valves (17, 26). The inspiratory valve (17) is opened and the expiratory valve (26) is closed. The closing of the contacts (12) starts the electric motor (2), and the closing of the contacts (11) provides an additional circuit for the relay (14) through the contacts (6).

As the cam (8) is turned by the motor (2) the contacts (4) are opened and the photo-electric-cell circuit is rendered unresponsive to any further inspiratory effort. Rotation of the cam (8) also closes the contacts (5) providing an alternative circuit for the motor (2). Further rotation of the cam allows the contacts (6) to open.

The holding-circuit for the relay (14) is broken and the relay is no longer energized. The pairs of contacts (11, 12, 13) now spring open. The solenoids are no longer energized and the positions of the inspiratory and expiratory valves (17, 26) are reversed. The circuit to the motor through the contacts (12) is broken, but since the motor is still being supplied through the contacts (5) the cam continues to rotate until it reaches its rest position. At this point the contacts (5) open, the motor stops, and the contacts (4) close. By this time the contacts (6) are also closed and the machine is again ready to respond to an inspiratory effort.

To set the machine for automatic operation the switch (10) is closed. This shorts out the contacts (9) in the triggering circuit and inflation commences as soon as the cam (8) reaches its rest position, because the relay (14) is now energized through the switch (10) as soon as the contacts (4) close.

When the machine is set for assisted respiration, a further electrical circuit ensures that the switch (10) is closed automatically if the patient fails to take a breath within a set time fixed by the manufacturers. The machine will then stay on 'automatic' until a reset button is pressed, reopening the switch (10).

The inflating pressure is limited by the safety-valve (19) which can be set for either 'child' or 'adult'. The limit is nominally 18 cmH$_2$O for children and 30 cmH$_2$O for adults. The speed with which the lungs are inflated depends on the flow of fresh gas

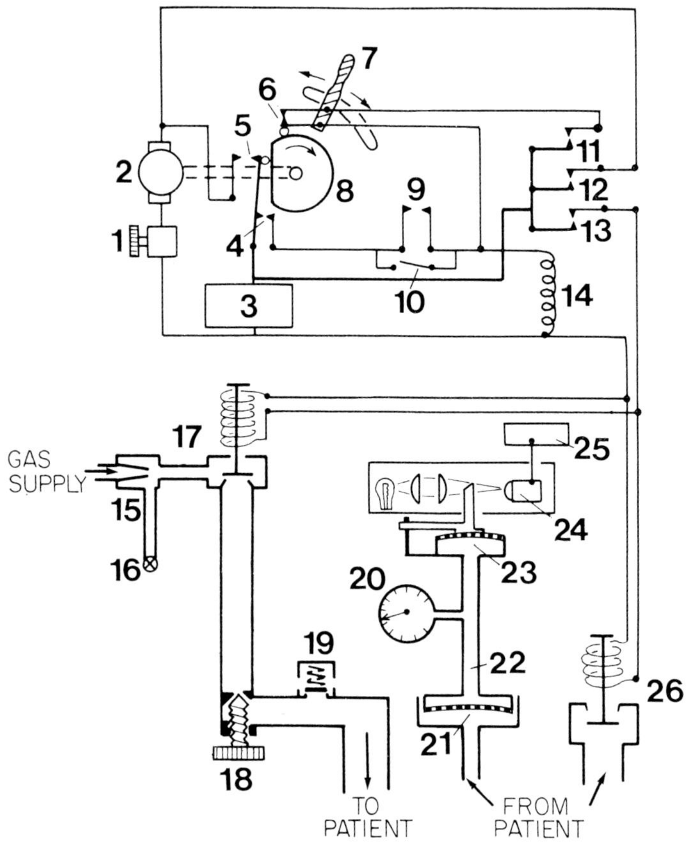

Fig. 78.2. Diagram of the 'Pneumotron'.

1. Respiratory-frequency control
2. Electric motor
3. Power pack
4. Contacts for starting-circuit of relay (14)
5. Contacts for holding-circuit of motor
6. Secondary contacts in holding-circuit of relay (14)
7. Control for adjusting the inspiratory-expiratory ratio
8. Cam driven by electric motor (2). This is shown in its 'rest' position
9. Contacts operated by relay (25)
10. 'Auto/Demand' switch. This is shown open for 'Demand'
11. Contacts for holding-circuit of relay (14)
12. Contacts for motor circuit
13. Contacts for solenoid-valve circuits
14. Relay for contacts (11), (12), and (13)
15. Injector-operated sucker
16. Schrader valve
17. Solenoid-operated inspiratory valve
18. Needle valve controlling flow of inflating gas
19. Safety-valve (dual range)
20. Manometer
21. 'Germ barrier'
22. Tube transmitting negative pressure to diaphragm of patient-trigger unit
23. Diaphragm
24. Photo-electric cell
25. Relay operating contacts (9)
26. Solenoid-operated expiratory valve

which is controlled by the needle valve (18). When set to 'automatic' the frequency is set by the control (1), which regulates the speed of the motor (2). The inspiratory-expiratory ratio is set by the control (7) which alters the position of the contacts (6) on the periphery of the cam (8) relative to the resting position of the cam. When set to 'demand' the setting of the control (1) limits the maximum frequency at which the ventilator can be patient-triggered since triggering can only occur when the cam is in the 'rest' position. The settings of the controls (1) and (7) in combination determine the duration of the inspiratory phase.

A 'germ barrier' (21) prevents the apparatus being contaminated by the patient. Pressures are indicated on the manometer (20). An injector-operated sucker (15) is available for use in clearing the respiratory tract. The sucker is brought into action by plugging a connector into the Schrader valve (16) which at other times closes the outlet.

FUNCTIONAL ANALYSIS

Inspiratory phase

In this phase the ventilator operates fundamentally as a constant-flow generator owing to the constant high pressure of the inflating gas applied to the resistance of the needle valve (18) (fig. 78.2). However, the safety-valve (19) is always partly open thereby constituting a leak in parallel with the constant-flow generator so that the complete system operates as a constant-pressure generator (see p. 85).

Change-over from inspiratory phase to expiratory phase

This change-over is time-cycled: the duration of the phase is determined by the rotation of the cam (8) and the position of the contacts (6).

Expiratory phase

In this phase the ventilator operates as a constant, atmospheric, pressure generator: the expired gas passes freely to atmosphere at the expiratory valve (26).

Change-over from expiratory phase to inspiratory phase

On 'Auto' this change-over is time-cycled: the duration of the expiratory phase is determined by the rotation of the cam (8) and the position of the contacts (6).

On 'Demand' this change-over is patient-cycled: an inspiratory phase is initiated only when an inspiratory effort by the patient produces sufficient negative pressure under the diaphragm (23) to actuate the patient-cycling mechanism and when the cam is in the 'rest' position.

CHAPTER 79

The 'R.P.R. Portable Volumetric Respirator, RP3'[1,2,3]

DESCRIPTION

This development (figs. 79.1 and 79.2) of the R.P.R. ventilator described in the first edition of this book incorporates two main modifications: (a) in the operation of the inspiratory and expiratory valves, and, (b) in the mechanism of compression of the concertina bag.

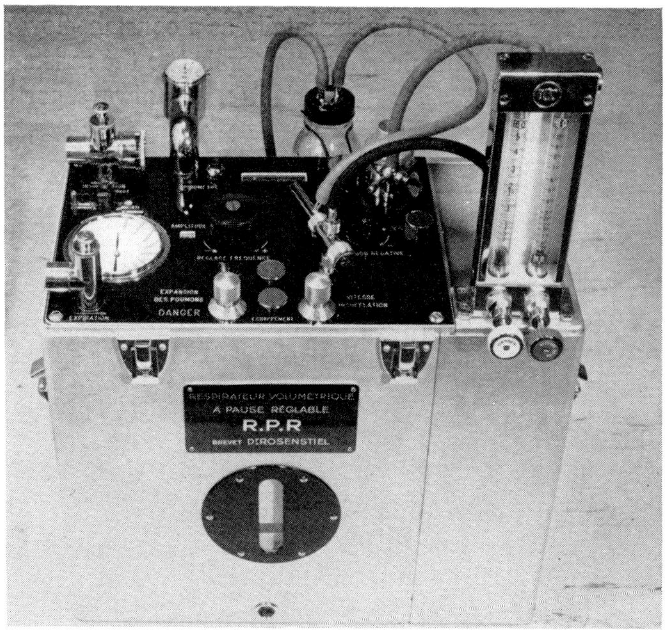

Fig. 79.1. The 'R.P.R. Portable Volumetric Respirator, RP3'.

Courtesy of R. Pesty.

This ventilator, which is a 'minute-volume divider' (see p. 140), is for anaesthetic or ward use. Oxygen or compressed air at a pressure of 45 lb/in^2 enters at the inlet (34) (fig. 79.3). This supply is connected to the cylinders (18, 25) and provides the pressure

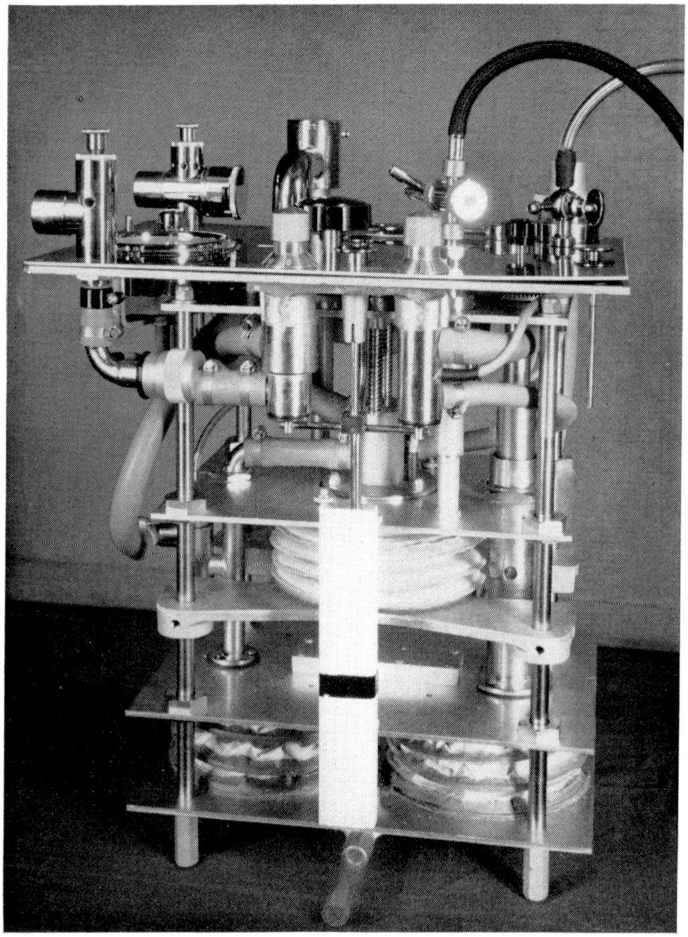

Fig. 79.2. The mechanism of the 'R.P.R. Portable Volumetric Respirator, RP3'.
Courtesy of Department of Medical Illustration, Cardiff Royal Infirmary.

needed to compress the concertina bags (31, 35) during the inspiratory phase. The gas which is ultimately delivered to the patient flows through the flowmeter (26), and is used to expand the positive-pressure bag (31). The latter flow may be supplemented with other gases supplied through the second flowmeter (27).

During the inspiratory phase, the pressure of the gas in the cylinders (18, 25) acts on the pistons and forces them down, together with the interconnected moveable top-plates (33, 37) of the positive-pressure concertina bag (31) and the twin negative-pressure concertina bags (35, 35). The dual-action valve (23), fitted to the top-plate (33), is held in the 'down' (inspiratory) position by the magnet (29), and the gas contained in the bag (31), together with inflating gas entering it, is forced, past the inspiratory-flow

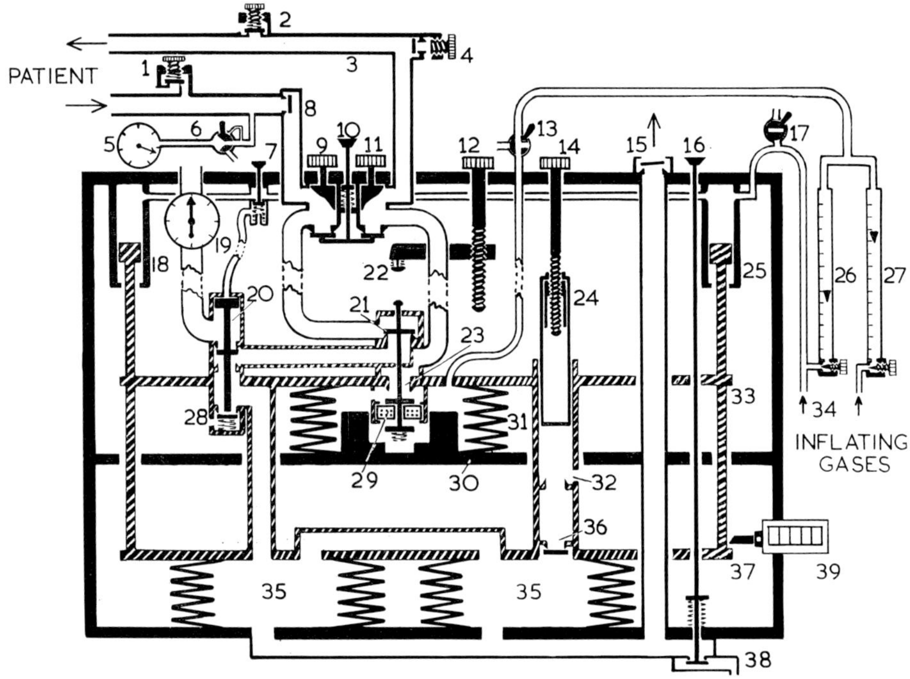

Fig. 79.3. Diagram of the 'R.P.R. Portable Volumetric Respirator, RP3'.

1. Negative-pressure safety-valve
2. Positive-pressure safety-valve
3. Inspiratory tube
4. 'Free-inspiration' valve
5. Manometer
6. Manometer tap
7. 'Spirometer' push-button
8. One-way valve
9. 'Expansion of the lungs' (resistance-to-expiration) control
10. 'Pressure release' control
11. 'Speed of inflation' control
12. 'Amplitude' control
13. Tap
14. 'Pause' control
15. One-way valve
16. 'Purge' push-button
17. Tap
18. Cylinder and piston
19. Wright respirometer
20. Spirometer valve
21. Expiratory valve
22. Spring-loaded stop
23. Inspiratory valve
24. Piston
25. Cylinder and piston
26. Flowmeter
27. Flowmeter
28. Air-inlet valve
29. Magnet
30. Base-plate
31. Positive-pressure concertina reservoir bag
32. Port
33. Top-plate
34. Gas inlet
35, 35. Negative-pressure concertina bags
36. One-way valve
37. Top-plate
38. Drain
39. Stroke counter

('speed of inflation') control valve (11), through the inspiratory tube (3), to the patient. At the same time expired gas stored in the negative-pressure bags (35, 35) is voided to atmosphere through the one-way valve (15).

When the top-plates (33, 37) have reached the lower limit of their travel, the positive-pressure bag (31) is virtually empty. The spring on the bottom of the stem of the dual valve (23) is now compressed against the fixed base-plate (30). When the force which the spring exerts on the valve stem is sufficient, the valve assembly (21, 23) snaps into the 'up' (expiratory) position, in which it is held by the magnet (29). The inspiratory valve (23) is closed, and the expiratory valve (21) is opened. Expired gas now flows from the patient, past the one-way valve (8), the resistance-to-expiration ('expansion of the lungs') control (9), and through the expiratory valve (21), to the bags (35, 35). The flow of fresh gas into the bag (31) raises the pressure within it until the force, exerted by the relatively-low pressure acting over the large area at the top of the bag, is sufficient to overcome the effect of the high pressure acting on the small area of the pistons (18, 25). The top-plates (33, 37) now move up until the top of the stem of the dual-action valve (21) strikes the spring-loaded stop (22). Further upward movement compresses the spring until the force exerted by the spring overcomes the pull of the magnet (29), the positions of the valves (21, 23) are reversed, and the expiratory phase ends.

The upward movement of the top-plate (37), during the expiratory phase, expands the concertina bags (35, 35) and produces a negative pressure within them which is transmitted to the expiratory pathway. Whether this negative pressure is transmitted during the whole of the expiratory phase depends on the setting of the 'pause' control (14), which is calibrated in 'mm excursion'. When the control (14) is in its lowest position, the piston (24) is free to rest at all times on the valve seating (32), and no air can be drawn in through the port (32). In the intermediate positions of the control (14), the piston (24) only rests on the valve (32) after the top-plate (33) has moved up sufficiently; until this occurs, air is drawn into the bags (35, 35), through the port (32) and the one-way valve (36), and no negative pressure is transmitted to the expiratory pathway; there is therefore a period of atmospheric pressure at the beginning of the expiratory phase. In the extreme setting of the control (14), the inlet (32) is not closed at all. The 'expansion of the lungs' (resistance-to-expiration) control (9) may be adjusted to limit the amount of negative pressure transmitted to the expiratory pathway. The maximum negative pressure is limited by the safety-valve (1). Maximum positive pressure is limited by the safety-valve (2).

The 'spirometer' push-button (7) allows high-pressure gas, from the supply to the cylinders (18, 25), to reverse the position of the valve (20) and open the valve (28). The reversal of the valve (20) diverts the expired gas through the Wright respirometer (19); at the same time, should the valve (32) be closed by the piston (24), air can be drawn freely through the open valve (28) into the negative-pressure concertina bags (35, 35) thereby ensuring that their expansion is not hindered. However, while the Wright respirometer is in circuit no negative pressure can be applied to the patient.

A 'free-inspiration' valve (4) may be opened so that, if the patient makes a spontaneous inspiratory effort at any time, air can be drawn in through it. The one-way valve (8) in the expiratory pathway prevents rebreathing of expired gas.

In one position of the tap (6), the manometer (5) indicates the fluctuating pressure in the breathing circuit. In another position, a resistance is interposed and the manometer indicates the mean pressure in the breathing circuit. A third position allows the zero reading of the manometer to be checked.

A tap (17) allows high-pressure gas to be delivered to an injector for suction.

Water which accumulates in the negative-pressure bags (35, 35) may be drained through the port (38) which is opened by pressing the 'purge' button (16).

The tap (13) allows inflating gas to be directed to a separate circuit for manual inflation. If, before the positive-pressure concertina bag (31) is completely collapsed, the inspiratory flow into the patient has fallen to less than the inflating-gas flow, the ventilator cannot cycle to expiration, and pressure in the circuit rises to safety-valve pressure. This situation can be relieved by depressing the 'pressure release' control (10), which opens both the inspiratory and expiratory pathways to atmosphere.

The 'amplitude' control (12), which is calibrated in 'mm excursion', determines the height of the stop (22), and hence the stroke volume (approx 35–700 ml) of the positive-pressure bag (31). The tidal volume of course always exceeds this volume by the volume of inflating gas which enters during the inspiratory phase. With an inspiratory-expiratory ratio of about 1:2 this agrees with the tidal volume range of 54–1100 ml quoted by the manufacturers.

So that very small volumes can be delivered effectively, the compliance of the bag (31) is reduced by filling up most of its minimum volume by a circular block.

The duration of the inspiratory phase is the time taken for the bag (31) to be compressed. It may be extended by adjusting the 'speed of inflation' control (11) so as to reduce the inspiratory flow. The duration of the expiratory phase is the time taken for the inflating-gas supply to refill the bag (31).

A counter (39) records the total number of respiratory cycles completed by the ventilator.

FUNCTIONAL ANALYSIS

Inspiratory phase

This ventilator contains a pressure transformer (see p. 89): the high supply pressure in cylinders (18) and (25) is transformed into a lower pressure in the positive-pressure concertina bag (31). Fundamentally, therefore, it operates as a constant-pressure generator. However, in the first place, owing to the elasticity of the bag material and to the force required to operate the valves (21, 23) the pressure in the bag declines as it empties, particularly at the start of its downstroke (fig. 79.4). In the second place, the pressure is always high (greater than 80 cmH_2O) and is applied to the patient through the resistance of the inspiratory pathway. Therefore in practice the ventilator approximates to a flow generator, with the flow declining somewhat as the bag empties. It can be seen in fig. 79.6 that halving the compliance (b) or doubling the airway resistance (c) has a negligible effect on the flow pattern, compared with that shown under standard

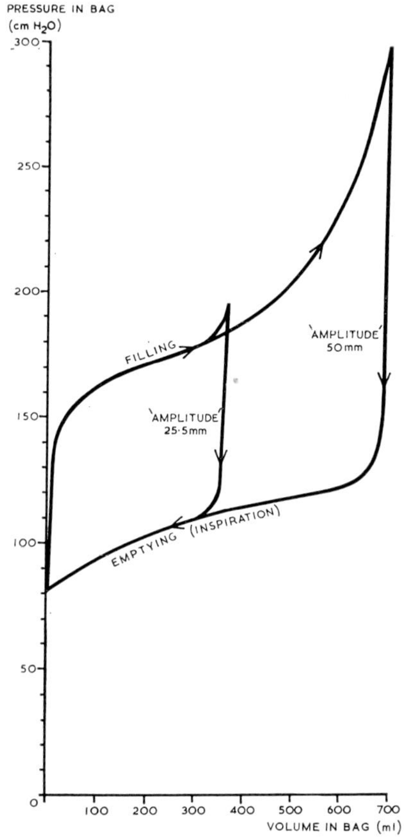

Fig. 79.4.

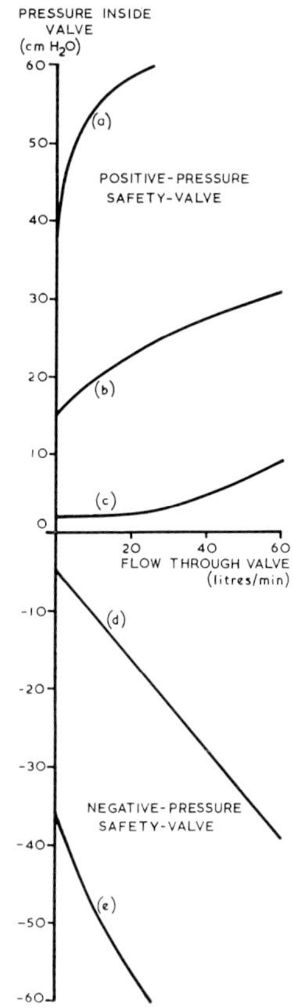

Fig. 79.5.

Fig. 79.4. 'R.P.R. Portable Volumetric Respirator, RP3'. Pressure-volume characteristics of the positive-pressure concertina reservoir bag. Volume is expressed in terms of the volume which the contents of the bag would occupy when expanded to atmospheric pressure without change of temperature. Conditions: driving gas at 45 lb/in^2; 'pause', at maximum, so that there was no 'load' on the negative-pressure concertina bags.

Fig. 79.5. 'R.P.R. Portable Volumetric Respirator, RP3'. Pressure-flow characteristics of the safety-valves.

Positive-pressure safety-valve:

(a) Maximum ($5\frac{1}{2}$ turns from minimum).
(b) Intermediate ($2\frac{3}{4}$ turns from minimum).
(c) Minimum.

Negative-pressure safety-valve:

(d) Minimum.
(e) Intermediate (3 turns from minimum).

At the maximum setting ($5\frac{3}{4}$ turns from the minimum) the opening pressure of the negative-pressure safety-valve was more negative than -60 cmH_2O.

conditions (a), but that the pattern of pressure at the mouth is substantially altered. The initial peak in the flow waveform is accounted for by the very high pressure which exists in the positive-pressure bag immediately after the change-over from the previous expiratory phase (fig. 79.4).

It is possible that the positive-pressure safety-valve (2) could come into action during the phase to impose some kind of pressure limit (see fig. 79.5) but if this were allowed to occur the minute-volume-dividing action (see the 'Controls' section below) would be destroyed. The safety-valve did not operate in the tracings of figs. 79.6 and 79.7.

Change-over from inspiratory phase to expiratory phase

This occurs when the positive-pressure concertina bag (31) has been compressed by a preset volume and the change-over is therefore best regarded as volume-cycled. But, since inflating gas enters the bag at a constant rate throughout the inspiratory phase, the tidal volume exceeds the stroke volume of the bag by an amount equal to the inflating-gas flow multiplied by the inspiratory time. Since the ventilator approximates to a flow generator during the inspiratory phase the inspiratory flow is little affected by changes in lung characteristics. Therefore, the time taken for the positive-pressure concertina bag to empty, i.e. the inspiratory time, is also little affected by such changes and the change-over from the inspiratory phase to the expiratory phase can be considered to be effectively time-cycled as well as volume-cycled. It can be seen in fig. 79.6 that the inspiratory phase always ends immediately a preset volume has entered the lungs in a preset time.

Expiratory phase

During the 'pause' part of the phase (before valve (32) is closed) the pressure in the negative-pressure concertina bags (35) must be atmospheric. This is because, if the expiratory flow from the patient is greater than the rate of expansion of the bags, the excess spills to atmosphere through one-way valve (15); if it is less, the difference is made up by air drawn in through one-way valve (36). In either case the ventilator operates as a constant, atmospheric, pressure generator throughout the 'pause' part of the phase. Atmospheric pressure is not recorded at the mouth because there is a substantial resistance in the ventilator (more than twice the standard airway resistance of the lung model) between the mouth and the one-way valve (15), even with the resistance to expiration control (9) set at '0'. This results in a rather slow decay in alveolar pressure and expiratory flow rate under standard conditions (fig. 79.6a) although the shorter time constant, consequent upon halving the compliance, is evident in fig. 79.6b. On the other hand, doubling the airway resistance produced only a small increase in time constant (fig. 79.6c) compared to the standard conditions (fig. 79.6a) because it represented only a relatively small increase in the total resistance of the system.

Later in the phase, when valve (32) is closed at the end of the 'pause', the patient's lungs and the negative-pressure concertina bags form a closed system except for the one-way valve (15). Therefore, there are two possibilities.

The first is that just before the valve (32) closes, the expiratory flow from the patient is less than the rate of expansion of the negative-pressure concertina bags. In this case, as soon as the valve does close, expiratory flow is immediately increased to equal the rate of expansion of the bags and is then maintained at that level for the rest of the phase. That is, the ventilator operates as a constant-flow generator. This is the situation in fig. 79.6 where, at the end of the 'pause', the expiratory flow rate is raised to a level which is constant for the rest of the phase and which is uninfluenced by changes in lung characteristics.

The second possibility is that, just before valve (32) closes, the expiratory flow is greater than the rate of expansion of the negative-pressure bags, the excess flow spilling

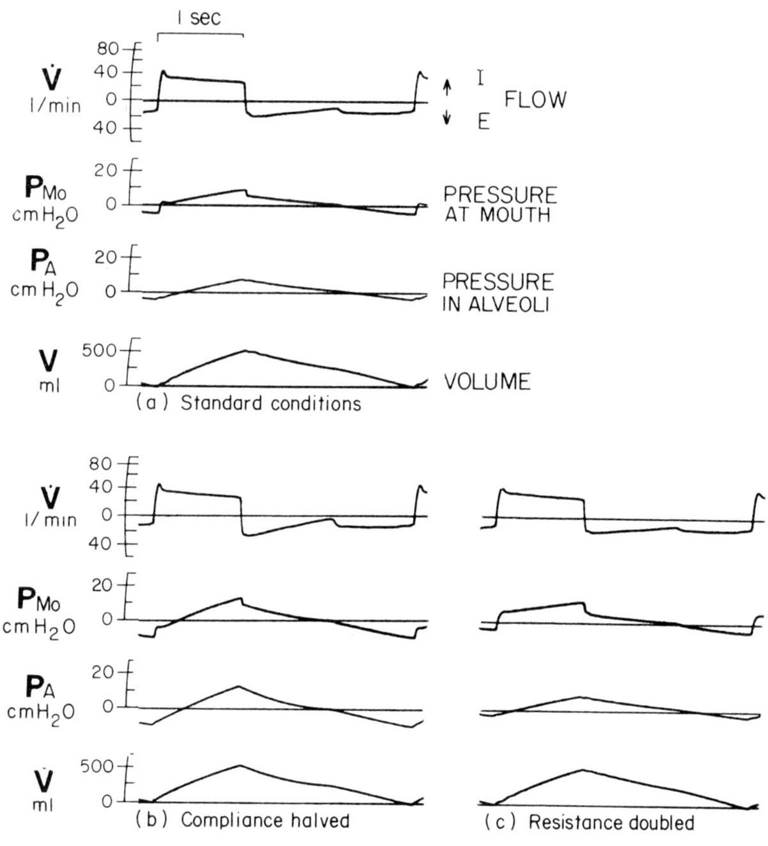

Fig. 79.6. 'R.P.R. Portable Volumetric Respirator, RP3'. Recordings showing the effects of changes of lung characteristics.

Standard conditions: driving gas, oxygen at 45 lb/in^2; safety-valves, set to maximum; 'expansion of the lungs' (resistance to expiration), set to '0'; inflating-gas flow, 10 litres/min (corrected to atmospheric pressure); 'amplitude', '25·5 mm', and 'speed of inflation', '3·8', to produce a tidal volume of 500 ml and an inspiratory-expiratory ratio of 1:2; 'pause', '13 mm' (half the 'amplitude').

to atmosphere through the valve (15). In this case excess gas continues to spill, and the ventilator continues to operate as a constant, atmospheric, pressure generator, until the expiratory flow has fallen to equal the rate of expansion of the bag. Then valve (15) will close and the expiratory flow will be maintained equal to the rate of expansion of the bags; the constant-flow-generating part of the phase will have commenced. This situation is illustrated in fig. 79.7b where the 'pause' was still set to half the 'amplitude', and therefore valve (32) must have closed half-way through the expiratory period, and yet the flow did not become steady until near the end of the phase.

Finally, it is possible that, towards the end of the phase, the negative-pressure safety-valve (1) may open. If it does, it is evident from the characteristics shown in fig. 79.5 that, even with the valve wide open (curve d), it will do no more than constitute a moderate leak in parallel with the patient; the pressure will *not* be limited to a specific value, independent of flow. For all the recordings of figs. 79.6 and 79.7 the negative-pressure safety-valve was kept tightly closed.

Change-over from expiratory phase to inspiratory phase

This occurs when the positive-pressure concertina bag (31) has been expanded by a preset volume by means of the preset inflating-gas flow; it therefore occurs at a preset time after the start of the expiratory phase. The change-over is therefore time-cycled. Fig. 79.6 shows that changes of lung characteristics have no effect on the duration of the expiratory phase.

CONTROLS

Total ventilation

Since this ventilator is a minute-volume divider (see p. 140) the total ventilation is directly controlled by the inflating-gas flow. However, the total ventilation is slightly more than the readings on the flowmeters because the gas within them is at a pressure appreciably above atmospheric. The total ventilation will be less than the inflating-gas flow if any gas escapes through the positive-pressure safety-valve (2). Provided that no such escape occurs the total ventilation is unaltered by changes in lung characteristics (fig. 79.6).

When the total ventilation is increased, by increasing the inflating-gas flow (fig. 79.7b), both tidal volume and respiratory frequency are increased. In addition, the inspiratory time occupies a bigger fraction of the reduced respiratory period. This is because the higher inflating-gas flow refills the concertina bag (31) more rapidly (shorter expiratory time) and adds a greater volume to the volume excursion of the bag to make up the increased tidal volume. This bigger tidal volume takes longer to deliver at the fixed inspiratory flow rate.

Under the conditions used to record fig. 79.7b increasing the inflating-gas flow by 50 per cent has resulted in a waveform of alveolar pressure which never falls to atmospheric.

This could be corrected by decreasing the resistance to inspiration by means of the 'speed of inflation' control (11) thereby shortening the inspiratory time and hence lengthening the expiratory time.

Tidal volume

This is primarily controlled by the 'amplitude' control (12). However, the tidal volume exceeds the volume excursion of the positive-pressure concertina bag (31) by the volume of inflating gas entering during the inspiratory phase. Therefore an increase in the inflating-gas flow (fig. 79.7b), or in the inspiratory time due to decreasing the setting of the 'speed of inflation' control (11) (i.e. increasing the resistance to inspiratory flow) (fig. 79.7d), increases the tidal volume. The tidal volume is not influenced by the changes of lung characteristics used in fig. 79.6.

When the tidal volume is increased by increasing the setting of the 'amplitude' control (12) (fig. 79.7c) the respiratory frequency decreases inversely since the total ventilation remains the same. The expiratory time is increased in the same proportion as the excursion of the concertina bag because the rate of refilling of the bag is constant. On the other hand, the degree of prolongation of the inspiratory phase needed to deliver the increased tidal volume depends on a number of factors and, unlike the prolongation of the expiratory phase, is not, in general, in the same proportion as the increase in bag excursion. Therefore the inspiratory-expiratory ratio is usually altered. In fig. 79.7c the inspiratory phase occupies a slightly-smaller fraction of the lengthened respiratory period.

Respiratory frequency

This is not directly controlled but is equal to the total ventilation (which is equal to the inflating-gas flow) divided by the tidal volume. Therefore any increase in total ventilation or decrease in tidal volume results in an increase in respiratory frequency. The changes of lung characteristics tried in fig. 79.6 did not affect the frequency.

Inspiratory-expiratory ratio

This is not directly controlled but, for a given total ventilation, is mainly influenced by the 'speed of inflation' control (11) (fig. 79.7d) and also, to a lesser extent, by the 'amplitude' control (12) (fig. 79.7c). The expiratory time is precisely determined by the volume excursion of the positive-pressure concertina bag (set by the 'amplitude' control), divided by the preset inflating-gas flow. But if the inspiratory time is increased, by adjusting the 'speed of inflation' control (11), in order to obtain a given inspiratory-expiratory ratio, then the tidal volume is also increased. This is because more inflating gas enters the positive-pressure concertina bag during the prolonged inspiratory phase. If the tidal volume is then reduced to the desired value by the 'amplitude' control this reduces the duration of both phases, but the inspiratory time is reduced slightly more than the expiratory time, and further adjustment of both 'speed of inflation' and 'amplitude' controls may be necessary to obtain exactly the required conditions. If the total ventilation should then be altered by adjusting the inflating-gas flow this will upset the inspiratory-expiratory ratio (fig. 79.7b, see above) and necessitate further adjust-

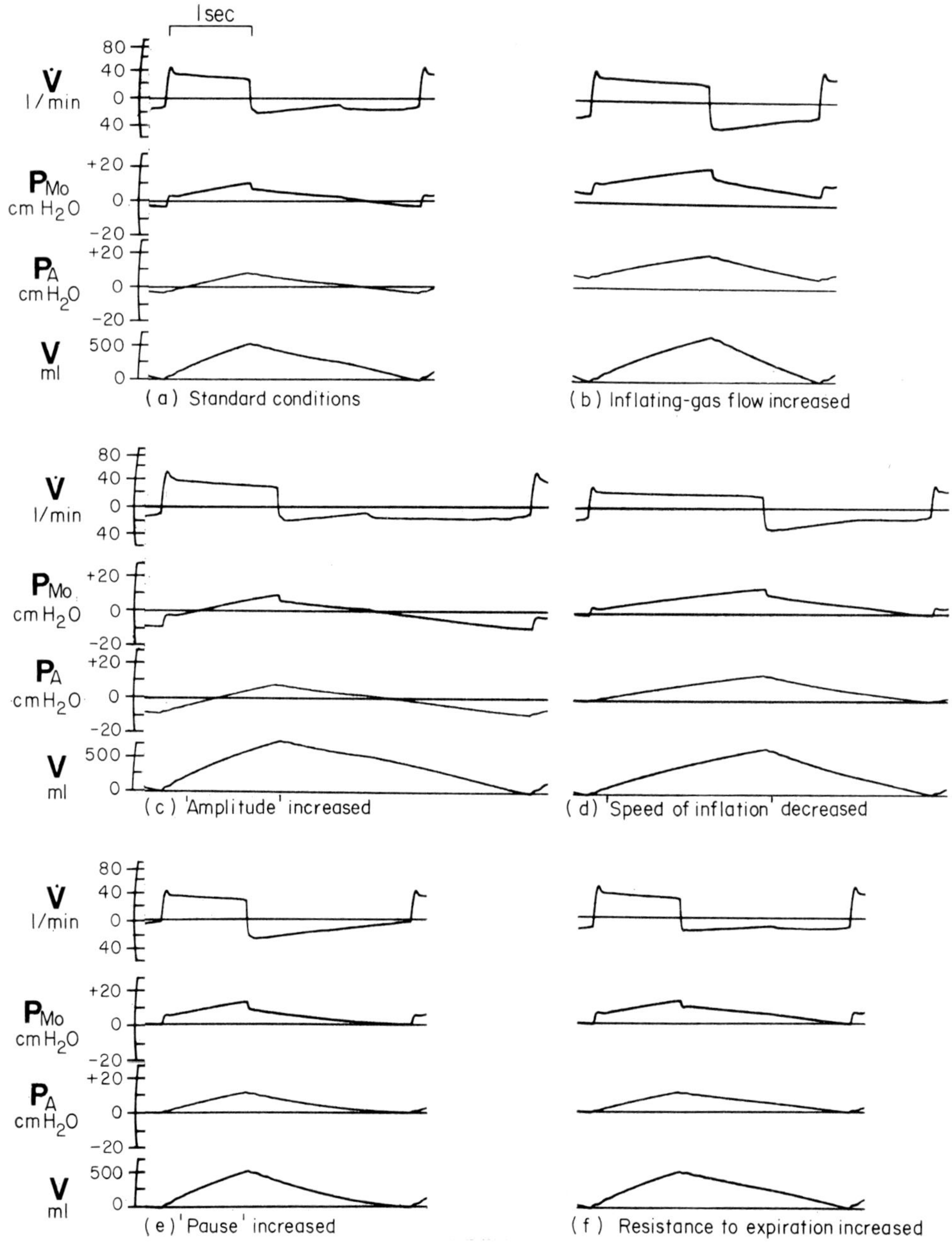

ment of the other controls. However, the instruction manual gives useful data which should make it possible to obtain values which are clinically satisfactory after only a single adjustment of each control and, once set, the tidal volume and inspiratory-expiratory ratio are little affected by the set of changes of lung characteristics tried here (fig. 79.6).

Inspiratory waveforms

Although the average flow rate during the inspiratory phase can clearly be modified by adjustment of the resistance to inspiration by control (11) this flow rate may already have been decided upon in order to deliver a given tidal volume in a given inspiratory time.

Expiratory waveforms

Here the operator has a wide choice, mainly by adjustment of the 'pause' control (14). The setting of this control, expressed as a fraction of the setting of the 'amplitude' control (12), indicates the fraction of the expiratory phase in which the ventilator operates as a constant, atmospheric, pressure generator before changing to a constant-flow generator. However, it should be remembered, as explained in the functional analysis, that the ventilator may continue to operate as a constant, atmospheric, pressure generator after the end of the 'pause' if this permits a greater expiratory flow than the flow being generated by the negative-pressure concertina bags.

Fig. 79.7e shows the effect of making the 'pause' as long as the expiratory time (setting the 'pause' control to the same or a greater setting than the 'amplitude' control) instead of the 'pause' being only half the expiratory time as in fig. 79.7a. Then, as can be seen in fig. 79.7e, the ventilator operates as a constant, atmospheric, pressure generator throughout the expiratory phase.

During the constant, atmospheric, pressure-generating part of the phase the initial flow rate can be reduced and the time constant of the exponential decay increased by increasing the resistance to expiration by means of the control (9) (fig. 79.7f), but the instruction manual recommends that this control be used only with an open thorax.

A rough negative-pressure limit can be brought into play at the end of the expiratory phase by setting the negative-pressure safety-valve (1) to its most sensitive position

---

Fig. 79.7. 'R.P.R. Portable Volumetric Respirator, RP3'. Recordings showing the effects of changes in the settings of the controls.

(a) Standard conditions as in fig. 79.6.
(b) Inflating-gas flow increased to 15 litres/min (corrected to atmospheric pressure).
(c) 'Amplitude' increased to '38 mm'.
(d) 'Speed of inflation' decreased to '2·8'.
(e) 'Pause' increased to greater than 'amplitude'.
(f) 'Expansion of the lungs' (resistance to expiration) increased to '7'.

(curve (d) in fig. 79.5), but the effect of this is marked only when a substantial negative pressure would otherwise develop. Its effect is not illustrated in fig. 79.7.

Pressure limits

The range of pressure in the alveoli is determined by the tidal volume divided by the patient's compliance. If the ventilator operates as a constant, atmospheric, pressure generator throughout the expiratory phase the alveolar pressure will approach atmospheric at the end of the phase. However, it may not reach atmospheric pressure if the time constant of the system is too high or the expiratory time is too short. When part of the expiratory phase is occupied with constant-flow generation this will reduce the alveolar pressure at the end of the phase, although in some circumstances, such as fig. 79.7b, there may still be a positive pressure at the end of the phase. In other circumstances, such as fig. 79.7c, the alveolar pressure may become sufficiently negative at the end of the phase to give a negative *mean* pressure. In extreme circumstances (not illustrated in fig. 79.7) it is even possible to obtain a waveform of alveolar pressure which is entirely negative. The positive-pressure and negative-pressure safety-valves can be used to set some limits to the mouth pressures but this is not illustrated in fig. 79.7.

The mean alveolar pressure can be deliberately raised by increasing the setting of the resistance-to-expiration control (9) (compare fig. 79.7f with 79.7a) or deliberately reduced by decreasing the setting of the 'pause' control (14) (compare fig. 79.7a with 79.7e). In addition, if the inspiratory-expiratory ratio has not been firmly decided on other grounds, the mean pressure can be reduced by increasing the setting of the 'speed of inflation' control (11), thereby shortening the inspiratory time in relation to the respiratory period. Fig. 79.7d shows the inverse of this: decreasing the 'speed of inflation' increases the mean pressure.

REFERENCES

1 Mollaret P. and Pocidalo J.J. (1956) Présentation d'un respirateur artificiel à pressions positive et négative avec pause réglable (R.P.R.) *C.R. Soc. Biol.* **150**, 1898.

2 Mollaret P. and Pocidalo J.J. (1957) Le respirateur R.P.R. du Centre de Réanimation Respiratoire de l'Hôpital Claude-Bernard (Paris). *Presse med.* **65**, 911.

3 Huguenard P. (1957) Premiers essais anesthésiologiques avec le respirateur R.P.R. *Anesth. Analg. Réanim.* **14**, 657.

4 Tremolières J. (1958) A new apparatus for artificial respiration. *J. Am. med. Ass.* **167**, 1086.

CHAPTER 80

The Rand-Wolfe Ventilator[1, 2]

DESCRIPTION

A flame-proof constant-speed electric motor (6) (fig. 80.2) working through a reduction

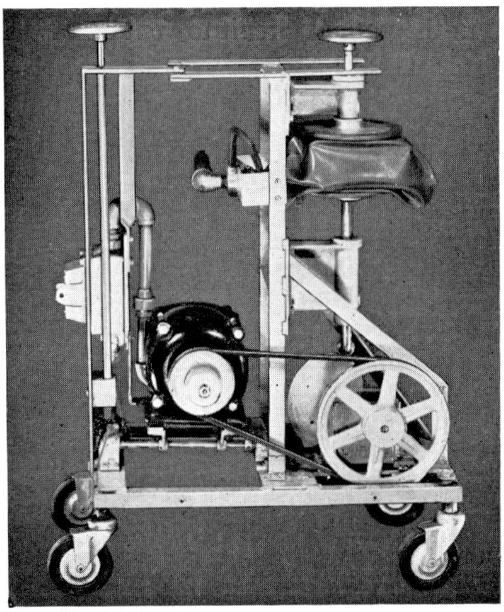

Fig. 80.1. The Rand–Wolfe ventilator.
Courtesy of K. Wolfe.

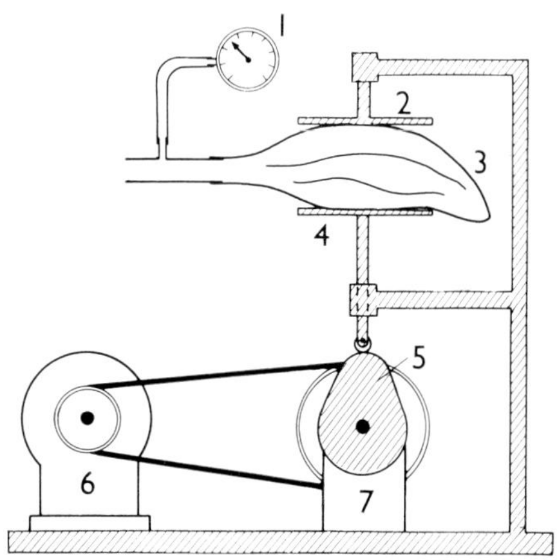

Fig. 80.2. Diagram of the Rand–Wolfe ventilator.

1. Manometer
2. Fixed plate
3. Reservoir bag
4. Moveable plate
5. Cam
6. Electric motor
7. Gear-box

gear (7) revolves a cam (5) which, by lifting a rod and plate (4), compresses the reservoir bag (3) against the stationary upper plate (2). The cam (5) is described[1] as being designed 'to produce a respiratory cycle similar to that of normal deep breathing. There is a gradual increase in pressure to a peak, a pause consisting of 25 per cent of the cycle, and then a sudden release of pressure. This is the mechanism produced by the anesthetist as she compresses and releases the rebreathing bag'. The continuously-variable reduction gear (7) provides respiratory frequencies between 14 and 28 per minute. The maximum pressure is varied by altering the flow of fresh gas and the setting of the expiratory valve on the anaesthetic apparatus. The inspiratory-expiratory ratio is fixed by the shape of the cam to approximately 1 : 1·5.

FUNCTIONAL ANALYSIS

This analysis is based on the assumption that the tidal volume delivered to the patient is appreciably less than the maximum of which the ventilator is capable.

Inspiratory phase

In this phase the ventilator operates as a non-constant-flow generator owing to the shape of the cam (5) and the constant speed of the driving motor (6). A pressure limit, due to the blow-off valve which must be incorporated in the patient circuit to vent excess gas, comes into operation during the inspiratory phase. Until then, the fresh-gas supply to the patient circuit acts as a small-constant-flow generator, supplementing the main flow generator.

Change-over from inspiratory phase to expiratory phase

This change-over is time-cycled owing to the constant speed of the electric motor (6), but it is only the time from the end of the previous expiratory phase which is rigidly determined by the ventilator (see below); the inspiratory time is somewhat dependent upon lung characteristics.

Expiratory phase

In this phase, assuming that the rapid descent of the plate (4) frees the reservoir bag (3) from restraint, the ventilator operates as a constant, atmospheric, pressure generator.

Change-over from expiratory phase to inspiratory phase

The upward movement of the plate (4) begins at a fixed time after the start of its descent because of the constant speed of the electric motor (6). To this extent the change-over is time-cycled, but inflation will not begin until the upward movement begins to compress the reservoir bag. Therefore, after the fixed time for the reversal of direction of the plate (4), there is a variable delay, dependent upon the setting of the blow-off valve, the fresh-gas flow, and the lung characteristics, before the change-over to the inspiratory phase occurs. Thus the expiratory time, and therefore the inspiratory time, are somewhat dependent upon lung characteristics even though (see above) the respiratory period is fixed.

REFERENCES

1 Wolfe K. and Rand H.J. (1950) Electro-mechanical aids in resuscitation and anesthesia. *Ohio St. med. J.* **46**, 39.

2 Falor W.H., Kelly T.R. and Reynolds C.W. (1954) Mechanical elimination of respiratory acidosis during open thoracic procedures. *Surg. Forum* (1954), p. 536.

CHAPTER 81

The 'Respirateur Artificiel Automatique SF4'[1, 2, 3]

DESCRIPTION

This ventilator (fig. 81.1) was originally developed for use in neurosurgical anaesthesia. The 24-volt electric motor (30) (fig. 81.2) runs continuously at a rate set by the volume control (29). The current is drawn from a battery which, when the ventilator is connected to the a.c. mains, is charged continuously. The motor drives the shaft (32) through a gear-box (31). The shaft carries two magnetic clutches (25) and (26). When the clutch (26) is energized the piston (21) is driven up by the arm (28) and the gas contained in the cylinder is driven to the patient, the valve (18) being open at the time.

When the clutch (25) is energized the piston (5) is driven down and gas is drawn into the cylinder from the expiratory pathway, the valve (1) being open at the time.

A second electric motor (34), the speed of which is set by the 'frequency' control (33), drives a timing mechanism (35, 36, 37, 38). This mechanism carries one fixed pair of contacts (35) and three moveable pairs (36, 37, 38). The positions of the moveable pairs are adjusted by their controls. As the plate on which these contacts are mounted rotates, each pair is operated in turn, once every revolution, the closure of each pair marking a stage in one complete respiratory cycle. The duration of one respiratory cycle therefore is the time taken for the plate to complete one revolution, and this is determined by the speed of the motor (34) which is set by the 'frequency' control (33).

When the fixed pair of contacts (35) is closed current is supplied to the magnetic clutch (26) and the piston (21) commences its compression stroke. At this time the solenoid of the inspiratory valve (18) is already energized and the valve is open. The active part of the inspiratory phase begins. When the second pair of contacts (38) is closed the supply of current to the solenoid (18) and to the magnetic clutch (26) is cut off. The inspiratory valve (18) is closed by its spring. The piston (21) is now drawn downwards by the spring (27) and fresh gas stored in the bag (14) is drawn into the cylinder. However, at the same time, the solenoid of the expiratory valve (1) is energized and the valve is opened. Passive expiration now begins, expired gas flowing to atmosphere through the one-way valve (6) and the spirometer tap (7), either direct to atmosphere or through the spirometer (9). When the third pair of contacts (37) is closed the magnetic clutch (25) is energized, and expired gas is now drawn into the cylinder by the downward movement of the piston (5). The expiratory negative-pressure limit is set by

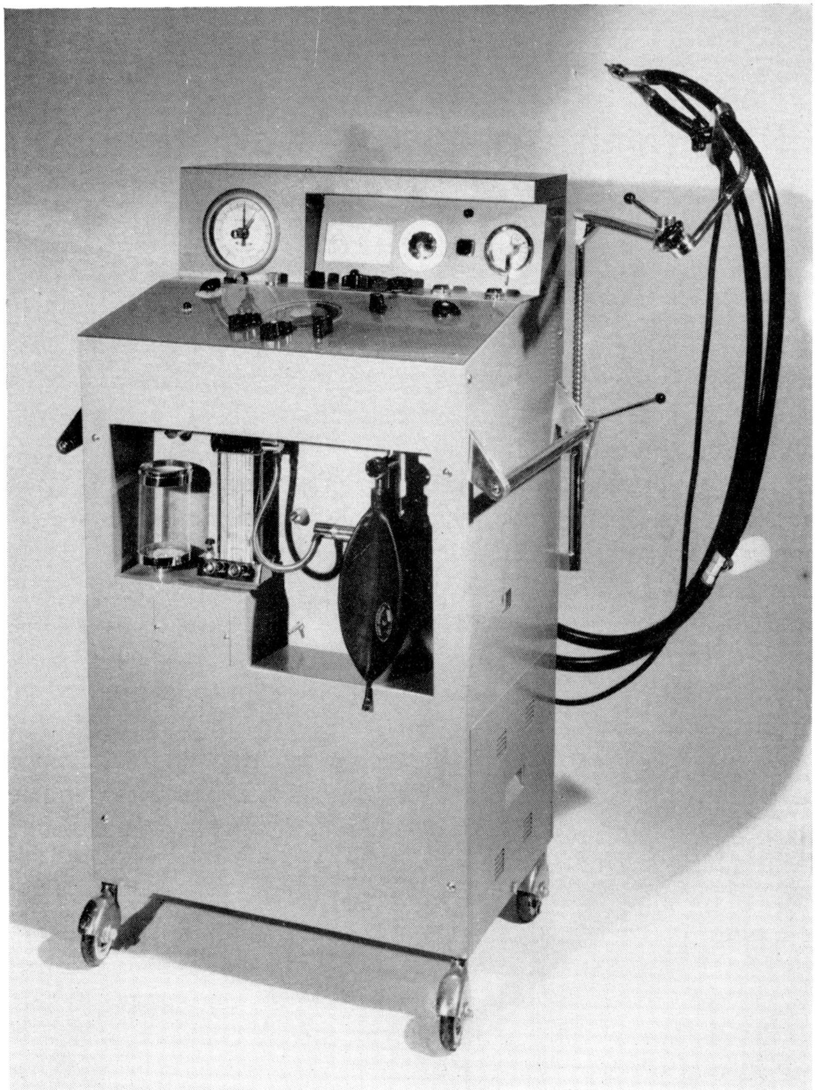

Fig. 81.1. The 'Respirateur Artificiel Automatique SF4'.
Courtesy of Société d'Exploitation des Laboratoires Robert et Carrière.

adjustment of the negative-pressure control (2). A resistance to expiratory flow may be introduced by means of the control (3). When the fourth pair of contacts (36) is closed, the supply of current to the solenoid (1) and the magnetic clutch (25) is cut off, and the valve (1) is closed by its spring. The piston (5) is now forced up by its spring and expired gas stored in the cylinder is discharged to atmosphere through the one-way valve (6), either directly to atmosphere or through the spirometer. The closure of the fourth pair

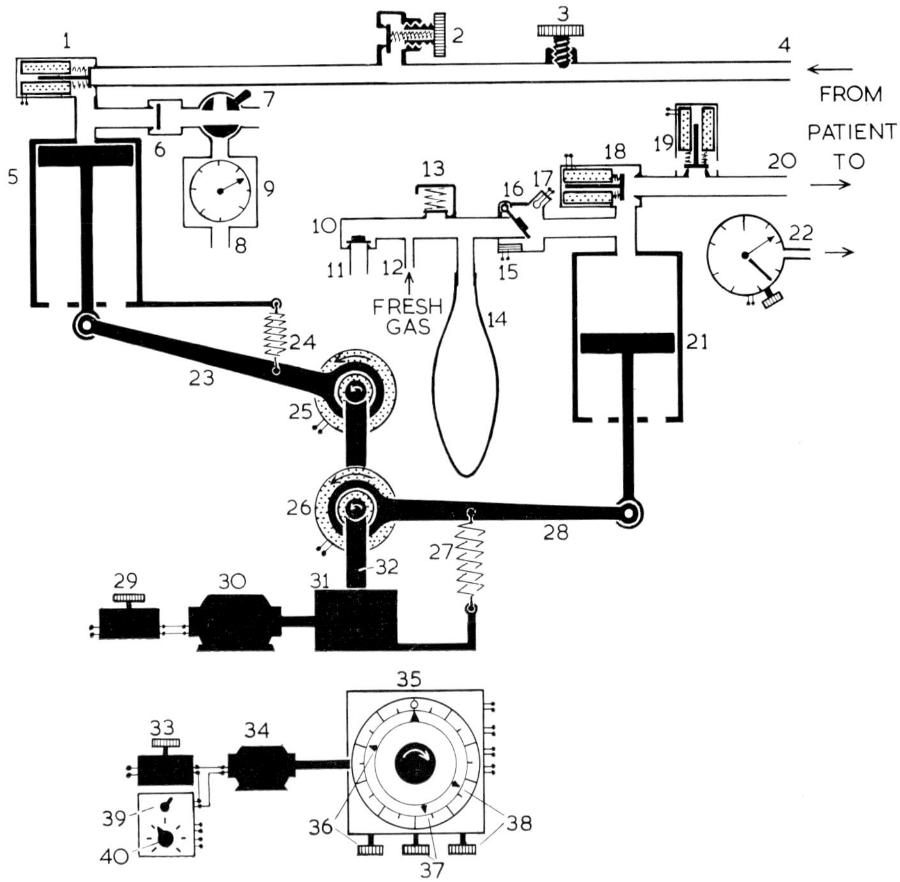

Fig. 81.2. Diagram of the 'Respirateur Artificiel Automatique SF4'.

1. Solenoid-operated expiratory valve
2. Negative-pressure control valve
3. Resistance-to-expiration control
4. Expiratory tube
5. Piston
6. One-way valve
7. Tap
8. Outlet port of spirometer
9. Spirometer
10. One-way valve
11. Air-inlet port
12. Fresh-gas inlet
13. Spill valve
14. Storage bag
15. Photo-electric cell
16. One-way valve
17. Lamp
18. Solenoid-operated inspiratory valve
19. Solenoid-operated safety-valve
20. Inspiratory tube
21. Piston
22. Manometer
23. Connecting arm
24. Spring
25. Magnetic clutch
26. Magnetic clutch
27. Spring
28. Connecting arm
29. Volume control
30. Electric motor
31. Gear-box
32. Shaft
33. Frequency control
34. Electric motor
35. Fixed contacts

36, 37, 38. Adjustable contacts

39. Patient-trigger switch
40. Time-delay control

of contacts, which allows the expiratory valve (1) to close, also energizes the solenoid of the inspiratory valve (18) which is therefore opened. This establishes free communication between the patient and the storage bag (14). If the alveolar pressure has been made negative during active expiration, passive flow into the lungs now takes place either from the storage bag (14) or, if this is empty, from the atmosphere, through valve (11).

If patient-triggering is desired the switch (39) is set to 'trigger'. Then, when one respiratory cycle is completed, i.e. the 'pre-inspiratory' phase is ended by the closure of the contacts (35), a new active inflation is *not* started immediately. Instead, the motor (34) is stopped until either the patient makes an inspiratory effort or until a time (which can be preset by the control (40) to between 1 and 10 sec) has elapsed.

When one or other of these events has occurred a normal cycle of operation is initiated: the motor (34) is restarted, the magnetic clutch (26) is energized and the piston (21) moves up. The patient trigger operates electrically: an inspiratory effort lifts the flap valve (16) deflecting the light of the lamp (17) towards the photocell (15), thereby sending a signal to the electrical circuit (39, 40). However, this circuit is operative only during the delay period after a complete respiratory cycle when the motor (34) is stopped. The ventilator cannot be triggered at any time during the preset respiratory cycle.

When the ventilator is set for patient-triggering the frequency set by the control (33) represents a maximum which will be approached only if the patient makes an inspiratory effort very soon after the preset respiratory cycle has been completed. The minimum frequency depends on the setting of the frequency control (33) and of the time delay (40). The manufacturers recommend that, when patient-triggering is in use, the fresh-gas flow should be set to equal the delivered total ventilation. If the fresh-gas flow appreciably exceeds this amount there is a risk that, during the delay after each cycle in which the ventilator is sensitive to inspiratory effort, the storage bag (14) may become distended and lift the flap (16) thereby triggering the ventilator. The manufacturers also recommend that the time interval between the fourth pair of contacts (36) and the first pair (35) should be set to equal at least one quarter of the preset respiratory period. This is to ensure that, if negative pressure is developed in the alveoli during active expiration, the flow from the storage bag (14) due to 'passive' inflation will have ceased by the end of this period.

A manometer (22) connected close to the patient indicates the pressure in the breathing circuit. A control on this manometer allows a pointer, which carries an electrical contact, to be set to the desired maximum pressure. When the manometer needle touches this contact it makes an electrical circuit which opens the solenoid valve (19). The setting of the control (2) determines the maximum negative pressure.

If desired a soda-lime canister may be fitted between the expiratory outlet (7) and the inspiratory inlet (11) converting the circuit to a closed one. Excess fresh gas then spills through the valve (13). Spillage through this valve occurs also when the non-rebreathing circuit is in use if the fresh-gas flow exceeds the total minute-volume ventilation.

The frequency may be adjusted between 8 and 60 per minute. Within the corresponding durations of a complete respiratory cycle (7·5 sec to 1 sec), the relative durations of each of the four phases of the cycle are infinitely variable. The maximum positive pressure is 100 cmH_2O and the maximum negative pressure is -100 cmH_2O.

The tidal volume is adjusted by the control (29) which alters the speed of the motor (30). This alters the rate at which the piston (21) drives gas into the lungs for the preset duration of the active part of the inspiratory phase. It also alters the rate at which the piston (5) draws gas out of the lungs during the active part of the expiratory phase. The total tidal volume exceeds the volume delivered by the piston (21) to the extent of any volume which enters the lungs directly from the bag (14) during the passive part of the inspiratory phase.

FUNCTIONAL ANALYSIS

In view of the design of this ventilator it is convenient to divide the respiratory cycle into four phases, with four change-overs, rather than the usual two.

Active part of inspiratory phase

During this part of the inspiratory phase, assuming the speed of the motor (30) to be constant for any given setting of the control (29), the ventilator operates as a flow generator due to the steady movement of the arm (28) driving the piston (21). If the relative dimensions of the arm and the piston are approximately as shown in fig. 81.2, the pattern of generated flow will constitute a small fraction of a sine wave, near the peak of the wave, and will therefore be nearly constant throughout the phase.

Change-over from active part of inspiratory phase to passive part of expiratory phase

This change-over is time-cycled: it occurs at a preset time after the start of the active inspiratory phase determined by the speed of the motor (34) and the setting of the contacts (38).

Passive part of expiratory phase

In this part of the expiratory phase the ventilator operates as a constant, atmospheric, pressure generator: the patient's expired gas passes to atmosphere through one of the ports (7) or (8). The series resistance may be adjusted by the control (3).

Change-over from passive part to active part of expiratory phase

Like the previous change-over this is time-cycled: it occurs when the contacts (37) are operated.

Active part of expiratory phase

In this part of the expiratory phase, again assuming the speed of the motor (30) to be constant, the ventilator operates as a flow generator due to the steady movement of the arm (23). Again the flow may well be nearly constant. The valve (2) sets a negative-pressure limit which is likely to be reached during the phase. Once it is reached, the ventilator operates as a constant, negative, pressure generator, with series resistance adjustable by the control (3).

Change-over from active part of expiratory phase to passive part of inspiratory phase
Like the previous change-overs this is time-cycled: it occurs when the contacts (36) are operated.

Passive part of inspiratory phase
If, in the previous phase, the alveolar pressure has fallen below the pressure in the bag (14) the ventilator now operates as a constant-pressure generator, the pressure being that in the bag (14). This pressure must be close to atmospheric because of the lightly-loaded inlet and outlet valves (11) and (13).

On the other hand if, at the start of this part of the inspiratory phase, the alveolar pressure is still above the pressure in the bag (14) no gas can flow into or out of the patient's lungs and the ventilator must be described as a zero-flow generator.

Change-over from passive part to active part of inspiratory phase
If the patient-trigger switch (39) is 'off' this change-over is purely time-cycled: it occurs when the contacts (35) are operated at a preset time which, in relation to the previous operation of these contacts (one complete respiratory cycle earlier), depends only on the setting of the frequency control (33).

If the patient-trigger switch (39) is 'on' this change-over is either patient-cycled or time-cycled. If the patient makes an inspiratory effort, causing light to fall on the photo-cell (15) during the delay period set by the control (40), active inflation will commence immediately and the change-over will be patient-cycled. If the patient fails to make an inspiratory effort during this period the change-over will be time-cycled: it will occur at the end of the delay period set by the control (40). The timing of this delay starts when the contacts (35) are operated. Therefore its end occurs at a time which is preset in relation to the change-over from the passive to the active part of the previous inspiratory phase, irrespective of the settings of the controls (36, 37, 38) which affect the timings of the other change-overs.

REFERENCES

1 TERRAC J. (1965) *Mille Heures de SF4. A propos de son utilisation en Neuro-Chirurgie chez l'Adulte.* (Thèse, Paris, 1965).

2 SABATHIE M., SEGUIN J. and BESSET CL. (1965) Utilisation per-opératoire du Respirateur SF4 chez le nouveau-né, le nourrisson et le jeune enfant. *Annales de l'anesthésiologie Française*, **6**, 333.

3 MAESTRACCI P. (1965) Le Respirateur SF4. Nouvel appareil de ventilation artificielle perfectionné. *Immex*, **3**, No. 7–8.

CHAPTER 82

The 'Respirateur Endo-tracheal MMS 104'

DESCRIPTION

This ventilator (fig. 82.1) is designed for ward or theatre use. An a.c. mains electric motor (23) (fig. 82.2) drives a variable-speed gear-box (24), the output shaft of which carries a crank-wheel (27). The crank-wheel (27) is connected by a system of levers to the

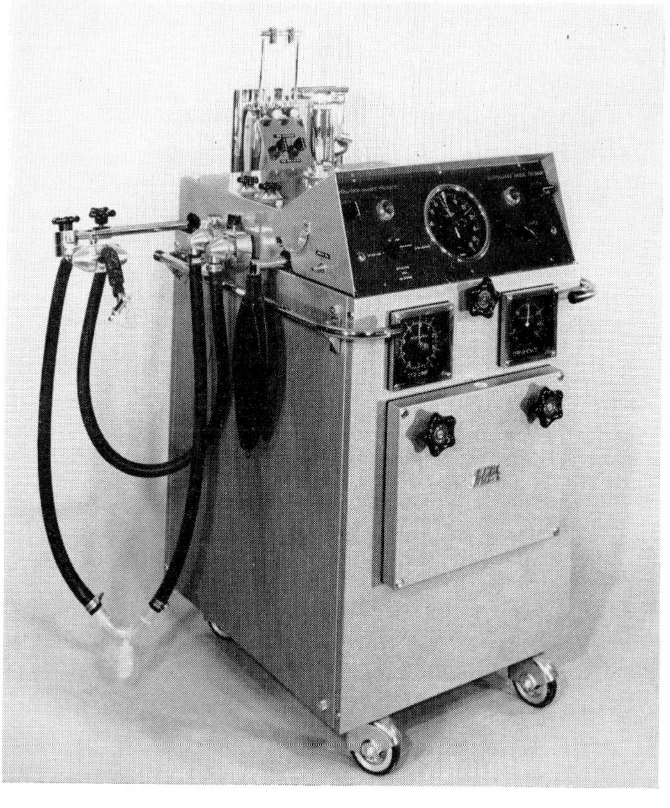

Fig. 82.1. The 'Respirateur Endo-tracheal MMS 104'.
Courtesy of Le Matérial Médical et Sanitaire.

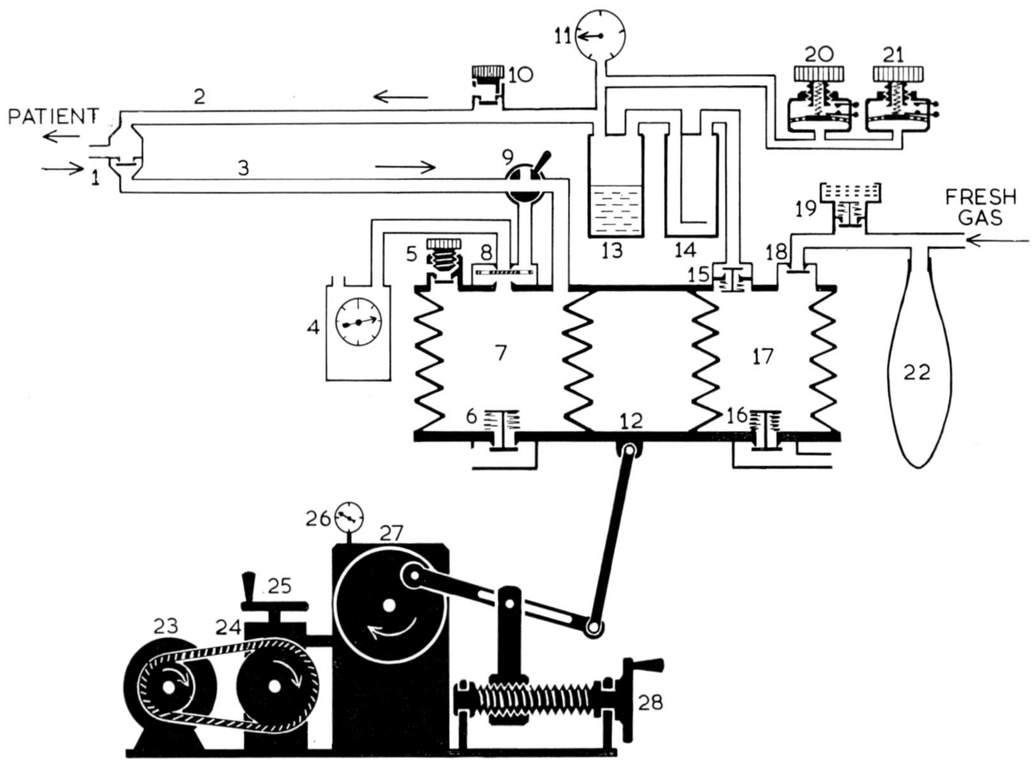

Fig. 82.2. Diagram of the 'Respirateur Endo-tracheal MMS 104'.

1. One-way valve
2. Inspiratory tube
3. Expiratory tube
4. Spirometer
5. Negative-pressure control
6. One-way valve
7. Concertina bag
8. Dual-action valve
9. Spirometer on/off tap
10. One-way inlet valve
11. Manometer
12. Base-plate
13. Humidifier
14. Chamber
15. One-way valve
16. Positive-pressure safety-valve
17. Concertina bag
18. One-way valve
19. Air inlet
20. 'Lowered pressure supervision' control
21. 'Raised pressure supervision' control
22. Storage bag
23. a.c. mains electric motor
24. Gear-box
25. Frequency control
26. Tachometer
27. Crank-wheel
28. Volume control

base-plate (12) of the two concertina bags (7) and (17) in such a way that this is forced up and down as the wheel rotates. When the base-plate moves up, the concertina bags (7) and (17) are compressed. The contents of the reservoir bag (17) are forced, through the one-way valve (15), the capacity chamber (14), the humidifier (13), and the inspiratory tube (2), to the patient. The simultaneous compression of the gas in the concertina bag (7) ensures the closure of the valve (1). The pressure in the inspiratory circuit is indicated by the manometer (11) and limited by the safety-valve (16). This is normally set at

50 cmH_2O but can be adjusted to any value between 20 and 55 cmH_2O. To ensure that the one-way valve (1) in the Y-piece remains closed throughout the inspiratory phase the valve (6), through which the concertina bag (7) empties during this phase, is set to open at a higher pressure than the safety-valve (16). When the upward movement of the base-plate (12) is completed, the inspiratory phase ends.

During the downward movement of the base-plate (12), the bag (17) fills with gas drawn in through the air inlet and filter (19) or stored in the bag (22). Expired gas flows, through the expiratory tube (3) and the tap (9), into the bag (7). The negative pressure produced in the expiratory pathway can be adjusted by the setting of the control (5) which allows air to be drawn into the bag (7). The magnitude of the negative pressure also depends on the stroke volume of the bag and the respiratory frequency. The maximum negative pressure is -30 cmH_2O. The tap (9) allows expired gas to be directed through the spirometer (4), in which case negative pressure is not produced in the expiratory pathway. The dual-action valve (8) ensures closure of the valve (1) during the inspiratory phase when the tap (9) is set to 'spirometer', and also prevents the contents of the bag (7) being forced through the spirometer during the inspiratory phase.

The valve (10) can be opened to allow the patient to inspire from atmosphere. It must be closed if negative pressure is to be developed in the expiratory phase.

When automatic ventilation has been satisfactorily established, the 'supervision' controls (20) and (21) are adjusted. These adjust two pressure-sensitive switches connected in the inspiratory pathway. One, the 'lowered pressure supervision' control, is adjusted so that its pressure switch is just operated by the peak pressure in each inspiratory phase causing a blue light to flash. Thus, if, after a time, the peak pressure falls, the blue light ceases to flash. Furthermore, if the cessation of flashing continues for 15 seconds an alarm bell sounds. The 'raised pressure supervision' control is adjusted so that its pressure switch is just not operated by the peak inspiratory pressure. Then, if, after a time, the peak pressure is raised, a red light begins to flash in each inspiratory phase.

The tidal volume can be adjusted by the control (28) to any value between 300 and 1400 ml. The respiratory frequency, which is displayed on the tachometer (26), can be adjusted to between 8 and 50/min by the control (25). The inspiratory-expiratory ratio is fixed at 1:1·6.

A separate battery-operated alarm system gives audible warning of a failure of the electrical supply. An elapsed-time indicator is provided. A variable expiratory resistance is available for connexion to the inlet of the 3-way tap (9).

FUNCTIONAL ANALYSIS

Inspiratory phase

During this phase the ventilator operates as a flow generator due to the constant speed of the electric motor (23). The pattern of flow generated is non-constant and its exact form is determined by the mechanical linkage between the gear-box (24) and the moving plate (12).

Change-over from inspiratory phase to expiratory phase

This change-over is volume-cycled and time-cycled: it occurs when a preset volume has been expelled from the concertina reservoir bag (17) in a preset time.

Expiratory phase

With the tap (9) set to 'spirometer' the ventilator operates as a constant, atmospheric, pressure generator: the patient's expired gas passes to atmosphere through the spirometer.

With the tap (9) set to direct the patient's expired gas into the concertina bag (7), the ventilator operates primarily as a flow generator due to the constant speed of the electric motor (23). The pattern of flow generated is non-constant and its exact form is determined by the mechanical linkage between the gear-box (24) and the moving plate (12). Initially this may well result in a positive pressure in the concertina bag (7) but when the pressure there falls to atmospheric the one-way valve of the negative-pressure control opens and puts a leak (adjustable by the negative-pressure control (5)) in parallel with the flow generator which therefore becomes a negative-pressure generator (see p. 85). The waveform of generated pressure will be similar in shape to the waveform of generated flow except that, if the negative-pressure control (5) is wide open, the generated pressure will be constant and atmospheric.

Change-over from expiratory phase to inspiratory phase

This change-over is time-cycled: it occurs when the concertina bags (7, 17) recommence their upward movement in a preset time.

CHAPTER 83

The 'Roswell Park' Ventilator[1]

DESCRIPTION

In this ventilator (fig. 83.1) a Trico windscreen-wiper motor provides the motive power. The square-shaped moulded rubber reservoir bag (1) is 8 inches across. One end is

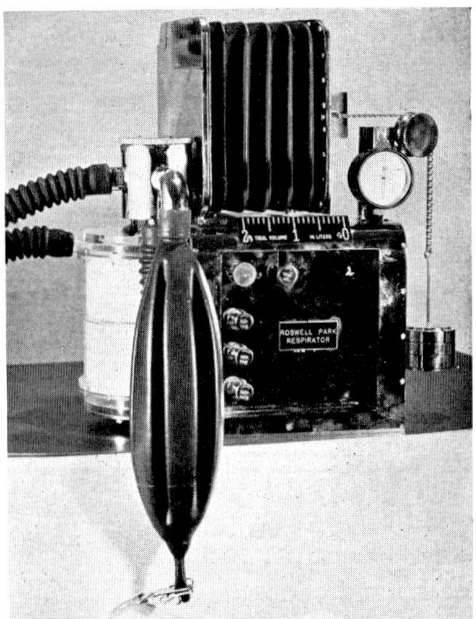

Fig. 83.1. The 'Roswell Park' ventilator.

Courtesy of Dr. J.O. Elam.

fixed and the other is attached to the plate (3), which is hinged at the fulcrum (2). Oxygen or compressed air, at a pressure of 30–55 lb/in^2, drives the Trico windscreen-wiper motor (9), operating the arm (5) which runs on the plate (3). The arm (5) has a 50° swing. The counterweight (10), if used, assists the expansion of the bag (1) and gives negative pressure during the expiratory phase.

The volume delivered by the apparatus is varied by rotating the whole motor about its shaft, in the direction A–A, thus bringing the arm (5) to bear on a different segment of the plate (3). When the motor is rotated in an anti-clockwise direction the volume is decreased; when in a clockwise direction the volume is increased. A pointer (4) attached

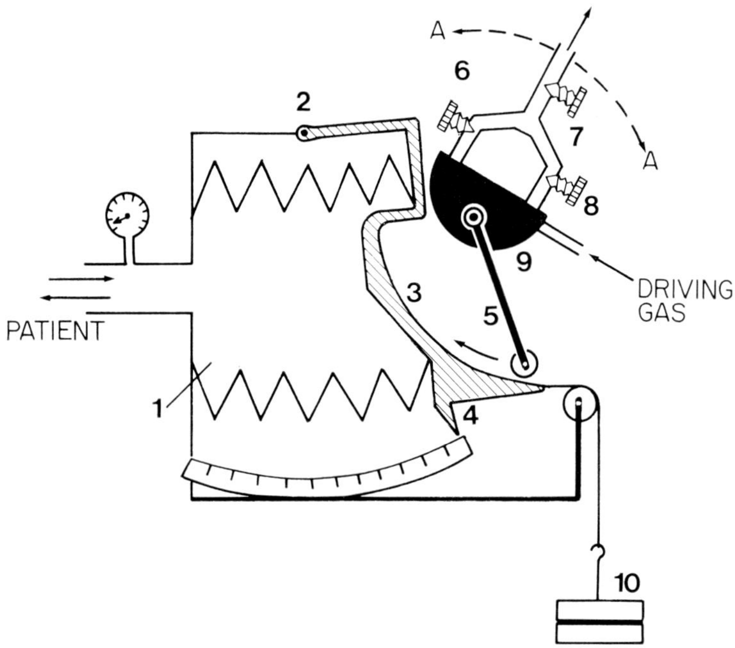

Fig. 83.2. Diagram of the 'Roswell Park' ventilator.

1. Concertina reservoir bag
2. Fulcrum of (3)
3. Hinged plate
4. Pointer indicating tidal volume
5. Moving arm
6. Control for varying expiratory time
7. Exhaust control of motor
8. Control for varying inspiratory time
9. Trico windscreen-wiper motor
10. Removeable counterweight

to the concertina bag (1) indicates on the scale the volume delivered by the apparatus. This can be varied between 400 and 1800 ml. The maximum pressure attained depends upon the amount of gas admitted to the anaesthetic circuit and on the setting of the expiratory valve of the anaesthetic apparatus, and can be as high as 50 cmH_2O. A negative pressure as low as -20 cmH_2O can be produced during the expiratory phase. The respiratory frequency is controlled by varying the speed with which driving gas escapes from the wiper motor through the exhaust tap (7). The durations of the inspiratory and the expiratory phases can be separately varied by the two valves (8) and (6).

FUNCTIONAL ANALYSIS

This ventilator contains a pressure transformer (see p. 89) with adjustable resistance (6), (7), and (8) (fig. 83.2) and a constant driving pressure at (9) on the input side. It therefore operates as a pressure generator with a substantial series resistance between it and the patient. However, since the mechanical advantage of the drive between the wiper motor and the concertina bag varies as the arm (5) moves over the plate (3), the generated pressure and the series resistance vary similarly. Thus, in the main, patterns of pressure are generated, in both the inspiratory and expiratory phases, which are entirely determined by the ventilator, but which are not constant. Furthermore the patterns of pressure are determined in relation to the volume in the concertina bag rather than in relation to time (see p. 112).

Inspiratory phase

In this phase the ventilator operates as a non-constant pressure generator with substantial series resistance which varies in a similar manner to the pressure; this is due to the pressure-transformer characteristics. A pressure limit, due to the blow-off valve which must be incorporated in the patient circuit to vent excess gas, comes into operation during the phase. Until then, the fresh-gas supply to the patient circuit acts as a small-constant-flow generator, supplementing the main pressure generator.

Change-over from inspiratory phase to expiratory phase

This change-over is volume-cycled: the phase ends when the driving mechanism reaches the end of its stroke and a preset volume has been expelled from the concertina bag. Since the supply of anaesthetic gas is continuous, but its escape, through the blow-off valve, is restricted to the inspiratory phase, the patient's tidal volume is less than the stroke volume of the bag, by an amount equal to the volume of fresh gas supplied during the expiratory phase.

Expiratory phase

In this phase the ventilator operates as a non-constant, negative-pressure generator, with substantial series resistance which varies in a similar manner to the pressure, owing to the pressure-transformer characteristics. The fresh-gas flow now slightly impedes the main pressure-generator action. A negative-pressure limit is set, in the concertina bag (1), by the action of the weights (10).

Change-over from expiratory phase to inspiratory phase

This change-over is volume-cycled: the phase begins when the driving mechanism reaches the beginning of its stroke and a preset volume has been either drawn into, or allowed to enter, the bag. The volume leaving the patient's lungs is less than this, by an amount equal to the volume of fresh gas which enters the patient circuit during the expiratory phase.

REFERENCE

1 Elam J.O., Brown E.S. and Janney C.D. (1956) A ventilator. *Anesthesiology*, **17**, 504.

CHAPTER 84

The Starling Pump

DESCRIPTION

This ventilator (fig. 84.1) was originally designed for animal use in the laboratory,[1] and subsequently found a place in clinical practice for the ventilation of infants.[2] It is now available in three sizes which differ in the maximum tidal volumes which they can deliver (250, 500, and 800 ml).

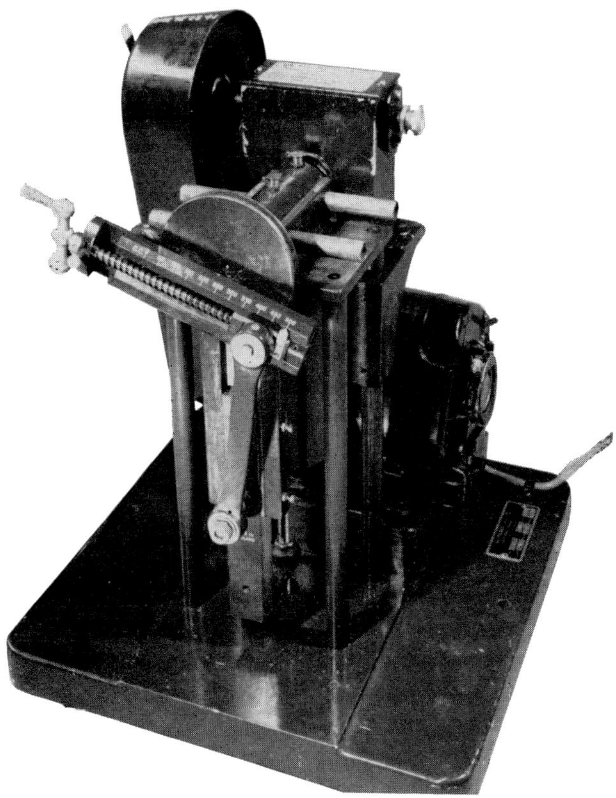

Fig. 84.1. The Starling pump.
Courtesy of Department of Medical Illustration, Cardiff Royal Infirmary.

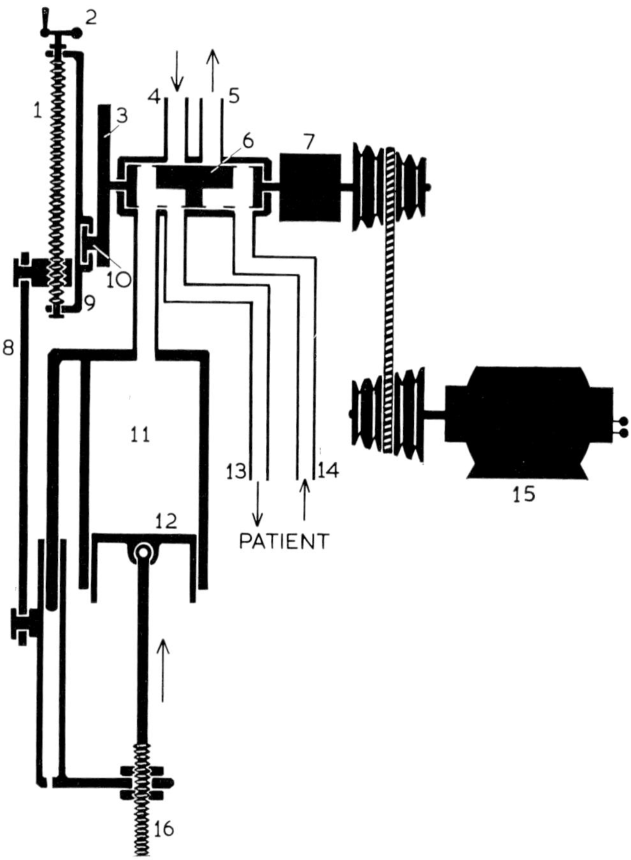

Fig. 84.2. Diagram of the Starling pump.

1. Screw rod
2. Volume control
3. Crank-wheel
4. Inlet port
5. Outlet port
6. Rotary valve
7. Gear-box
8. Connecting rod
9. Lever
10. Crank pin
11. Cylinder
12. Piston
13. Inspiratory tube
14. Expiratory tube
15. a.c. mains electric motor
16. Screw rod

A constant-speed a.c. mains electric motor (15) (fig. 84.2) drives a gear-box (7) through a five-step pulley system, which allows frequencies of 14, 20, 26, 36, and 45 per minute to be selected. The output shaft of the gear-box (7) is connected to a rotary valve (6) and a crank-wheel (3) which is linked, through the lever (9) and the connecting rods (8) and (16), to the piston (12). In this way the movement of the piston is synchronized with the rotation of the valve (6).

During the inspiratory phase the piston (12) is driven upwards and the valve (6) moves through that part of its cycle during which the cylinder (11) is connected to the inspiratory tube (13), and the expiratory tube (14) is occluded. Therefore the gas stored in the cylinder (11) is delivered to the patient. The inspiratory phase ends when the piston completes its compression stroke, this being coincident with the valve (6) having rotated as far as the point at which the pathway between the cylinder (11) and the inspiratory tube (13) is closed, and the pathway between the expiratory tube (14) and the expiratory outlet (5) is opening. Expired gas therefore flows, through the outlet (5), to atmosphere. At the same time the expansion stroke of the piston (12) draws in air from the atmosphere, or gas from a reservoir, through the inlet port (4). The expiratory phase ends when the rotation of the valve (6) and the crank-wheel (3) is completed and the next respiratory cycle commences. The inspiratory-expiratory ratio is fixed at approximately 1:1·2.

The crank-wheel pin (10) drives the lever (9) which carries the top bearing of the connecting rod (8). The position of this bearing in relation to the crank pin (10) is set by adjustment of the screw-rod (1), by the control (2). This mechanism, which constitutes a lost-motion device, determines the magnitude of the motion imparted through the connecting rod (8) to the piston and hence sets the tidal volume.

When the ventilator is set to deliver less than the maximum tidal volume, the setting of the screw (16) may be adjusted to ensure that the piston moves over the upper part of its stroke and that there is no dead space in the cylinder at the end of the inspiratory phase.

FUNCTIONAL ANALYSIS

Inspiratory phase

In this phase the ventilator operates as a flow generator owing to the constant speed of the electric motor. The pattern of generated flow approximates to a half cycle of a sine wave due to the nature of the linkage from the crank-wheel (3) to the piston (12).

Change-over from inspiratory phase to expiratory phase

This change-over is both volume-cycled and time-cycled: it occurs when the piston (12) has delivered a preset volume in a preset time due to the constant speed of the motor (15).

Expiratory phase

In this phase the ventilator operates as a constant, atmospheric, pressure generator: the patient's expired gas passes to atmosphere through the outlet port (5).

Change-over from expiratory phase to inspiratory phase

This change-over is time-cycled: it occurs when the pathway from the cylinder (11) to the inspiratory tube (13) is reopened in a preset time.

REFERENCES

1 STARLING E.H. (1926) An improved method of artificial respiration. *J. Physiol., Lond.* **61**, 14.

2 MONRO J.A. and SCURR C.F. (1961) The Starling pump as a ventilator for infants and children. *Anaesthesia*, **16**, 151.

CHAPTER 85

The Stephenson 'Controlled Respiration Unit'

DESCRIPTION

Ventilation is brought about by the compression of a large concertina reservoir bag. A variable blow-off valve limits the maximum positive pressure. Should the setting of this valve be too low to drive the desired volume into the lungs, that part of the preset tidal volume which blows off through the valve is collected in the reserve concertina bag. The movements of the arm of the blow-off valve and of the reserve bag therefore give immediate information as to how much the ventilation of the patient falls short of that desired, and also indicates when sufficient pressure is being used to push in the desired volume. Cycling occurs when the preset volume has been delivered from the main bag.

During the expiratory phase the main bag is forcibly expanded creating a negative pressure, the limit of which is set by the adjustment of an inlet valve. If the lungs do not empty quickly enough, air from the reserve bag is drawn in and this gives an indication that the negative pressure is too little. Towards the end of the expansion of the main bag a subsidiary mechanism comes into play which delays cycling for a controllable period of time. Eventually the main bag is filled, at which point cycling occurs and an inspiratory phase begins. The tidal volume may be varied between 200 and 1800 ml. The maximum positive pressure obtained during inflation may be varied up to 47 cmH_2O and the negative pressure during expiration between 0 and -26 cmH_2O. The ventilator is driven by compressed air or oxygen at approximately 40–60 lb/in^2.

1. The Power Circuit

(a) *Inspiratory phase.* Driving gas enters at (31) (fig. 85.1) and is led directly to the upper ends of the cylinders (3, 3) and through the needle valve (32) to the cycling mechanism (25). The needle valve (32) regulates the inflation speed and hence the duration of the inspiratory phase for a given tidal volume. During inflation the cycling mechanism diverts gas to the lower ends of the cylinders (24, 24). The driving gas is also within the upper parts of the cylinders above the pistons (23, 23). However, the underneath surface of the piston is of larger effective area than the upper surface. The pistons are therefore forced upwards. The base-plate (22) of the main concertina bag (21) is connected to the pistons and the bag is therefore compressed. As the base-plate rises, its striking pin (19) meets the pin (16), the position of which on the rod (20) determines the tidal volume.

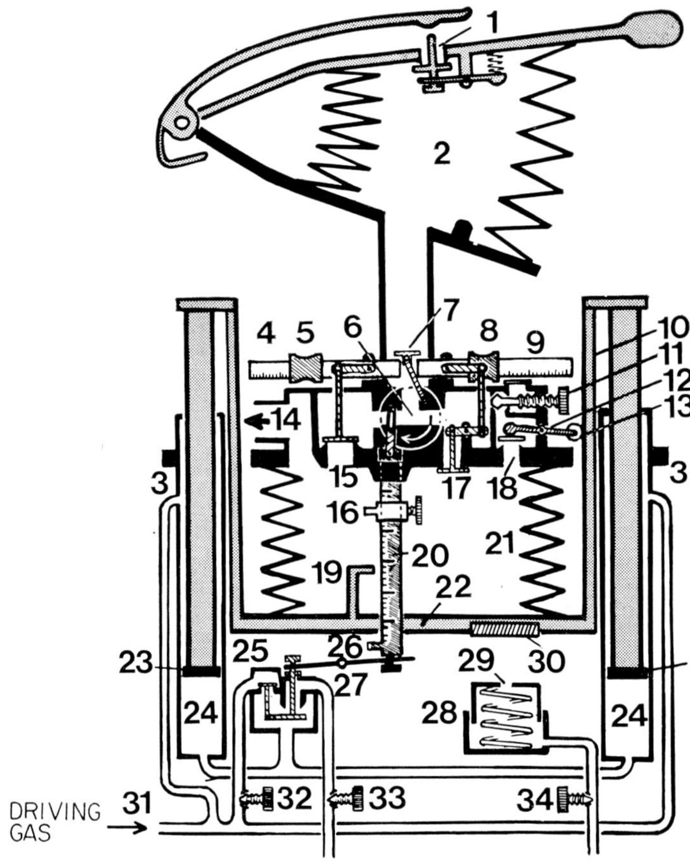

Fig. 85.1. Diagram of the Stephenson 'Controlled Respiration Unit'.

1. Double-action spill valve
2. Reserve concertina bag
3, 3. Upper ends of cylinders
4. Beam
5. Sliding weight
6. 'Manual/Auto' control
7. Lever
8. Sliding weight
9. Beam
10. Connecting rod
11. Exhaust valve
12. Pivoted rod
13. Friction shoe
14. Port for connexion to patient
15. Blow-off valve
16. Adjustable pin
17. Inlet valve
18. One-way valve
19. Striking pin
20. Rod carrying tidal-volume scale
21. Main concertina reservoir bag
22. Base-plate
23, 23. Pistons
24, 24. Lower ends of cylinders
25. Cycling mechanism
26. Fixed pin
27. Lever
28. Pneumatic cylinder
29. Pneumatic-cylinder vent
30. Rubber disc
31. Driving-gas inlet
32. Inflation-speed control valve
33. Needle valve
34. Needle valve

The rod (20) is lifted and, through the snap-over mechanism (27), operates the cycling mechanism.

(b) *Expiratory phase.* The lower ends of the cylinders are now cut off from the driving-

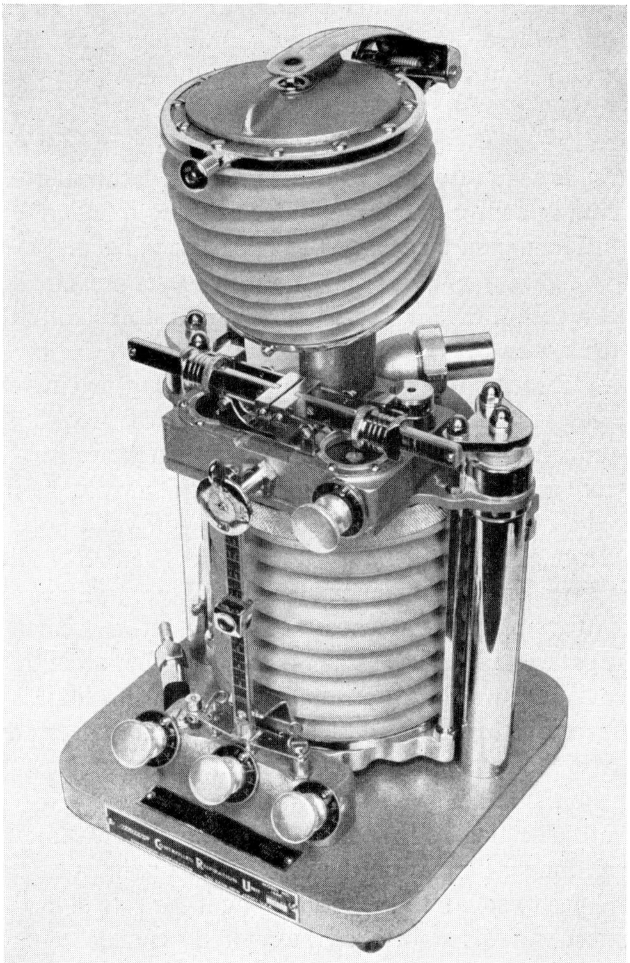

Fig. 85.2. The Stephenson 'Controlled Respiration Unit'.
Courtesy of the Stephenson Corporation.

gas supply and are connected to atmosphere through the needle valve (33). This valve (33) regulates the speed of expansion of the bag and hence the duration of this portion of the expiratory phase. The pistons are forced down by the pressure in the upper ends of the cylinders. Just before the base-plate reaches the limit of its downward motion, a rubber disc (30) on it makes contact with a small pneumatic cylinder (28), sealing off the cylinder vent (29). The air in the cylinder (28) is now compressed and is forced out through the needle valve (34). The setting of this valve regulates the time delay between the end of the expansion of the bag (21) and the next inspiratory phase.

When the pneumatic cylinder (28) is compressed to a certain point the striking pin

(19) on the base-plate meets the pin (26) on the lower end of the rod (20) and the cycling mechanism is again operated, starting the next inspiratory phase. A light spring in the pneumatic cylinder (28) now refills it with air.

2. The Patient Circuit

As the main bag (21) is compressed its contents are forced, through the tube (14), to the patient. The maximum positive pressure within it during inflation is controlled by the blow-off valve (15). The pressure necessary to open this valve may be varied by adjustment of the sliding weight (5) on the beam (4). If this preset pressure is reached the valve opens and, during the rest of the inspiratory phase, gas is forced into the reserve bag (2). During inflation the expiratory valve (18) is kept closed by the pivoted rod (12), the outer end of which is forced up by the friction of a shoe (13) against the connecting rod (10). If the reserve bag becomes fully distended, gas escapes through the safety-valve (1). A detachable weight can be placed on the handle of the reserve bag to maintain a constant positive pressure of up to 5 cmH_2O within it. The tidal volume is set by the position of the pin (16) on the calibrated rod (20). If the blow-off valve (15) is set at too low a pressure, it lifts before the desired tidal volume is delivered. The lungs will be held inflated at this pressure for the remainder of the inspiratory phase.

When the expiratory phase commences the downward movement of the main bag draws gas from the patient, the valve (15) being closed. The limit of the negative pressure is set by adjustment of the weight (8) on the beam (9). If this limit is reached, the inlet valve (17) from the reserve bag opens and gas is drawn through it from the reserve bag into the main bag. If the reserve bag is emptied, the safety-valve (1) opens and air is drawn in to complete the refilling of the main bag.

As soon as the connecting rod (10) begins to move downwards, the lever (12) is moved so that it no longer presses on the disc of the one-way valve (18). This allows some of the expired gas to spill into the reserve bag if the rate of expansion of the main bag is not sufficient. A variable amount of the expired gas may be vented to atmosphere by adjustment of the exhaust valve (11).

3. Manual Control

For manual operation the 'Manual/Auto' control (6) is turned. This lifts the rod (20) and the power circuit is held with the pistons at the lower ends of the cylinders. At the same time the lever (7) is drawn down and the valves (15, 17), which limit the positive and negative pressures, are held open. Movement of the reserve bag (2) is now transmitted freely to the lungs.

4. Patient-triggering

A patient-triggered unit for assisted respiration has been designed. When an inspiratory effort is made, the negative pressure produced acts on a large diaphragm, the movement of which switches on an injector. The greater negative pressure from this source rapidly sucks air out of the cylinder (28). Cycling can therefore only be triggered by the patient during the second or passive part of the expiratory phase.

FUNCTIONAL ANALYSIS

This ventilator contains a pressure transformer (see p. 89) with adjustable resistances (32) and (33) (fig. 85.1) and a constant driving pressure at (31) on the input side. It therefore acts mainly as a pressure generator with substantial series resistance between it and the patient.

Inspiratory phase
In this phase the ventilator operates as a constant-pressure generator, with substantial series resistance, owing to the pressure-transformer characteristics. The generated pressure is probably high enough for the action to approximate to that of a constant-flow generator. The fresh-gas supply to the patient circuit acts as a small-constant-flow generator, supplementing the action of the main generator. The blow-off valve (15) sets a pressure limit, but, if this is allowed to come into operation, the tidal volume is not controlled by the ventilator.

Change-over from inspiratory phase to expiratory phase
This change-over is volume-cycled: the phase ends when the striking pin (19) has travelled from the lower to the upper limit and a preset volume has been expelled from the main concertina bag. The volume entering the patient's lungs exceeds this by an amount equal to the volume of fresh gas which enters the patient circuit during the phase.

Expiratory phase, Part I. (Expansion of the main concertina bag)
In this part of the phase the ventilator operates approximately as a constant-flow generator, owing to the pressure-transformer characteristics, but with an atmospheric pressure limit set by the valve (18) and a negative-pressure limit set by the valve (17) (see p. 120).

Change-over from Part I of expiratory phase to Part II
This change-over may be regarded as either volume-cycled or time-cycled, although neither view is exactly true in the conventional sense. The change-over is volume-cycled in the sense that it occurs when a preset volume has been drawn into the main concertina bag; however, the volume leaving the lungs differs from this because of the fresh-gas inflow, and because of the spillage that may have occurred to or from the reserve bag (2). The volume of this spillage, and therefore the tidal volume, is partly dependent on lung characteristics,

The change-over can be regarded as approximately time-cycled since the ventilator operates approximately as a constant-flow generator in Part I of the expiratory phase and therefore the main concertina bag will be driven through its preset stroke volume in a time which varies only slightly with lung characteristics.

Expiratory phase, Part II. (Main concertina bag almost at rest in the expanded position) In this part of the 'expiratory' phase the very slow expansion of the main concertina bag constitutes a small, expiratory, constant-flow generator, while the fresh-gas flow to the patient circuit constitutes a small, inspiratory, constant-flow generator. The net effect will be that of a small-constant-flow generator, either expiratory or inspiratory depending on whether the fresh-gas flow is small or large. In the latter case the one-way valve (18) will set an upper (atmospheric) pressure limit.

Change-over from expiratory phase to inspiratory phase

This change-over is either time-cycled or patient-cycled, whichever comes first: cycling occurs when sufficient gas has escaped from the cylinder (28). This may occur either gradually, through the needle valve (34) in a preset time after the end of Part I of the expiratory phase, or suddenly, into the injector which is brought into operation by the patient-cycling mechanism, when the patient makes an inspiratory effort.

CHAPTER 86

The Takaoka Ventilator[1]

DESCRIPTION

This ventilator (fig. 86.1) was devised in circumstances in which nitrous oxide was not readily available. It is designed for both theatre and ward use. It is intended that oxygen

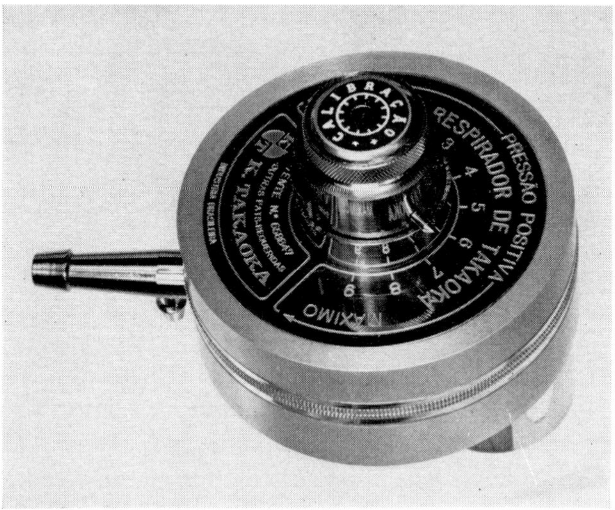

Fig. 86.1. The Takaoka ventilator.

Courtesy of Dr. K. Takaoka.

alone should be used as the inflating gas, and anaesthesia, when required, be maintained by non-inhalation agents. This consideration does not preclude the addition of other gases.

The oxygen to be delivered to the patient flows continuously through an injector (6) (fig. 86.2). During the inspiratory phase this gas passes directly to the patient; during the expiratory phase it escapes to atmosphere along with the expired gas which the injector (6) then entrains. The expired gas all passes through the ventilator, which must therefore be placed close to the patient so as to reduce mechanical dead space to a minimum; the dead space of the ventilator itself is only 7 ml.

The oxygen is supplied through the inlet (3) and the jet (6) of the injector at a flow

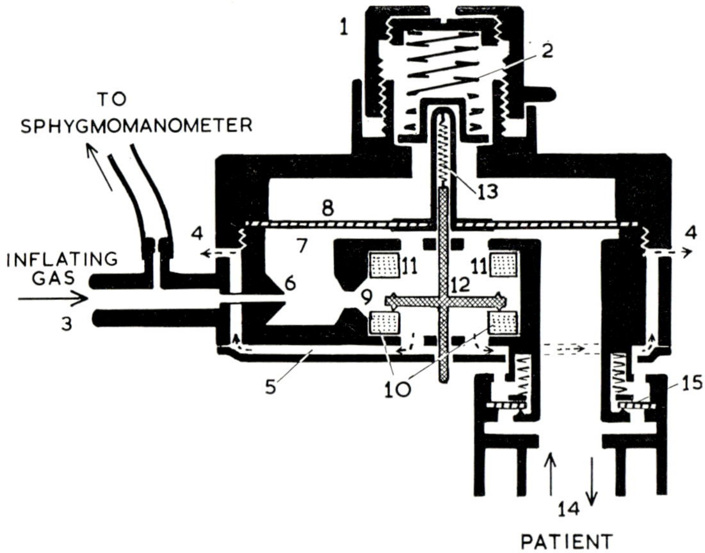

Fig. 86.2. Diagram of the Takaoka ventilator.

1. 'Positive pressure' control
2. Spring
3. Inflating-gas inlet
4, 4. Expiratory slit
5. Space
6. Jet of injector
7. Entrainment port
8. Diaphragm
9. Outlet of injector
10. Ring magnet
11. Ring magnet
12. Soft-iron valve
13. Spring
14. Breathing tube
15. Safety-valve

of between 3 and 15 litres/min. The pressure behind the jet is measured on a sphygmomanometer which must be connected to the side-arm of the inlet (3). Since the size of the jet (6) is fixed, the pressure recorded on the manometer is a direct indication of the magnitude of the gas flow. When oxygen flows at 12 litres/min the reading on the sphygmomanometer is 200 mmHg (3·5 lb/in^2). These figures will vary somewhat if other gases having different densities are used.

During the inspiratory phase the soft-iron valve (12) is held down by the attraction of the ring magnet (10), which also acts as its lower seating, and thus establishes a free connexion between the outlet (9) of the injector and the entrainment port (7), rendering the injector ineffective. The gas therefore flows, through the main chamber and the breathing tube (14), to the patient. The pressure in the main chamber rises and the rubber diaphragm (8) is forced upwards against the force of the spring (2). This upward movement expands the spring (13) until its tension is sufficient to overcome the pull of the magnet (10) on the soft-iron valve (12). The valve flicks upwards and is held by the ring magnet (11), which is its upper seating. Inflation ceases.

The pathway between the outlet (9) of the injector and the entrainment port (7) is now blocked, and the breathing tube (14) is connected only with the entrainment port

(7); the injector therefore becomes effective. The inflating gas now flows beneath the soft-iron valve (12) and through felt pads, which fill the space (5) and act as silencers. The gas then passes, through channels in the main casing of the ventilator, to the slit (4, 4) where it escapes to atmosphere. The consequent fall in pressure in the main chamber allows the spring (2) to force the diaphragm (8) downwards. As expiration proceeds the pressure in the main chamber continues to fall, eventually becoming negative owing to the action of the injector (6). This continuing fall of pressure leads to a continuing downward movement of the diaphragm (8) which compresses the spring (13) until the pull of the upper magnet (11) is overcome, and the soft-iron valve (12) flicks down to be held in the inflating position by the lower magnet (10). The next inspiratory phase commences.

A safety-valve (15) limits the pressure within the ventilator to 52 cmH_2O.

Respiratory cycling depends on the changes in position of the soft-iron valve (12). During the inspiratory phase the attraction of the ring magnet (10) for the valve (12) is constant and hence the tension which must be exerted by the spring (13) in order to initiate the expiratory phase is also constant. This tension of the spring (13) is produced by the upward movement of the diaphragm (8) through a fixed distance. But, as the upward movement of the diaphragm is opposed by compression of the spring (2), the pressure required beneath the diaphragm to produce this fixed amount of upward movement can be varied by rotation of the 'positive pressure' control (1) which alters the force exerted by the spring (2). The tidal volume delivered to the patient depends on the cycling pressure set in this way, and on the lung characteristics of the patient. Hence, for any tidal volume the duration of the inspiratory phase depends on the inflating-gas flow. In a similar way the expiratory phase ends when the diaphragm (8) has moved downwards through a fixed distance producing sufficient compression of the spring (13) to overcome the attraction of the magnet (11) for the soft-iron valve (12), and so reverse its position. The duration of the expiratory phase therefore is the time necessary for the pressure within the ventilator to fall sufficiently for this to occur. This depends essentially on the characteristics of the injector; these are such that, over the recommended range of inflating flows (3–15 litres/min) and within the pressure range set by the safety-valve (15), the entrainment factor is approximately 1:1. Therefore the time taken for one tidal volume of expired gas to be entrained is approximately the time taken for one tidal volume of inflating gas to be delivered, and the durations of the inspiratory and expiratory phases are almost equal under any conditions. For this reason the total minute-volume ventilation is approximately half the inflating-gas flow, and depends almost solely on this flow. So long as there is no change in the compliance of the patient, the respiratory frequency depends, for any given inflating-gas flow, on the setting of the control (1). If the setting of the control (1) is not altered, the frequency is varied by changing the inflating-gas flow. If the patient's compliance alters then the tidal volume, and hence the frequency, alters.

In summary, adjustment of the 'positive pressure' control (1) varies the tidal volume without change of total ventilation. Adjustment of the inflating-gas flow varies the total minute-volume ventilation without change in the tidal volume.

As the flow of gas into the patient is that at which inflating gas is supplied to the ventilator, and this is not intended to exceed 15 litres/min, the duration of the inspiratory phase is somewhat prolonged. For example, at a flow of 15 litres/min and a tidal volume of 500 ml, the inspiratory phase lasts 2 seconds, the expiratory phase lasts 2 seconds, the respiratory frequency is 15 per minute, and the total minute-volume ventilation is 7·5 litres/min.

Furthermore, as the gas flow into and from the patient is relatively low, the pressure drop across the airway is also low. Therefore, so long as no untoward obstruction occurs, the pressures within the main chamber of the ventilator and the patient's lungs are nearly equal at all times. If the airway becomes obstructed this will no longer be true and the ventilator will cycle when a smaller tidal volume has been delivered. Conversely, if a leak develops between the ventilator and the patient, the pressure rise inside the ventilator will be limited and may be insufficient to cycle it.

FUNCTIONAL ANALYSIS

Inspiratory phase

In this phase the ventilator operates as a constant-flow generator due to the constant high pressure at the inlet (3) and the high resistance of the jet (6) of the injector.

Change-over from inspiratory phase to expiratory phase

This change-over is pressure-cycled: it occurs when the pressure on the underside of the diaphragm (8), which is the same as the pressure at the mouth, has risen high enough to produce sufficient movement of the diaphragm against the force of the spring (2) to pull the soft-iron valve (12) away from the lower ring magnet (10).

Expiratory phase

In this phase the ventilator operates as a constant, negative, pressure generator with substantial series resistance owing to the characteristics of the injector. The generated pressure and the resistance are high enough for the system to make a fair approximation to a constant-flow generator.

Change-over from expiratory phase to inspiratory phase

This change-over also is pressure-cycled: it occurs when the pressure below the diaphragm (8) has fallen far enough to produce sufficient movement of the diaphragm to push the soft-iron valve (12) away from the upper ring magnet.

REFERENCE

1 Dobkin A.B. (1961) The Takaoka respirator for automatic ventilation of the lungs. *Can. Anaesth. Soc. J.* **8**, 556.

CHAPTER 87

The U.S. Army Volume-cycled Ventilator

DESCRIPTION

This ventilator (fig. 87.1) is intended for anaesthetic or ward use. It is a development of

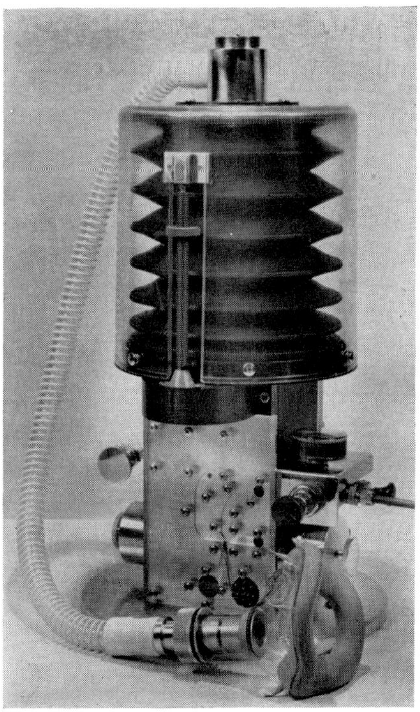

Fig. 87.1. The U.S. Army volume-cycled ventilator.
Courtesy of Medical Audio Visual Dept. Walter Reed Army Inst. of Research, Washington 12, D.C.

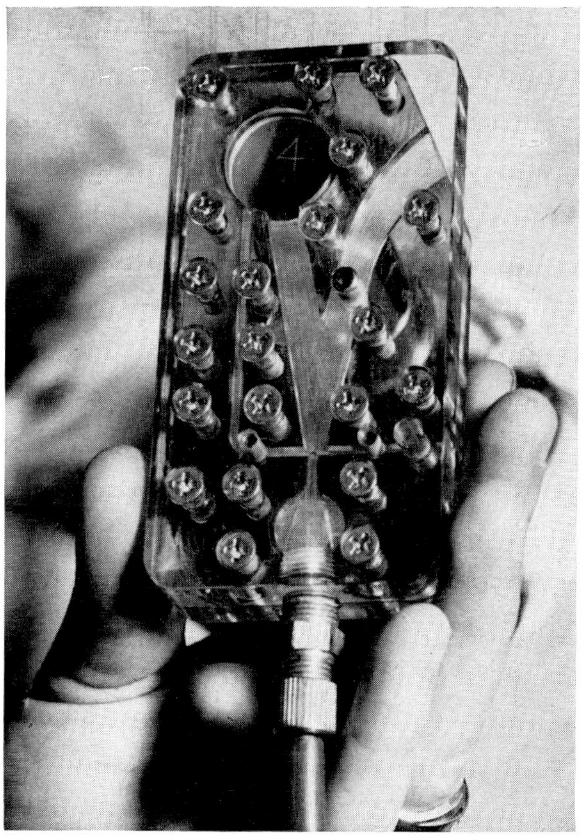

Fig. 87.2. The U.S. Army 'Emergency Respirator'.
Courtesy of Medical Audio Visual Dept. Walter Reed Army Inst. of Research, Washington 12, D.C.

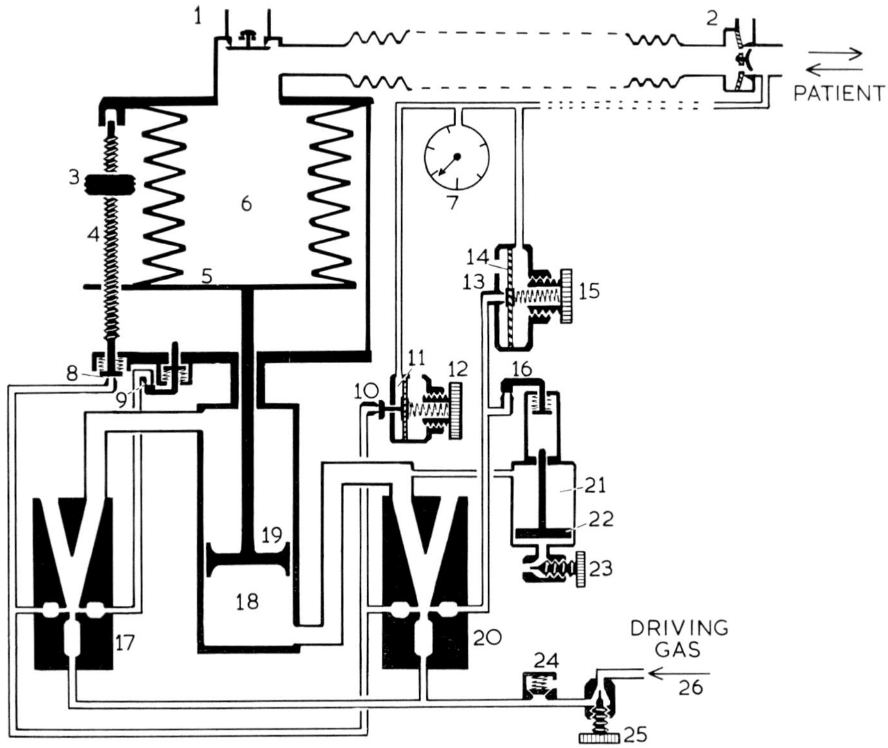

Fig. 87.3. Diagram of the U.S. Army volume-cycled ventilator.

1. One-way valve
2. Inflating valve
3. Adjustable-stop volume control
4. Screwed rod
5. Base-plate
6. Concertina bag
7. Manometer
8. Air-inlet valve
9. Air-inlet valve
10. Air-inlet valve
11. Chamber
12. Inspiratory-pressure control
13. Air-inlet valve
14. Diaphragm
15. Patient-trigger control
16. Air-inlet valve
17. Fluid amplifier
18. Cylinder
19. Piston
20. Fluid amplifier
21. Chamber
22. Piston
23. Expiratory-time-control needle valve
24. Safety-valve
25. Inspiratory-time-control needle valve
26. Driving-gas inlet

the U.S. Army 'Emergency Respirator'[1] (fig. 87.2) which consists essentially of a single 'fluid amplifier'[2] which directs a flow of compressed gas alternately through one channel to the patient or through the other to atmosphere. It is driven by compressed gas which does not go to the patient. The power control units are bi-stable fluid amplifiers and have no moving parts.

Driving gas, at a pressure not higher than 50 lb/in^2, is supplied at the inlet (26) (fig. 87.3) and passes, at a flow controlled by the 'inspiratory time' control (25), to the two fluid amplifiers (17) and (20). This flow of driving gas issuing from the 'power-stream jets' of the amplifiers exerts a venturi effect in the side ports of each amplifier. During the inspiratory phase the driving gas issuing from the 'power-stream jets' flows through the left-hand channels of both amplifiers. The flow through the amplifier (17) escapes to atmosphere and, since the valves (8), (9), and (10) are held closed by their springs, the venturi effect produces a negative pressure in both side ports. The flow of driving gas through the left-hand channel of the amplifier (20) passes to the lower part of the cylinder (18) and forces the piston (19) upwards, thereby compressing the concertina reservoir bag (6) and driving the gas contained in it, through the inflating valve (2), to the patient. At the same time, since the valves (8), (10), (13), and (16) are closed, a negative pressure is produced in both side ports of the amplifier (20). The driving gas contained in the cylinder above the piston (19) flows to atmosphere as it is entrained by the driving gas flowing through the amplifier (17). If the ventilator is being used in the volume-cycled mode, the inspiratory phase continues until the base-plate (5) has risen sufficiently for it to strike the adjustable stop (3) and so lift the screw-rod (4) and open the valve (8).

The left-hand ports of both amplifiers are now connected to atmosphere; the pressure within them rises above that in the right-hand ports, and the stream of driving gas coming from the main jet of each amplifier is deflected to the right. The stream through the right-hand amplifier (20) now escapes to atmosphere; the stream through the left-hand amplifier passes through the right-hand channel to the upper part of the cylinder (18) and forces the piston (19) downwards. The gas contained in the cylinder below the piston is entrained by the flow of driving gas through the amplifier (20). The change of direction of the driving-gas streams, therefore, marks the end of the inspiratory phase. As the piston moves downwards, fresh gas is drawn in through the one-way valve (1), whilst expired gas flows to atmosphere through the expiratory ports of the inflating valve (2).

As soon as the reservoir bag has begun to move down, the base-plate (5) comes away from the stop (3) and the valve (8) is closed by its spring. This results in the restoration of negative pressure in the left-hand ports of each amplifier, but the main streams remain in the right-hand channels of both amplifiers—they are said to be 'stabilized'. When the bag reaches the lower limit of its travel the base-plate (5) strikes the pin of the valve (9) and opens it. The right-hand port of the amplifier (17) is now connected to atmosphere and pressure in this port rises. This results in the stream of driving gas from the main jet of this amplifier being redirected through the left-hand channel of the amplifier to atmosphere. Compressed gas in the upper part of the cylinder is released to atmosphere as it is entrained by the driving gas. A similar entrainment effect is being exerted on the underside of the piston (19) by the amplifier (20) so that a pressure balance is established.

Meanwhile air contained in the chamber (21) above the piston of the 'expiratory time' control is being entrained by the 'jet-stream flow' of the amplifier (20) and flowing to atmosphere through the right-hand channel. This produces a pressure difference across the piston (22) which moves upwards at a rate dependent on the setting of the 'expiratory time' control (23) which determines the rate at which air can enter the chamber below the piston. When the piston (22) has risen sufficiently, its stem lifts the valve (16) against the force of its spring and the right-hand port of the amplifier (20) is connected to atmosphere. The pressure in this port now exceeds that in the left-hand port and the main stream of driving gas through this amplifier is redirected to the left-hand channel of the amplifier. The next inspiratory phase begins as the piston (18) is again driven upwards.

Since the left-hand channel of the amplifier is connected to the chamber (21) above the piston (22) of the 'expiratory time' control, the pressure above the piston (22) increases, forcing down the piston, and the valve (16) is closed by its spring. The negative-pressure balance between the two ports of the amplifier (20) is restored and the gas stream is again 'stabilized'.

If the ventilator is to be pressure-cycled, the inspiratory phase is terminated as follows. Positive pressure at the mouth is transmitted to the chamber (11) of the 'pressure cycle' control mechanism and the diaphragm is pushed over against the force of the spring, opening the valve (10), and thereby connecting the left-hand ports of both amplifiers to atmosphere and ending the inspiratory phase. The pressure required to do this depends on the force exerted by the spring which is set by adjustment of the control (12). As soon as the valve is opened, the stream of driving gas in both amplifiers is deflected to the right-hand channel and the ventilator cycles to the expiratory position.

If the ventilator is to be patient-triggered, the control (15) is set so that, when the patient makes an inspiratory effort during that part of the expiratory phase after the concertina bag has reached the lower limit of its travel, the diaphragm (14) is drawn over against the force exerted by the spring and the valve (13) is opened, thus connecting the right-hand port of the amplifier (20) to atmosphere and so redirecting the main stream through this amplifier into the left-hand channel and initiating a new inspiratory phase. If the patient fails to make an inspiratory effort the expiratory phase is terminated after a time set by the 'expiratory time' control (23).

If the patient makes an inspiratory effort before the concertina bag has completed its re-expansion, the main stream of the amplifier (20) will be deflected to the left-hand channel while the main stream of the amplifier (17) is still directed towards the right-hand channel. The regular cycling of the ventilator will therefore be altered in some way.

The safety-valve (24) prevents excessive driving-gas pressure being exerted on the fluid amplifiers.

If air is to be used for inflation of the patient the valve inlet (1) is left open to atmosphere. Attachments are available for enriching the air with oxygen or for replacing it by an anaesthetic mixture.

FUNCTIONAL ANALYSIS

Inspiratory phase

In this phase the patient is connected to a pressure transformer (see p. 89) comprising the concertina reservoir bag (6) on the low-pressure side and the piston and cylinder (19 and 18) on the high-pressure side. The driving pressure at the inlet (26) is high and there is an adjustable resistance at the needle valve (25). The functioning will also be influenced by the characteristics of the two fluid amplifiers (17, 20). It seems likely that the combined effect will be that of a constant-pressure generator with series resistance; the magnitude of the generated pressure is uncertain but it is probably quite high.

Change-over from inspiratory phase to expiratory phase

This change-over is either volume-cycled or pressure-cycled whichever occurs first: it occurs when the pressure in the left-hand side ports of the fluid amplifiers (17, 20) is raised to atmospheric, either by the opening of valve (8) when a preset volume has been delivered from the concertina reservoir bag (6), or by the opening of the valve (10) when a preset pressure has been built up at the mouth. Commonly the cycling-volume (3) and cycling-pressure (12) controls will be set so that only one or the other of these modes of cycling normally occurs.

Expiratory phase

In this phase the ventilator operates as a constant, atmospheric, pressure generator: the patient's expired gas passes to atmosphere through the expiratory port of the inflating valve (2).

Change-over from expiratory phase to inspiratory phase

This change-over is either time-cycled or patient-cycled whichever occurs first: it occurs when the pressure in the right-hand side port of the right-hand amplifier (20) is raised to atmospheric, either by the opening of the valve (16) when the piston (22) has been sucked up far enough at a rate controlled by the needle valve (23), or by the opening of valve (13) when an inspiratory effort by the patient overcomes the force of the spring acting on the diaphragm (14)—always providing that the inspiratory effort does not occur before the concertina bag (6) has completed its re-expansion and caused the main stream of the amplifier (17) to be directed to the left by the opening of the valve (9).

REFERENCES

1 STRAUB H.H. and MOSLEY E. (1964) A respirator without moving parts. 17th Annual Conference on Engineering in Medicine and Biology, Cleveland, Ohio. November 16–18, 1964.

2 ANGRIST S.W. (1964) Fluid control devices. *Scient. Am.* **211**, No. 6, 80.

CHAPTER 88

The Van Bergen Ventilator[1]

DESCRIPTION

A constant-speed electric motor with a variable-speed transmission drives a piston, whose stroke is variable, up and down a cylinder. The movement of the piston within the cylinder, and hence the pattern of flow in the inspiratory phase, is governed by the shape of the cam by which the piston is driven. This shape is designed to give a rapid rise of pressure to a peak.

During the inspiratory phase (fig. 88.2) air passes from the cylinder, through a cam-operated inspiratory valve and a non-distensible tube, to the patient.

At the end of the inspiratory phase the cam of the inspiratory-expiratory valve has rotated so that the inspiratory valve shuts and the expiratory valve opens (fig. 88.3). Expired gas then passes to atmosphere through the expired-gas outlet.

A short period of negative pressure occurs immediately preceding the inspiratory phase. The negative pressure occupies one-sixth of the entire cycle and can be varied

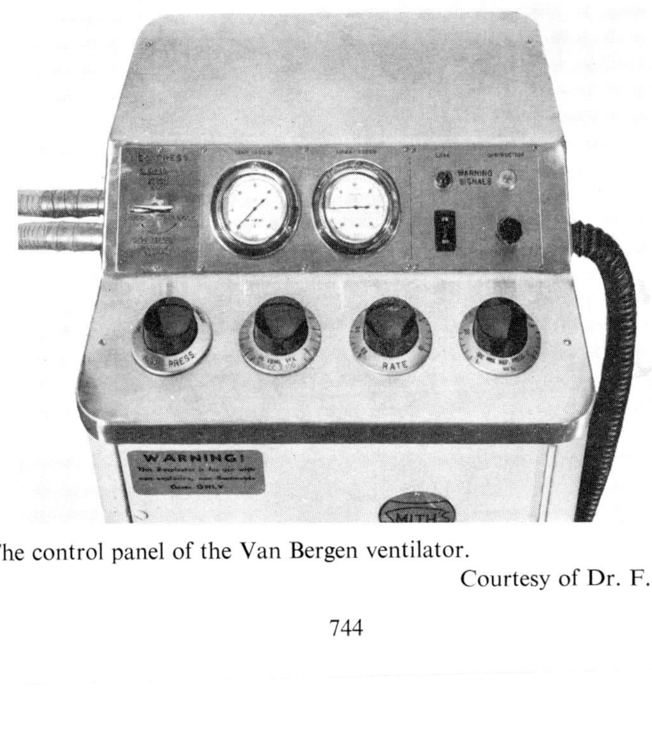

Fig. 88.1. The control panel of the Van Bergen ventilator.

Courtesy of Dr. F. H.Van Bergen.

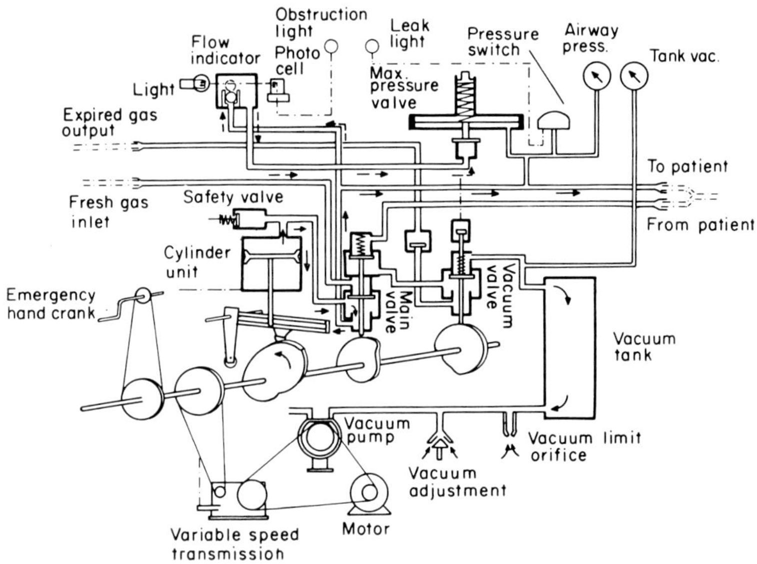

Fig. 88.2. Diagram of the Van Bergen ventilator—inspiratory phase.
Courtesy of *Anesthesiology*.[1]

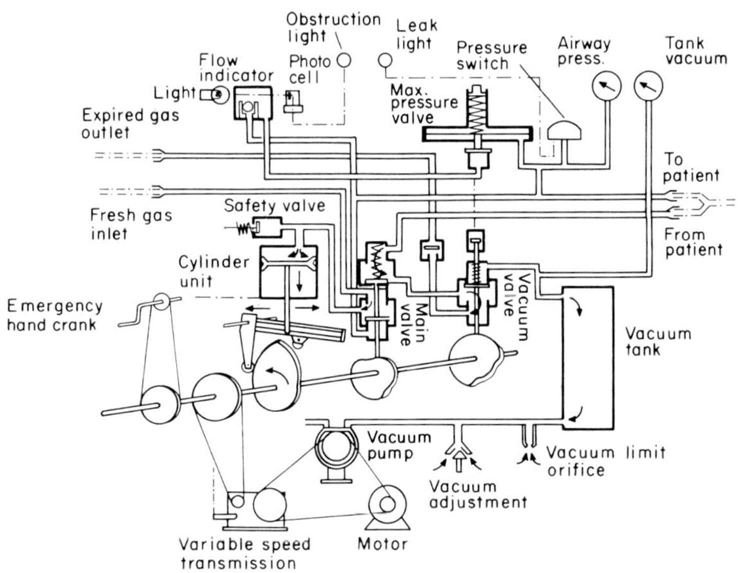

Fig. 88.3. Diagram of the Van Bergen ventilator—expiratory phase.
Courtesy of Smith Welding Equipment Corporation.

between 0 and -15 cmH_2O. Its source is a vacuum tank evacuated by a vacuum pump driven by the main motor. A third cam operates a valve which connects the expiratory tube to the vacuum tank at the proper time.

The maximum positive pressure can be varied by a spring-loaded diaphragm valve. When this pressure is exceeded, the escaping gas passes through a flow indicator and lights a warning light. This is labelled in figs. 88.2 and 88.3 as the 'Obstruction Light', since it would indicate an increase in the respiratory resistance. Either a removal of the cause of the obstruction is indicated, or an adjustment of the 'maximum pressure' valve to increase the delivery pressure to a point at which spillage ceases and the total ventilation is maintained. On the other hand, should the inflating pressure be less than 9 cm H_2O, a red warning signal lights up. This is called the 'Leak Light', since a common cause for its action is a break in the connexion between the apparatus and the patient. The maximum inspiratory pressure is 45 cmH_2O. The negative pressure is limited to -15 cmH_2O, by the 'vacuum limit orifice'. The inspiratory-expiratory ratio is fixed at 1 : 2.

FUNCTIONAL ANALYSIS

Inspiratory phase

In this phase the ventilator operates as a non-constant-flow generator owing to the constant speed of the electric motor. The pattern of flow is determined by the shape of a cam.

Change-over from inspiratory phase to expiratory phase

This change-over is volume-cycled and time-cycled: the constant-speed motor expels a preset volume of gas from the cylinder in a preset time. Provided the fresh-gas supply arrangements are such that no gas enters the cylinder during the inspiratory phase, then the volume entering the lungs will be exactly equal to that expelled by the piston, since normally no gas escapes during the phase.

Expiratory phase

In this phase the ventilator operates first as a constant, atmospheric, pressure generator: the expired gas passes freely to atmosphere at the 'expired gas outlet'.

Later, when the 'vacuum valve' connects the patient to the 'vacuum tank', the ventilator operates as a 'charging compliance' (see pp. 112 and 98).

Change-over from expiratory phase to inspiratory phase

This change-over is time-cycled: the duration of the expiratory phase is determined by the rotation of the cams.

REFERENCE

1 Van Bergen F.H., Buckley J.J., Weatherhead D.S.P., Schultz E.A. and Gordon J.R. (1956) A new respirator. *Anesthesiology*, **17**, 708.

CHAPTER 89

The 'Vellore' Ventilator[1, 2]

DESCRIPTION

This ventilator (fig. 89.1) was designed as a simple, reliable, and inexpensive apparatus for ward or anaesthetic use in tropical countries.

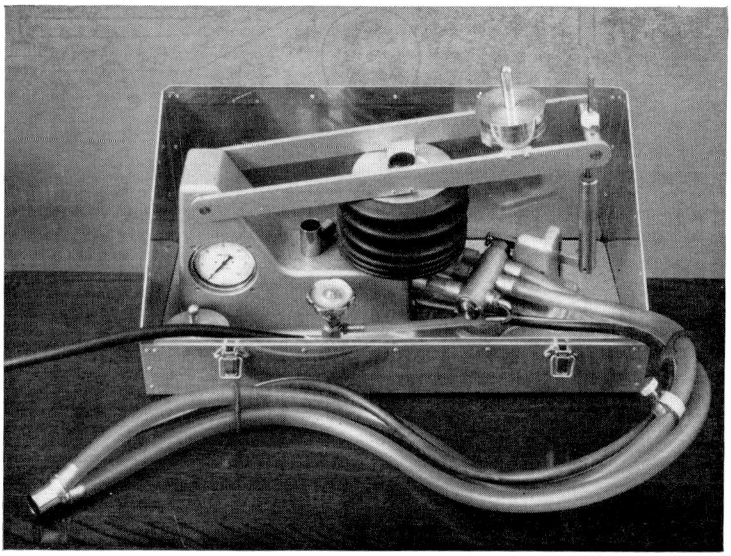

Fig. 89.1. The 'Vellore' ventilator.
Courtesy of Department of Medical Illustration, Cardiff Royal Infirmary.

The compressed gas which operates the ventilator is also delivered to the patient. Because the cyling valve (8) (fig. 89.2) has to be free to move easily, there is a small leakage of gas around it during the inspiratory phase, and the flow of gas required is slightly greater than the total minute-volume ventilation.

The compressed gas is supplied at a pressure of between 3 and 30 lb/in^2 at the inlet (6). During the expiratory phase it flows, through the cycling valve (8), into the concertina reservoir bag (1), at a rate determined by the setting of the 'minute volume' valve (7). The bag (1) is expanded, lifting the hinged beam (2) and the weights (3). The beam moves

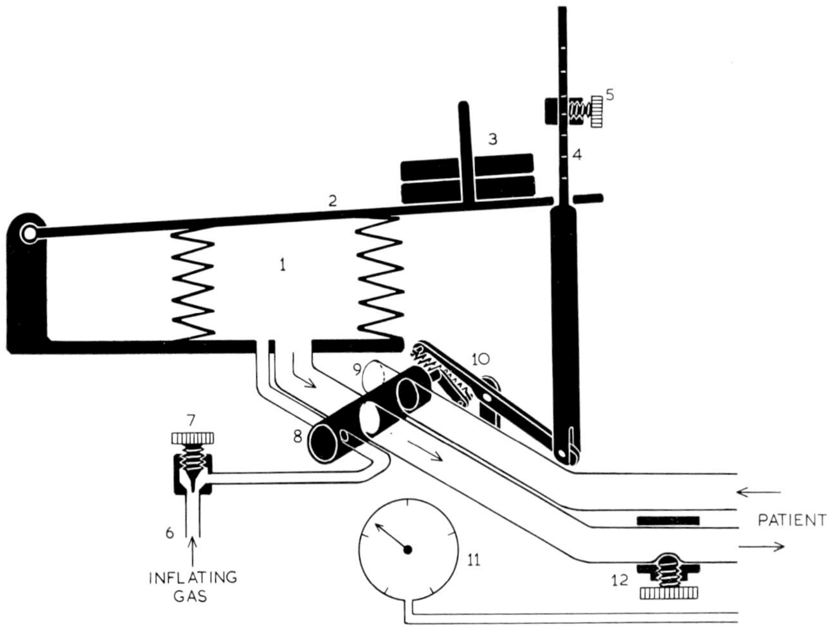

Fig. 89.2. Diagram of the 'Vellore' ventilator.

1. Concertina reservoir bag
2. Hinged beam
3. Weights
4. 'Respiratory volume setting' rod
5. 'Respiratory volume adjuster'
6. Inflating-gas inlet
7. 'Minute volume' control
8. Cycling valve
9. Expiratory port
10. Toggle
11. Manometer
12. Screw clip 'ratio valve'

upwards until its free end contacts the adjustable stop (5) ('respiratory volume adjuster') on the 'respiratory volume setting' rod (4), which is now also raised. This takes with it one end of the spring-loaded toggle lever (10), until, when this reaches its critical point, the spring flicks over, rotating the cycling valve (8) to the inspiratory position. The flow of compressed gas into the bag (1) is cut off, and free connexion is established between the bag (1) and the inspiratory tube. The force exerted by the weights (3) compresses the concertina bag (1) and the gas contained in it flows to the patient. As the beam (2) moves down it contacts the fixed stop on the rod (4). The rod (4) now moves down until the critical point is reached at which the click mechanism operates again. The position of the cycling valve (8) is reversed and inflation ceases. Expired gas now passes freely through the port (9) of the cycling valve (8) to atmosphere, and fresh gas again flows into the concertina bag (1).

The total minute-volume ventilation is controlled between 2 and 20 litres/min by the needle valve (7). The tidal volume is set by the stop (5) between 200 and 1200 ml. An infant-size concertina bag may be fitted, in which case the tidal volume is variable between 50 and 300 ml. Eight 10-ounce weights are provided, and these allow the inflation pressure to be adjusted between 10 and 30 cmH_2O. A screw clip (12) is fitted on the inspiratory tube and may be used to limit the inspiratory flow, and hence prolong the inspiratory time.

For economy, the basic unit has no instrumentation but provision is made for the addition of a manometer (11) to indicate inflation pressure. A Wright respirometer may be fitted to the expiratory port (9). There is no provision for manual ventilation. If this is required the ventilator must be disconnected.

FUNCTIONAL ANALYSIS

Inspiratory phase

During this phase the ventilator operates fundamentally as a constant-pressure generator owing to the constant force exerted by the weights (3) on the constant cross-sectional area of the concertina reservoir bag (1). However, the waveforms of pressure at the mouth in fig. 89.4 are considerably different from those of an ideal constant-pressure generator for the following reasons.

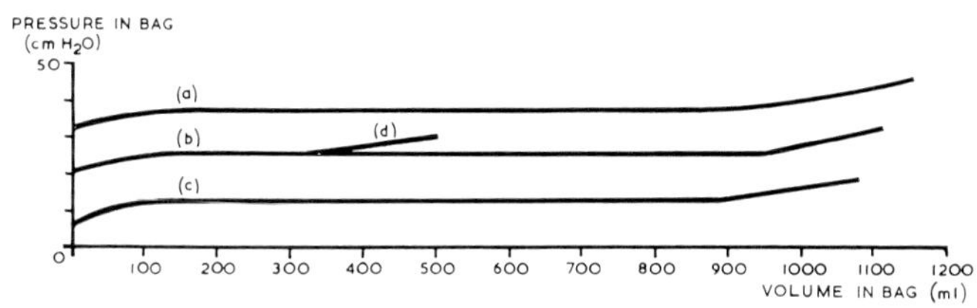

Fig. 89.3. The 'Vellore' ventilator. Pressure-volume characteristics of the concertina reservoir bag.

(a) With 8 weights added to the beam and the 'respiratory volume adjuster' set to maximum, i.e. to '10'.

(b) As (a) but with only 4 weights.

(c) As (a) but with no weights.

(d) With 4 weights, and the 'respiratory volume adjuster' set, not to '10', but to '3·9' as for the recordings in fig. 89.4 and fig. 89.5a, b, c, and e.

Firstly, the force acting on the bag is not constant throughout the phase: at the beginning of the phase the spring of the cycling-valve reversing mechanism (10) helps to compress the bag while, at the end of the phase, it opposes the action of the weights. However, the pressure is much more nearly constant over most of the volume excursion of the bag than is the case with many weighted or spring-loaded concertina bags.

Secondly, the inertia of the weights imposes some oscillation on the pressure in the bag.

Thirdly, there is inevitably some resistance between the bag, where the pressure is generated, and the mouth, where pressure is recorded. This resistance was moderately high when the recordings of fig. 89.4 were made because, with the generated pressure set high enough to ensure cycling in the face of a halved compliance (fig. 89.4b), the 'ratio valve' had to be screwed well down to obtain the 'standard' inspiratory time of 1 sec with the 'standard' values of compliance and resistance (fig. 89.4a).

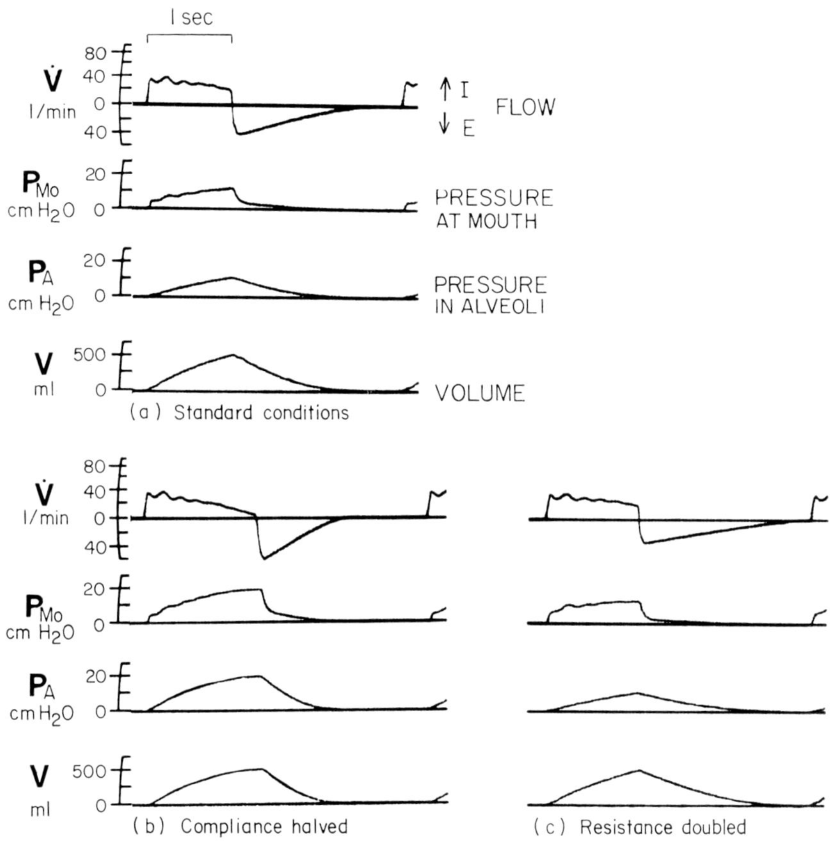

Fig. 89.4. The 'Vellore' ventilator. Recordings showing the effects of changes of lung characteristics.

Standard conditions: inflating gas, oxygen at 5 lb/in^2; 'respiratory volume adjuster', set to '3·9' for a tidal volume of 500 ml; 4 weights on the beam; 'ratio valve', set to give an inspiratory time of 1 sec and 'minute volume valve' set to give an expiratory time of 2 sec, and hence a respiratory frequency of 20/min and an inspiratory-expiratory ratio of **1:2.**

However, the generated pressure and inspiratory resistance used for fig. 89.4 were not so high as to convert the ventilator to a flow generator since the flow waveform is very much modified when the compliance is halved (fig. 89.4b). Therefore the ventilator must be regarded as a near-constant-pressure generator in this phase, with substantial series resistance. Nevertheless, if the maximum number of weights (eight) is applied, the generated pressure ranges between 32 and 45 cmH_2O (fig. 89.3a) and the ventilator does then make a fair approximation to a flow generator providing the compliance does not become too low.

Change-over from inspiratory phase to expiratory phase

This is volume-cycled; it occurs when a preset volume has been discharged from the concertina bag. In fig. 89.4 it can be seen that, when the lung characteristics are changed, the change-over always occurs immediately a given volume has been driven into the lungs, not when some critical pressure has been reached at the mouth nor after a fixed time. Since the inflating-gas flow is shut off during the inspiratory phase, and since the connecting tubes to the patient are non-distensible, the tidal volume will equal the stroke volume of the bag apart from any losses through leaks.

Expiratory phase

In this phase the 'Vellore' operates as a constant, atmospheric, pressure generator because the patient's lungs are connected to the atmosphere at the port (9). There is some resistance between this point and the mouth, at which pressure is recorded, so the pressure at the mouth (fig. 89.4) does not fall to the generated pressure until the flow has fallen to a low level. However, it is clear from fig. 89.4 that the flow waveform in the expiratory phase is considerably influenced by changes in lung characteristics: the decay is more rapid when the compliance is halved (fig. 89.4b) and more gradual when the resistance is doubled (fig. 89.4c).

Change-over from expiratory phase to inspiratory phase

This is time-cycled. It occurs when the concertina bag has been expanded through a preset volume excursion by means of a preset flow of inflating gas and therefore in a preset time. In fig. 89.4 it can be seen that the change-over occurs at a fixed time after the start of the expiratory phase, irrespective of changes of lung characteristics, and not immediately a given pressure has been reached at the mouth, nor immediately a given volume has come out of the lungs.

CONTROLS

Total ventilation

Despite some similarities of the 'Vellore' to the minute-volume dividers this ventilator does not operate in that way; the total ventilation cannot be directly controlled because the inflating gas does not flow continuously, but is shut off during the inspiratory phase. Therefore the tidal volume and respiratory frequency must be controlled separately.

Tidal volume

This is directly controlled by the 'respiratory volume adjuster' (5) and is not influenced by changes in the settings of the other controls (fig. 89.5). Since the ventilator is volume-cycled the tidal volume is not influenced by changes of lung characteristics (fig. 89.4). Even the small variation of tidal volume with compliance, which sometimes arises from the variable loss of volume in the compliance of the breathing tubes, is absent here, because the compliance of the smooth thick-walled tubing supplied with the ventilator is so small.

There are only two circumstances (apart from leaks) in which the tidal volume can vary inadvertently. One of these is when the initial flow rate out of the concertina bag is very high because of a combination of a heavy weight on the beam and a low total resistance to inflation (patient's respiratory resistance plus ventilator resistance). In these circumstances the 'respiratory volume setting rod' (4) falls freely at the start of the

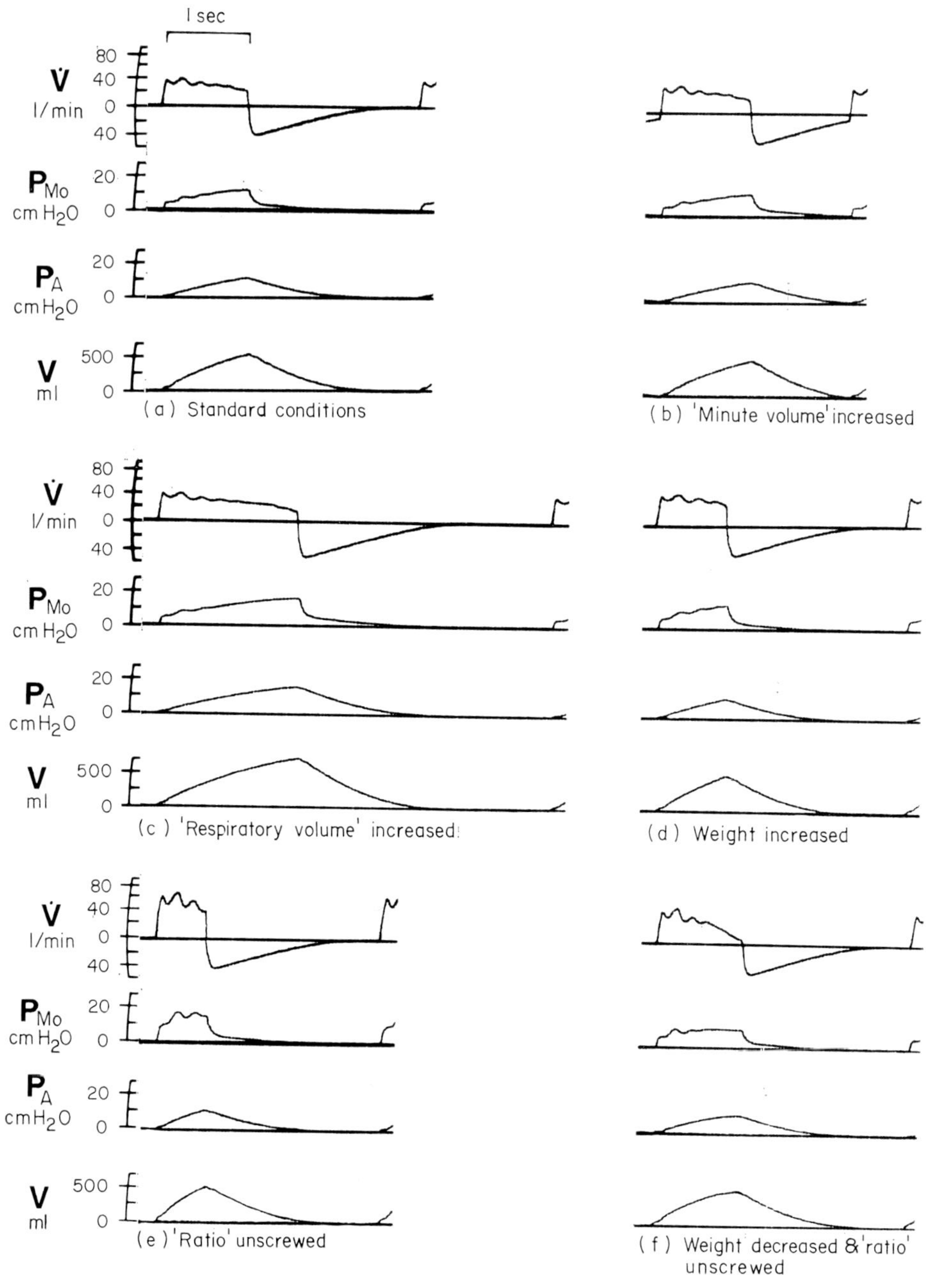

phase and its inertia is sufficient to reverse the cycling valve to expiration before the concertina bag has emptied. The other circumstance is when the weights are decreased, or when the compliance falls, to such an extent that the generated pressure is not sufficient to drive the preset tidal volume into the lungs. The ventilator then becomes arrested in the inspiratory phase.

Respiratory frequency and inspiratory-expiratory ratio

These cannot be directly controlled but are both determined by the separately-variable inspiratory and expiratory times.

The inspiratory time is the time taken to deliver the tidal volume. It can be decreased either by increasing the generated pressure, by means of adding weights to the beam (fig. 89.5d), or by decreasing the inspiratory resistance, by means of unscrewing the 'ratio valve' (fig. 89.5e). However, the extent to which the inspiratory time may be shortened is limited by the risk of premature cycling to expiration, by the inertia of the 'respiratory volume setting' rod (4) as explained under 'tidal volume' above. Thus in fig. 89.5e the 'ratio valve' was unscrewed as far as possible without introducing premature cycling.

The inspiratory time is incidentally-increased when the tidal volume is increased (fig. 89.5c) unless the weights or the 'ratio valve' are also adjusted to compensate. The inspiratory time is also influenced by changes of lung characteristics (fig. 89.4), particularly of compliance, although the influence is small if the maximum weight is used, and the 'ratio valve' is well screwed down, so that the ventilator approximates to a flow generator.

The expiratory time is the time taken to refill the concertina bag and therefore is directly controlled by the setting of the 'minute volume valve' (7). The expiratory time is incidentally-changed in exact proportion to any change in tidal-volume setting (fig. 89.5c), unless a compensating change of the 'minute volume valve' is made; but the timing is not influenced by changes of lung characteristics (fig. 89.4). Increasing the weight on the beam (fig. 89.5d) slightly increases the expiratory time because the leakage of inflating gas around the cycling valve is thereby increased.

Fig. 89.5. The 'Vellore' ventilator. Recordings showing the effects of changes in the settings of the controls.

(a) Standard conditions as in fig. 89.4.

(b) 'Minute volume valve' unscrewed one turn.

(c) 'Respiratory volume adjuster' increased from '3·9' to '6·2' to produce a tidal volume of 750 ml.

(d) Weights on the beam increased to 8.

(e) 'Ratio valve' unscrewed as far as was possible without introducing premature cycling to expiration.

(f) Weights on the beam decreased to one, the 'ratio valve' unscrewed to maintain an inspiratory time of 1 sec, and the 'minute volume valve' adjusted slightly to maintain an expiratory time of 2 sec.

Thus the respiratory frequency may be primarily controlled by the 'minute volume valve' but it is also influenced by changes in the settings of all the other controls (fig. 89.5) and, at least to some extent, by changes of lung characteristics (fig. 89.4). Similarly, the inspiratory-expiratory ratio may be primarily controlled by the 'ratio valve' (12), but is also influenced by all the other controls and by lung characteristics. However, a change of tidal volume does not have much effect on the inspiratory-expiratory ratio because it tends to change both the inspiratory and expiratory times in the same proportion (fig. 89.5c) especially if the ventilator is approximating to a flow generator in the inspiratory phase.

Inspiratory waveforms

This ventilator provides some degree of real choice of inspiratory waveforms for a given tidal volume and a given inspiratory time. If a small weight is used, and the 'ratio valve' is unscrewed the generated pressure is small, but the flow rate is initially high and declines rapidly (fig. 89.5f). On the other hand if a large weight is used, and the 'ratio valve' is well screwed down, the ventilator approximates to a flow generator and the initial flow is smaller but declines much less during the phase. The 'standard conditions' of fig. 89.5a go some way in this direction and may be compared with fig. 89.5f. However, the range of variation is rather small in practice since, if a small weight is used, quite a small decrease in compliance is sufficient to arrest the ventilator in an inspiratory phase. The four weights used for the 'standard conditions' of fig. 89.5a were the minimum necessary to ensure cycling when the compliance was halved.

Expiratory waveforms

There is no choice of expiratory waveforms; they are determined by the effect of the atmospheric pressure, generated at (9), on the lungs.

Pressure limits

Since the ventilator operates as a constant, atmospheric, pressure generator during the expiratory phase, the alveolar pressure normally falls to this level by the end of the phase. It does so in all the recordings in figs. 89.4 and 89.5, except for fig. 89.5b where the expiratory time is a little too short. The pressure will also fail to reach atmospheric if the respiratory resistance is very high. The peak alveolar pressure, at the end of the inspiratory phase cannot be directly controlled; whatever the minimum alveolar pressure at the end of the expiratory phase happens to be, the peak alveolar pressure exceeds it by an amount equal to the tidal volume divided by the compliance.

REFERENCES

1 Milledge J.S. (1963) Proceedings International Tetanus Conference, Bombay.
2 Milledge J. S. (1967) A simple automatic respirator. *Lancet*, **1**, 1090.

CHAPTER 90

The Williams 'Pneumoflator'[1, 2]

DESCRIPTION

This compact device plugs into the outlet from a continuous-flow type anaesthetic apparatus (e.g. the Boyle) (fig. 90.1) and is connected to the patient by a single breathing tube.

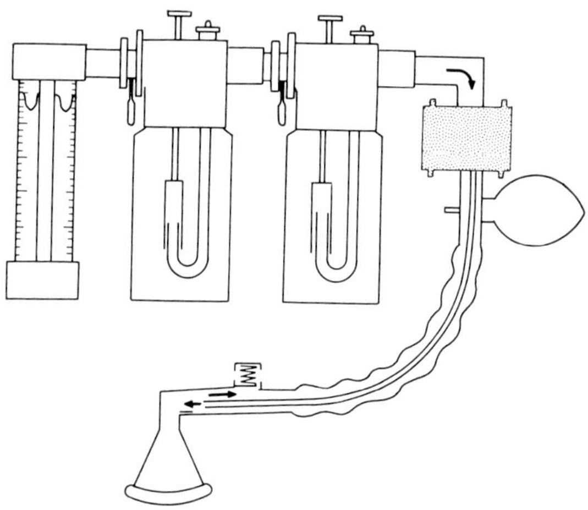

Fig. 90.1. Diagram of the Williams 'Pneumoflator' in position on a Boyle's anaesthetic apparatus. Note that the reservoir bag is switched out of circuit.

Courtesy of *British Journal of Anaesthesia.*[2]

The ventilator is driven by the anaesthetic gases from the flowmeters. The apparatus contains two stout rubber diaphragms (1) and (8) connected by a metal thrust rod (3). Lateral movement of this rod actuates the toggle trip switch (7), moving it from one extreme position to the other. The piston commutator of the gas valve (2) is attached to the trip switch.

In the inspiratory phase (fig. 90.2) the anaesthetic gases flow from the anaesthetic apparatus through the narrow tube (5), which lies within the corrugated breathing tube, to the patient. Meanwhile the pressure exerted behind the diaphragm (8) gradually rises and moves the diaphragm and the thrust rod (3) to the left until the trip switch (7) flicks over into the expiratory position.

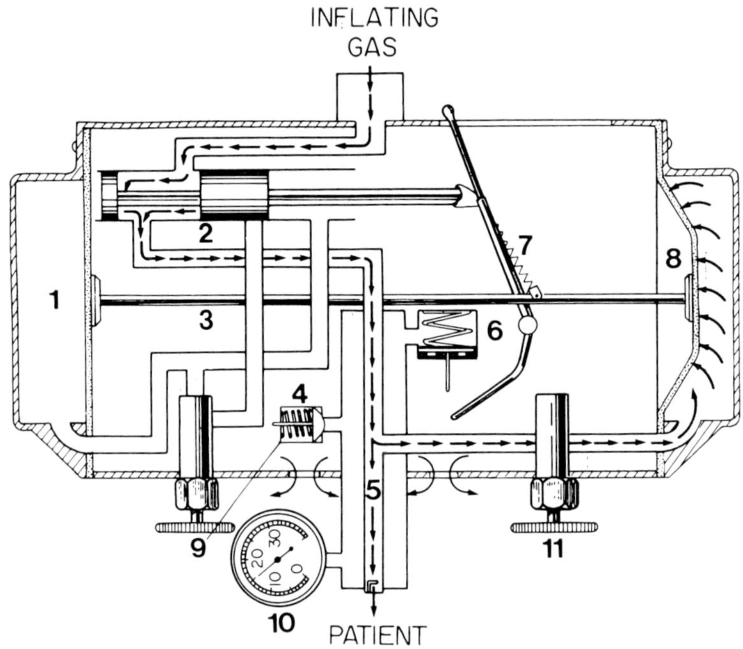

Fig. 90.2. Diagram of the Williams 'Pneumoflator'—inspiratory phase.

1. Stout rubber diaphragm
2. Gas valve with piston commutator
3. Metal thrust rod
4. Safety-valve
5. Narrow gas-delivery tube to patient
6. Expiratory valve
7. Toggle trip switch
8. Stout rubber diaphragm
9. Needle valve
10. Manometer
11. Needle valve

Courtesy of *British Journal of Anaesthesia.*[2]

In the expiratory phase (fig. 90.3) the gas supply to the patient is cut off by the movement of (2), and the large expiratory valve (6) is opened by the trip switch (7). The expired gas returns along the corrugated tubing from the patient and out through this valve. The circuit is thus unidirectional, no rebreathing taking place.

The inspiratory phase commences when the gas passing through the left-hand side of the valve (2) has built up enough pressure behind the diaphragm (1) to reverse the position of the trip switch (7). The maximum pressure during the inspiratory phase and the duration of the expiratory phase are controlled by the two needle valves (9, 11). The needle valve (11) controls the flow of gas to the chamber on the right of the diaphragm (8) and therefore influences the time taken for the pressure in the chamber to reach its critical value. It therefore helps to determine the duration of the inspiratory phase. This time is also influenced by the main flow of gas, and the characteristics of the lungs, which builds up pressure in the tube (5) on the left of the needle valve. The needle valve

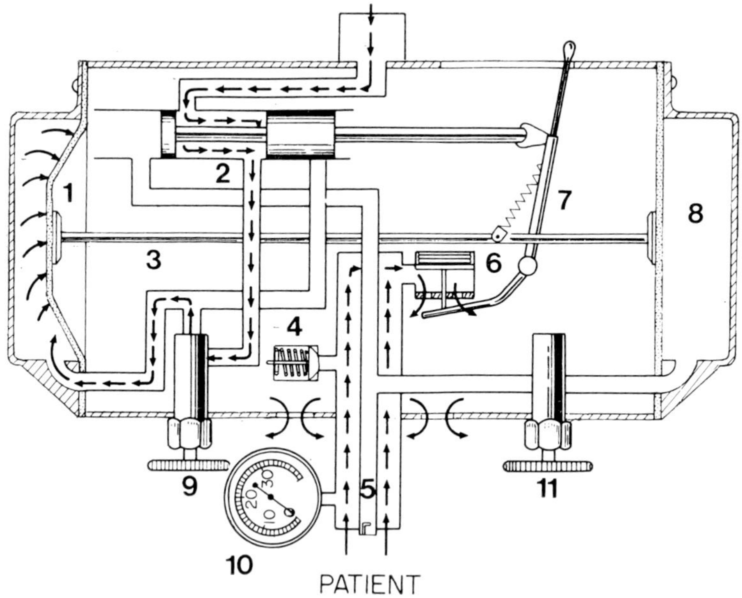

Fig. 90.3. Diagram of the Williams 'Pneumoflator'—expiratory phase.

1. Stout rubber diaphragm
2. Gas valve with piston commutator
3. Metal thrust rod
4. Safety-valve
5. Narrow gas-delivery tube to patient
6. Expiratory valve
7. Toggle trip switch
8. Stout rubber diaphragm
9. Needle valve
10. Manometer
11. Needle valve

Courtesy of *British Journal of Anaesthesia*.[2]

(9) controls the time taken for the pressure in the chamber on the left of the diaphragm (1) to reach its critical pressure, i.e. the duration of the expiratory phase.

It should be noted that the flow of gas into the ventilator, and hence the inspiratory flow, is limited to the output of the Boyle's apparatus, which, at the time when this ventilator was produced, was some 15 litres/min of metered gases. The total ventilation of the patient was therefore limited to about 8 litres/min.

FUNCTIONAL ANALYSIS

Inspiratory phase

In this phase the ventilator operates as a constant-flow generator owing to the constant high pressure from the reducing valves, applied to the resistances of the flow controls on the anaesthetic machine.

Change-over from inspiratory phase to expiratory phase

This change-over is a hybrid mixture of time-cycled and pressure-cycled (see p. 108). Cycling occurs when the pressure in the tube (5) (fig. 90.2), acting across the resistance of the needle valve (11), has raised the pressure behind the diaphragm (8) to the cycling value. If the pressure in (5) increases more rapidly, due to a change in the supply flow or to a change in the lung characteristics, cycling occurs after a shorter time but at a higher mouth pressure than before.

Expiratory phase

In this phase the ventilator operates as a constant, atmospheric, pressure generator: the expired gas passes freely to atmosphere at the expiratory valve (6).

Change-over from expiratory phase to inspiratory phase

This change-over is time-cycled: the expiratory phase ends when the pressure behind the diaphragm (1) has increased to the cycling value at a rate, and therefore in a time, which depends on characteristics of the ventilator and anaesthetic machine and is uninfluenced by the patient.

REFERENCES

1 WILLIAMS T.M. (1952) An automatic breathing attachment to Boyle's apparatus. *Br. J. Anaesth.* **24**, 222.

2 MUSHIN W.W. and RENDELL-BAKER L. (1954) Modern automatic respirators. *Br. J. Anaesth.* **26**, 131.

CHAPTER 91

Manual Controlled Ventilation: Manually-operated Ventilators

MANUAL CONTROLLED VENTILATION

Although this book is mainly concerned with the automatic ventilator it is not the authors' intention to give the impression that such a device is essential for the proper conduct of controlled respiration. It cannot be emphasized too strongly that efficient ventilation can be ensured by the rhythmic squeezing of a reservoir bag by hand. This method, indeed, is still very commonly used throughout the world. The expired gas is dealt with, either by passing it through the soda-lime canister of a closed circuit, or by discharging it to the atmosphere. The former is still a very-widely-used practice because of the great economy of gas and vapour usage which it achieves. However, in the case of the to-and-fro absorber, the position of the heavy canister is inconvenient, and soda-lime dust cannot altogether be excluded as partly responsible for post-operative tracheobronchitis. In any case, inefficient absorption, due to imperfect packing or exhaustion of the absorbent, may be more frequent than is generally realized. The uncontrolled production of water vapour and heat, once hailed as an advantage, has on one occasion at least been accused of leading to heat stroke and water intoxication![1] Where economy of gases and vapours is not a paramount consideration, therefore, an increasing number of anaesthetists now deal with expired carbon dioxide by discharging all expired gas to atmosphere, i.e. by using a non-rebreathing circuit.

Inflating valves

If a non-rebreathing circuit is to be used it is clearly necessary to ensure that, when the reservoir bag is compressed, the lungs are inflated, and that when no longer compressed, the bag refills with fresh gas while expired gas passes freely to atmosphere. This can be achieved by the use of an inflating valve.*

Pressure-equalizing valves

When fresh gas continues to enter any ventilator, manual or automatic, and rhythmic

* Some of these valves are sometimes referred to as 'non-rebreathing valves'. We feel that the term 'inflating valve' is less likely to lead to any confusion.

inflation is discontinued, an inflating valve may be forced into the 'closed' or inflating position. If a safety-valve is incorporated in the circuit, the pressure in the lungs increases to the limit set by this valve, and then remains at that limit indefinitely. If there is no safety-valve, the pressure can rise to a dangerous level. This risk can be entirely avoided either by delivering the fresh gas to a reservoir, open to the atmosphere, from which the ventilator takes the tidal volume,[2] or by incorporating a 'pressure-equalizing valve'. A pressure-equalizing valve permits the lungs to be inflated in the usual way, but prevents the pressure in the breathing circuit rising more than a few cmH_2O above atmospheric if rhythmic compression of the bag ceases.

Both inflating valves and pressure-equalizing valves are described in the next chapter.

MANUALLY-OPERATED VENTILATORS[3,4]

THE KREISELMAN 'BELLOWS RESUSCITATOR'
Figs. 91.1, 91.2, and 91.3

A concertina reservoir bag (1) is mounted on a face mask (2). The lungs are inflated by compressing the bag. When this is done (fig. 91.2) the inspiratory valve (8) does not open until the pressure in the bag forces the base-plate (5) and the inner tube (6) downwards. The inner tube now occludes the expiratory ports (7) and the inspiratory valve (8) is opened. A safety-valve (10) limits the pressure in the bag to 25 cmH_2O.

When compression of the bellows ceases (fig. 91.3), the spring (9) forces up the base-plate (5) and the inner tube (6) of the sliding valve. The valve (8) is closed and expired gas escapes freely to atmosphere through the expiratory port (7). At the same time, during the expiratory phase, the expansion of the bellows draws in air through the one-way valve (3). Oxygen may be added at the inlet (4) which incorporates a non-return valve.

A modified form of the Kreiselman 'Resuscitator', similar in appearance and mode of action, has been designed by the Chemical Defence Experimental Establishment in Great Britain[5,6] (fig. 91.4).

THE 'OXFORD' INFLATING BELLOWS[7]
Figs. 91.5, and 91.6

This apparatus consists of the concertina reservoir bag of the Connell anaesthetic apparatus[8] with a spiral spring inside, the function of which is to expand, and so refill, the bag during the expiratory phase. An inlet tube and tap allow oxygen to be added.

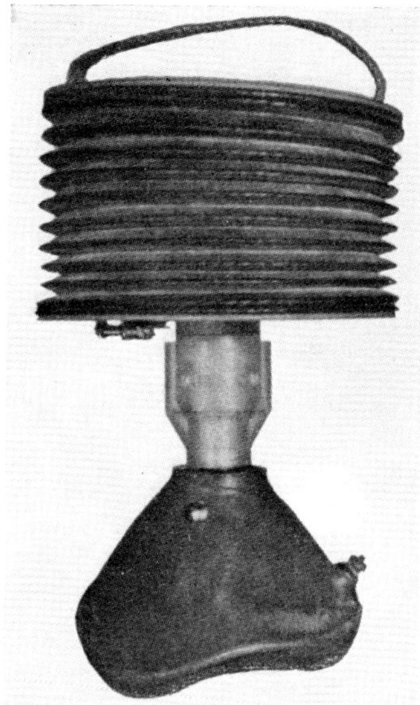

Fig. 91.1.

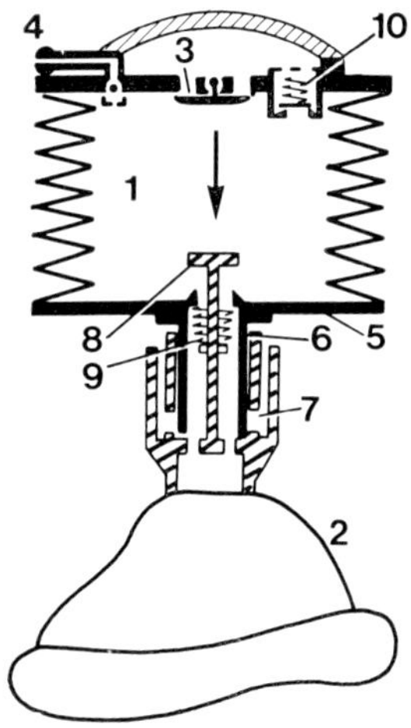

Fig. 91.2.

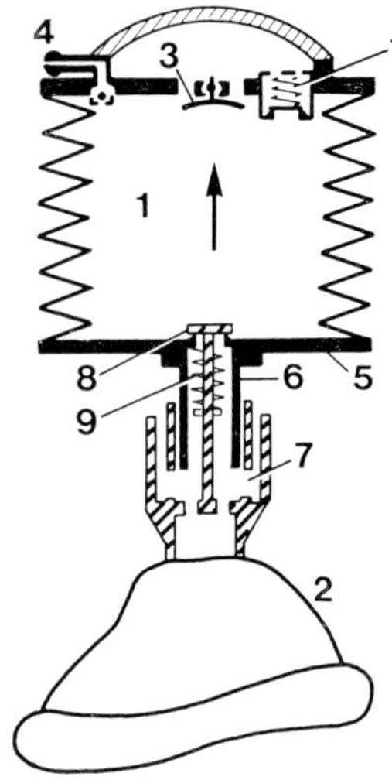

Fig. 91.3.

Fig. 91.1. The Kreiselman 'Bellows Resuscitator'.

Courtesy of *Anesthesiology*.[3]

Fig. 91.2. Diagram of the Kreiselman 'Bellows Resuscitator'—inspiratory phase.
Fig. 91.3. Diagram of the Kreiselman 'Bellows Resuscitator'—expiratory phase.

1. Concertina reservoir bag
2. Face mask
3. One-way air-inlet valve
4. Oxygen inlet
5. Base-plate of concertina reservoir bag
6. Inner tube of sliding valve
7. Expiratory ports of sliding valve
8. Inspiratory valve
9. Compression spring
10. Safety-valve

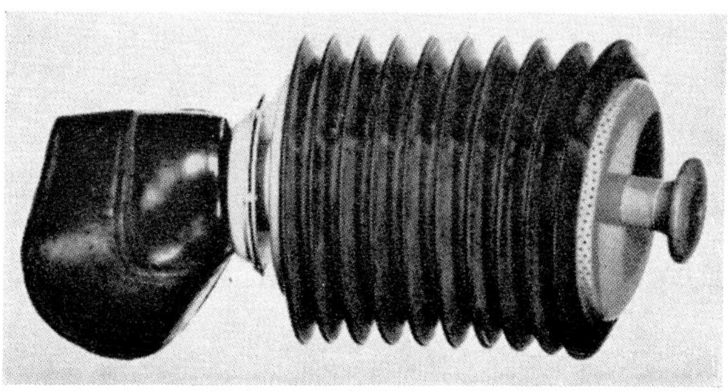

Fig. 91.4. The 'Chemical Defence Resuscitator'.

Courtesy of *British Medical Journal*.[6]

Two gravity-operated valves ensure unidirectional flow so that rebreathing is avoided. When the bag is compressed, the lungs are inflated.

The apparatus is connected to the patient by a standard corrugated breathing tube. When it is used with a face mask, slightly raising the mask allows passive expiration to

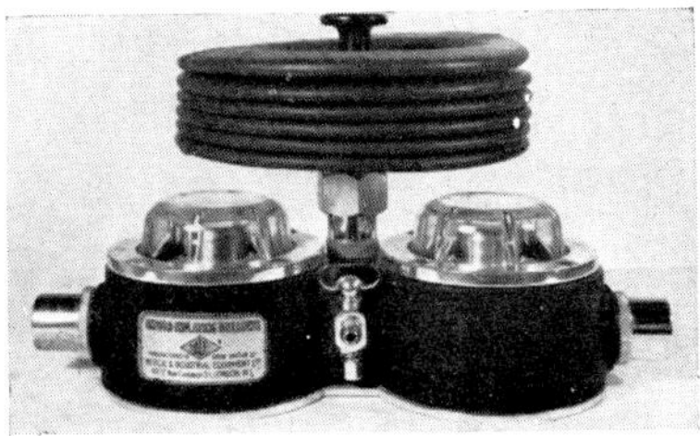

Fig. 91.5. The 'Oxford' Inflating Bellows.

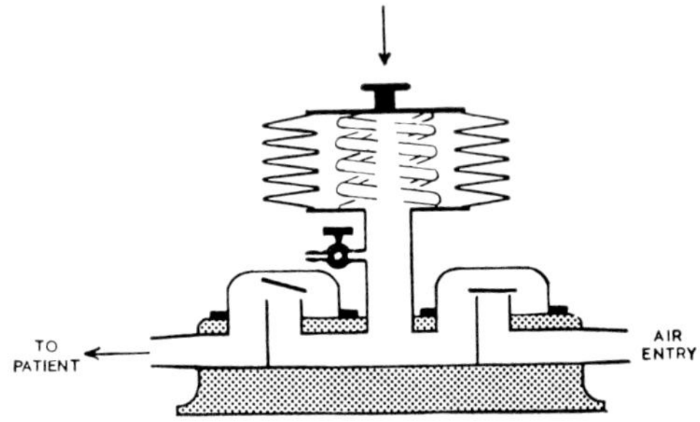

Fig. 91.6. Diagram of the 'Oxford' Inflating Bellows.

take place. When it is used with an endotracheal tube, an inflating valve is necessary, and the one-way outlet valve of the bellows must be put out of action. This may be done by removing the disc of the outlet valve, or by holding it off its seating with the magnet provided.

THE RUBEN 'AMBU' BAG[9,10]

Figs. 91.7, and 91.8

When the bag of this apparatus is squeezed the gas within it is forced, through the Ruben valve (2) (see p. 790), into the patient's lungs. When pressure on the bag is released, the elastic recoil of the sponge rubber with which it is lined re-expands the bag and fresh air is drawn in through the one-way valve (3). At the same time expired gas escapes freely through the expiratory port of the Ruben valve.

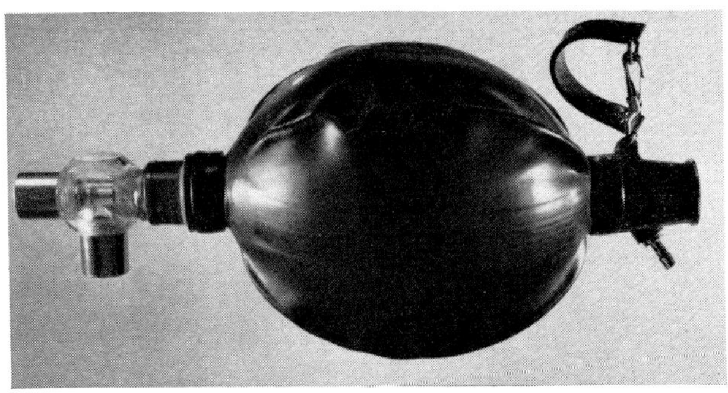

Fig. 91.7. The Ruben 'Ambu' Bag.

Courtesy of Department of Medical Illustration, Cardiff Royal Infirmary.

The sponge-rubber lining of the bag is not uniformly thick but is strengthened towards each 'pole' and round the 'equator' of the bag.

Many variations of the original 'Ambu' self-filling bag have been developed. A large

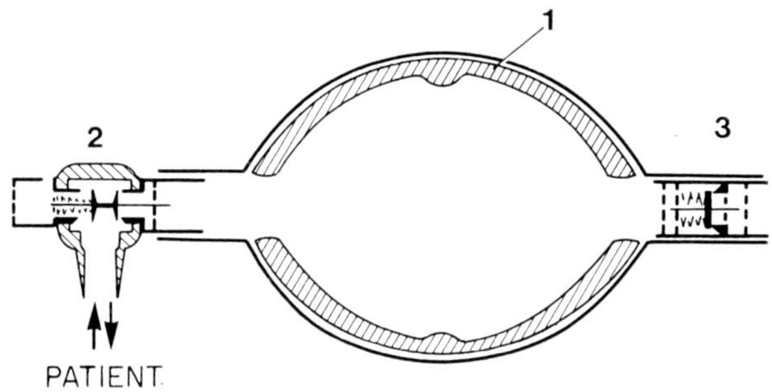

Fig. 91.8. Diagram of the Ruben 'Ambu' bag.
1. Reservoir bag with sponge-rubber lining 2. Ruben inflating valve 3. One-way valve

proportion of these are unlined and rely for refilling on the elastic recoil of the bag itself. This may mean that the bag is made of quite firm rubber or plastic and that some of the sense of pressure felt by the hand is therefore lost. Most manufacturers supply an inflating valve of their own design for use with their own particular bag.

THE ETSTEN VENTILATOR[11]
Figs. 91.9, and 91.10

This is one of the few manually-operated ventilators in which negative pressure can be applied during the expiratory phase. The operator's elbow rests on the platform (1) and his hand on the knob (2). Downward movement of the hinged plate (3) compresses the concertina reservoir bag (4), forcing its contents, through the corrugated tubing (5), to the patient. During the expiratory phase gas flows back into the bag (4) until the upward movement of the plate (3) is arrested by the fixed stop (6). Just before the plate reaches this point the chain (7) inside the bag is fully stretched and the valve (8) to which it is attached is lifted, allowing any excess of expired gas to flow into the reserve bag (9). The spring (10), attached to one end of the hinged plate (3), assists the expansion of the bag (4). The tension of this spring may be adjusted by the control (11). If the tension is set high enough, the bag (4) expands faster than expired gas flows from the patient and a negative pressure is produced within the bag (4). The volume of gas delivered from the bag (4) is indicated on the scale (12) and depends on the position of the adjustable stop (13) which limits the downward movement of the plate (3). The pressure is indicated on the manometer (14). An adjustable spring-loaded blow-off valve (15) limits the positive pressure and, in closed-circuit use, allows the escape of excess gas.

If desired, the plate (3) may be allowed to remain in its top position, in which case the reserve bag (9) functions as an ordinary reservoir bag. Spontaneous breathing can

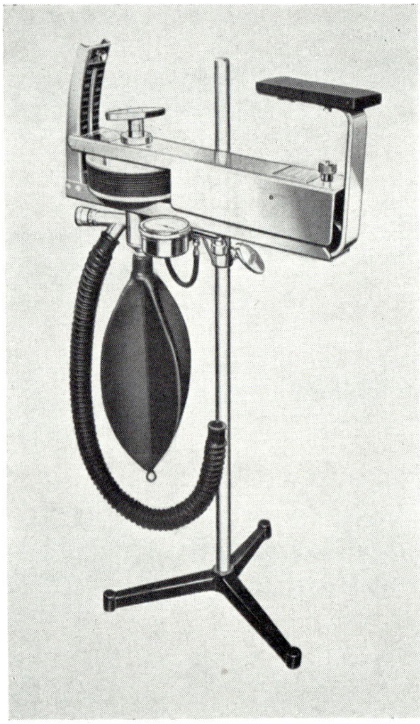

Fig. 91.9.

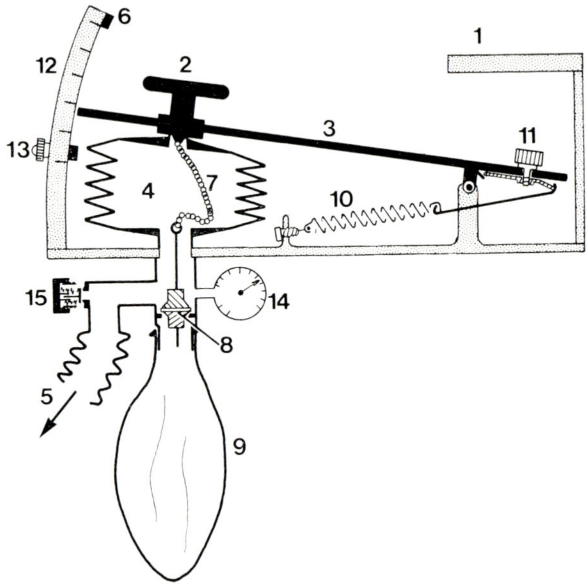

Fig. 91.10.

Fig. 91.9. The Etsten ventilator.

Courtesy of Ohio Chemical & Surgical Equipment Co.

Fig. 91.10. Diagram of the Etsten ventilator.

1. Elbow rest
2. Hand grip
3. Hinged plate
4. Concertina reservoir bag
5. Corrugated breathing tube
6. Fixed stop
7. Chain
8. Valve
9. Reserve bag
10. Expansion spring
11. Negative-pressure control
12. Volume scale
13. Adjustable stop
14. Manometer
15. Adjustable blow-off valve

then take place, or, alternatively, controlled respiration can be performed by squeezing the bag (9). If the fresh-gas flow is high, the reserve bag (9) may be detached, in which case the valve (8) acts as a spill valve, venting excess gas to atmosphere at the end of the expiratory phase.

Some basic similarity will be seen between the Etsten ventilator and the simple adaptation of the 'Oxford' Inflating Bellows[12] illustrated in fig. 91.11.

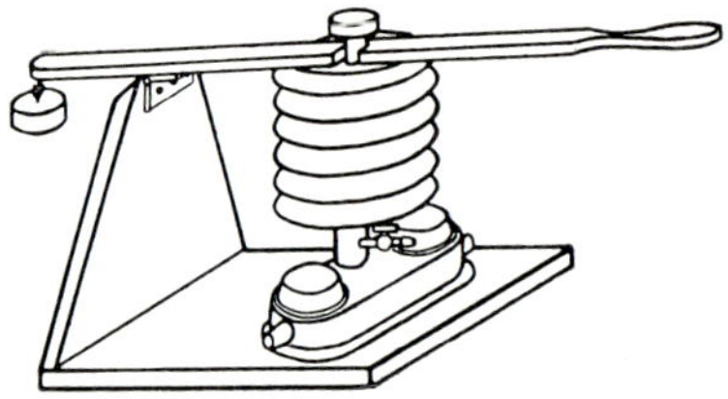

Fig. 91.11. The Hillard adaptation of the 'Oxford' Inflating Bellows.

THE POPPELBAUM VENTILATOR[13]

Figs. 91.12, and 91.13

The ventilator consists of a double concertina bag. When this bag is compressed the contents of the outer chamber (1) are forced, through the one-way valve (4) and the

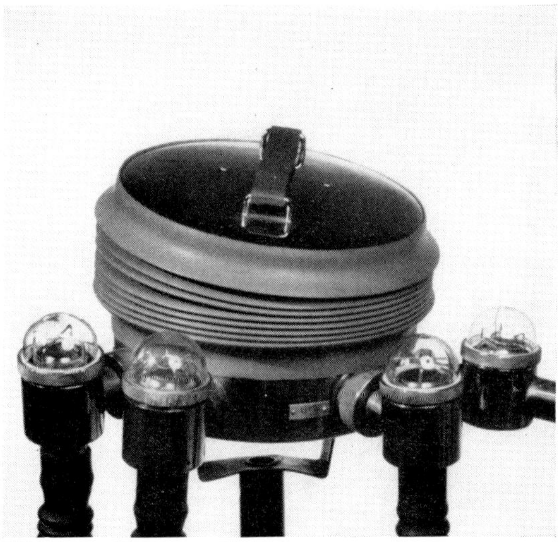

Fig. 91.12.

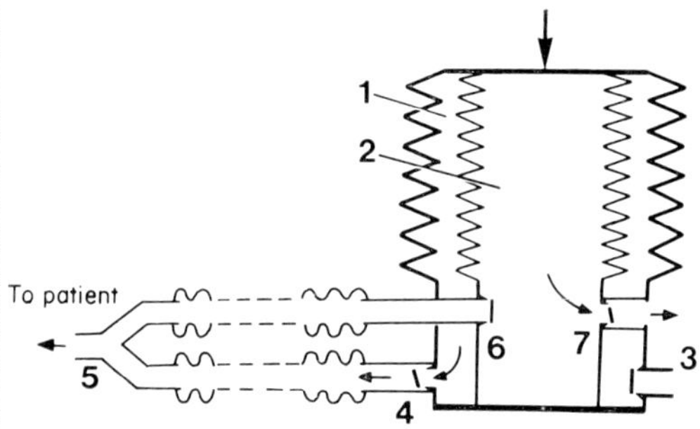

Fig. 91.13.

Fig. 91.12. The Poppelbaum ventilator.

Courtesy of Dr. F. Poppelbaum.

Fig. 91.13. Diagram of the Poppelbaum ventilator—inspiratory phase.

1. Outer chamber of double concertina bag
2. Inner chamber of double concertina bag
3. One-way inlet valve
4. One-way inspiratory valve
5. Y-connexion to patient
6. One-way expiratory valve
7. One-way outlet valve

Y-connexion (5), to the patient. At the same time the contents of the inner chamber (2) are forced, through the one-way valve (7), to atmosphere. When the top-plate of the bag is pulled up expired gas is drawn through the one-way valve (6) into the inner chamber (2), and fresh air or anaesthetic gas is drawn through the one-way valve (3) into the outer chamber (1). The negative pressure produced during the expiratory phase depends on the force used to pull up the top-plate.

Poppelbaum also described a manually-operated ventilator[14] consisting of a calibrated concertina bag in a closed circuit. The bag is so strengthened that during the expansion stroke a negative pressure of up to -5 cmH_2O can be produced. A pressure-sensitive switch starts a small sampling pump towards the end of the expiratory phase, so that the end-expiratory carbon dioxide can be estimated. This simple arrangement is similar to one described by MacKay[15] in which the reservoir bag of a Coxeter-Mushin absorber,[19] though still connected to the absorber, is mounted on the anaesthetic table.

THE 'CARDIFF' INFLATING BELLOWS[16]

Figs. 91.14, 91.15, and 91.16

This apparatus incorporates the 'Cardiff' inflating valve (see p. 779). In other respects it is similar to the Kreiselman 'Bellows Resuscitator' (see p. 760).

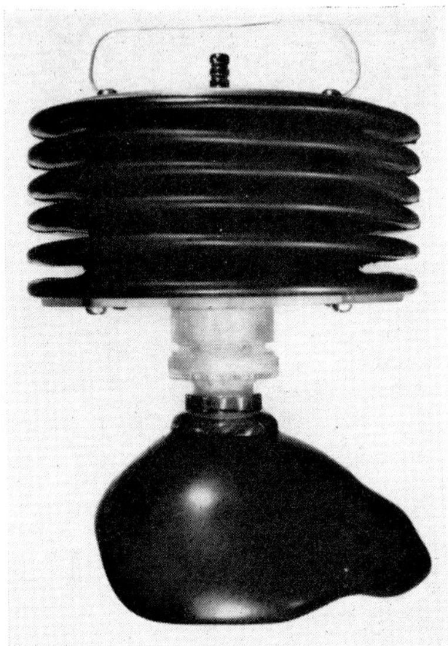

Fig. 9.14.

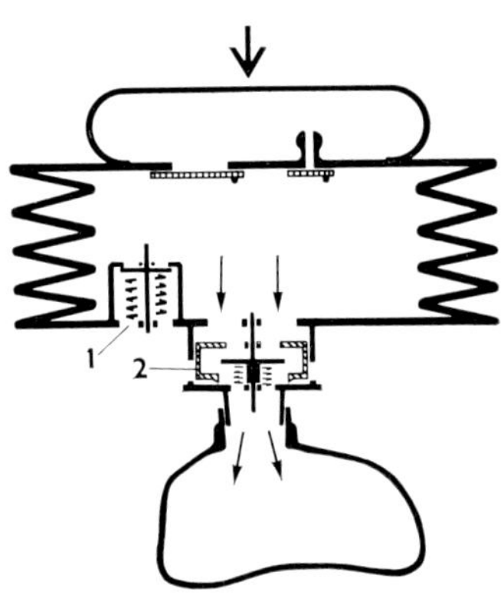

Fig. 91.15.

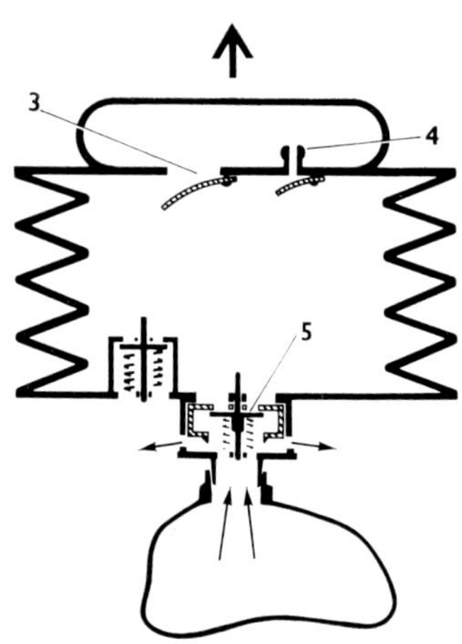

Fig. 91.16.

Fig. 91.14. The 'Cardiff' Inflating Bellows.

Courtesy of Department of Medical Illustration, Cardiff Royal Infirmary.

Fig. 91.15. Diagram of the 'Cardiff' Inflating Bellows—inspiratory phase.

Fig. 91.16. Diagram of the 'Cardiff' Inflating Bellows—expiratory phase.

1. Safety-valve
2. Piston
3. Air-inlet valve
4. Oxygen inlet
5. One-way valve

THE CLUTTON-BROCK MANUAL VENTILATOR[17]

Figs. 91.17, and 91.18

This apparatus is a 'weighted-bag-in-bottle' arrangement designed to introduce a phase of negative pressure into manually-performed controlled respiration with a closed

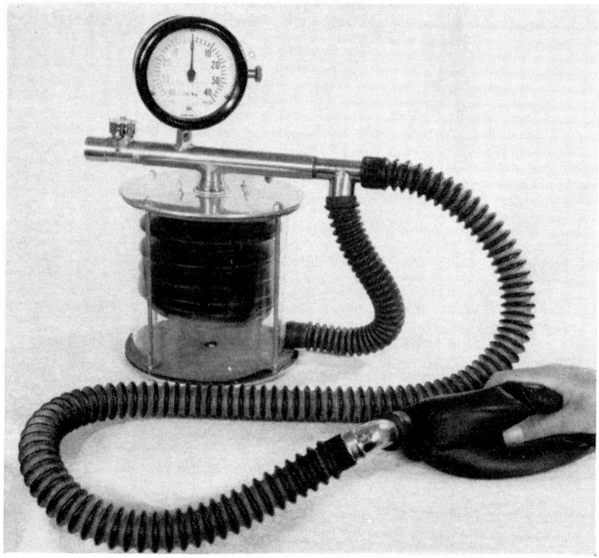

Fig. 91.17. The Clutton-Brock manual ventilator.

Courtesy of Professor J. Clutton-Brock.

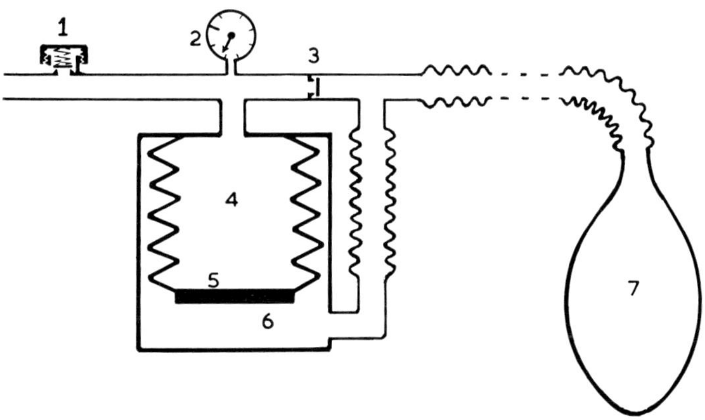

Fig. 91.18. Diagram of the Clutton-Brock manual ventilator.

1. Adjustable blow-off valve
2. Manometer
3. One-way valve
4. Concertina reservoir bag
5. Weight
6. Rigid plastic pressure chamber
7. Bag

circuit. When the bag (7) is squeezed, pressure rises in the rigid plastic pressure chamber (6) and the contents of the weighted concertina bag (4) are forced to the patient. When the bag (7) is released, the weight (5) aids the expansion of the concertina bag (4). This produces a negative pressure within the bag (4) and a positive pressure in the chamber (6). The one-way valve (3) is therefore held closed, and expired gas flows into the bag (4). At the same time the gas in the chamber (6) is forced back into the bag (7). If negative pressure is to be maintained throughout the expiratory phase the concertina bag (4) must not be allowed to 'bottom' and excess gas must be blown off through the valve (1) during the inspiratory phase. In these circumstances the one-way valve (3) is held closed throughout the respiratory cycle. If the bag (4) is fully expanded before the end of the expiratory phase, the negative pressure within it decays rapidly and any excess gas spills through the one-way valve (3) to the bag (7). This process can be used to prime the bag (7) and to top it up as necessary to compensate for any leakage. A manometer (2) indicates the pressure in the breathing circuit.

THE 'CARDIFF' INFANT INFLATING BAG[18]

Figs. 91.19, and 91.20

This small inflating bag was designed for safe manual artificial ventilation of the new-

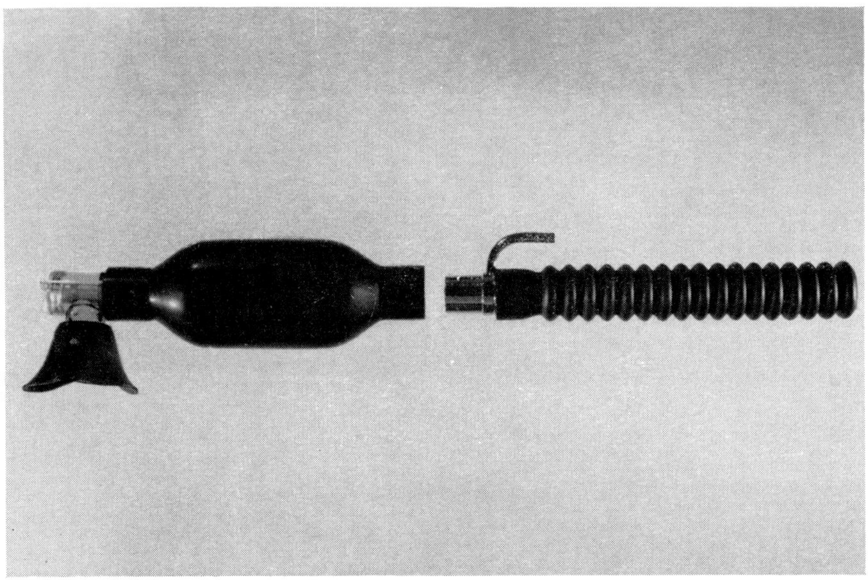

Fig. 91.19. The 'Cardiff' Infant Inflating Bag.

Courtesy of *British Medical Journal*.[18]

born. When the bag (2) is squeezed its contents are forced, through the inflating valve (1), to the baby.

A small leak-hole in the cap of the inflating valve (1) allows some escape of gas during inflation. The pressure produced in the lungs, therefore, depends not only on the volume displaced from the bag and the compliance of the lungs but also on the speed of

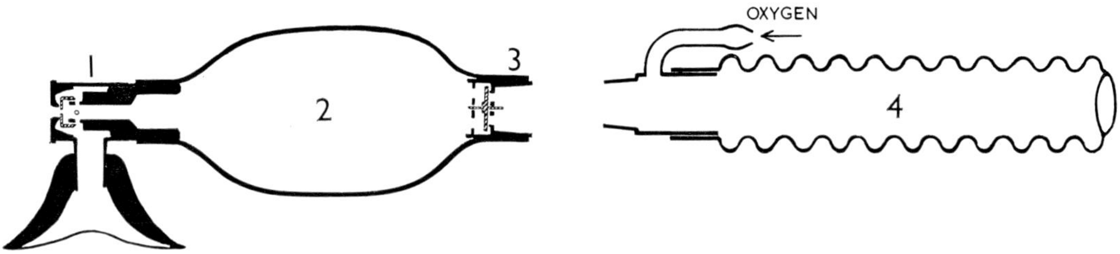

Fig. 91.20. Diagram of the 'Cardiff' Infant Inflating Bag.

1. Inflating valve
2. Self-expanding bag
3. One-way inlet valve
4. Reservoir tube

inflation and the airway resistance. The volume of the bag and the size of the leak-hole is such that when the bag is squeezed very rapidly a maximum pressure of about 150 cm H_2O is produced when the compliance of the lungs is zero, and a maximum pressure of only 10 cmH_2O when the compliance is 5 ml/cmH_2O. When the bag (2) is released, gas escapes, through the inflating valve (1), to atmosphere, and, as the bag re-expands, fresh gas is drawn in through the one-way valve (3).

A separate reservoir tube (4) with an oxygen inlet can be attached to the bag. This ensures that, no matter what flow of oxygen is supplied, the pressure in the inflating bag cannot be increased inadvertently.

REFERENCES

1 Clark R.E., Orkin L.R. and Rovenstine E.A. (1954) Body temperature studies in anesthetized man. Effect of environmental temperature, humidity and anesthesia system. *J. Am. med. Ass.* **154**, 311.

2 Saklad M. and Gulati R. (1963) Adaptation of Ambu respirator for high oxygen concentration. *Anesthesiology*, **24**, 877.

3 Kreiselman J. (1943) A new resuscitation apparatus. *Anesthesiology*, **4**, 608.

4 Report of Council on Physical Medicine. (1944) Kreiselman Resuscitator bellows type, Model 110, acceptable. *J. Am. med. Ass.* **126**, 99.

5 Chief characteristics of nerve gas. Notes on first aid treatment. (1952) *Br. med. J.* **2**, 334.

6 Lucas B.G.B. and Whitcher H.W. (1958) Artificial respiration. Comparison between manual and intermittent positive-pressure methods. *Br. med. J.* **2**, 887.

7 Macintosh R.R. (1953) Oxford inflating bellows. *Br. med. J.* **2**, 202.

8 Macintosh R.R., Mushin W.W. and Epstein H.G. (1963) *Physics for the Anaesthetist*, 3rd ed., p. 210. Oxford: Blackwell.

9 Ruben H. and Ruben A. (1957) Apparatus for resuscitation and suction. *Lancet*, **2**, 373.

10 Ruben H., Knudsen E.J., Winkel E. and Hjorth, Aa. (1958) Eine narkosemethode, dic auch in katastrophensituationen gebraucht werden kann. *Anaesthesist*, **7**, 161.

11 Dobkin A.B. (1958) Evaluation of a ventilator with fixed volume control and variable regulated pressure. *Can. Anaesth. Soc. J.* **5**, 288.

12 Hillard E.K. (1954) A lever for the Oxford bellows. *Anaesthesia*, **9**, 121.

13 POPPELBAUM H.F. (1957) Die wechseldruckbeatmung unter apnoe bei geschlossenem und offenem thorax und zur reanimation. *Anaesthesist*, **6**, 25.

14 POPPELBAUM H.F. (1956) Uber wechseldruckbeatmung in der transpleuralen lungenschirurgie. *Dtsch. Gesundht.-Wes.* **11**, 890.

15 MACKAY I.M. (1956) A new manual respirator. *Can. Anaesth. Soc. J.* **3**, 113.

16 HILLARD E.K. and MUSHIN W.W. (1960) The Cardiff inflating bellows. *Br. med. J.* **2**, 729.

17 CLUTTON-BROCK J. (1962) A device for introducing a phase of subatmospheric pressure into manually performed IPPR. *Br. J. Anaesth.* **34**, 746.

18 MUSHIN W.W. and HILLARD E.K. (1967) A neonatal inflating bag. *Br. med. J.* **1**, 416.

19 MUSHIN W.W. (1943) A new circle type carbon dioxide absorber. *Br. J. Anaesth.* **18**, 97.

CHAPTER 92

Valves for use in Controlled Ventilation

INFLATING VALVES

The basic features of a true inflating valve (fig. 92.1) are an inspiratory port (1), an expiratory port (2), and a third port (3) for connexion to the patient, all interconnected

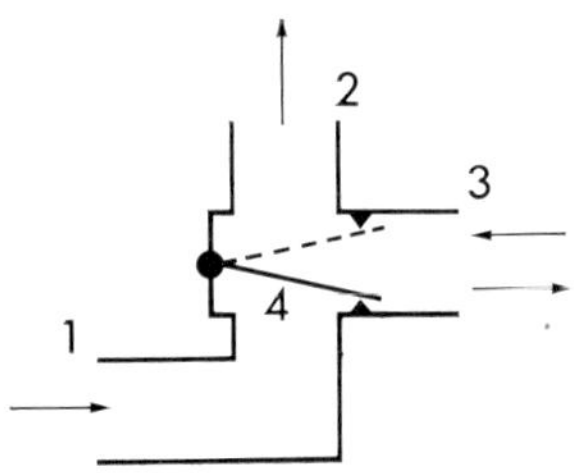

Fig. 92.1. Diagram showing the basic features of an inflating valve.
1. Inspiratory port
2. Expiratory port
3. Port for connexion to patient
4. Valve mechanism

by some valve mechanism (4). The function of this mechanism is to ensure (a) that during the inspiratory phase the expiratory port is blocked and all the inflating gas, delivered at the inspiratory port from a ventilator or a manually-compressed reservoir bag, is delivered to the patient, and (b) that during the expiratory phase the expiratory port is unblocked to permit free expiration and, in most cases, the inspiratory port is blocked, thereby eliminating rebreathing.[1]

Although the number of inflating valves is large, the number of mechanical principles on which they work is relatively limited. It is therefore possible to group the valves broadly according to their mode of operation. For instance, the rubber flap in the Lewis-Leigh valve, the rubber disc in the Aga 'Polyvalve', the disc in the Tashiro-Wakai valve, the disc in the 'Ambu Magnet' valve, and the loosely-held leaves of the one-way valves in the 'Ambu E' valve, all perform the same function as the hinged flap in the original Neff valve. Nevertheless, each valve differs in detail.

We have listed the inflating valves according to their mode of operation, and, within each group, arranged them chronologically and according to their date of publication. However, the subsequent descriptions are given in alphabetical order for convenience of reference.

Type A (fig. 92.2)

The Neff valve[2]
The Lewis-Leigh valve[3]
The Aga 'Polyvalve'
The Tashiro-Wakai valve[4]
The 'Ambu Magnet' valve

A free-moving flap or disc (4) is forced away from the inspiratory port (1) onto the expiratory port (2) during inflation. During the expiratory phase the flap or disc reseats on the inspiratory port; the inspiratory port is now closed and the expiratory port is open.

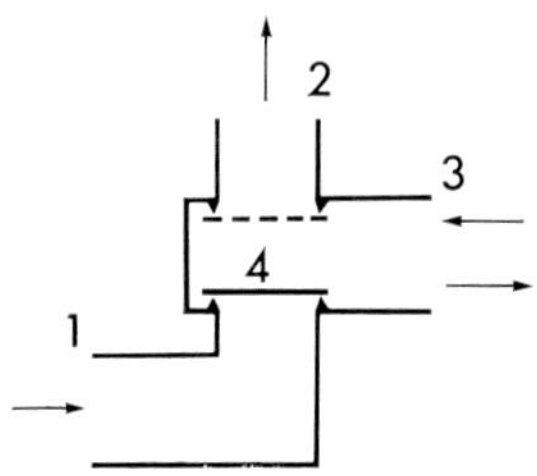

Fig. 92.2. Diagram of inflating valve, type A.
1. Inspiratory port
2. Expiratory port
3. Port for connexion to patient
4. Flap or disc

Type B (fig. 92.3)

The Stott 'ping-pong ball' valve[5]
The Ruben valve[6,7]
The 'Magnetic POI' valve[8]

A ball or bobbin (4) performs the same function as the flap or disc of a type A valve.

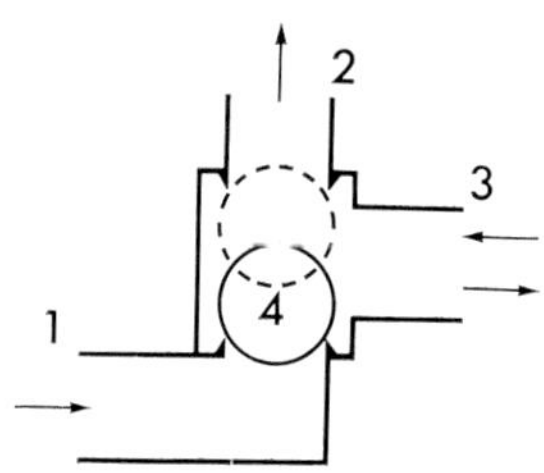

Fig. 92.3. Diagram of inflating valve, type B.
1. Inspiratory port
2. Expiratory port
3. Port for connexion to patient
4. Ball or bobbin

Type C (fig. 92.4)

The 'Cardiff' valve[9]
The Newton valve[10]
The 'Dewsbury' valve[11]
The Zuck valve[12]

A freely-moving piston (4) performs the same function as the flap or disc of a type **A** valve.

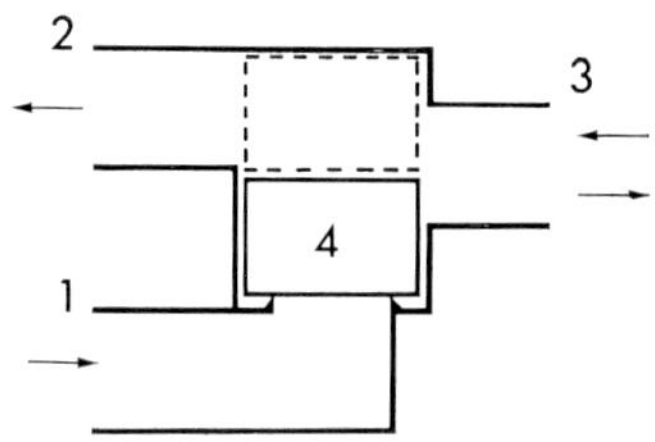

Fig. 92.4. Diagram of inflating valve, type C.
1. Inspiratory port
2. Expiratory port
3. Port for connexion to patient
4. Piston

Type D (fig. 92.5)

The Beaver valve
The Stott valve[13]
The Flach-Voss valve [14]
The Fink valve[15]
The Aga valve[16]
The Shuman valve[17]
The Etheridge valve[18]
The Frumin valve[19]
The 'Ranima' valve
The 'Ambu E' valve

During inflation gas is delivered to the patient through a one-way valve (5) and the inflating pressure distends a diaphragm (4) which occludes the expiratory port (2). When inflation ceases and the pressure at the inspiratory port (1) falls, the one-way valve (5) closes, the diaphragm (4) relaxes, and the expiratory port (2) is opened. In some of these valves the one-way valve (5) is an integral part of the diaphragm (4).

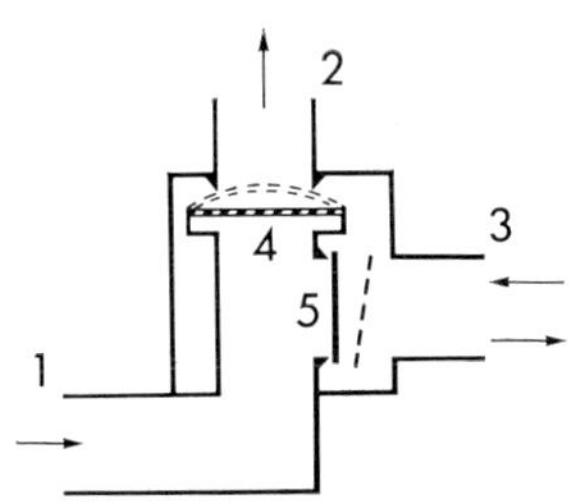

Fig. 92.5. Diagram of inflating valve, type D.
1. Inspiratory port
2. Expiratory port
3. Port for connexion to patient
4. Diaphragm
5. One-way valve

THE AGA INFLATING VALVE[16]

Figs. 92.6, and 92.7

This valve was fitted to the original Aga 'Pulmospirator'. The ports (6 and 9) are connected to the patient through two wide-bore tubes and a Y-piece.

During the inspiratory phase (fig. 92.6) the diaphragm (4) is expanded against the force exerted by the spring (7) and, by means of a rod fixed to it, holds the expiratory valve (8) closed. Inflating gas now flows, through the open inspiratory valve (3) and the spring-loaded one-way valve (5), to the patient. When inflation ceases and pressure at the inspiratory port falls (fig. 92.7), the diaphragm (4) is forced downwards by the spring (7) and the inspiratory valve (3) is closed. The rod no longer bears on the expiratory valve (8); expired gas flows, through the valve (8) and the expiratory port (2), to atmosphere.

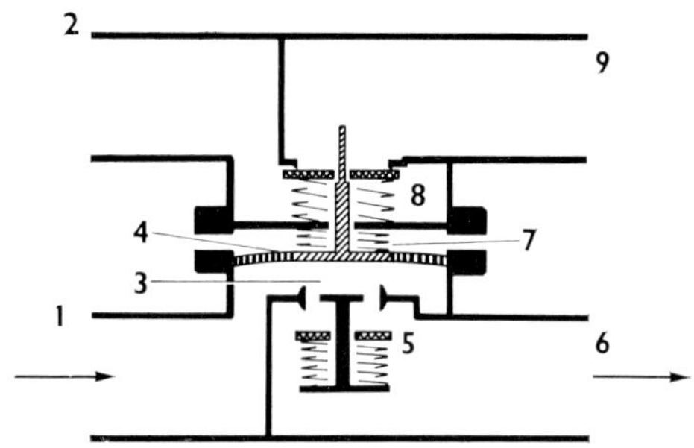

Fig. 92.6. Diagram of the Aga inflating valve—inspiratory phase.

1. Inspiratory port
2. Expiratory port
3. Inspiratory valve
4. Diaphragm
5. One-way valve
6. Port for connexion to patient
7. Spring
8. One-way valve
9. Port for connexion to patient

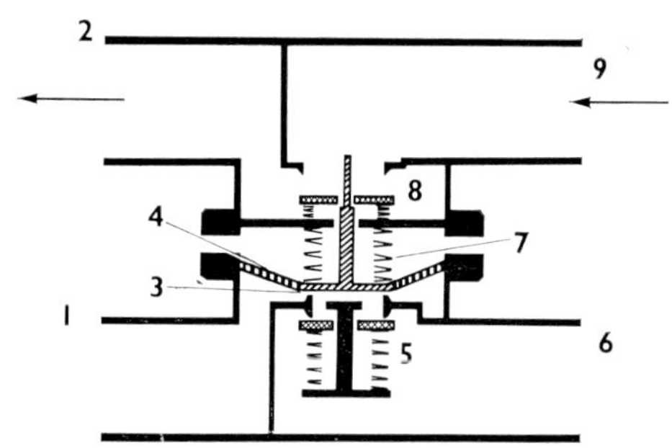

Fig. 92.7. Diagram of the Aga inflating valve—expiratory phase.

THE AGA 'POLYVALVE'
Fig. 92.8

This valve is used with the Aga 'Spiropulsator' when a non-rebreathing circuit is desired. It is also intended for resuscitation and a self-expanding bag is supplied for use in this way. The valve is unusual in that it incorporates an inlet through which fresh gas is drawn into the reservoir bag.

A moulded rubber disc (4) is held in position by 'fingers' which extend into the expiratory port (6). When the self-expanding reservoir bag (1) is compressed, the one-way valve (3) is closed and the disc (4) is forced onto its seating on the expiratory port (6). Inflating gas from the bag (1) flows, through the port (5), to the patient. When the reservoir bag (1) is released, the higher pressure at the port (5) forces the disc (4) over, the connexion with the bag is closed, and the expiratory port (6) is opened. Expired gas

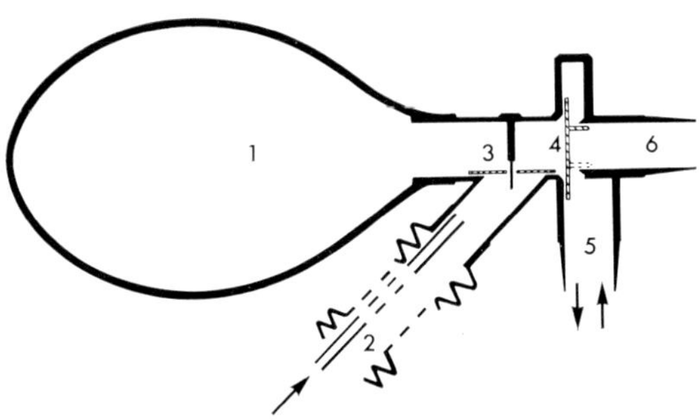

Fig. 92.8. Diagram of the Aga 'Polyvalve'.
1. Self-expanding reservoir bag
2. Reservoir tube
3. One-way inlet valve
4. Rubber disc with 'fingers'
5. Port for connexion to patient
6. Expiratory port

now flows, past the 'fingers' on the disc (4), to atmosphere. At the same time fresh gas is drawn from the reservoir tube (2), past the one-way valve (3), into the bag (1). An oxygen supply tube lies inside the open-ended reservoir tube (2) and this allows any oxygen percentage up to 100 to be delivered without risk of raising the pressure in the breathing circuit.

THE 'AMBU E' INFLATING VALVE

Fig. 92.9

The leaves of the moulded rubber one-way valves (3, 5) are attached to their bodies at two points on their circumference. When the reservoir bag connected to the port (1) is compressed the leaf of the inspiratory valve (3) is forced against one end of the chimney

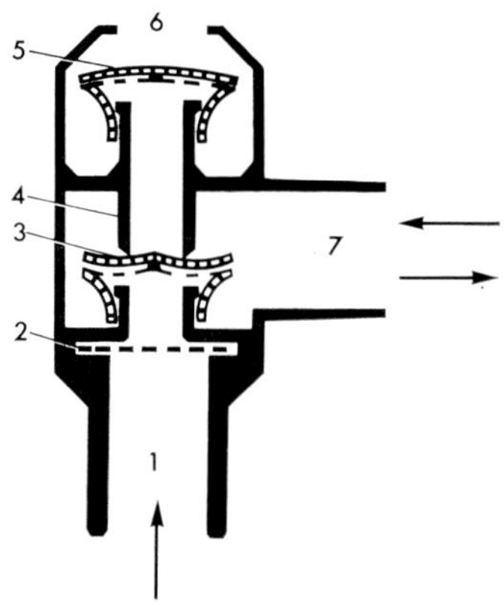

Fig. 92.9. Diagram of the 'Ambu E' inflating valve.
1. Inspiratory port
2. Wire-gauze filter
3. One-way inspiratory valve
4. Chimney
5. One-way expiratory valve
6. Expiratory port
7. Port for connexion to patient

(4) and inflating gas flows, through the wire-gauze filter (2) and the valve (3), to the patient. When the bag is released and pressure at the inspiratory port (1) falls, the valve (3) closes and expired gas flows, through the chimney (4) and the one-way expiratory valve (5), to atmosphere.

If the patient is breathing spontaneously, his inspiratory effort closes the expiratory valve (5) and gas is drawn in through the inspiratory valve (3). During expiration, the inspiratory valve (3) is closed and expired gas flows, through the expiratory valve (5), to atmosphere.

THE 'AMBU MAGNET' INFLATING VALVE

Fig. 92.10

This valve is similar to the 'Ambu E' inflating valve, the moulded rubber one-way valves being replaced by magnets (3 and 6) and discs (4 and 7).

The valve discs (4 and 7) are held in their closed positions by the two ring magnets

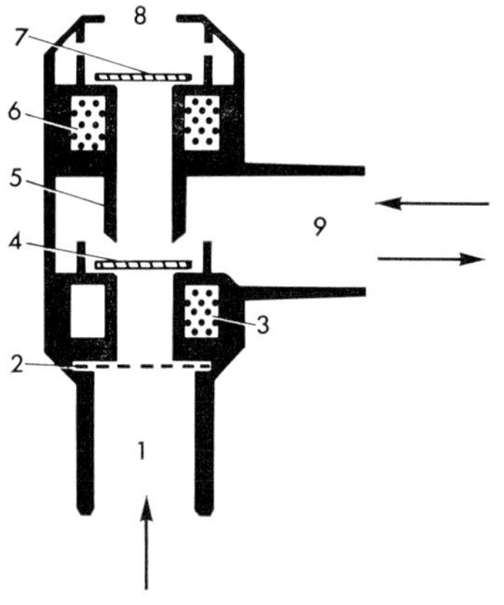

Fig. 92.10. Diagram of the 'Ambu Magnet' inflating valve.

1. Inspiratory port
2. Wire-gauze filter
3. Magnet
4. Inspiratory valve
5. Chimney
6. Magnet
7. Expiratory valve
8. Expiratory port
9. Port for connexion to patient

(3 and 6) which are sealed in the plastic casing. When the reservoir bag connected to the inspiratory port (1) is compressed, the inspiratory valve disc (4), is forced away from its magnet (3) onto one end of the chimney (5). Inflating gas from the bag flows, through the wire-gauze filter (2), the valve (4), and the port (9), to the patient. When the bag is released the disc is drawn back by its magnet, closing the inspiratory port (1). Expired gas now flows, through the chimney (5) and the one-way expiratory valve (7), to atmosphere.

The magnet (3) surrounding the inspiratory port is cut away on one side. Therefore, if the flow of fresh gas is excessive and the pressure in the bag rises, the disc (4) tilts without seating on the chimney, and the excess gas escapes to atmosphere. The attraction of the magnets is such that the valves operate easily with spontaneous respiration.

THE BEAVER INFLATING VALVE

Figs. 92.11, and 92.12

This valve was originally designed for use with the Beaver ventilator (see p. 313).

During the inspiratory phase (fig. 92.11) the pressure in the inspiratory port (1) forces the rubber diaphragm (5) onto its seating, and the pathway between the patient and the expiratory port (2) is closed. Inflating gas now flows, through the one-way valve (4) in the centre of the diaphragm (5) and the port (3), to the patient. When inflation ceases (fig. 92.12) and pressure at the inspiratory port (1) falls, the one-way valve (4) closes, blocking the inspiratory port (1), and the diaphragm (5) relaxes, allowing expired gas to flow, through the port (3) and the expiratory port (2), to atmosphere.

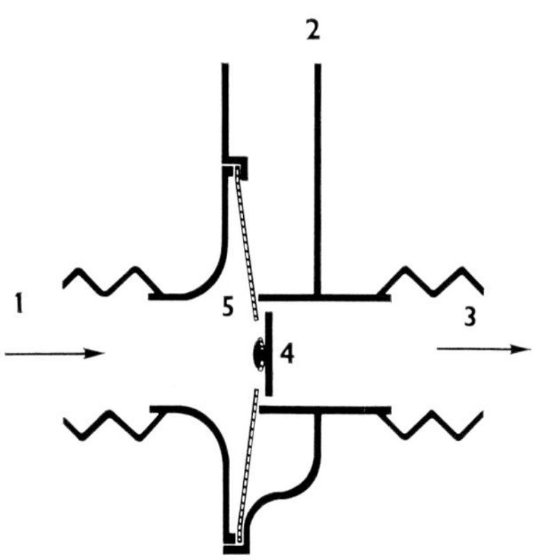

Fig. 92.11.

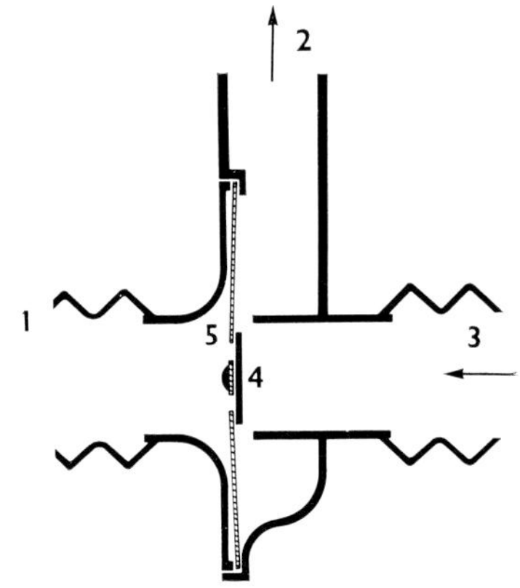

Fig. 92.12.

Fig. 92.11. Diagram of the Beaver inflating valve—inspiratory phase.

Fig. 92.12. Diagram of the Beaver inflating valve—expiratory phase.

1. Inspiratory port
2. Expiratory port
3. Port for connexion to patient
4. One-way valve
5. Diaphragm

This valve is designed in such a way that it can be taken to pieces for drying, cleaning, and sterilization. When replacing the diaphragm care must be taken that the one-way valve faces in the correct direction. Studs on the diaphragm fit into slots in the valve housing and make it obvious which way round it should go. Accidents have occurred when the diaphragm was incorrectly fitted.[20]

THE 'CARDIFF' INFLATING VALVE[9]

Figs. 92.13, and 92.14

During inflation (fig. 92.13) the piston (4) and its valve (3) move towards the port (8), until the valve seating (6) on the piston reaches the end-plate and the expiratory slots (5) are sealed off. The valve (3) continues its travel, the ports (2) in the piston are opened,

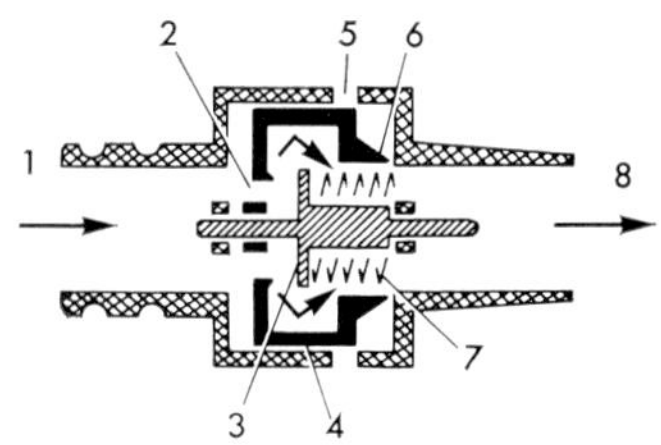

Fig. 92.13. Diagram of the 'Cardiff' inflating valve—inspiratory phase.

1. Inspiratory port
2. Ports in piston
3. One-way valve in piston
4. Piston
5. Expiration slots
6. Valve seating on piston
7. Spring
8. Port for connexion to patient

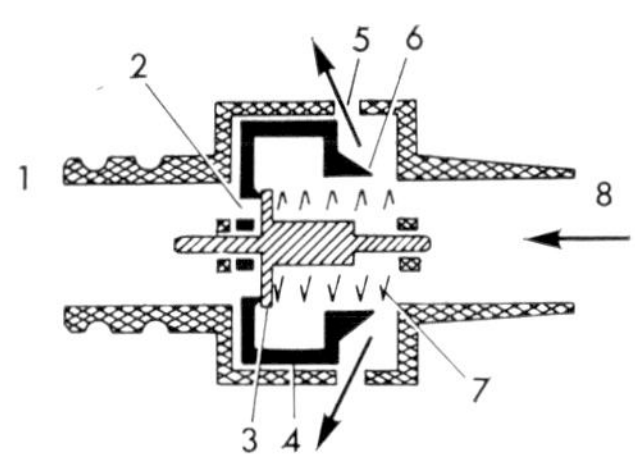

Fig. 92.14. Diagram of the 'Cardiff' inflating valve—expiratory phase.

and inflating gas flows, through the ports (2) and the port (8), to the patient. When inflation ceases (fig. 92.14) the higher pressure in the port (8) and the force exerted by the light spring (7) close the valve (3) and move the piston (4) in the reverse direction. The expiratory ports (5) are opened, and expired gas flows through them to atmosphere.

THE 'DEWSBURY' INFLATING VALVE[11]

Fig. 92.15

A loose-fitting piston (3) can move freely between its seating on the inspiratory port (1) and the stop (5). During inflation it is forced against the stop (5), closing two expiratory

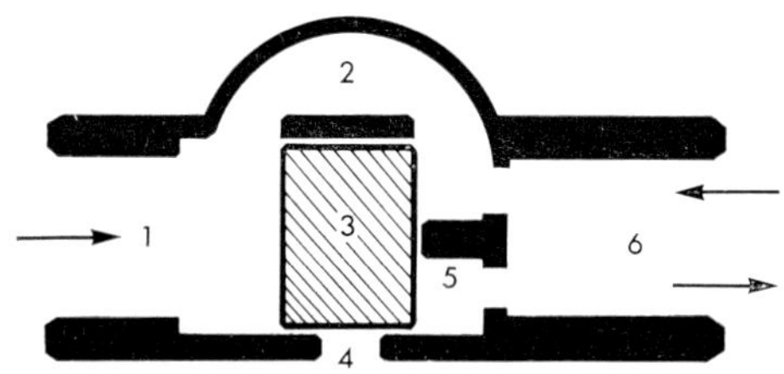

Fig. 92.15. Diagram of the 'Dewsbury' inflating valve.

1. Inspiratory port
2. By-pass tubes
3. Piston
4. Expiratory ports
5. Stop
6. Port for connexion to patient

ports (4) in opposite sides of the valve. Inflating gas flows, through two by-pass tubes (2), set at right angles to the expiratory ports (4), and the port (6), to the patient. When inflation ceases and pressure in the inspiratory port (1) falls, the piston (3) is forced back onto its seating, closing the inspiratory port (1) and opening the expiratory ports (4) through which expired gas flows to atmosphere.

THE ETHERIDGE INFLATING VALVE[18]

Figs. 92.16, and 92.17

When the reservoir bag (1) is compressed (fig. 92.16), pressure is transmitted, through the open tap (2) and the narrow tube (3), to a small thin-walled rubber balloon (6), which is inflated, occluding the expiratory outlet (7). Inflating gas now flows, through the

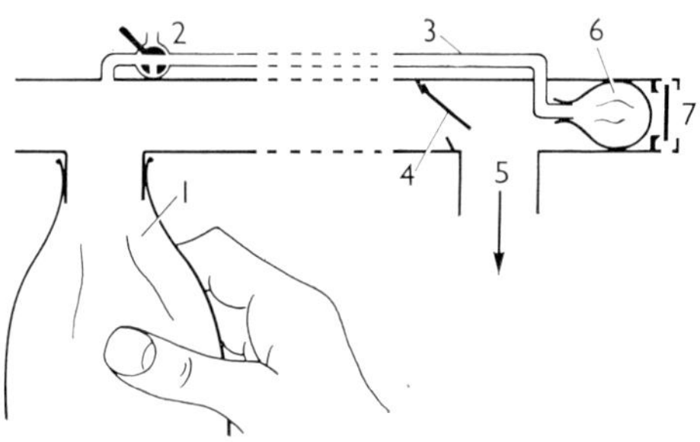

Fig. 92.16. Diagram of the Etheridge inflating valve—inspiratory phase.

1. Reservoir bag
2. Tap
3. Narrow-bore tube
4. One-way valve
5. Port for connexion to patient
6. Thin-walled rubber balloon
7. Expiratory valve

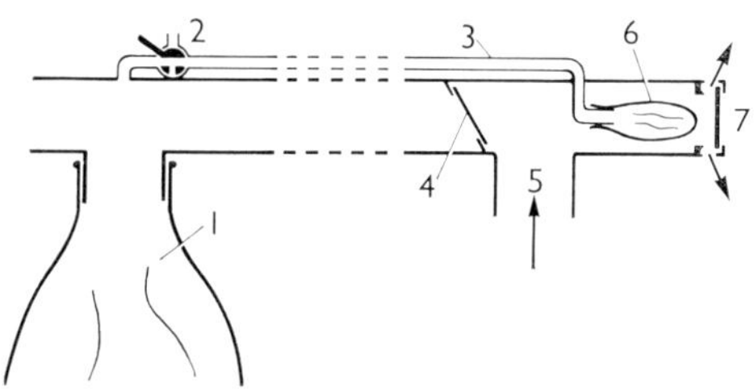

Fig. 92.17. Diagram of the Etheridge inflating valve—expiratory phase.

one-way valve (4) and the port (5), to the patient. When inflation ceases (fig. 92.17) the balloon (6) collapses and expired gas flows, past the balloon (6) and through the expiratory valve (7), to atmosphere.

If the patient is breathing spontaneously the balloon (6) becomes distended if the fresh-gas flow is excessive. This difficulty may be overcome by closing the tap (2).

THE FINK INFLATING VALVE[15]

Fig. 92.18

During inflation, pressure at the inspiratory port (1) is transmitted, through the narrow-bore tube (2), to the chamber above the diaphragm (6). The diaphragm (6) expands and holds the rubber-mushroom expiratory valve (4) closed. Inflating gas flows, through the

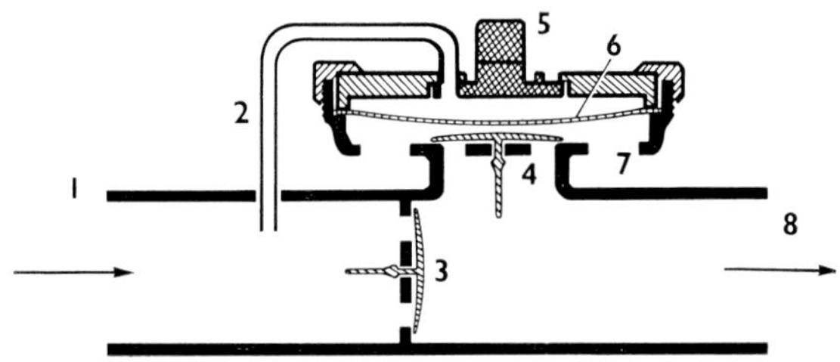

Fig. 92.18. Diagram of the Fink inflating valve.

1. Inspiratory port
2. Narrow-bore tube
3. Rubber-mushroom valve
4. Rubber-mushroom valve
5. Rotatable knob
6. Diaphragm
7. Expiratory ports
8. Port for connexion to patient

rubber-mushroom valve (3) and the port (8), to the patient. When inflation ceases and pressure at the inspiratory port (1) falls, the one-way valve (3) closes, the diaphragm (6) relaxes, and expired gas flows, through the one-way valve (4) and the expiratory ports (7), to atmosphere.

Rotation of the knob (5) in the centre of the diaphragm housing occludes the narrow-bore tube (2) and opens a port connecting the chamber above the diaphragm (6) to atmosphere. The diaphragm (6) is now inoperative and pressure in the circuit cannot rise above atmospheric. It is advisable to have the knob (5) in this position during spontaneous breathing to avoid any possibility of the expiratory valve (4) being held closed if the fresh-gas flow is excessive.

THE FLACH-VOSS INFLATING VALVE[14]
Fig. 92.19

During spontaneous respiration the valve (2) prevents rebreathing, and expired gas flows to atmosphere through the lightly-loaded expiratory valve (6). During inflation the pressure at the inspiratory port (1) is transmitted, through the narrow-bore tube (4), to the chamber behind the diaphragm (5). The diaphragm (5) is distended and the plunger

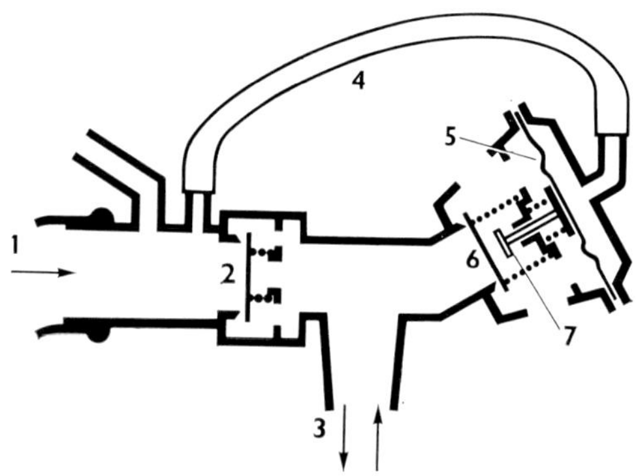

Fig. 92.19. Diagram of the Flach-Voss inflating valve.

1. Inspiratory port
2. One-way valve
3. Port for connexion to patient
4. Narrow-bore tube
5. Diaphragm
6. One-way valve
7. Plunger

Courtesy of *Der Anaesthesist*.

(7) is pushed down. Since the area of the diaphragm (5) is larger than that of the valve (6) the latter is held closed.

When inflation ceases pressure at the inspiratory port (1) falls and the diaphragm (5) relaxes. Expired gas now flows through the expiratory valve (6) to atmosphere.

THE FRUMIN 'NON-REBREATHING' VALVE[19]

Fig. 92.20

During inflation the pressure in the inspiratory port (1) distends the capsule (5) closing the expiratory port (4). Inflating gas flows, past the rubber disc valve (2) and through

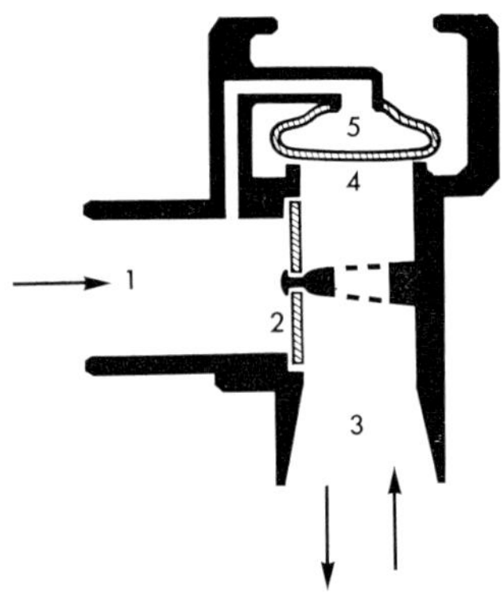

Fig. 92.20. Diagram of the Frumin 'non-rebreathing' inflating valve.

1. Inspiratory port
2. One-way rubber disc valve
3. Port for connexion to patient
4. Expiratory port
5. Capsule

the port (3), to the patient. When inflation ceases pressure at the inspiratory port (1) falls, the rubber disc valve (2) closes, and the capsule (5) collapses. Expired gas now flows, through the port (3) and the expiratory port (4), to atmosphere. During spontaneous respiration the capsule (5) remains relaxed and acts as a one-way expiratory valve.

THE LEWIS-LEIGH INFLATING VALVE[3]

Figs. 92.21, and 92.22

During inflation the rubber flap (2) (fig. 92.21) is forced against one end of the chimney (4), closing the expiratory pathway. Inflating gas flows, past the chimney and through

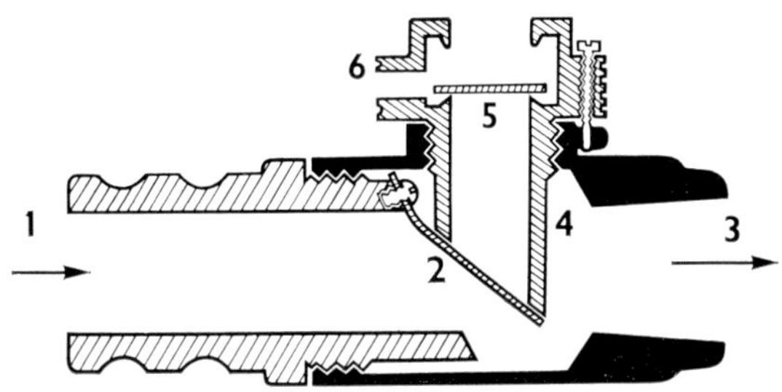

Fig. 92.21. Diagram of the Lewis-Leigh inflating valve—inspiratory phase.

1. Inspiratory port
2. Rubber flap
3. Port for connexion to patient
4. Chimney
5. One-way valve
6. Expiratory ports

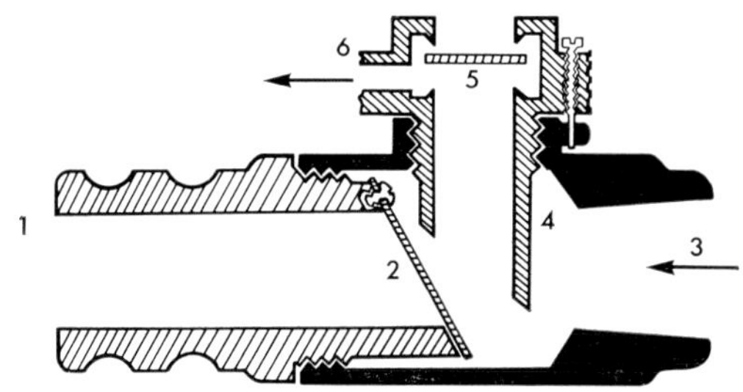

Fig. 92.22. Diagram of the Lewis-Leigh inflating valve—expiratory phase.

the port (3), to the patient. When inflation ceases, pressure at the inspiratory port (1) falls, the flap (2) returns to its resting position (fig. 92.22), and expired gas flows, through the chimney (4), past the one-way valve (5), and through the expiratory ports (6), to atmosphere. Rotation of the chimney (4) prevents its lower end being occluded by the flap (2); pressure in the circuit cannot rise above atmospheric. The disc valve (5) in the chimney prevents inhalation of air during spontaneous breathing.

THE 'MAGNETIC POI' INFLATING VALVE[8]

Fig. 92.23

This valve incorporates two magnets (5 and 7). One is fitted in the expiratory port (8) and the other in the bobbin (2). They are arranged so that like poles are adjacent. In

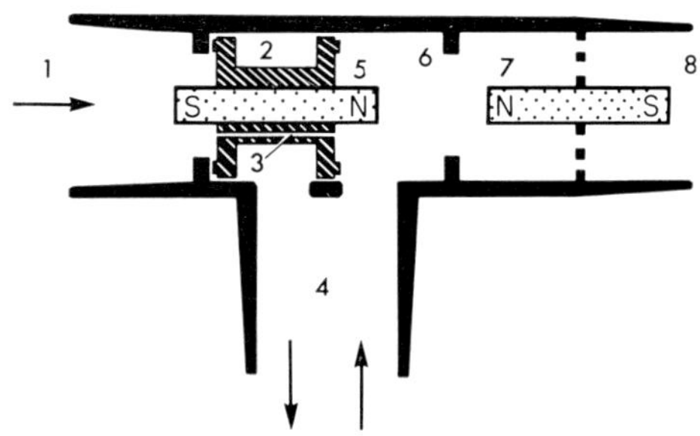

Fig. 92.23. Diagram of the 'Magnetic POI' inflating valve.

1. Inspiratory port
2. Bobbin
3. Leak channel
4. Port for connexion to patient
5. Magnet
6. Bobbin seating
7. Fixed magnet
8. Expiratory port

the resting position, the bobbin (2) is forced against the inspiratory port (1) by the repelling magnetic force. During inflation the pressure in the inspiratory port (1) overcomes the repulsion of the magnets, and the piston is forced onto the seating (6), the expiratory port (8) is closed, and inflating gas flows through the port (4) to the patient. When inflation ceases, pressure at the inspiratory port (1) falls, the bobbin (2) is forced back, closing the inspiratory port (1). Expired gas now flows, past the fixed magnet (7) and through the expiratory port (8), to atmosphere.

A leak channel (3) through the bobbin allows gas to leak slowly from the inspiratory port (1). This reduces the risk of the pressure at the inspiratory port (1) rising sufficiently to hold the bobbin (2) in the inflating position.

THE NEFF INFLATING VALVE[2]

Figs. 92.24, and 92.25

This valve was devised to enable controlled respiration to be carried out with the concertina bag of the 'Oxford' Ether Vaporizer during World War II. It consists of a 3-inch diameter circular metal box, inside which is a light hinged metal strip (2). During inflation (fig. 92.24) one end of the metal strip (2) is forced away from the inspiratory port (1), and the other end onto the expiratory port (4). Inflating gas now flows, through the inspiratory port (1) and the port (3), to the patient. A disc (6), containing a number of different-sized holes, can be rotated to provide a rough limit to the inflating pressure. When inflation ceases (fig. 92.25) pressure falls at the inspiratory port (1), and the end of hinged valve flap (2), which is weighted with a blob of solder, falls away from the expiratory port (4). The inspiratory port (1) is now closed and expired gas flows, through

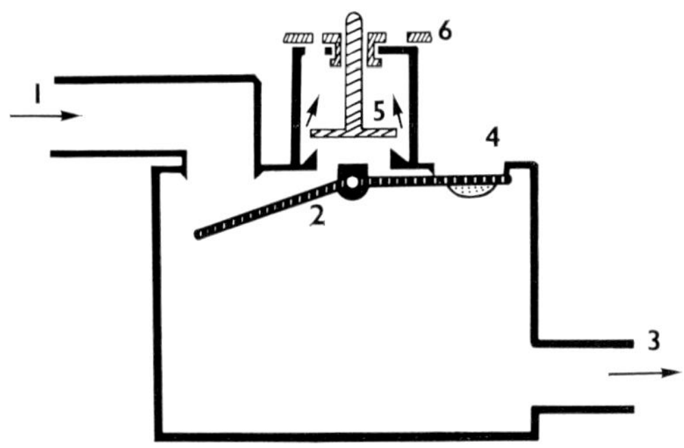

Fig. 92.24.

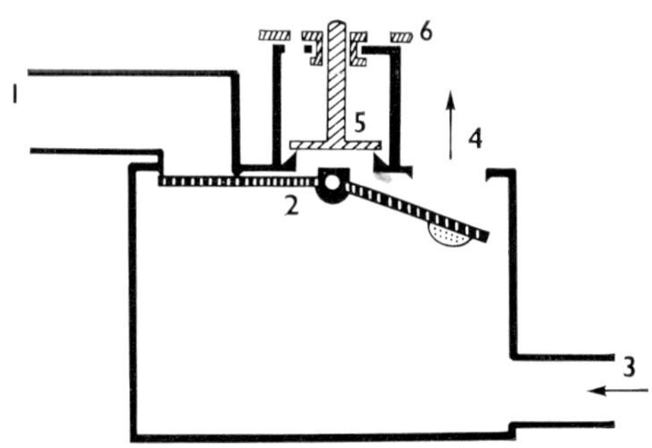

Fig. 92.25.

Fig. 92.24. Diagram of the Neff inflating valve—inspiratory phase.

Fig. 92.25. Diagram of the Neff inflating valve—expiratory phase.

1. Inspiratory port
2. Hinged strip
3. Port for connexion to patient
4. Expiratory port
5. One-way valve
6. Rotatable disc

the port (3) and the expiratory port (4), to atmosphere. The hinged valve (2) is so balanced that it moves during spontaneous breathing; the patient inhales through the inspiratory port (1) and expired gas flows, through the expiratory port (4), to atmosphere. A one-way valve (5) prevents the inhalation of air through the holes in the rotatable disc (6).

THE NEWTON INFLATING VALVE[10]

Figs. 92.26, and 92.27

At rest this valve is in the inflating position (fig. 92.26), the plastic piston (5) being held over the expiratory ports (6, 6) by the light beryllium-copper spring (3). During inflation

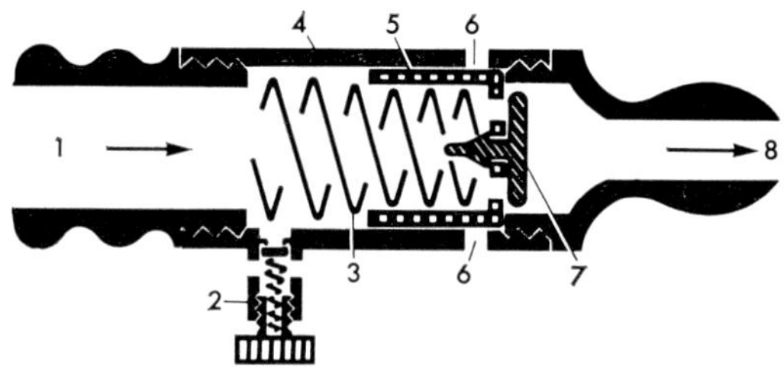

Fig. 92.26. Diagram of the Newton inflating valve—inspiratory phase.

1. Inspiratory port
2. Adjustable safety-vavel
3. Light beryllium-copper spring
4. Valve body
5. Plastic piston
6, 6. Expiratory ports
7. Rubber-mushroom valve
8. Port for connexion to patient

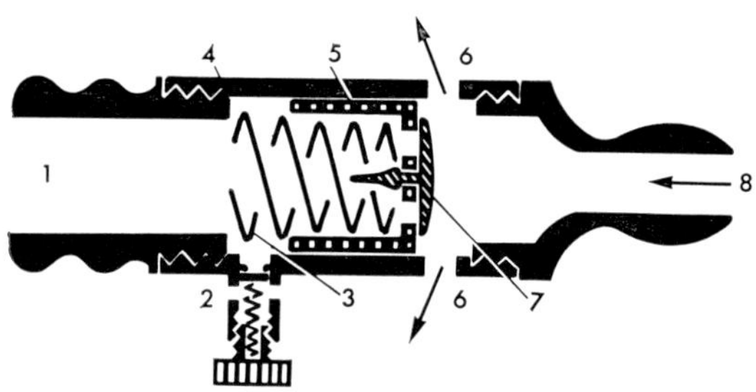

Fig. 92.27. Diagram of the Newton inflating valve—expiratory phase.

gas flows, through the rubber-mushroom valve (7), to the patient. An adjustable safety-valve (2) limits the inflating pressure. At the end of inflation (fig. 92.27) pressure at the inspiratory port (1) falls and the one-way valve (7) closes. The pressure of gas in the port (8) overcomes the force exerted by the spring (3) and drives the piston (5) back. The expiratory ports (6, 6) are now open and expired gas flows to atmosphere.

THE 'RANIMA' INFLATING VALVE
Fig. 92.28

This valve was designed as an integral part of the manually-operated Ranima Insufflator'.

During inflation the concertina valve (7) is held on its seating and the light spring-loaded one-way valve (6) opens. Inflating gas flows, through the inspiratory port (1), the one-way valve (6) and the port (8), to the patient. A safety-valve (4) limits the inflation pressure to 35–50 cmH_2O. When the concertina bag of the 'Insufflator' is expanded,

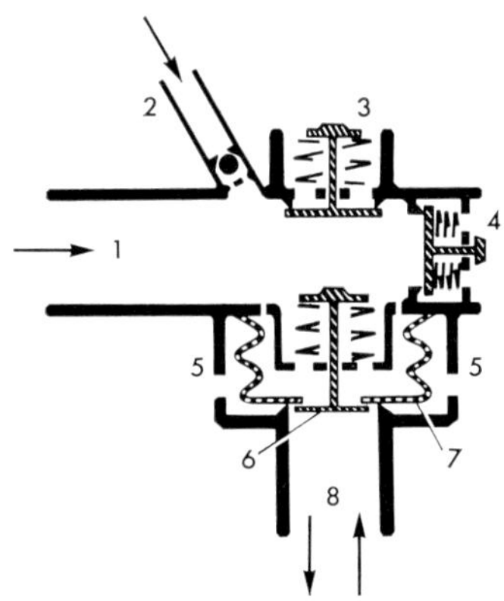

Fig. 92.28. Diagram of the 'Ranima' inflating valve.

1. Inspiratory port
2. Oxygen inlet
3. Air-inlet valve
4. Safety-valve
5, 5. Expiratory ports
6. One-way valve
7. Concertina valve
8. Port for connexion to patient

pressure at the inspiratory port (1) falls, and the one-way valve (6) closes. The concertina valve (7) collapses and expired gas flows, through the port (8) and the expiratory ports (5, 5), to atmosphere. At the same time the concertina bag of the 'Insufflator' refills with air drawn in through the lightly-loaded one-way valve (3). Oxygen can be added through a side tube (2) which contains a one-way ball valve.

THE RUBEN INFLATING VALVE[6, 7]

Figs. 92.29, and 92.30

This valve is constructed of clear plastic. At rest the bobbin (2) is held against the inspiratory port (1) by the light spring (5). During inflation (fig. 92.29) the bobbin (2) is forced onto the expiratory port (4) and inflating gas flows, through the inspiratory port (1) and the port (3), to the patient. When inflation ceases (fig. 92.30), pressure at the

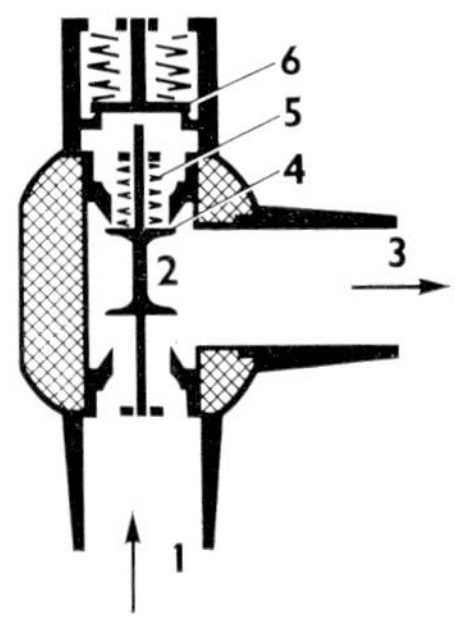

Fig. 92.29. Diagram of the Ruben inflating valve—inspiratory phase.

1. Inspiratory port
2. Bobbin
3. Port for connexion to patient
4. Expiratory port
5. Spring
6. One-way valve

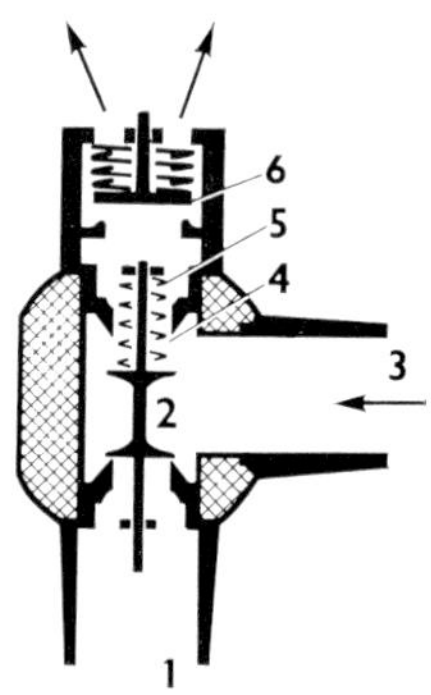

Fig. 92.30. Diagram of the Ruben inflating valve—expiratory phase.

inspiratory port (1) falls and the spring (5) returns the bobbin (2) to its resting position. The inspiratory port (1) is closed, and expired gas flows, through the port (3), the expiratory port (4), and the one-way valve (6), to atmosphere. During spontaneous respiration the bobbin moves in the same way as during controlled ventilation.

When this valve is combined with a self-expanding bag for resuscitation, the one-way valve (6) is not fitted. Then any spontaneous inspiration draws in air from the atmosphere, through the expiratory port (4).

THE SHUMAN INFLATING VALVE[17]

Figs. 92.31, and 92.32

During inflation (fig. 92.31) the thin-rubber tube (5), which covers the apertures in the side of the inspiratory tube (1), is distended, occluding the expiratory port (3). Inflating gas flows, through the inspiratory tube (1), the rubber-mushroom valve (6), and the port (7), to the patient. When inflation ceases (fig. 92.32), pressure at the inspiratory

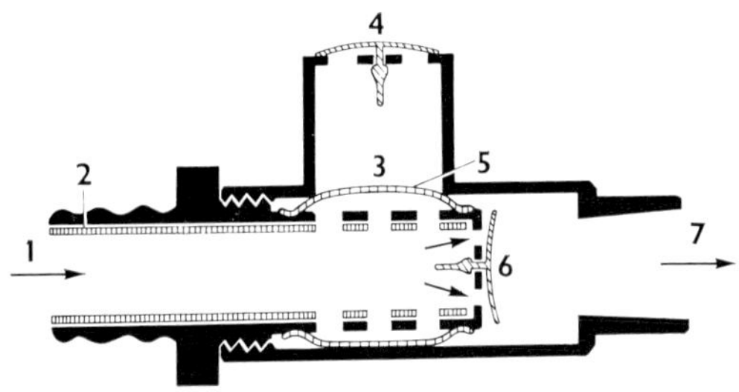

Fig. 92.31. Diagram of the Shuman inflating valve—inspiratory phase.

1. Inspiratory port and tube
2. Inner sleeve of inpiratory tube
3. Expiratory port
4. Rubber-mushroom valve
5. Thin-rubber tube
6. Rubber-mushroom valve
7. Port for connexion to patient

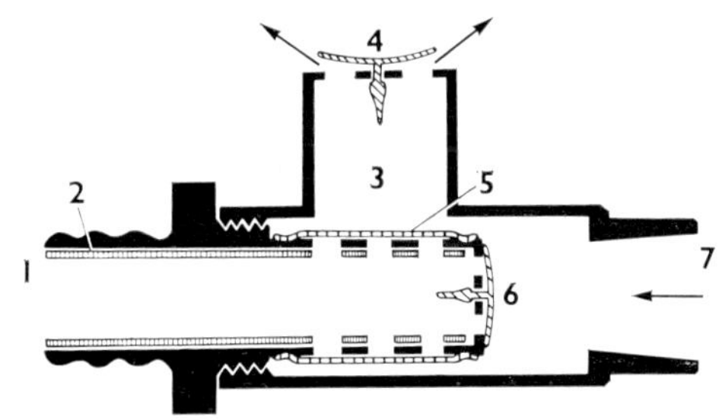

Fig. 92.32. Diagram of the Shuman inflating valve—expiratory phase.

port (1) falls, the one-way valve (6) closes, the thin-rubber tube (5) collapses, and expired gas flows, through the port (3) and the rubber-mushroom valve (4), to atmosphere.

The inner sleeve (2) of the inspiratory tube (1) can be rotated to close the apertures in the tube. This prevents distension of the thin-rubber tube (5) and the pressure in the circuit cannot rise above atmosphere.

THE STOTT INFLATING VALVE[13]

Figs. 92.33, and 92.34

The two circular rubber leaves (3) are loosely connected at points on their circumference. During inflation (fig. 92.33) the upper leaf occludes the expiratory port (2) and inflating gas flows, through the inspiratory port (1), between the rubber leaves (3), and through

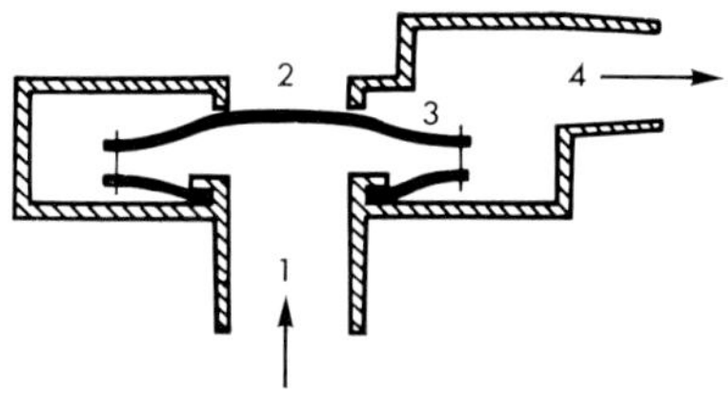

Fig. 92.33. Diagram of the Stott inflating valve—inspiratory phase.

1. Inspiratory port
2. Expiratory port
3. Rubber leaves
4. Port for connexion to patient

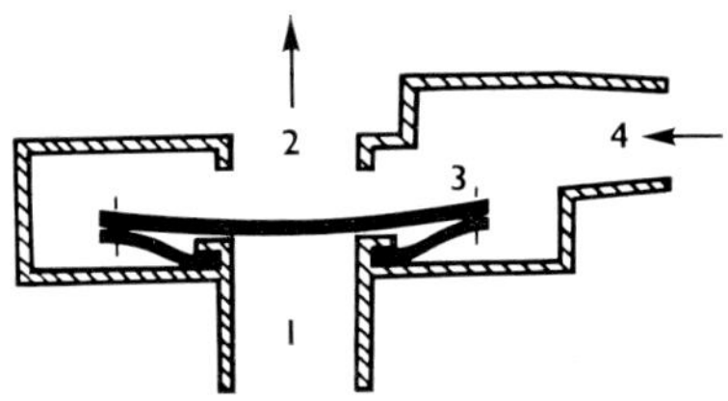

Fig. 92.34. Diagram of the Stott inflating valve—expiratory phase.

the port (4), to the patient. When inflation ceases (fig. 92.34), pressure at the inspiratory port (1) falls, the upper rubber leaf relaxes against the lower leaf, occluding the inspiratory port (1) and opening the expiratory port. Expired gas flows, through the port (4) and the expiratory port (2), to atmosphere.

THE STOTT 'PING-PONG BALL' INFLATING VALVE[5]

Figs. 92.35, and 92.36

A vertical cylinder contains a ping-pong ball (2). During inflation (fig. 92.35) this ball is forced up to occlude the expiratory port (3) and inflating gas flows, through the inspiratory port (1) and the port (4), to the patient. When inflation ceases (fig. 92.36), pressure

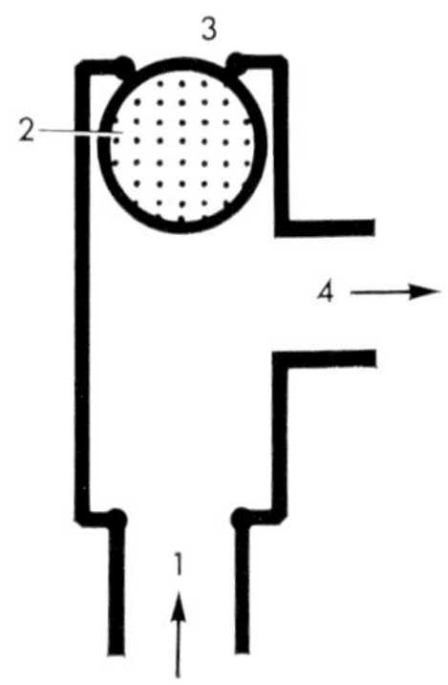

Fig. 92.35. Diagram of the Stott 'ping-pong ball' inflating valve—inspiratory phase.

1. Inspiratory port
2. Ping-pong ball
3. Expiratory port
4. Port for connexion to patient

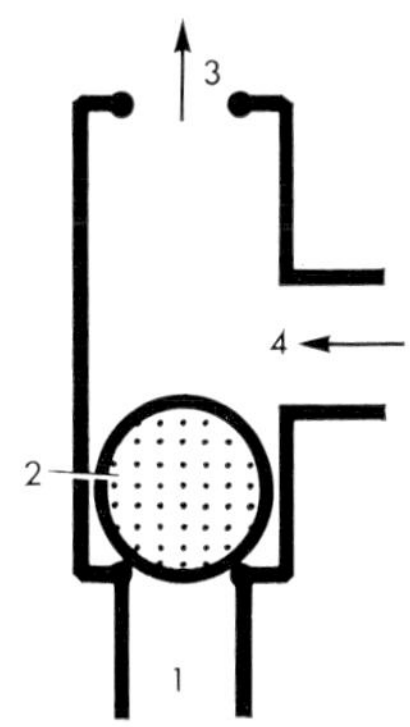

Fig. 92.36. Diagram of the Stott 'ping-pong ball' inflating valve—expiratory phase.

at the inspiratory port (1) falls, and the ball drops under the influence of gravity, closing the inspiratory port (1). Expired gas flows, through the port (4) and the expiratory port (3), to atmosphere.

THE TASHIRO-WAKAI INFLATING VALVE[4]

Fig. 92.37

During inflation the light flexible valve disc (2) is forced off its lower seating and held on its upper seating at the bottom of the central tube (3). Inflating gas flows, through the inspiratory port (1), the one-way valve (2), and the port (7), to the patient. When

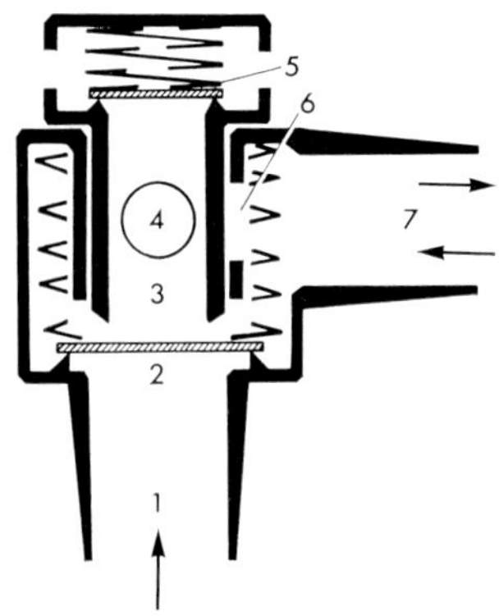

Fig. 92.37. Diagram of the Tashiro-Wakai inflating valve.

1. Inspiratory port
2. Valve disc
3. Central tube
4. Orifice
5. One-way valve in expiratory port
6. Port
7. Port for connexion to patient

inflation ceases, pressure at the inspiratory port (1) falls, the valve disc (2), which has a much larger diameter than the tube (3), moves down onto its lower seating, and expired gas flows, through the central tube (3) and the one-way valve (5), to atmosphere.

During spontaneous respiration the inner tube (3) should be turned so as to bring the orifice (4) in line with the port (6). This prevents the pressure in the circuit rising above atmospheric.

THE ZUCK PAEDIATRIC INFLATING VALVE[12]
Fig. 92.38

This small inflating valve is designed for paediatric use. At rest the loose-fitting piston (2) is held against the inspiratory port (1) by the light spring (3). During inflation the piston (2) is moved away from the inspiratory port (1) and occludes the expiratory port

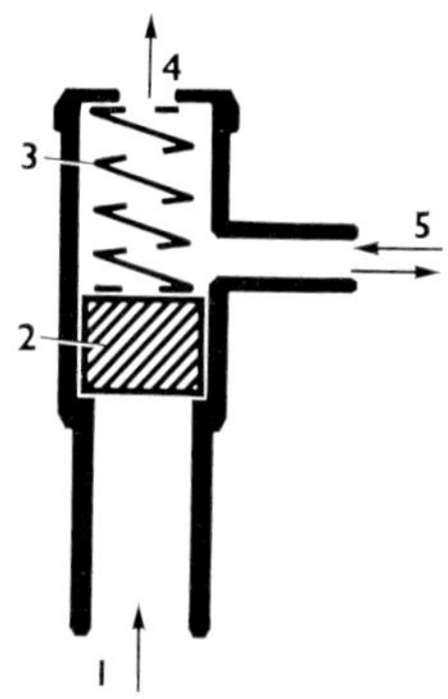

Fig. 92.38. Diagram of the Zuck paediatric inflating valve.

1. Inspiratory port
2. Piston
3. Light spring
4. Expiratory port
5. Port for connexion to patient

(4). Inflating gas flows, through the inspiratory port (1) and the port (5), to the patient. When inflation ceases, pressure at the inspiratory port (1) falls, the piston is returned by the spring (3), and expired gas flows, through the port (5) and the expiratory port (4), to atmosphere.

PRESSURE-EQUALIZING VALVES[21,22]

If, in a breathing circuit which includes an inflating valve, the fresh-gas flow exceeds the total minute-volume ventilation, either because the flow is excessive or because squeezing of the bag is interrupted, a dangerous situation may arise. The pressure in the breathing circuit increases steadily until it is high enough to hold the inflating valve in its inspiratory position and no gas can escape from the circuit since the expiratory port is closed. The lungs are now held inflated and, as fresh gas continues to enter the circuit, the pressure within them continues to rise and a potentially-dangerous level may be reached. The 'pressure-equalizing' valves described here were designed to obviate this hazard.

THE HORN PRESSURE-EQUALIZING VALVE[23]

Fig. 92.39

This valve is designed to fit into the tail of a reservoir bag (1). A small rise in pressure in the bag (1) moves the valve disc (2) from its inner seat against the force of the light spring (4) and gas flows, through the valve and the ports in the rotatable disc (5), to atmosphere.

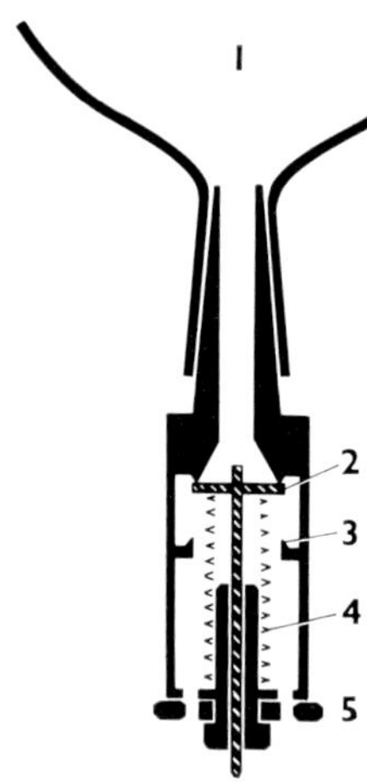

Fig. 92.39. Diagram of the Horn pressure-equalizing valve.

1. Tail of reservoir bag
2. Valve disc
3. Lower valve seat
4. Spring
5. Disc with outlet ports

Rapid compression of the bag forces the valve disc (2) against its outer seat (3), so closing the pathway to atmosphere. The disc (5) can be rotated to occlude the outlet ports, thus putting the valve out of action.

THE LEE PRESSURE-EQUALIZING VALVE[24]

Fig. 92.40

This valve is designed to be fitted into the tail of a reservoir bag (1). A small rise in pressure in the reservoir bag moves the valve (3) from its inner seat against the force of the spring (2) and excess gas spills around it to atmosphere. When inflating the lungs the reservoir bag is sharply compressed, forcing the valve against its outer seat (4) and

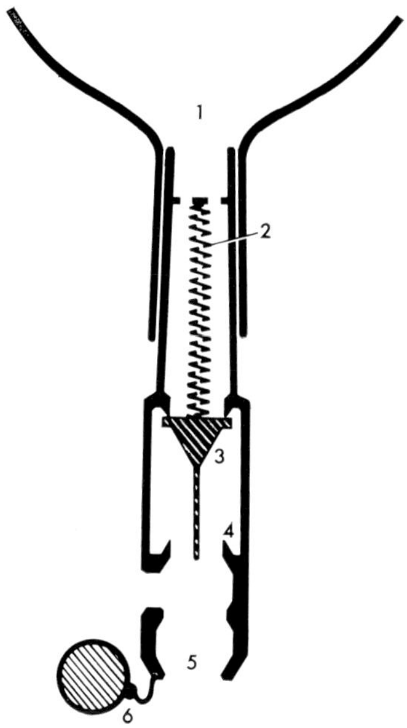

Fig. 92.40. Diagram of the Lee pressure-equalizing valve.

1. Tail of reservoir bag
2. Spring
3. Valve
4. Outer seat
5. Housing for ball
6. Ball

closing the pathway to atmosphere. If the fresh-gas flow is particularly excessive, as might occur if the circuit is flushed, the ball (6) can be fitted into the end of the valve (5). This prevents the valve (3) reaching its outer seating (4) and allows gas to escape to atmosphere continuously. The valve (3) can be held in its closed position by pushing the ball (6) further in.

THE MAXWELL-GRANT PRESSURE-EQUALIZING VALVE[25]

Fig. 92.41

This valve was derived from the Steen pressure-equalizing valve. It may be used as a pressure-equalizing valve in a non-rebreathing circuit which includes an inflating valve, or as a valve for disposing of excess gas from a closed circuit. When used as a pressure-equalizing valve its mode of operation is similar to that of the Steen valve.

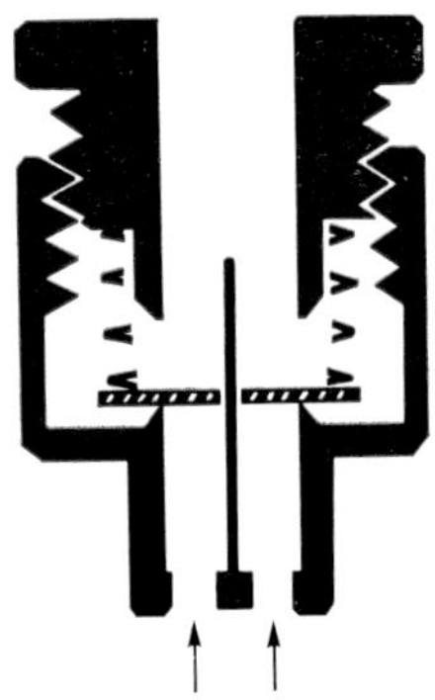

Fig. 92.41. Diagram of the Maxwell-Grant pressure-equalizing valve.

When used for disposing of excess gas from a closed circuit, spill occurs while the valve disc is moving from its lower to its upper seating. The distance between the upper and lower seats of the valve can be varied by adjusting the position of the top seat. This allows the amount of gas spilled at each inflation to be adjusted to match the fresh-gas flow.

THE SMITH-VOLPITTO PRESSURE-EQUALIZING VALVE[26]

Fig. 92.42

This valve is designed to fit into the tail of a reservoir bag (1). At rest the piston (2) is held in the position shown in fig. 92.42 by a light spring (5). Gas from the reservoir bag

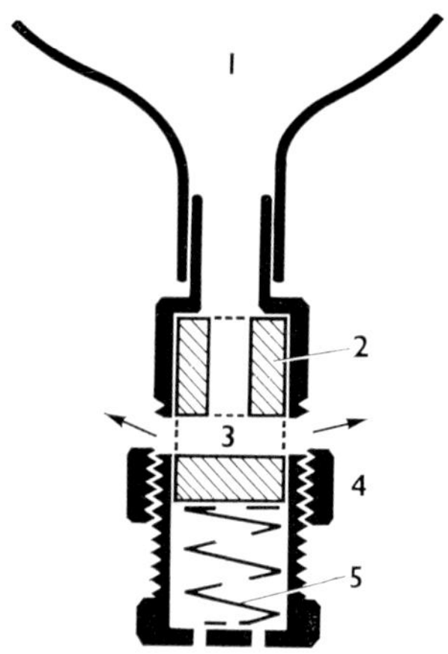

Fig. 92.42. Diagram of the Smith-Volpitto pressure-equalizing valve.

1. Tail of reservoir bag
2. Piston
3. Ports
4. Screw ring
5. Spring

can flow, through the piston (2) and the ports (3), to atmosphere. The ports (3) may be partially covered by the screw ring (4), the setting of which should be adjusted so that for any given fresh-gas flow the reservoir bag just becomes fully-distended during the expiratory phase.

In order to inflate the lungs the reservoir bag is compressed sharply and the rise in pressure moves the piston (2) downwards against the force of the spring (5). The ports (3) are now occluded, preventing any escape of gas through the valve to atmosphere. When inflation ceases and the pressure in the bag has fallen sufficiently, the piston is returned to its resting position by the force of the spring (5) and excess fresh gas again escapes to atmosphere.

THE STEEN PRESSURE-EQUALIZING VALVE[19, 21, 22]

Fig. 92.43

This valve was first introduced for use with the Frumin inflating valve (see p. 784). A square piece of Teflon (1) is held by the light spring (2) on the lower of its two seatings. When the pressure in the breathing circuit rises above 1·5 cmH_2O, the pressure in a full

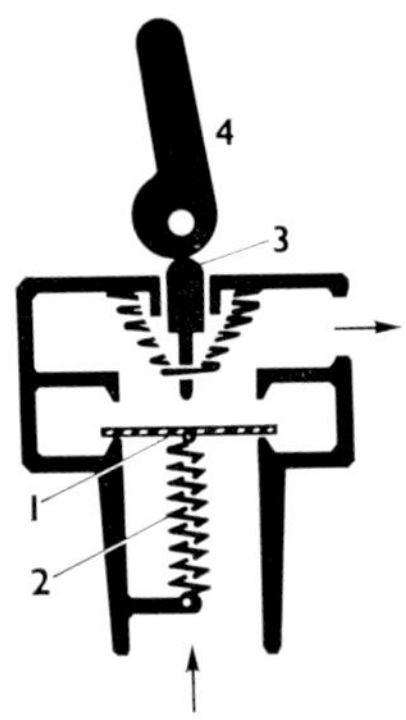

Fig. 92.43. Diagram of the Steen pressure-equalizing valve.

1. Square piece of Teflon
2. Spring
3. Spring-loaded pin
4. Lever

reservoir bag, the valve flap (1) is lifted and any excess fresh gas leaks past it to atmosphere. To inflate the lungs the reservoir bag is compressed sharply. The resulting rapid increase in pressure in the breathing circuit forces the valve flap (1) onto its upper seating and gas can no longer escape to atmosphere. When the lever (4), attached to the top of the valve, is depressed, the spring-loaded pin (3) extends below the upper seating. The valve flap (1) is thereby prevented from occluding the expiratory port. With the lever (4) in this position it is not possible to control respiration.

OTHER VALVES FOR USE IN CONTROLLED VENTILATION

The three types of valve described here do not conform to our definition of an inflating valve in that they do not necessarily ensure that rebreathing is eliminated by the closure of an inspiratory port during the expiratory phase. In one of them the expiratory port is not automatically closed during the inspiratory phase.

Type E

These valves are adaptations of standard expiratory valves and operate as such during the expiratory phase. During inflation the valve disc is forced onto a second seating to occlude the expiratory port.

The Lee valve[27]
The Searle valve[28]

Type F

The primary function of this type of valve is to operate as an adjustable safety-valve. Once the valve has been opened, an additional mechanism holds it open for a set time.

The Holger Hesse valve

Type G

This valve operates as a standard expiratory valve unless the expiratory port is closed manually by remote control in order to allow inflation to be performed.

The 'Cardiff' remote-control expiratory valve[29]

THE LEE INFLATING VALVE[27]

Fig. 92.44

This valve is designed for use during anaesthesia with controlled or spontaneous respiration. During controlled respiration, the sleeve (1) is turned to occlude the expiratory ports (2) in the valve body. When the reservoir bag is compressed sharply the valve

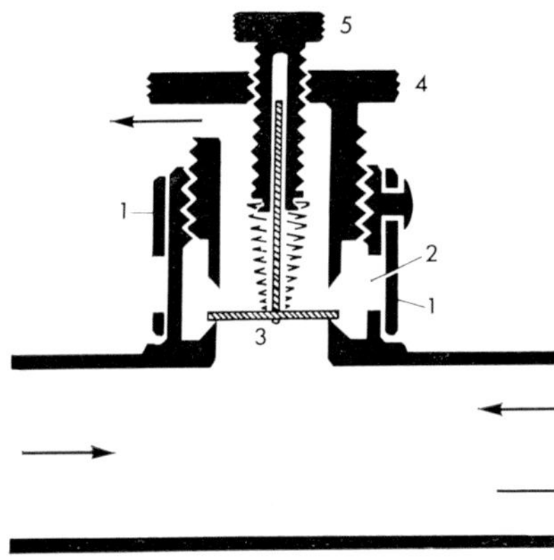

Fig. 92.44. Diagram of the Lee inflating valve.
1. Sleeve
2. Expiratory ports
3. One-way valve
4. Screw cap
5. Screw

(3) is forced up and seats against the lower end of the screw cap (4), closing the pathway through the cap to atmosphere. Inflating gas from the bag flows to the patient. When the bag is released, the valve (3) moves down slightly and expired gas passes around it and through the screw cap (4) to atmosphere.

The pressure required to lift the valve onto its upper seating is set by adjusting the compression of its light spring with the central screw control (5) and the distance the valve must travel before closing against the top seating is set by adjusting the screw cap (4). These settings, and the compression of the reservoir bag, must be so balanced that, while only a small volume of gas is spilled at the beginning of inflation, there is little resistance to expiration.

When the valve is used for spontaneous respiration, the sleeve (1) is turned to the position where the holes in it correspond with the ports (2) in the valve body. It then acts as a normal expiratory valve.

Provided the fresh-gas flow is at least equal to the total minute-volume ventilation rebreathing will be largely eliminated since the pattern of gas flow in this circuit with controlled respiration is similar to that in the Magill attachment in spontaneous respiration.

THE SEARLE VALVE[28]

Fig. 92.45

Externally this valve closely resembles the commonly-used Heidbrink-type expiratory valve except that the expiratory ports (2) are in the top of the adjustable cap instead of

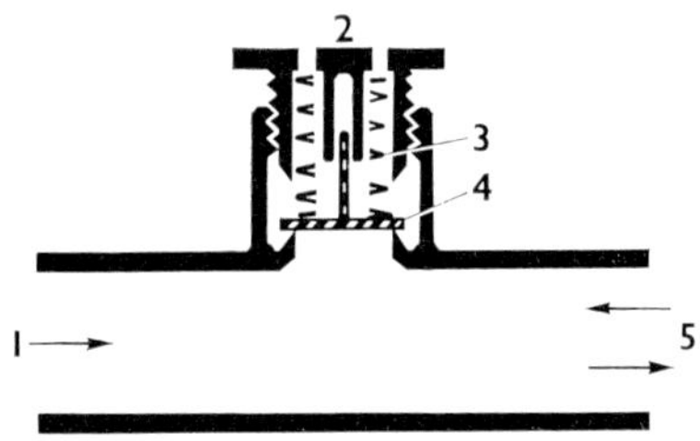

Fig. 92.45. Diagram of the Searle inflating valve.
1. Inspiratory port
2. Expiratory ports
3. Spring
4. Valve disc
5. Port for connexion to patient

in the side of the valve body. During spontaneous respiration the valve acts as a normal expiratory valve. When it is desired to inflate the patient's lungs the reservoir bag is compressed sharply. This forces the valve disc (4) against its top seat on the adjustable cap, thus closing the expiratory ports (2). When the reservoir bag is released the valve disc is forced down from the top seat by the force of its spring (3) and gas flows, around the valve (4) and through the expiratory ports (2), to atmosphere.

As in the Lee inflating valve rebreathing will occur unless the fresh-gas flow is adequate.

THE HOLGER HESSE 'DEBLOCKING' VALVE
Fig. 92.46

During inflation, the metal disc (5), which forms the base of a capsule, is held on its seating by the attraction of the magnet (4). When the pressure in the breathing circuit has increased sufficiently to overcome this attraction, the disc (5) is forced up, gas escapes to atmosphere through the ports (2), and the pressure in the circuit falls. As the disc (5) moves up, the capsule is compressed and air contained in it flows, past the freely-lifting disc (3) in the upper chamber, to atmosphere. When the pressure in the circuit falls and the capsule is no longer compressed, the disc (3) reseats. The capsule then re-expands, but only slowly in a time determined by the small orifice in the valve disc (3)

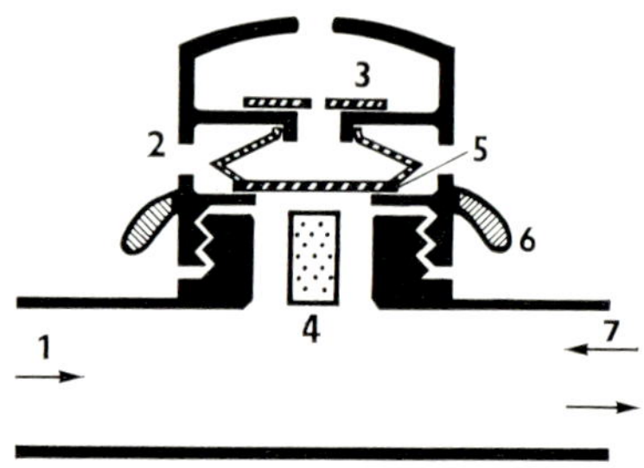

Fig. 92.46. Diagram of the Holger Hesse 'deblocking' valve.

1. Inspiratory port
2. Expiratory ports
3. Light disc with small hole
4. Magnet
5. Valve disc at base of capsule
6. Rubber ring
7. Port for connexion to patient

which restricts the flow of air into the capsule. Until the capsule is full and the valve disc (5) has reseated the expiratory pathway is open, and the next inflation cannot begin.

The pressure at the end of inflation can be set by rotating the valve housing. This adjusts the distance between the magnet (4) and the valve disc (5) and so determines the force of attraction. Calibrations on the housing enable this pressure to be set between 20 and 60 cmH_2O. When a higher inflating pressure is desired, a rubber ring (6) around the valve can be flicked up to occlude the expiratory ports (2) completely.

This valve differs from most other inflating valves in that compression of the valve must *not* be commenced sharply since this would open the valve prematurely. Instead, the bag should be squeezed evenly so that there is a progressive build-up of pressure in the valve.

THE 'CARDIFF' REMOTE-CONTROL EXPIRATORY VALVE[29]

Fig. 92.47

This valve is useful when artificial ventilation may be needed occasionally during an anaesthetic and access to the 'expiratory valve' is difficult. It is intended for use with a

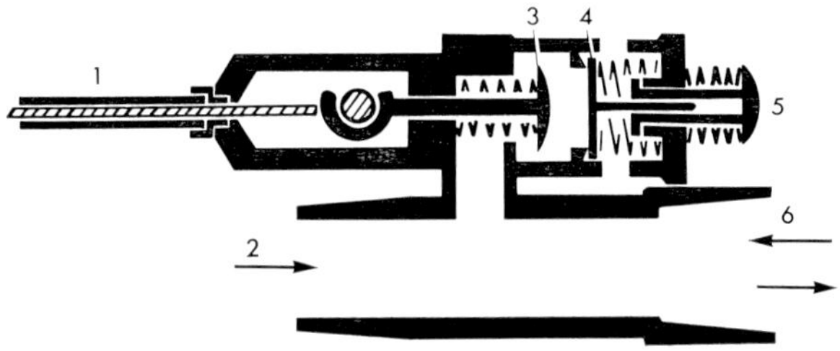

Fig. 92.47. Diagram of the 'Cardiff' remote-control expiratory valve.

1. Bowden cable
2. Inspiratory port
3. Disc occluding the expiratory port
4. Expiratory valve
5. Plunger
6. Port for connexion to patient

semi-closed circuit such as the Magill attachment. The Bowden cable (1) is operated by a hand control situated near the reservoir bag on the anaesthetic apparatus. When this control is pulled, the disc (3) closes the expiratory port and the lungs can be inflated by squeezing the bag. When the control is released, expired gas flows, past the valve (3) and the lightly-spring-loaded expiratory valve (4), to atmosphere. The valve (4) also acts as an expiratory valve during spontaneous breathing. It can be shut by pressing the plunger (5).

REFERENCES

1 LOEHNING R.W., DAVIS G. and SAFAR P. (1964) Rebreathing with 'nonrebreathing' valves. *Anesthesiology*, **25**, 854.

2 NEFF W. and LIND S. (1945) Ether anesthesia with improvised apparatus for intrathoracic operations under emergency circumstances. *Anesthesiology*, **6**, 337.

3 LEWIS G. (1956) Nonrebreathing valve. *Anesthesiology*, **17**, 618.

4 TASHIRO M. and WAKAI I. (1965) An automatic nonrebreathing valve of new design. *Anesthesiology*, **26**, 232.

5 STOTT F.D. (1951) Personal communication.

6 BECK M. (1964) Uber ein neues ventil zur verhindenung von rückmatung bei künstlichen atmung. *Anaesthesist*, **2**, 240.

7 RUBEN H. (1955) A new nonrebreathing valve. *Anesthesiology*, **16**, 643.

8 MITCHELL J.V. and EPSTEIN H.G. (1966) A pressure-operated inflating valve. *Anaesthesia*, **21**, 277.

9 MUSHIN W.W. (1953) Cardiff inflating valve. *Br. med. J.* **2**, 202.

10 NEWTON G.W., NOWILL W.K. and STEPHEN C.R. (1955) A piston-type nonrebreathing valve. *Anesthesiology*, **16**, 1037.

11 REES D.F. (1960) Automatic unidirectional flow valve. *Anaesthesia*, **15**, 79.

12 ZUCK D. (1964) A non-return valve for use with intermittent positive pressure respiration in paediatric surgery. *Br. J. Anaesth.* **36**, 674.

13 SMITH A.C., SPALDING J.M.K. and RUSSELL W.R. (1954) Artificial respiration by intermittent positive pressure in poliomyelitis and other diseases. *Lancet*, **1**, 939.

14 FLACH A. VON and VOSS G. (1954) Zur künstlichen beatmung im halboffenen system. *Anaesthesist*, **3**, 210.

15 FINK B.R. (1954) A nonrebreathing valve of new design. *Anesthesiology*, **15**, 471.

16 RATTENBORG C. (1954) A non-return-valve, designed to ventilate polio patients with respiratory paralysis by manual positive pressure ventilation. *Acta med. scand.* **147**, 431.

17 SHUMAN R.C. (1956) Modified nonrebreathing valve. *Anesthesiology*, **17**, 749.

18 ETHERIDGE F.G. (1958) Automatic non-rebreathing valve. *Br. J. Anaesth.* **30**, 245.

19 FRUMIN M.J., LEE A.S.J. and PAPPER E.M. (1959) New valve for nonrebreathing systems. *Anesthesiology*, **20**, 383.

20 FRANKS E.H. (1959) A hazard in the use of the Beaver pulmonary ventilator. *Br. med. J.* **2**, 92.

21 STEEN S.N. and LEE A.S.J. (1960) Prevention of inadvertent excess pressure in closed systems. *Anesth. Anal. curr. Res.* **39**, 264.

22 STEEN S.N. and CHEN J.L. (1963) Automatic nonrebreathing valve circuits: some principles and modifications. *Br. J. Anaesth.* **35**, 379.

23 HORN B. (1960) Valve for assisted or controlled ventilation. *Anesthesiology*, **21**, 83.

24 LEE S. (1964) A universal valve for anaesthetic circuits. *Br. J. Anaesth.* **36**, 318.

25 MAXWELL D.C. and GRANT G.C. (1960) An inflating spill valve for controlled respiration in a semi-closed circuit. *Br. J. Anaesth.* **32**, 616.

26 SMITH R.H. and VOLPITTO P.P. (1959) Volume ventilation valve. *Anesthesiology*, **20**, 885.

27 LEE S. (1964) A new pop-off valve. *Anesthesiology*, **25**, 240.

28 SEARLE J.B. (1958) Inflating valve. *Anaesthesia*, **13**, 345.

29 HILLARD E.K. (1953) The 'Cardiff' remote control expiratory valve. *Br. J. Anaesth.* **25**, 268.

CHAPTER 93

Concluding Remarks

Automatic ventilators have come to stay. Few will doubt their utility in the conduct of even short anaesthetics, to say nothing of the prolonged treatment of respiratory insufficiency which may go on for weeks, months, or even years.

Automatic ventilators have now become essential in any highly-developed hospital where modern anaesthesia and medicine are practised. Nevertheless, no mechanical device can altogether take the place of sensitive and skilled hands squeezing a reservoir bag. To believe, as some may do, that a machine, however elaborate, can 'give' an anaesthetic or treat respiratory insufficiency, is a point of view which cannot be accepted. We think it is still worthwhile, therefore, to set down what, in our opinion, are the indications for, and the advantages of, using an automatic ventilator rather than squeezing a bag by hand.

1. It sets free the hands of the anaesthetist who is working alone, and it enables him to perform other tasks connected with the care of the patient.
2. With an automatic ventilator the anaesthetist generally has more exact data about the ventilation of his patient. Tidal volume, respiratory frequency, minute-volume ventilation, positive- and negative-pressure limits, and the ratio of inspiratory to expiratory times, may all be available to him, and it may be possible to vary some or all of them over a wide range.
3. Where the anaesthetist is not wholly skilled in manual ventilation an automatic ventilator provides the surgeon with an operating field which moves to a more uniform rhythm, facilitating delicate dissections, particularly within the thorax.
4. In cases of long-continued respiratory insufficiency, and particularly when a number of cases are being treated at the same time, an automatic ventilator effects an obvious economy in the time of skilled personnel.
5. With certain exceptions manual ventilation cannot provide a negative-pressure phase. Many automatic ventilators do; and one must therefore be used if negative pressure is wanted.
6. It relieves the physical fatigue of the anaesthetist's hands and arms during long cases.
7. It relieves the mental fatigue (the boredom of monotony) of squeezing the bag during such long cases.

The value of an automatic device when ventilation must be carried on for days or weeks is obvious. The purely clinical reasons for using a ventilator during anaesthesia have been given, justifying the automatic device in place of the well-trained hand. The list of advantages of the automatic ventilator given above is impressive, the second one being perhaps the most important. Nevertheless, hazards are introduced, and some information is lost by this substitution.

1. The information which the anaesthetist gains from his handling of the bag is lost. Almost subconsciously, for example, the experienced anaesthetist compensates for the compression of the lung by surgical retraction. He quickly senses, from the increased resistance to his efforts, when further doses of relaxants are needed. The presence or otherwise of respiratory obstruction and accumulated secretions are easily detected. Every flicker of the diaphragm and every embryo cough are felt. By constantly watching the lungs, the action of the hands is correlated with the effects produced inside the chest. None of these things is necessarily done by the automatic ventilator. These virtues of bag squeezing at one time seemed all important, and they led anaesthetists in the past to refer to the 'educated hand'. We are increasingly dubious and anxious over this supposed attribute of the anaesthetist's hand. The 'educated hand', however much it may have existed in the past, is nowadays exposed as largely an illusion, for its discrimination and quantitation of respiratory phenomena is comparatively crude.[1] The 'educated hand' is giving way to the educated anaesthetist, whose intellectual activity interprets the more exact and reliable information from an automatic ventilator. It is the anaesthetist, and no other agency, that 'gives' the anaesthetic.

2. The anaesthetist may be lulled into a false sense of security. He may assume that because the machine clicks regularly the patient is being adequately ventilated. On more than one occasion we have seen patients exhibiting obvious cyanosis and cardiovascular depression without these effects exciting any concern on the part of the anaesthetist or the surgeon, because the machine connected to the patient was apparently working well. This situation only arises in an environment in which uninformed opinion takes the view that a machine is all that is necessary for good thoracic or any other anaesthesia. In fact, a machine can never be more than a tool of, and not a substitute for, a trained and experienced anaesthetist.

3. Mechanical failure may occur at any time and without warning. Unless such failure is quickly detected, and skilled manual ventilation substituted, the patient, if he remains apnoeic, will quickly die.

The mechanical design of the automatic ventilator has passed out of the hands of the anaesthetist into those of the expert mechanical, pneumatic, and electrical, engineer with all the resources of industry behind him. Nevertheless, the ingenuity and efficiency of automatic ventilators described in the literature of a past generation[2] have by no means been excelled, and it is possible that the present demand will bring to light inventions long buried in old papers. Inventors are well advised to study these papers.

There is no doubt that refinement of design can enhance the ease and delicacy with which the various parameters involved in automatic ventilation can be adjusted. Particularly from a research and study point of view is it valuable to be able to adjust any one without altering the others. Whether in the present state of our knowledge the patient has gained from recent rapid and striking mechanical development in ventilator design is another matter.

Without good biochemical and other physiological and clinical evidence, therefore, too much stress should not, at this stage in the development of automatic ventilation, be placed on the need for still further refinement in the mechanical design of ventilators; a development which in any case might well bring in its train an increased liability to breakdown.

For nearly twenty years anaesthetists with little more than their hands, a reservoir bag, and clinical acumen have most effectively conducted anaesthesia for thoracic and other complex surgical operations, and most successfully treated patients with respiratory insufficiency due to other causes for long periods of time. With more exact information of the patients' ventilatory requirements and with more readily-available biochemical checks, still better results will be obtained. It would be a pity if in these circumstances less reliance came to be placed on clinical judgment, and if some of the skills of the present generation of anaesthetists came to be lost to the next. This would be deplorable. Even in the best of circumstances, occasions will undoubtedly arise when reliance will have to be placed on careful clinical appraisal of the patient, and on such data as blood pressure, pulse rate, and colour, easily observable in every hospital operating theatre.

The automatic ventilator is clearly an undoubted boon to the anaesthetist and his patient. If these benefits are to be realized and still further enlarged, the machine must never be allowed to master the anaesthetist. The latter will always need to be a highly-trained individual, well-versed in the basic physiological working of his patient's body and familiar with the reasons for, and the upsets resulting from, such a disturbance of nature as the institution of controlled respiration. Only then can the patient derive the greatest benefit from the use of the automatic ventilator.

That this instrument is no more than a tool, albeit useful and rapidly becoming, if not already, essential, is our present contention. Well understood and wisely used it is another milestone in the march of anaesthetic progress.

REFERENCES

1 Egbert L.D. and Bisno D. (1967) The educated hand of the anesthesiologist. *Anesth. Anal. curr. Res.* **46**, 195.

2 Mushin W.W. and Rendell-Baker L. (1953) *The Principles of Thoracic Anaesthesia.* Oxford: Blackwell.

APPENDIX I

Functional Characteristics of Ventilators

The table at the back of the book presents the functional characteristics of the ventilators in concise tabular form. It necessarily involves some simplification of the more-complex ventilators and the individual accounts should be consulted for further information. On the other hand, this table was compiled after the main text had been completed and the opportunity was taken, in the case of some ventilators, to include additional modes of operation not mentioned in the text. Even so, the list of modes is not exhaustive. Generally a separate line is used for each mode. The choice of mode is largely within the control of the anaesthetist but, in some circumstances, the ventilator may change from one mode to another (e.g. from volume cycling to pressure cycling) as a result of a change of lung characteristics.

For this table a low-pressure generator is regarded as one in which the generated pressure is little more than that required in the alveoli. The dividing line between a high-pressure generator and a flow generator is somewhat arbitrary but, generally, if the generated pressure is greater than 100 cmH_2O the ventilator is classed as a flow generator.

The table may be found useful as a means of obtaining a summary of the action of a particular ventilator, but perhaps more so as a means of finding a ventilator with a particular combination of characteristics.

The 'Controls' section should be helpful in conjunction with the butterfly diagram (see fig. 5.1): a copy of this diagram is provided on a card surfaced so that it may be written on in pencil and the writing easily erased. The reader may find it helpful to mark this diagram (in the manner described in Chapter 5) in accordance with the information given in the 'Controls' section of the table. It should be borne in mind, however, that the butterfly diagram is not sufficiently comprehensive to express all relationships in all ventilators. In particular it does not show the action of discharging compliances.

Symbols—Ventilators, Circuits, and Modes

* = ventilators which have been investigated in the laboratory (see Chapter 7).

NRB = non-rebreathing.

FGF = fresh-gas flow.

MVD = minute-volume divider.

Symbols—Functional Analysis

† usually with substantial series resistance.

X indicates the presence of a particular mode of operation.

1, 2, 3, 4 indicate successive modes of operation within one phase. Not all such successive modes are necessarily present in all circumstances.

Where X or a figure occurs more than once between a pair of vertical lines this indicates one of two things. Firstly there may be alternative, mutually exclusive, modes of operation (e.g. time-cycling or patient-cycling). In this case, which mode occurs is usually largely within the control of the anaesthetist but may be dependent upon the patient. Secondly, there may be alternative ways of describing the same mode (e.g. discharging compliance or decreasing-pressure generator).

HH indicates a hybrid mixture of two types of cycling.

SS indicates simultaneous time and volume cycling.

Y indicates a cycling mechanism or an adjustable pressure or volume limit which, for the rest of the line in which the symbol occurs, is assumed not to operate. Non-adjustable safety-valves are generally not indicated.

Z indicates valves used for the disposal of excess gas from the patient circuit which operate somewhat differently from the conventional spill or blow-off valves.

Symbols in *italics* indicate that the action is not fully determined by the ventilator but is somewhat influenced by lung characteristics.

Superior suffixes have the following meanings:

^{F}: the generated flow is only the fresh-gas or inflating-gas flow to the patient circuit.

^{Z}: the generated flow is zero.

^{D}: decreasing.

^{I}: increasing.

^{S}: approximately sine-wave.

^{U}: unspecified waveform.

Symbols—'Controls'

A = determined by the ventilator and directly adjustable.

F = determined by the ventilator but fixed.

I = determined by the ventilator but only indirectly adjustable—as can be deduced from the butterfly diagram: e.g. if frequency f and I/E ratio are determined and directly adjustable then the inspiratory and expiratory times, T_I and T_E, are also determined but can be adjusted only indirectly.

A F I = as above, i.e. primarily determined by the ventilator, but slightly influenced by lung characteristics and therefore only approximately determined by the ventilator. In the case of the flow waveform it is comparatively rare for there to be any real choice open to the anaesthetist. Therefore the italic forms *A*, *F*, *I*, are used if the waveform, although not primarily determined by the ventilator, and although very much dependent on lung characteristics, can be influenced to an appreciable degree by the ventilator controls.

– = not determined by the ventilator; much dependent upon lung characteristics.

A′A′, A″A″ or A‴A‴ = two factors which are simultaneously adjusted by a single control and therefore cannot be independently adjusted.

^{1}A ^{2}A ^{3}A and so on = factors which are separately adjustable but are determined for only the first, second, third and so on, parts of the phase respectively. In some instances it is impracticable to represent all parts of a phase in the 'Controls' columns.

A_i $_iA$ = two factors which are separately adjustable but when the factor represented by A_i is adjusted it has some influence on the factor represented by $_iA$. Subscripts $_{i\ j\ k\ l}$ are used to indicate separate influences within the same ventilator. By no means all cross-influences have been indicated. In particular the influences of changes of fresh-gas flow and of any nebulizer flow have been omitted. The effects of fresh-gas flow are discussed in general terms in Chapter 4 and in the individual accounts of those ventilators which were tested in the laboratory. Influences on flow waveform, and on factors which are only indirectly adjustable, are not indicated.

The symbols for factors have essentially the same significance as in Chapter 5:

$\dot{V}$ = total minute-volume ventilation.

V_T = tidal volume.

f = frequency.

T_I = inspiratory time.

T_E = expiratory time.

$\dot{V}_{\bar{I}}$ = mean magnitude of flow in the inspiratory phase.

$\dot{V}_{I'}$ = instantaneous value of flow at the end of the inspiratory phase.

P_{GI} = generated pressure in the inspiratory phase.

$P_{MoI'}$ = pressure at the mouth at the end of the inspiratory phase.

R_I = resistance of the ventilator during the inspiratory phase. Note that, in this column, the presence of a — is highly significant: it indicates that the resistance of the *ventilator* is dependent upon lung characteristics.

$\dot{V}_I$ w/f = waveform of flow during the inspiratory phase.

$\dot{V}_{\bar{E}}$, $\dot{V}_{E'}$, P_{GE}, $P_{MoE'}$, R_E, $\dot{V}_E$ w/f represent the corresponding factors during the expiratory phase.

C_R = compliance of reservoir (bag or rigid vessel) in the ventilator.

$P_{C_RI'}$, $P_{C_RE'}$ = pressure in the reservoir compliance at the end of the inspiratory or expiratory phase respectively.

P_{ET,CO_2} = partial pressure of CO_2 in end-tidal gas.

APPENDIX II

Glossary

Artificial ventilation (synonym, **controlled respiration**). Any form of intermittent artificial inflation of the lungs, whether carried out manually or automatically, and whether intermittent positive or alternating positive and negative pressure is used. Inflation is not necessarily synchronous with any spontaneous respiratory activity of the patient.

Assisted respiration. A form of artificial ventilation which is synchronized with the patient's spontaneous inspiratory efforts.

Blow-off valve. A valve in the patient circuit which vents excess gas as the pressure rises to a critical level towards the latter part of the inspiratory phase.

Closed circuit. A breathing circuit in which gas passes to-and-fro between a reservoir bag and the patient. Carbon-dioxide absorption by soda-lime is effected in either the inspiratory or the expiratory stream, or in both. Fresh gas, containing at least sufficient oxygen for metabolic needs, enters the circuit. Any flow in excess of metabolic requirements is vented by some means. How 'closed' the circuit is, therefore, depends on the flow of fresh gas. If there is no excess flow of fresh gas the circuit is 'totally closed'.

Driving (power) circuit. A pneumatic circuit in a ventilator used to drive gas contained in the patient circuit to the patient. The driving or power circuit is normally separated from the patient circuit by at least the wall of a rubber bag.

Driving gas. The gas supplied to the driving circuit of a ventilator. This gas powers the ventilator but is not delivered to the patient.

Exhaust valve. A valve communicating with a pressure chamber which is opened to lower the pressure in the chamber and bring about expiration.

Expiratory phase. That part of the respiratory cycle between the commencement of expiratory flow and the commencement of inspiratory flow. Any 'expiratory pause' is therefore regarded as part of the expiratory phase.

Expiratory time. The duration of the expiratory phase.

Expiratory valve. A valve which is opened so that the expired gas from the patient can pass through it during the expiratory phase.

Fresh gas. Gas which is supplied to the patient circuit for delivery to the patient. It does not power the ventilator.

Inflating gas. Gas which powers a ventilator and which constitutes at least a substantial part of the gas supplied to the patient.

Inflating valve. A valve which, when pressure is applied, permits inflation of the lungs by occluding an expiratory outlet. When the expiratory phase commences, the expiratory outlet communicates with the patient (see Chapter 92).

Inspiratory phase. That part of the respiratory cycle between the commencement of inspiratory flow and the commencement of expiratory flow. Any 'inspiratory pause', during which the lungs are held inflated, is therefore regarded as part of the inspiratory phase.

Inspiratory time. The duration of the inspiratory phase.

Inspiratory valve. A valve which is opened so that gas can pass through it to the patient during the inspiratory phase.

Inspiratory-expiratory ratio.[1] The ratio of the inspiratory time to the expiratory time.

Inspiratory-expiratory valve. A valve which combines the functions of an inspiratory and an expiratory valve.

Non-rebreathing circuit. A breathing circuit in which all the expired gas passes to the exterior and is not rebreathed.

Patient circuit. The gas pathways of a ventilator which, in at least some part of the respiratory cycle, are in direct communication with the patient's lungs.

Pressure chamber. A chamber not communicating with the patient's lungs, but enclosing a reservoir bag which is compressed or expanded by fluctuations in pressure produced in the pressure chamber.

Pressure-equalizing valve. A valve designed to prevent the patient being accidentally inflated by the fresh-gas flow. It opens to limit any slow build-up of pressure in the breathing circuit, but closes when a sudden build-up of pressure occurs in the breathing circuit (see Chapter 92).

Pressure-limiting valve (positive or negative). A valve which limits the pressure in either direction, in either the patient circuit or the driving circuit. The valve may have the additional function of a safety-valve. A positive-pressure-limiting valve in the patient circuit may act as a blow-off valve.

Reservoir bag. A bag in direct communication with the patient's lungs which is compressed by some means in order to inflate them.

Respiratory frequency.[1] The number of breathing cycles per minute.

Respiratory period. The duration of a complete respiratory cycle. The sum of the inspiratory time and the expiratory time. The reciprocal of the respiratory frequency.

Resuscitator.[1] A portable device used in emergency situations to provide lung ventilation in individuals whose breathing is inadequate.

Safety-valve. A pressure-limiting valve intended to protect the patient or the ventilator from excessive positive or negative pressure. It normally remains closed throughout the respiratory cycle.

Spill valve (synonym, **dump valve**). A valve in a closed circuit which opens during some part of the expiratory phase, usually the end, to allow excess gas to escape from the circuit.

Storage bag. A bag in which gas is stored during one part of the cycle to be withdrawn for use during another. The gas may be stored at a near-atmospheric pressure to be drawn into a reservoir bag from which it is then driven to the patient, or at higher pressures to provide energy for inflating the lungs.

REFERENCE

1 Specification for breathing machines for medical use. (1964) British Standard 3806:1964. British Standards Institution: London.

APPENDIX III

Manufacturers

MANUFACTURERS OF VENTILATORS

'Adelaide' ventilator	'Delwyn' Lane End Close Bembridge Isle of Wight ENGLAND
Aga 'Spiropulsator' ME-2440	Aga Medical Division Lidingö 1 SWEDEN
Aika 'Respirator R-100'	Ichikawa Shiseido & Co Ltd Tokyo JAPAN
'Aintree' ventilator	Medical & Industrial Equipment Ltd P.O. Box 2AD 26–40 Broadwick Street London W1 ENGLAND
Air-Shields ventilators	Air-Shields Inc Hatboro Pennsylvania U.S.A.
Almeida 'Pulmo-Ventilador Universal'	Narcosul Ind. & Com. S.A. Rua Luzitana 661 Porto Alegre Rio Grande do Sul BRAZIL

Ventilator	Manufacturer
'Amsterdam Infant Ventilator'	G. L. Loos & Co's Fabrieken N.V. Postbus 663 Amsterdam HOLLAND
'Autoanestheton'	Invengineering Inc P.O. Box 360 Belmar New Jersey U.S.A.
'Autovent'	H. G. East & Co Ltd Sandy Lane West Littlemore Oxford ENGLAND
'Barnet' ventilators	W. Watson & Sons Ltd Barnet Herts ENGLAND
Beaver Mark III ventilator	The British Oxygen Co Ltd Medical Dept Hammersmith House London w6 ENGLAND
Bennett ventilators	Bennett Respiration Products Inc 1639 Eleventh Street Santa Monica California U.S.A.
Bird ventilators and attachments	Bird Corporation Mark 3 Respirator Lane Palm Springs California 92262 U.S.A.

Blease ventilators	Blease Medical Equipment Ltd Deansway Chesham Bucks ENGLAND
Bourns 'Pediatric Respirator'	Bourns Inc 300 Airport Road Ames Iowa 50011 U.S.A.
Cape-Waine 'Anaesthetic' and Cape ventilators	Cape Engineering Co Ltd The Cape Warwick ENGLAND
Cardiff Inflating Bellows	Medical & Industrial Equipment Ltd P.O. Box 2 AD 26–40 Broadwick Street London W1 ENGLAND
Cardiff Infant Inflating Bag	Longworth Scientific Co Ltd Radley Road Abingdon Berkshire ENGLAND
'Clevedon' ventilator	Willcocks (Clevedon) Ltd Clevedon Somerset ENGLAND
'Cyclator' 'Cyclator Combined Automatic Ventilator Unit' ('Cyclator CAV')	The British Oxygen Co Ltd Medical Dept Hammersmith House London W6 ENGLAND

Ventilator	Manufacturer
Dräger ventilators	Drägerwerk (Heinr. & Bernh. Dräger) Lübeck GERMANY
'E.G.C. Paediatric' ventilator	J. F. Eardley Ltd 63 Stalker Lees Road Sheffield 11 ENGLAND
East-Freeman ventilator East-Radcliffe ventilators	H. G. East & Co Ltd Sandy Lane West Littlemore Oxford ENGLAND
Emerson ventilators	J. H. Emerson Company 22 Cottage Park Avenue Cambridge Massachusetts U.S.A.
Engström ventilators	Mivab Elektro-Medicinska Apparater Luntmakargatan 12 Stockholm SWEDEN
Etsten ventilator	Ohio Chemical & Surgical Equipment Co 1400 East Washington Avenue Madison 3 Wisconsin U.S.A.
'Fazakerley' ventilator	Elliotts (Liverpool) Ltd Buckland Street Aigburth Liverpool 17 ENGLAND

Frumin ventilator	Invengineering Inc P.O. Box 360 Belmar New Jersey U.S.A.
Gullberg 'Positive-Pressure Attachment'	Kifa Banvaktsvagen 20 Solna 3 SWEDEN
Howells ventilator	W. Watson & Sons Ltd Barnet Herts ENGLAND
Jefferson ventilator	Air-Shields Inc Hatboro Pennsylvania U.S.A.
Kreiselman 'Bellows Resuscitator'	Ohio Chemical & Surgical Equipment Co 1400 East Washington Avenue Madison 3 Wisconsin U.S.A.
Lundia 'Special' ventilator Model B	Kifa Solna 1 SWEDEN
Manley ventilator	Blease Medical Equipment Ltd Deansway Chesham Bucks ENGLAND
Mautz ventilator	Ohio Chemical & Surgical Equipment Co 1400 East Washington Avenue Madison 10 Wisconsin U.S.A.

'Minivent'	The Acme Instrument Co P.O. Box 3474 Johannesburg SOUTH AFRICA
Mörch 'Surgical' ventilator	Distributed by Liquid Carbonic Division of General Dynamics Corporation Dept 911 135 South La Salle Street Chicago 3 Illinois U.S.A.
Mörch 'Piston' ventilator	V. Mueller & Co 1840 W. Van Buren Street Chicago Illinois 60612 U.S.A.
Mortimer ventilator	Coventry & Jeffs Ltd Stafford Street off Mill Lane Bristol 3 ENGLAND
Ohio (Monaghan) ventilators	Ohio Chemical & Surgical Equipment Co 1400 East Washington Avenue Madison 3 Wisconsin U.S.A.
Oxford Inflating Bellows	Supplied by all British anaesthetic equipment firms
'Pneumotron'	The British Oxygen Co Ltd Medical Dept Hammersmith House London W6 ENGLAND
R.P.R. 'Portable Volumetric Respirator, RP3'	R. Pesty 7–13 Rue des Cascades Paris XXe FRANCE

Rand-Wolfe ventilator	H. J. Rand Foundation 13 600 Deise Road Cleveland Ohio U.S.A.
'Respirateur Artificiel Automatique SF4'	Société d'Exploitation des Laboratoires Robert et Carrière 1 & 1bis Avenue de Villars Paris 7e FRANCE
'Respirateur Endo-trachéal MMS 104'	Le Matériel Médical et Sanitaire 5 Avenue de la Trentaine 77-Chelles FRANCE
Ruben 'Ambu' bag	Ambu International (Testa-Laboratorium a/s) 32 Marielundvej Copenhagen-Herlev DENMARK
Starling pump	C. F. Palmer (London) Ltd Myographic Works Effra Road Brixton London SW2 ENGLAND
Stephenson 'Controlled Respiration Unit'	The Stephenson Corporation Red Bank New Jersey U.S.A.
Takaoka ventilator	K. Takaoka AV. Bosque de Saúde 519 São Paulo SP BRAZIL

U.S. Army Volume-cycled ventilator	Department of the Army Harry Diamond Laboratories Washington DC U.S.A.
Van Bergen ventilator	The Smith Welding Equipment Corporation 2619-33 Fourth Street, South East Minneapolis 14 Minnesota U.S.A.
'Vellore' ventilator	Longworth Scientific Co Ltd Radley Road Abingdon Berkshire ENGLAND

MANUFACTURERS OF VENTILATION METERS

Bennett ventilation meter	Bennett Respiration Products Inc 1639 Eleventh Street Santa Monica California U.S.A.
Dräger 'Volumeter'	Drägerwerk (Heinr. & Bernh. Dräger) Lübeck GERMANY
Wright respirometer	The British Oxygen Co Ltd Medical Dept Hammersmith House London W6 ENGLAND under licence from: National Research Development Corporation 1 Tilney Street London W1 ENGLAND

Parkinson and Cowan dry gas meters	Parkinson Cowan Industrial Products Dolphin Works Fitzalan Street London SE11 ENGLAND

MANUFACTURERS OF INFLATING VALVES

Aga inflating valve Aga 'Polyvalve'	Aga Medical Division Lidingö 1 SWEDEN
'Ambu E' inflating valve 'Ambu Magnet' inflating valve	Ambu International (Testa-Laboratorium a/s) 32 Marielundvej Copenhagen-Herlev DENMARK
Beaver inflating valve	The British Oxygen Co Ltd Medical Dept Hammersmith House London W6 ENGLAND
'Cardiff' inflating valve	Supplied by all British anaesthetic equipment firms
'Cardiff' remote-control expiratory valve	Medical & Industrial Equipment Ltd P.O. Box 2 AD 26–40 Broadwick Street London W1 ENGLAND
'Dewsbury' inflating valve	C. F. Thackray Ltd 10 Park Street Leeds 1 ENGLAND

Etheridge inflating valve	Medical & Industrial Equipment Ltd P.O. Box 2 AD 26–40 Broadwick Street London W1 ENGLAND
Fink inflating valve	Ohio Chemical & Surgical Equipment Co 1400 East Washington Avenue Madison 3 Wisconsin U.S.A.
Flach-Voss inflating valve	Drägerwerk (Heinr. & Bernh. Dräger) Lübeck GERMANY
Frumin 'non-rebreathing' valve	Invengineering Inc P.O. Box 360 Belmar New Jersey U.S.A.
Holger Hesse 'deblocking' valve	Ambu International (Testa-Laboratorium a/s) 32 Marielundvej Copenhagen-Herlev DENMARK
Lewis-Leigh inflating valve	G. I. Dundas 329 Pope Street Menlo Park California U.S.A.
'Magnet POI' inflating valve	H. G. East & Co Ltd Sandy Lane West Littlemore Oxford ENGLAND

'Ranima' inflating valve	R. Pesty 7–13 Rue des Cascades Paris XXe FRANCE
'Ruben' inflating valve	Ambu International (Testa-Laboratorium a/s) 32 Marielundvej Copenhagen-Herlev DENMARK
Steen pressure-equalizing valve	Invengineering Inc P.O. Box 360 Belmar New Jersey U.S.A
Tashiro-Wakai inflating valve	Dept of Anaesthesia Nagoya University School of Medicine Showa-ku Nagoya JAPAN
Zuck paediatric inflating valve	Talley Anaesthetic Equipment Ltd 505 Liverpool Road London N7 ENGLAND

Index

The Table of Functional Characteristics of Ventilators in the back pocket serves as an index to the modes of operation of the individual ventilators.

J

K

L

M

Z